SIGNAL TRANSDUCTION AND CARDIAC HYPERTROPHY

PROGRESS IN EXPERIMENTAL CARDIOLOGY

Edited by Naranjan S. Dhalla, Ph.D., M.D. (Hon.), D. Sc. (Hon.)

SIGNAL TRANSDUCTION AND CARDIAC HYPERTROPHY

Editors

NARANJAN S. DHALLA, PhD, MD (Hon), DSc (Hon)
Distinguished Professor and Director
Institute of Cardiovascular Sciences
St. Boniface General Hospital Research Centre
Faculty of Medicine, University of Manitoba
Winnipeg, Canada

LARRY V. HRYSHKO, PhD
Associate Professor
Institute of Cardiovascular Sciences
St. Boniface General Hospital Research Centre
Faculty of Medicine, University of Manitoba
Winnipeg, Canada

ELISSAVET KARDAMI, PhD
Professor
Institute of Cardiovascular Sciences
St. Boniface General Hospital Research Centre
Faculty of Medicine, University of Manitoba
Winnipeg, Canada

PAWAN K. SINGAL, PhD, DSc
Professor
Institute of Cardiovascular Sciences
St. Boniface General Hospital Research Centre
Faculty of Medicine, University of Manitoba
Winnipeg, Canada

KLUWER ACADEMIC PUBLISHERS
BOSTON / DORDRECHT / LONDON

Distributors for North, Central and South America:
Kluwer Academic Publishers
101 Philip Drive
Assinippi Park
Norwell, Massachusetts 02061 USA
Telephone (781) 871-6600
Fax (781) 681-9045
E-Mail: kluwer@wkap.com

Distributors for all other countries:
Kluwer Academic Publishers Group
Post Office Box 322
3300 AH Dordrecht, THE NETHERLANDS
Telephone 31 786 576 000
Fax 31 786 576 474
E-Mail: services@wkap.nl

 Electronic Services < http://www.wkap.nl >

World Heart Congress (17th : Winnipeg, Man.)
   Signal transduction and cardiac hypertrophy / editors, Naranjan S. Dhalla ... [et al.].
     p. ; cm. -- (Progress in experimental cardiology ; 7)
   "World Heart Congress held on July 6-11th, 2001 in Winnipeg, Canada"--Pref.
   Includes bibliographical references and index.
   ISBN 1-4020-7218-X (alk. paper)
   1. Heart--Hypertrophy--Congresses. 2. Cellular signal transduction--Congresses. I.
Dhalla, Naranjan S. II. Title. III. Series.
   [DNLM: 1. Cardiomegaly--physiopathology--Congresses. 2. Gene Expression
Regulation--physiology--Congresses. 3. Signal Transduction--physiology--Congresses.
WG 210 W927s 2003]
   RC685.H9 W67 2001
   616.1'207--dc21

               2002030072

Contents

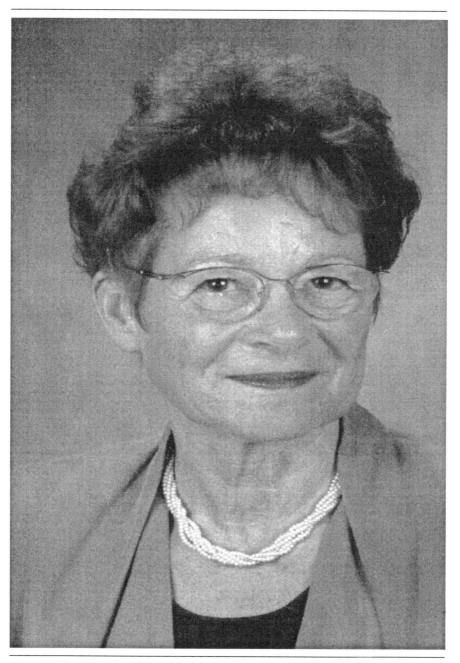

PROFESSOR DR. JUTTA SCHAPER, MD, PhD
Bad Nauheim, Germany

A Tribute to Professor Dr. Jutta Schaper, MD, PhD

This book is dedicated to Professor Dr. Jutta Schaper to recognize her capable leadership and superior scientific achievements in the field of Cardiovascular Sciences. Prof. Schaper received her MD degree from the School of Medicine in Dusseldorf in 1961 and her PhD degree from Justus-Liebig University, Giessen in 1980. She started her professional career at the Janssen Research Foundation in Belgium and was appointed on the Faculty of the University of Antwerp in 1970. She moved to Max-Planck Institute for Physiological and Clinical Research in 1972 as Head of the Department of Cardiovascular Cell Biology in Bad Nauheim and has been serving as Professor of Experimental Cardiology at the University of Giessen since 1980.

Three major fields of Cardiovascular Sciences in which Dr. Jutta Schaper has made major contributions include Collateral Circulation of the Heart, Ischemic Tolerance of the Human Heart During Cardiac Surgery, and the Structural Basis of Human Heart Failure. She has studied the structure and ultrastructure as well as the protein expression in normal and growing coronary arteries. Together with her husband, Prof. Dr. Wolfgang Schaper, Dr. J. Schaper has published many articles and 3 books on arteriogenesis. Dr. Schaper has clarified and standardized the ultra-structural characteristics of ischemic injury; this work was original and has been cited frequently. Dr. Schaper was the first to describe structural defects in failing human hearts and to determine multiple factors involved in structural remodeling. She evaluated the importance of transcriptional and translational disturbances. The studies by Dr. Schaper represent the most complete and a completely new investigation of human failing hearts available in the scientific literature. She has published a total of 166 peer-reviewed full length articles, in addition to numerous abstracts and book chapters. Dr. Schaper has been invited to present her work on all three topics at numerous international conferences during the past 25 years.

Professor Schaper has received several honours and awards including Arthur-Weber Prize of the German Cardiac Society, Purkyne Honorary Medal of the Academy of Sciences of the Czech Republic, and Honorary Doctorate from the University of Strathclyde, Glasgow. She has been serving on the editorial boards of different journals such as the Journal of Molecular and Cellular Cardiology, Circulation and Circulation Research. Dr. Schaper served the International Society for Heart Research first as Secretary of the European Section and then as President with great distinction. Her strength lies in handling complex issues with great ease and she is known for her efforts in promoting young cardiovascular scientists.

Naranjan S. Dhalla
Larry V. Hryshko
Elissavet Kardami
Pawan K. Singal

Preface

Cellular signaling in cardiac muscle refers to the myriad of stimuli and responses that direct and control the physiological operation of this organ. Our understanding of these complex signaling cascades has increased dramatically over the past few decades with the advent of molecular tools for their dissection. Moreover, this information is beginning to provide tangible targets towards manipulating cardiac function in the setting of cardiovascular disease. The mechanisms and factors that regulate cardiac cell growth are of particular interest as both adaptive and maladaptive responses can occur during cardiac hypertrophy.

Cardiac hypertrophy describes the increase in individual cardiac myocyte size that is accomplished through the series and/or parallel addition of sarcomeres. The ability of cardiac muscle to increase in size through hyperplasia becomes highly restricted or negligible shortly after birth. Consequently, the increase in heart size associated with development and growth of an individual occurs through hypertrophy. In response to a chronic increase in workload, cardiac muscle cells can dramatically increase in size to face their increasing contractile demands. While this plasticity is clearly a beneficial response under many conditions, it can be highly deleterious and inappropriate under others. For example, cardiac hypertrophy associated with endurance exercise clearly enhances athletic performance. In contrast, the hypertrophy associated with chronic hypertension, stenotic or regurgitant heart valves, or following a myocardial infarction often continues far beyond the period where this adaptive response is beneficial. Progressive cardiac hypertrophy and remodeling in these situations becomes maladaptive and directly contributes to the development of heart failure.

The numerous cell signaling pathways that contribute to or produce cardiac hypertrophy are becoming increasingly understood. Intense interest in this area derives from the clinical observation that cardiac hypertrophy and remodeling usually precede overt heart failure. Furthermore, the specific pattern of hypertrophy observed is unique for distinct triggering stimuli. For example, concentric hypertrophy is usually associated with chronic pressure overload such as that occurring due to hypertension or stenotic cardiac valves. In contrast, eccentric hypertrophy is often seen with volume overload such as that associated with regurgitant valves. It seems likely that these distinct hypertrophic phenotypes will become amenable to pharmacological regulation once the associated signaling pathways become progressively better understood.

This collection of 35 chapters was selected from talks presented at the World Heart Congress held on July 6–11th, 2001 in Winnipeg, Canada. An exceptional breadth of topics was presented by leading experts in the fields of cellular signaling and cardiac hypertrophy. These range from the fundamental processes essential for physiological cardiac functioning to the maladaptive responses that ultimately can lead to overt heart failure. Progress in this area offers great potential for reducing the pathophysiology associated with maladaptive cardiac hypertrophy and remodeling.

Naranjan S. Dhalla
Larry V. Hryshko
Elissavet Kardami
Pawan K. Singal

Winnipeg, Canada

Acknowledgments

We are grateful to the following corporations and granting agencies for their generous donations in support of the XVII World Heart Congress of the International Society for Heart Research, the first Public Heart Health Forum as well as publication of this book:

PATRONS:
Government of Canada (Dept. of Western Diversification)
Government of Manitoba (Depts. of Industry Trade and Mines; Health;
   Post-Secondary Education; Culture Heritage and Tourism)
Merck Frosst Canada, Ltd.
Mitsubishi-Tokyo Pharmaceuticals Inc.

PARTNERS:
American Section of the International Society for Heart Research
AstraZeneca
Aventis Pharmaceuticals Inc.
Bayer Canada, Inc.
City of Winnipeg
International Academy of Cardiovascular Sciences
International Society for Heart Research (Kaito Fund, Bayer Yakuhin Fund and
   Canon Fund)
Kowa Pharmaceuticals
Pfizer Canada
St. Boniface General Hospital Research Foundation

COLLABORATORS:
CanWest Global Foundation
CIHR Institute of Circulatory and Respiratory Health
Eli Lilly
Great West Life and London Life
Manitoba Liquor Control Commission
Mars Incorporated
Medicure, Inc.

Myles Robinson Memorial Heart Fund
Safeway Food and Drug
University of Manitoba (Faculty of Medicine; Departments of Physiology and
   Human Anatomy & Cell Science)

BENEFACTORS:
ATL Canada
Beckman Coulter Canada Inc.
Canadian Cardiovascular Society
Canadian Institutes of Health Research
Cardiovascular Solutions, Inc.
Dairy Farmers of Canada
De Fehr Foundation
Faculty of Health Sciences, University of Western Ontario
Heart and Stroke Foundation of Manitoba
Institute of Biodiagnostics, National Research Council of Canada
Japanese Working Group on Cardiac Structure and Metabolism
Manitoba Hydro
Merck KGaA (Germany)
Pulsus Group Inc.
St. Boniface General Hospital Research Centre
Wawanesa Mutual Insurance Company
World Heart Corporation

The collaboration of Ms. Eva Little, Ms. Janet Labarre, Ms. Diane Stowe, Ms.
Florence Willerton and Ms. Susan Zettler in coordinating diverse editorial activities
associated with this book is gratefully acknowledged. Special thanks are due to Mr.
Zachary Rolnik, Ms. Mimi T. Breed, Ms. Melissa Ramondetta and their editorial
staff at Kluwer Academic Publishers for their patience, interest and hard work in
assembling this volume.

SIGNAL TRANSDUCTION AND CARDIAC HYPERTROPHY

I. Cardiac Adaptation and Remodeling

Signal Transduction and Cardiac Hypertrophy,
edited by N.S. Dhalla, L.V. Hryshko,
E. Kardami & P.K. Singal
Kluwer Academic Publishers, Boston, 2003

Molecular Changes of the Myocardium after Mechanical Circulatory Support

Florian Grabellus,[1] Bodo Levkau,[2] Hans-H. Scheld,[3] Atsushi Takeda,[4] Michael Erren,[5] Jörg Stypmann,[2] and Hideo A. Baba[1]

From the [1] Institute of Pathology
University of Essen
Hufelandstrasse 55, 45122 Essen
Germany
[2] Department of Cardiology and Angiology
University of Münster
Albert-Schweitzer Strasse 33
48149 Münster, Germany
[3] Department of Thoracic- and Cardiovascular Surgery
University of Münster
Albert-Schweitzer Strasse 33
48149 Münster, Germany
[4] Department of Internal Medicine
Aoto Hospital, Jikei University
Tokyo, Japan
[5] Institute of Clinical Chemistry and Laboratory Medicine University of Münster
Albert-Schweitzer Strasse 33, 48149 Münster
Germany

Summary. Left ventricular assist devices (LVAD) have been used to "bridge" patients with end-stage heart failure to transplantation. Although several reports have suggested that the native ventricular function recovers after long-term LVAD support, a process called "reverse remodeling", the underlying biological mechanisms are still unclarified.

Various molecular pathways of the human myocardium associated with apoptosis; response to stress, or matrix changes are known to be altered under conditions of heart failure and some of them have been shown to be reversibly regulated during left ventricular mechanical support suggesting that the descriptive term of "reverse remodeling" is actualy, at least in parts, a reversed mechanisms.

Address for Correspondence: Dr. H. A. Baba, Institute of Pathology, University of Essen, Hufelandstrasse 55, 45122 Essen, Germany. E-mail: hideo.baba@medizin.uni-essen.de, Fax: +49-201-723 3926, Phone: +49-201-72335 77.

The reduction of volume and pressure overload with a decrease of ventricular wall stress leading to an improvement of myocardial blood supply under mechanical circulatory assist may be one explanation for the molecular myocardial changes and may reflect one possible cause for the phenomenon reverse remodeling.

Key words: Reverse remodeling, myocardium, heart failure.

INTRODUCTION

Morbidity and mortality rates due to end-stage myocardial failure continue to escalate. Today, heart transplantation is only one reliable way to treat patients with terminal heart failure. The limitation in number of donor hearts led to the establishment of alternative treatments like the introduction of left ventricular assist devices (LVAD) (1).

Left ventricular assist devices have been used successfully to "bridge" patients with end-stage heart failure while on the waiting list for heart transplantation. The mechanical circulatory support improves the overall hemodynamics, leading to increased cardiac output, normalization of systemic blood pressure, and improved end-organ function (2).

In addition to these short-term benefits, several reports have also suggested recovery of native ventricular function after long-term mechanical support with a reversal of chronic ventricular dilation (2,3). In single patients LVAD support reverses the complex process of chronic left ventricular remodeling to the point where these patients could be weaned from the device and recover normal cardiac function (4–6). The underlying process is called "reverse remodeling".

Examination of hearts during long-term LVAD support revealed alterations of left ventricular geometry and myocardial structure. LV-geometry showed a reduction of chamber size and mass (1) as well as an increased LV-wall thickness after mechanical unloading. On histological and morphometrical examination of the myocardium after LVAD support a reduction of myocytes diameter (Figure 1D), volume, and elongation as an indicator of structural reverse remodeling was present (7–9). The reduction of myocardial interstitial (replacement-) fibrosis under LVAD therapy is disscussed controversialy (4,5,10,11). In our cohort the measurement of interstitial fibrosis before and after mechanical unloading showed no significant reduction (Figure 1A–C).

Besides this morphologic changes of the heart and myocardium recent investigations point to a complex change in the biology of myocardial cells in correlation with "reverse remodeling".

Myocardial gene expression of regulators of myocyte apoptosis have been shown to be altered under hemodynamic unloading by LVAD in patients with end-stage heart failure since loss of myocytes via apoptosis was identified to be one basic mechanism in the development of cardiac failure (12). Programmed cell death of cardiomyocytes occurs in failing hearts (13) and is accompanied with specific DNA fragmentation and changes in the expression of apoptosis related genes like those of the BCL-2 family. The expression of the antiopoptotic member BCL-2 is enhanced during heart failing whereas its proapoptotic opponent BAX remains

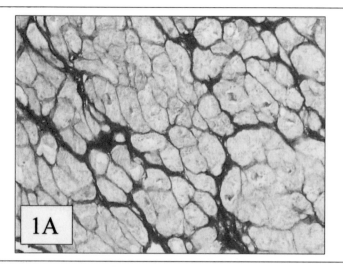

Figure 1A. Measurement of interstitial and perivascular fibrosis in the left ventricular myocardium of one patient with heart failure before LVAD support using Sirius Red staining (fibrous tissue = dark, cardiomyocytes = pale). Quantification was performed with a computer-assisted image analysis system (KS-300, Zeiss, Germany). Scars were excluded from the measurements.

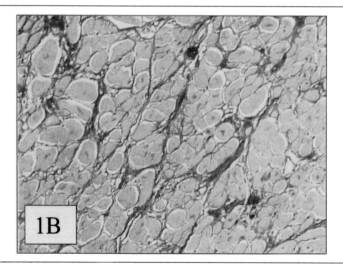

Figure 1B. Same heart after LVAD support.

constant, which can be interpreted as a possible compensatory mechanism to maintain cell survival (12). The downregulation of BCL-x_L, another gene of the BCL-2 family, is reversed in failing hearts after mechanical circulatory support suggesting a decreased susceptibility of the myocardium to apoptosis (14).

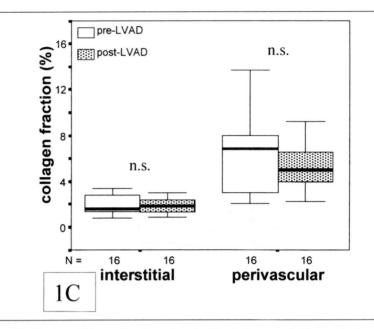

Figure 1C. The interstitial as well as the perivascular fibrosis shows no significant reduction after mechanical unloading in 16 patients.

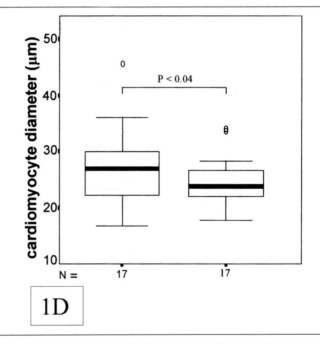

Figure 1D. Morphometric measurement of left ventricular cardiomyocyte diameter (μm) before and after mechanical support showing a reduction after LVAD support. Analysis was performed with a computer-assisted image analysis system (KS-300, Zeiss, Germany). "Reprinted from J Heart Lung Transplant 19(7), Baba HA et al., Reversal of metallothionein expression is different throughout the human myocardium after prolonged left ventricular mechanical support. 668–674, 2000, with permission from Elsevier Science".

The cardiac Fas (APO-1/CD95) system, a further apoptosis regulating pathway of the heart, is closely related to hemodynamic loading conditions (15). Moreover recent investigations of certain antiapoptotic Fas isoforms (FasExo6Del) in failing hearts are related with a normalization of their mRNA levels under unloading therapy (14).

A well known signal-transduction pathway is the family of mitogen-activated protein kinases (MAPKs) which are involved in the regulation of cell growth and apoptosis. Different members of the cardiac set of MAPKs are known to be upregulated in patients with dilated or ischemic cardiomyopathy (16,17). After long-term mechanical support the failing hearts showed a differential regulation of this cardiac subset in combination with a decrease in myocyte apoptosis and cell volume indicating a possible role of MAPKs in the regulation of myocardial structure and viability (18).

Besides these changes in cardiomyocyte function and biology alterations in the components of extracellular matrix might play a fundamental role in the development of heart failure, particularly ventricular dilation (19,20). Extracellular matrix turnover with degradation of collagens, the major components of myocardial extracellular matrix, is regulated by matrix metalloproteinases (MMPs) and a family of tissue inhibitors of metalloproteinases (TIMPs). Together, these proteins are suspected to contribute to myocardial remodeling in heart failure. After LVAD support the ratio of a subset of these opponents is changed with a downregulation of damaging MMPs (MMP-1 and MMP-9), an increase of TIMPs (TIMP-1 and TIMP-3) and an alteration of collagen quality with increased levels of undamaged collagen (21). Interestingly, the administration of MMP inhibitors in mice hearts after experimental myocardial infarction or in pigs with congestive heart failure due to rapid pacing, attenuates left ventricular dilation (22,23) and may provide a therapeutic target for controlling myocardial matrix remodeling in the setting of developing heart failure (24). This results suggest that remodeling of myocardial extracellular matrix may play a significant role in left ventricular plasticity in heart failure and that failing heart may benefit from matrix reverse remodeling after left ventricular support.

Another fundamental mechanism that is linked with heart failure is the altered expresssion of genes encoding for proteins involved in Ca^{2+} handling. Since the contractile strength of the intact myocardium is associated with increasing intracellular Ca^{2+} the compromised cardiac contractility during heart failure seems to be caused by an abnormal coordination of Ca^{2+} release from and reuptake in the sarcoplasmic reticulum. SERCA (sarcoplasmic Ca^{2+}-ATPase) and its endogenous regulator phospholamban, the sarcolemmal Na+-Ca2+ exchanger, or the sarcoplasmireticular ryanodine receptor (RyR) are members of this set of Ca2+ regulating proteins and their expression has been shown to be altered in failing hearts (25–28). LVAD support can improve the contractile function of the failing myocardium and one known mechanism is the reversible regulation of genes encoding for Ca2+ cycling proteins (29).

Other individual genes of hormones or cytokines such as atrial natriuretic peptide/brain natriuretic peptide (ANP/BNP)(7), interleukin-6 (IL-6) (30), and tumor necrosis factor-α (TNF-α) (31) have been shown to be reversibly regulated under LVAD as well.

The variable changes going along with heart failure conditions have been shown to be straight stressful events on the myocardium leading to an upregulation of stress-induced factors in cardiomyocytes and other cells of the myocardium. A reversible activation under mechanical support was described in the stress-associated proteins treated below.

MECHANICAL CIRCULATORY SUPPORT AND THE TRANSCRIPTION FACTOR NF-κB

The transcription factor nuclear factor kappa B (NF-κB) is an important regulator of numerous cytokines, acute phase response proteins, and adhesions molecules and function as a cellular protector against apoptosis (32,33). Activation of NF-κB has recently been observed in the myocardium of patients with congestive heart failure (34). NF-κB is localized in the cytoplasm in a complex with inhibitory proteins (IκBs), which mask its nuclear localisation signal and prevent its translocation to the nucleus. Site-specific phosphorylation and proteasomal degradation of IkBs after a specific stimulus allows NF-κB to translocate to the nucleus, bind DNA, and activate the transcription of specific genes (35).

Examination of the NF-κB activity in 16 patients with end-stage heart failure due to different causes before and after mechanical circulatory support demonstrated abundant activity of NF-κB in cardiomyocytes of failing hearts (Figure 2A). The activity decreased dramatically after mechanical unloading (Figure 2B–D). Thus, NF-κB is the first transcription factor that was identified to be negatively regulated under LVAD (36).

The stimuli leading to NF-κB activation in the failing heart and to its inactivation after LVAD-mediated unloading are still unknown. However, we have observed a gradient in the activity of NF-κB in the failing heart with higher activity in the subendocardium than in the subepicardium, which disappears after LVAD (Figure 5B). The subendocardium is the least well-perfused region of the myocardium in failing hearts (37) and the most vulnerable region to reduction of blood supply due to abnormally high wall stress in heart failure. The resulting local tissue hypoxia may contribute to the high NF-κB activity we observe in the subendocardium, since hypoxia has been shown to activate NF-κB (38). A similar transmural gradient has been observed previously for ANP/BNP (1), cyclooxygenase-2 (34), metallothionein (8) and heme oxygenase-1 (39), some of which are transcriptionally regulated by NF-κB. LVAD decreases the ventricular filling pressure as well as the ventricular wall stress, and improves myocardial O_2-supply most effectively in the subendocardium. This correlates with the observation of a decrease of cardiomyocyte hypertrophy specially in the subendocardial area (8), the region with the greatest reduction of wall stress. Thus, reduction of local tissue hypoxia in the subendocardium may result in decreased NF-κB activity.

As NF-κB is a transcription factor which plays a crucial role in the regulation of

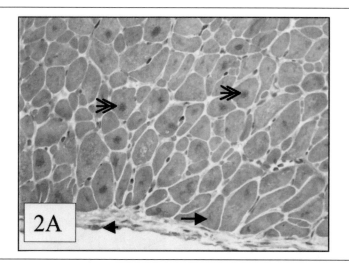

Figure 2A. Immunolocalization of activated NF-κB in cardiomyocyte nuclei (double arrows) in the subendocardial area of an end-stage failing heart due to dilated cardiomyopathy with only few NF-κB negative nuclei (arrow). Endocardial endothelial cells are activated as well (arrowhead) × 200.

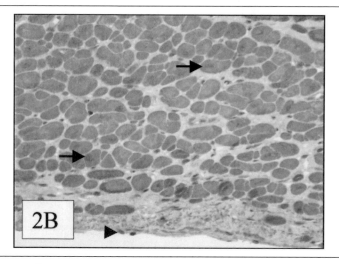

Figure 2B. Tissue from the same heart at the time of LVAD explantation with negative NF-κB nuclei in cardiomyocytes (arrows) and endocardial cells (endo, arrowhead) × 200.

genes involved in the protective response against cell stress and apoptosis, its activation in the failing heart may reflect this purpose. NF-κB's activation in the failing myocardium and the reversibility during LVAD support indicates that NF-κB may be involved in the process of "reverse remodeling".

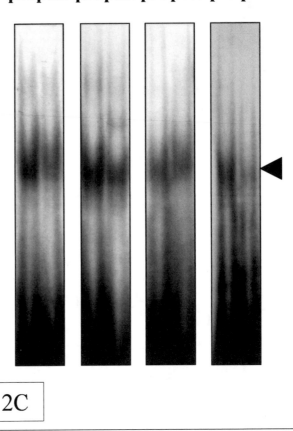

Figure 2C. Gel-shifts for NF-κB's DNA-binding activity in myocardial tissue from four patients at the time of LVAD implantation (pre-) and LVAD explantation (post-), respectively. Decrease of the activity after mechanical unloading. Arrow indicates the mobility of the NF-κB complex.

MECHANICAL CIRCULATORY SUPPORT AND HEME OXIGENASE-1

Heme oxygenase-1 (HO-1, HSP 32) catalyzes the degradation of heme to biologically active molecules: iron, a gene regulator; biliverdin, an antioxidant; and carbon monoxide, a heme ligand. HO-1 is inducible by a diverse variety of conditions including hypoxia, and belongs to the heat shock protein family. Heme oxygenase-1 is expected to have a central role in the regulation of many physiological and pathophysiological processes besides its established function in heme catabolism and its expression has been suggested as a marker to detect an imbalance of the intracellular homeostasis (40–42).

The expression of HO-1 in left ventricular tissue of 23 patients transplantation

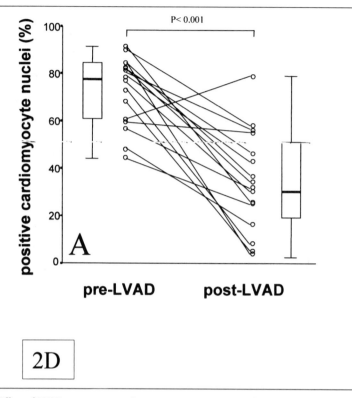

Figure 2D. Effect of LVAD support on cardiomyocyte NF-κB activity in 16 patients hearts. Box plots contain the median (black bold horizontal bar) as well as the 25th and 75th percentile (fine horizontal bar).

was analysed before and after LVAD support (39). The failing myocardium showed elevated levels of HO-1 expression mainly in cardiomyocytes, but also in endothelial cells, some smooth muscle cells and fibroblasts (Figure 3A). The hearts of patients with ischemic heart disease (IHD) showed significantly higher amounts of HO-1 than hearts with dilated cardiomyopathy (DCM) or myocarditis/congenital heart disease. After LVAD support the HO-1 content decreased significantly in the DCM and IHD group (Figure 3B,C). The distribution of HO-1 activity throughout the left ventricular wall showed a similar pattern to the NF-kB and MT data with higher activity in the subendocardium than in the subepicardium (Figure 5B). In an in vitro model with neonatal rat cardiomyocytes an increase of HO-1 protein content up to 6-fold above the normal level was seen in cell culture under hypoxia. HO-1 levels returned to normal values after reoxygenation conditions (Figure 3D).

MECHANICAL CIRCULATORY SUPPORT AND METALLOTHIONEIN

Metallothioneine (MT) is a cytokine-inducible low molecular weight protein with a high content of cystein (43). One function of MT is to detoxificate heavy metals

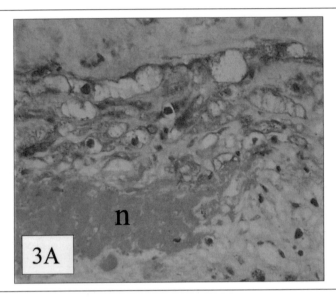

Figure 3A. Immunolocalization of HO-1 (dark staining) in subendocardial cardiomyocytes of one patient with end-stage heart failure due to ischemic heart disease. Several immunopositive cardiomyocytes with signs of degeneration (vacuolization) next to a focal necrosis (n).

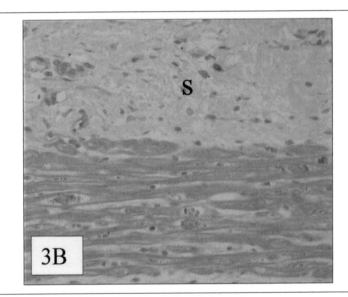

Figure 3B. Negative HO-1 immunoreactivity after mechanical unloading. Scartissue (s).

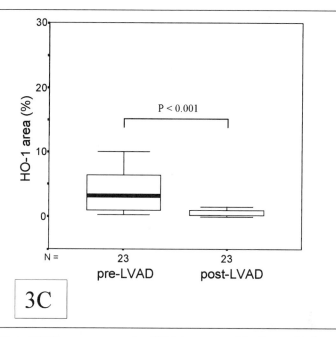

Figure 3C. Effect of LVAD support concerning HO-1 immunoreactivity illustrated in box plots.

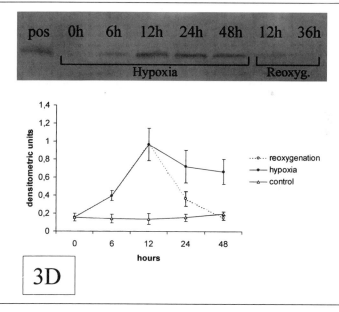

Figure 3D. Representative HO-1 western blot of neonatal rat cardiomyocytes after hypoxia and reoxygenation (top panel). Pos = positive control (protein extract from rat spleen). HO-1 values of rat cardiomyocytes after hypoxic cultivation (filled circles) and after reoxygenation (open circles with dotted line). Control cells under normoxic cultivation at the corresponding time points (open triangle). The activation of HO-1 due to hypoxic conditions is reversibly regulated after reoxygenation of the neonatal rat cardiomyocytes.

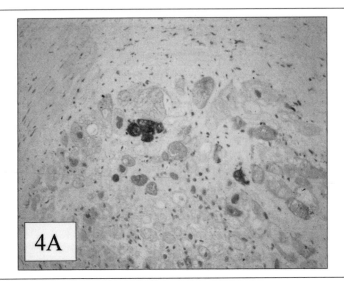

Figure 4A. Immunhistochemical staining for MT (dark staining). Myocardial left ventricular tissue of one patient with end-stage heart failure. The immunopositive cardiomyocytes show vacuolized cytoplasm.

by binding metal ions (44). Overexpressed MT may act as a free radical scavenger and protect against radical-induced lipid peroxidation (45). The biosynthesis of MT can be induced by a wide variety of stress factors including bivalent heavy metals, cytokines, growth factors, tumor promotors, and glucocorticoids.

In failing hearts of 17 patients with end-stage heart failure, who received a LVAD as a bridge to transplantation, MT was located mainly in subendocardial cardiomyocytes, which often showed signs of degeneration like perinuclear vacuolization (Figure 4A). Other cells of the myocardium in particular the endothelium and smooth muscle cells of small vessels throughout the myocardium had an elevated MT expression just as the myocytes. During mechanical support the MT expression of all above mentioned cells decreased (Figure 4B). In addition to the down regulation of MT expression in cardiomyocytes, their cell diameter and the signs of degeneration were significant lower after unloading. This preferential reduction of MT in the subendocardial myocardium is comparable with the concept of greatest reduction of wall stress with improvement of blood flow and oxygen supply.

CORONARY BLOOD FLOW IN FAILING HEARTS AND STRESS FACTORS

The investigation of the stress associated proteins NF-kB, MT, and HO-1 had similar results. First, the activation of stress factors were demonstrable before mechanical support. This was reversibly regulated after mechanical ventricular unloading by LVAD. Second, the activation due to heart failure was strongest in the subendocardial cardiomyocytes (Figure 5A,B).

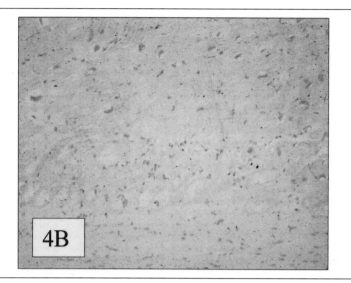

Figure 4B. The same heart after LVAD support with MT negative myocardium.

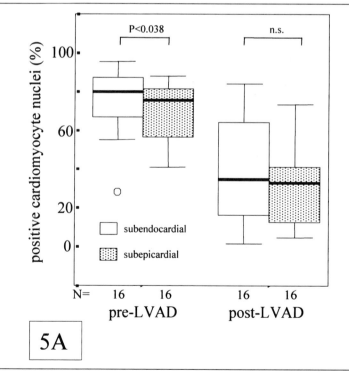

Figure 5A. NF-kB immunopositivity in cardiomyocyte nuclei in percent before and after LVAD subdivided in subepicardial and subendocardial myocardium. Before LVAD a significant gradient throughout the myocardium, with higher NF-kB activation in the subendocardium, is observed. This gradient is not longer present after LVAD therapy.

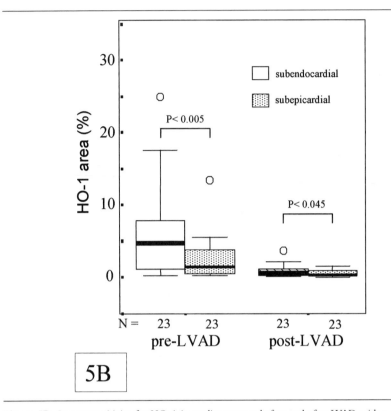

Figure 5B. Immunopositivity for HO-1 in cardiomyocytes before and after LVAD with a gradient of positive cells (subendocardial > subepicardial) throughout the myocardium. This gradient is strongly attenuated after mechanical unloading.

Under heart failing conditions several stressful events have effects on the myocardium. One is the altered coronary blood flow going along with myocardial hypertrophy (46) and volume/pressure overload with an increased ventricular wall stress. In healthy hearts the subendocardial regions of the myocardium show a higher perfusion than subepicardial areas. This is reversed in failing hearts, making the subendocardium the least well perfused myocardial region (37).

The reduction of coronary blood flow with a chronic hypoxia of the myocardium in failing hearts and an improvement of blood supply under mechanical circulatory assist may be an explanation for the results and may reflect one facet of the phenomenon called reverse remodeling.

REFERENCES

1. Goldstein DJ, Oz MC, Rose EA. 1998. Implantable left ventricular assist devices. N Engl J Med 339:1522–1533.
2. Frazier OH, Benedict CR, Radovancevic B, Bick RJ, Capek P, Springer WE, Macris MP, Delgado R, Buja LM. 1996. Improved left ventricular function after chronic left ventricular unloading. Ann Thorac Surg 62:675–681.

3. Levin HR, Oz MC, Chen JM, Packer M, Rose EA, Burkhoff D. 1995. Reversal of chronic ventricular dilation in patients with end-stage cardiomyopathy by prolonged mechanical unloading. Circulation 91:2717–2720.
4. Mancini DM, Beniaminovitz A, Levin H, Catanese K, Flannery M, DiTullio M, Savin S, Cordisco ME, Rose E, Oz M. 1998. Low incidence of myocardial recovery after left ventricular assist device implantation in patients with chronic heart failure. Circulation 98:2383–2389.
5. Müller J, Wallukat G, Weng YG, Dandel M, Spiegelsberger S, Semrau S, Brandes K, Theodoridis V, Loebe M, Meyer R, Hetzer R. 1997. Weaning from mechanical cardiac support in patients with idiopathic dilated cardiomyopathy. Circulation 96:542–549.
6. Nakatani T, Sasako Y, Kobayashi J, Komamura K, Kosakai Y, Nakano K, Yamamoto F, Kumon K, Miyatake K, Kitamura S, Takano H. 1998. Recovery of cardiac function by long-term left ventricular support in patients with end-stage cardiomyopathy. ASAIO J 44:M516–M520.
7. Altemose GT, Gritsus V, Jeevanandam V, Goldman B, Margulies KB. 1997. Altered myocardial phenotype after mechanical support in human beings with advanced cardiomyopathy. J Heart Lung Transplant 16:765–773.
8. Baba HA, Grabellus F, August C, Plenz G, Takeda A, Tjan TD, Schmid C, Deng MC. 2000. Reversal of metallothionein expression is different throughout the human myocardium after prolonged left ventricular mechanical support. J Heart Lung Transplant 19:668–674.
9. Zafeiridis A, Jeevanandam V, Houser SR, Margulies KB. 1998. Regression of cellular hypertrophy after left ventricular assist device support. Circulation 98:656–662.
10. Nakatani S, McCarthy PM, Kottke-Marchant K, Harasaki H, James KB, Savage RM, Thomas JD. 1996. Left ventricular echocardiographic and histologic changes: impact of chronic unloading by an implantable ventricular assist device. J Am Coll Cardiol 27:894–901.
11. Scheinin SA, Capek P, Radovancevic B, Duncan JM, McAllister HA Jr, Frazier OH. 1992. The effect of prolonged left ventricular support on mycardial histopathology in patients with end-stage cardiomyopathy. ASAIO Journal 38:M271–M274.
12. Olivetti G, Abbi R, Quaini F, Kajstura J, Cheng W, Nitahara JA, Quaini E, Di Loreto C, Beltrami CA, Krajewski S, Reed JC, Anversa P. 1997. Apoptosis in the failing human heart. N Engl J Med 336:1131–1141.
13. Narula J, Haider N, Virmani R, DiSalvo TG, Kolodgie FD, Hajjar RJ, Schmidt U, Semigran MJ, Dec GW, Khaw BA. 1996. Apoptosis in myocytes in end-stage heart failure. N Engl J Med 335:1182–1189.
14. Bartling B, Milting H, Schumann H, Darmer D, Arusoglu L, Koerner MM, El-Banayosy A, Koerfer R, Holtz J, Zerkowski HR. 1999. Myocardial gene expression of regulators of myocyte apoptosis and myocyte calcium homeostasis during hemodynamic unloading by ventricular assist devices in patients with end-stage heart failure. Circulation 100:II216–II223.
15. Wollert KC, Heineke J, Westermann J, Ludde M, Fiedler B, Zierhut W, Laurent D, Bauer MK, Schulze-Osthoff K, Drexler H. 2000. The cardiac Fas (APO-1/CD95) receptor/FAS ligand system. Relation to diastolic wall stress in volume-overload hypertrophy in vivo and activation of the transcription factor AP-1 in cardiac myocytes. Circulation 101:1172–1178.
16. Cook SA, Sugden PH, Clerk A. 1999. Activation of c-Jun N-terminal kinases and p38-mitogen-activated protein kinases in human heart failure secondary to ischaemic heart disease. J Mol Cell Cardiol 31:1429–1434.
17. Haq S, Choukroun G, Lim H, Tymitz KM, del Monte F, Gwathmey J, Grazette L, Michael A, Hajjar R, Force T, Molkentin JD. 2001. Differential activation of signal transduction pathways in human hearts with hypertrophy versus advanced heart failure. Circulation 103:670–677.
18. Flesch M, Margulies KB, Mochmann HC, Engel D, Sivasubramanian N, Mann DL. 2001. Differential regulation of mitogen-activated protein kinases in the failing human heart in response to mechanical unloading. Circulation 104:2273–2276.
19. Li YY, Feldman AM, Sun Y, McTiernan CF. 1998. Differential expression of tissue inhibitors of metalloproteinases in the failing human heart. Circulation 98:1728–1734.
20. Mann DL, Spinale FG. 1998. Activation of matrix metalloproteinases in the failing human heart: breaking the tie that binds. Circulation 98:1699–1702.
21. Li YY, Feng Y, McTiernan CF, Pei W, Moravec CS, Wang P, Rosenblum W, Kormos RL, Feldman AM. 2001. Downregulation of matrix metalloproteinases and reduction of collagen damage in the failing human heart after support with left ventricular assist devices. Circulation 104:1147–1152.
22. Rohde LE, Ducharme A, Arroyo LH, Aikawa M, Sukhova GH, Lopez-Anaya A, McClure KF, Mitchell PG, Libby P, Lee RT. 1999. Matrix metalloproteinase inhibition attenuates early left ventricular enlargement after experimental myocardial infarction in mice. Circulation 99:3063–3070.

23. Spinale FG, Coker ML, Krombach SR, Mukherjee R, Hallak H, Houck WV, Clair MJ, Kribbs SB, Johnson LL, Peterson JT, Zile MR. 1999. Matrix metalloproteinase inhibition during the development of congestive heart failure. Effects on left ventricular dimensions and function. Circ Res 85:364–376.

24. Spinale FG, Coker ML, Bond BR, Zellner JL. 2000. Myocardial matrix degradation and metalloproteinase activation in the failing heart: a potential therapeutic target. Cardiovasc Res 46:225–238.

25. Solaro RJ. 1999. Is calcium the "cure" for dilated cardiomyopathy? NatureMed 5:1353–1354.

26. Marks AR. 2000. Cardiac intracellular calcium release channels. Role in heart failure. Circulation Res 87:8–11.

27. Minamisawa S, Hoshijima M, Chu G, Ward CA, Frank K, Gu Y, Martone ME, Wang Y, Ross J Jr, Kranias EG, Giles WR, Chien KR. 1999. Chronic phospholamban-sarcoplasmic reticulum calcium ATPase interaction is the critical calcium cycling defect in dilated cardiomyopathy. Cell 99:313–322.

28. Linck B, Boknik P, Eschenhagen T, Muller FU, Neumann J, Nose M, Jones LR, Schmitz W, Scholz H. 1996. Messenger RNA expression and immunological quantification of phospholamban and SR-Ca^{2+}-ATPase in failing and nonfailing hearts. Cardiovasc Res 31:625–632.

29. Heerdt PM, Holmes JW, Cai B, Barbone A, Madigan JD, Reiken S, Lee DL, Oz MC, Marks AR, Burkhoff D. 2000. Chronic unloading by left ventricular assist device reverses contractile dysfunction and alters gene expression in end-stage heart failure. Circulation 102:2713–2719.

30. Plenz G, Baba HA, Erren M, Scheld HH, Deng MC. 1999. Reversal of myocardial interleukin-6-mRNA expression following long-term left ventricular assist device support for myocarditis-associated low output syndrome. J Heart Lung Transplant 18:923–992.

31. Torre-Amione G, Stetson SJ, Youker KA, Durand JB, Radovancevic B, Delgado RM, Frazier OH, Entman ML, Noon GP. 1999. Decreased expression of tumor necrosis factor-alpha in failing human myocardium after mechanical circulatory support: A potential mechanism for cardiac recovery. Circulation 100:1189–1193.

32. Baichwal VR, Baeuerle PA. 1997. Activate NF-kappa B or die? Curr Biol 7: R94–R96.

33. Barnes PJ, Karin M. 1997. Nuclear factor-kappaB: a pivotal transcription factor in chronic inflammatory diseases. N Eng J Med 336:1066–1071.

34. Wong SC, Fukuchi M, Melnyk P, Rodger I, Giaid A. 1998. Induction of cyclooxygenase-2 and activation of nuclear factor-kappaB in myocardium of patients with congestive heart failure. Circulation 98:100–103.

35. Ghosh S, May MJ, Kopp EB. 1998. NF-κB and Rel proteins: evolutionarily conserved mediators of immune response. Annu Rev Immunol 16:225–260.

36. Grabellus F, Levkau B, Sokoll A, Welp H, Schmid C, Deng MC, Takeda A, Breithardt G, Baba HA. 2002. Reversible activation of nuclear factor-κB in human end-stage heart failure after left ventricular mechanical support. Cardiovasc Res 53:124–130.

37. Hoffman JI, Spaan JA. 1990. Pressure-flow relations in coronary circulation. Physiol Rev 70:331–390.

38. Koong AC, Chen EY, Mivechi NF, Denko NC, Stambrook P, Giaccia AJ. 1994. Hypoxic activation of nuclear factor-kappa B is mediated by a Ras and Raf signaling pathway and does not involve MAP kinase (ERK1 or ERK2). Cancer Res 54:5273–5279.

39. Grabellus F, Scmid C, Levkau B, Breukelmann D, Halloran PF, August C, Takeda A, Wilhelm M, Deng MC, Baba HA. 2002. Decreased expression of heme oxygenase-1 after prolonged left ventricular mechanical support. J Pathol (in press).

40. Elbirt KK, Bonkovsky HL. 1999. Heme oxygenase: recent advances in understanding its regulation and role. Proc Assoc Am Physicians 111:438–447.

41. Maines MD. 1997. The heme oxygenase system: a regulator of second messenger gases. Annu Rev Pharmacol Toxicol: 17–554.

42. Poss KD, Tonegawa S. 1997. Reduced stress defense in heme oxygenase 1-deficient cells. Proc Natl Acad Sci U S A 94:10925–10930.

43. Kagi JH, Schaffer A. 1988. Biochemistry of metallothionein. Biochemistry 27:8509–8515.

44. Karin M. 1985. Metallothioneins: proteins in search of function. Cell 41:9–10.

45. Markant A, Pallauf J. 1996. Metallothionein and zinc as potential antioxidants in radical-induced lipid peroxidation in cultured hepatocytes. J Trace Elem Med Biol 10:88–95.

46. Hittinger L, Shannon RP, Kohin S, Lader AS, Manders WT, Patrick TA, Kelly P, Vatner SF. 1989. Isoprterenol-induced alterations in myocardial blood flow, systolic and diastolic function in conscious dogs with heart failure. Circulation 80:658–668.

Signal Transduction and Cardiac Hypertrophy,
edited by N.S. Dhalla, L.V. Hryshko,
E. Kardami & P.K. Singal
Kluwer Academic Publishers, Boston, 2003

Reverse Molecular Remodeling of the Failing Human Heart Following Support with a Left Ventricular Assist Device

Paul M. Heerdt and Daniel Burkhoff

Departments of Anesthesiology and Pharmacology
Weill Medical College of Cornell
University and Department of Medicine
Laboratory of Circulatory Physiology
Columbia University
New York, NY

Summary. Accumulating evidence suggests that mechanical circulatory support with a left ventricular assist device (LVAD) can reverse some of the structural abnormalities associated with end-stage heart failure. Recent work from our laboratory and other investigators indicate that LVAD support may also reverse some of the subcellular abnormalities contributing to impaired excitation-contraction coupling in the failing heart. This chapter reviews data regarding LVAD-induced changes in the expression of genes and the proteins for which they encode, and relates these changes to functional aspects of myocyte calcium cycling and muscle strip contraction.

INTRODUCTION

Although it was generally believed in the past that the massively dilated and dysfunctional hearts of patients with severe end-stage heart failure are irrevocably damaged, in some patients circulatory support with a left ventricular assist device (LVAD) leads to reversal of chamber enlargement, reduction in LV mass, improved global pump function, and normalized *ex vivo* pressure-volume relations (1–4). This process has been termed *reverse structual remodeling*. Additional investigation of isolated myocytes (5) and intact isometric LV trabeculae (6) has demonstrated increased contractile function and an enhanced inotropic response to β–adrenergic stimulation following LVAD which occurs in conjunction with improved cytosolic Ca^{2+}

Address for Correspondence: Paul M. Heerdt, M.D., Ph.D., 525 East 68th. St, Lasdon 2, box 50, New York, NY 10021. Tel: 212-746-2701, Fax: 212-746-8316, E-mail: pmheerd@mail.med.cornell.edu

transients (5) and normalization of some aspects of mitochondrial energetics (7). Taken together, these data indicate that augmented left ventricular pump function is not simply the result of changes in chamber size, geometry, and compliance. Recent data indicate that LVAD support also produces other subcellular changes within myocytes that contribute to, or result from, normalized structure and/or function. This process has been termed *reverse molecular remodeling*. Evidence supporting the concept of reverse molecular remodeling and implications of this process will be reviewed.

The stimulus for reverse remodeling

The distortion of myocytes that accompanies increased pressure and volume within any heart chamber triggers a sequence of events, many of which are calcium-regulated, (8) that eventually lead to adaptive remodeling of individual cells. While the major stimulus is probably physical stretch of the myocardium, this process also involves autonomic neurotransmitters and intracardiac paracrine/autocrine mediators. These individual factors coalesce to produce a cascade of immediate and ultimately prolonged molecular and cellular events mediated in part by altered expression of a variety of genes within both myocytes and non-contractile elements of the myocardium (9). The capacity for LVADs to directly provide pressure and volume unloading of the left ventricle and indirectly normalize the neurohormonal mileu has been widely described (1,6,10).

In an effort to dissociate physical stimuli for reverse remodeling from neurohormonal, structural normalization of the left ventricle in LVAD-supported hearts was compared to that of the attendant right ventricle (6). As shown in Figure 1, a normally functioning LVAD effectively empties the left ventricle while volume load of the right ventricle is maintained. In comparison to non-failing hearts and those with chronic failure but no LVAD support, hearts that were supported with an LVAD for more than 30 days exhibited normalization of the *ex vivo* pressure-volume relationship in the left but not right ventricle (Figure 2). Furthermore, as also shown in Figure 2, myocyte size regressed in the left but not right ventricle. These data indicate that the primary stimulus for reverse structural remodeling is reduced pressure-volume stress. However, as noted below the stimulus for reverse molecular remodeling appears to involve not only the primary process of pressure-volume unloading but also a secondary alteration in neurohormonal input to the heart. Additional investigation has characterized the time-dependency of reverse structural remodeling (11). As shown in Figure 3, both the *ex vivo* pressure-volume relationship and myocyte diameter exhibit progressive changes during LVAD support that plateau ~40 days when fit to a monoexponential regression model.

Evidence for reverse molecular remodeling

Multiple lines of investigation indicate a range of subcellular changes produced by LVAD support. Facilitating this research is the fact that during implantation of most devices a significant amount of LV tissue is removed which can subsequently be

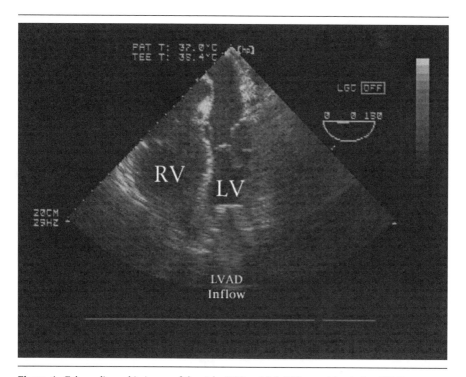

Figure 1. Echocardiographic image of the right (RV) and left (LV) ventricles during LVAD support. The apical cannula for inflow to the LVAD is evident as is decompression of the LV with continued volume loading of the RV and a shift of the interventricular septum. (From reference 6, used by permission).

used for both functional and biochemical study thus allowing for pre- and post-LVAD comparison within individual patients. In general, data have been reported to demonstrate LVAD-induced up-regulation of β-adrenergic and endothelin-A receptors (12,13) modulation of antiapoptotic genes (14), deactivation of nuclear factor-kappaB (15) normalization of mitochondrial ultrastructure (16), and down-regulation of matrix metalloproteinases, tumor necrosis factor-α, and β-tubulin (17–19). Work from our laboratory has focused primarily upon regulation of myocyte calcium cycling due to the fundamental abnormalities in excitation-contraction coupling that accompany end-stage heart failure.

Phenotypic changes in myocardial calcium cycling

Myocardial systolic and diastolic dysfunction in severe heart failure have been associated with abnormal calcium release from, and uptake into, the sarcoplasmic reticulum (SR) (20). Accordingly, data from isolated myocytes demonstrating improved cytosolic Ca^{2+} transients (increased peak, accelerated decay) and an increased

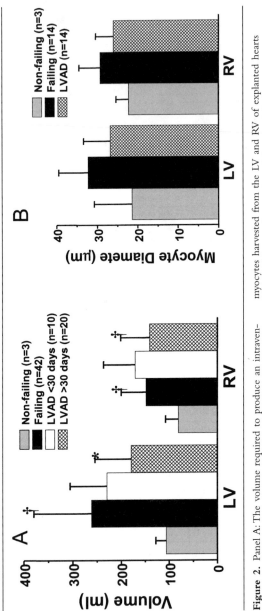

Figure 2. Panel A: The volume required to produce an intraventricular pressure of 30 mmHg in the left (LV) and right (RV) ventricles of explanted, non-beating hearts. Panel B: Diameter of myocytes harvested from the LV and RV of explanted hearts (Adapted from reference 6, used by permission).

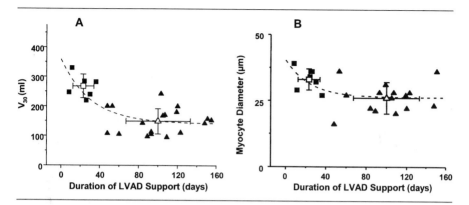

Figure 3. Panel A: The volume required to produce an intraventricular pressure of 30 mmHg (V_{30}) in the left ventricles of explanted, non-beating hearts plotted as a function of LVAD duration. Panel B: Diameter of left ventricular myocytes plotted as a function of LVAD duration. For both panels, squares depict <40 days and triangles >40 days. Open symbols represent mean ± SE. (adapted from reference 11, used by permission).

rate of shortening following LVAD (5) prompted further investigation into calcium uptake by isolated SR membranes and the intrinsic myocardial performance of intact, loaded muscle.

a. **Isolated SR membranes.** Both the release and uptake of calcium by isolated SR membranes has been reported to be impaired in patients with end-stage heart failure (4,20). As a means to determine if LVAD support improves this abnormality, calcium uptake by SR membranes isolated from non-failing, failing, and LVAD hearts was measured (4). As shown in Figure 4, relative to non-failing hearts, the amount of oxalate-supported Ca^{2+} uptake over 5 minutes (in nM/mg protein) was reduced by failure and restored by LVAD. Addition of ryanodine to the incubation medium to block concomitant release via the ryanodine-sensitve calcium release channel increased Ca^{2+} uptake in non-failing membranes by ~25% but only ~10% by SR membranes from *both* CHF and CHF + LVAD hearts.

b. **Isolated muscle strips.** For these studies, the contractile strength of endocardial trabeculae harvested from non-failing, non-LVAD transplant hearts ("failing"), the apical "core" tissue obtained at the time of LVAD implantation, and from LVAD-supported hearts were assessed (4). At 1 Hz stimulation frequency, absolute force generation by non-failing, pre-LVAD, post-LVAD and non-LVAD transplanted hearts (normalized to cross-sectional area) were similar to each other, consistent with prior reports (21). However, assessing the force-frequency relationship (FFR) of each preparation by using progressively higher rates of stimulation demonstrated that while force declined in muscle from the pre-LVAD and non-LVAD supported hearts (negative FFR), it increased in the non-failing and post-LVAD supported hearts (positive FFR). Representative force

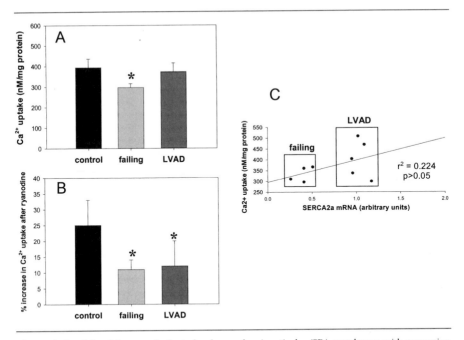

Figure 4. Panel A: calcium uptake by isolated sarcoplasmic reticular (SR) membranes with restoration of uptake following LVAD evident; *designates difference from non-failing. Panel B: The percent increase in calcium uptake by isolated SR membranes after addition of ryanodine to block simultaneous efflux via the RyR; *designates difference from non-failing. Panel C: calcium uptake by failing and LVAD-supported hearts plotted as a function of the mRNA for sarcoplasmic endoreticular calcium ATPase subtype 2a (SERCA2a); no significant correlation is evident.

tracings from the same patient both pre- and post-LVAD are shown in Figure 5. These investigations also demonstrated that in post-LVAD hearts, β-adrenergic responsiveness is restored not just in the unloaded LV but in the RV as well (Figure 6). Similar results with regard to FFR and β-adrenergic responsiveness have been obtained from LVAD patients with either ischemic (ICM) or idiopathic dilated cardiomyopathy (DCM). However, results of preliminary experiments indicate quantitative differences in some responses depending upon whether inotropic therapy was being administered prior to tissue harvest. This observation suggests that improved β-adrenergic responsiveness following LVAD may more closely reflect the withdrawal of inotropic support and improved neurohormonal status than chronic mechanical unloading of the LV (10). Nevertheless, these results indicate that although resting strength may not be significantly influenced, two important mechanisms regulating contractile strength—β-adrenergic responsiveness and frequency of contraction—are restored during LVAD support.

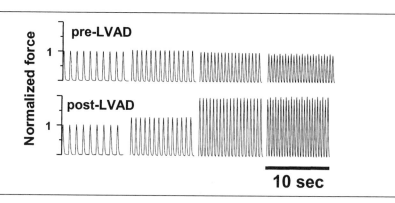

Figure 5. Force tracings from endocardial trabeculae from the same heart before (pre) and after (post) LVAD support. The response to pacing at increasing frequency shows progressively impaired systolic performance pre-LVAD but progressively improved performance post-LVAD. (Adapted from reference 4, used by permission).

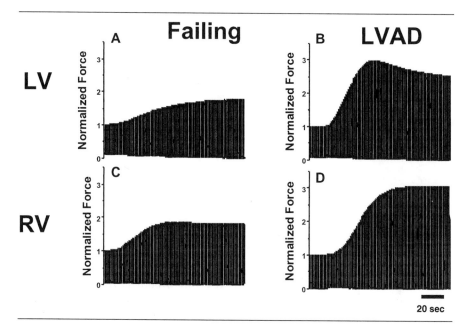

Figure 6. Force tracings from endocardial trabecuale harvested from failing and LVAD-supported hearts during isoproterenol stimulation. Panels A and B depict enhanced responsiveness in the left ventricle (LV). Panels C and D depict similar enhancement in the right ventricle (RV) despite maintenance of volume loading during LVAD support. (Adapted from reference 6, used by permission).

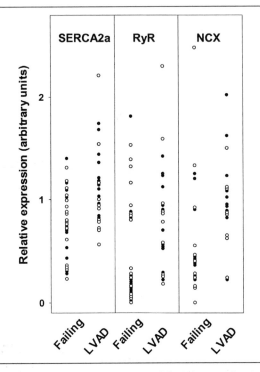

Figure 7. Individual mRNA values (normalized to non-failing) for sarcoplasmic endoreticular calcium ATPase subtype 2a (SERCA2a); the ryanodine receptor (RyR) and the sarcolemmal sodium: calcium exchanger (NCX). Open circles represent ischemic cardiomyopathy (ICM) and closed circles dilated cardiomyopathy (DCM).

Gene and protein evidence for reverse remodeling
of myocyte calcium cycling components

The findings of LVAD-induced improvement in isolated myocyte Ca^{2+} metabolism coupled with normalization of the FFR of loaded trabeculae supported the hypothesis that expression of genes encoding for proteins involved in Ca^{2+} handling are altered by LVAD support. To further test this hypothesis, expression of the sarcoplasmic endoreticular calcium-ATPase subtype 2a (SERCA2a), the ryanodine-sensitive calcium release channel (RyR), and the sarcolemmal sodium-calcium exchanger (NCX) was determined by Northern blotting. Alteration in the expression (reduced for SERCA2a; increased for NCX) and/or function (reduced for SERCA2a and RyR, increased for NCX) of each of these proteins appears to be associated with various aspects of contractile dysfunction in severe heart failure (22–26).

a. Gene expression in pooled and paired samples. As shown in Figure 7, there was marked variability and considerable overlap in the mRNA message for

SERCA2a, RyR and the NCX. In an attempt to limit the impact of variability by having each patient serve as his own control, tissue samples obtained from 20 individual hearts before and after LVAD support were compared to those harvested from non-failing hearts (4). As shown in Figure 8, there was, on average, increased expression of all 3 genes following LVAD support.

b. **mRNA-Protein relationship.** In order to determine whether there is a relationship between mRNA and protein, Western blotting for SERCA2a, RyR, and NCX protein was performed on a subset of patients (4). As shown in Figure 9, only SERCA2a exhibited a significant rise for both mRNA and protein. However, within individual patients there was no significant correlation between the two.

c. **Time-dependence.** Subsequent investigation evaluated the importance of LVAD duration on SERCA2a expression (11). Not surprisingly, plotting mRNA as a function of LVAD support days revealed a progressive rise that reached a plateau after ~40 days (Figure 10) when fit to a monoexponential regression equation.

d. **Physical *vs* neurohormonal stimuli.** Although the right and left ventricles share a common biochemical milieu, during LVAD support the left ventricle may be profoundly unloaded while the right is not (27). We therefore took advantage of this difference to test the hypothesis that altered hemodynamic load is the predominant stimulus for increased SERCA2a expression (6). Using samples taken from both ventricles of the same hearts, SERCA2a protein content was measured by Western blot analysis in 14 transplant hearts and 14 LVAD supported hearts. As shown in Figure 11, LVAD support more than doubled left ventricular SERCA2a protein content. In contrast, there was no significant change in SERCA2a protein within the right ventricle.

Significance and limitations

Gene-protein-function relationship

In that activity of SERCA2a has been linked with the FFR, down-regulation of the gene encoding for SERCA2a in heart failure (4,20) appears to be associated with the negative FFR. Consistent with these findings, our data suggest that improved force and FFR following LVAD were accompanied by SERCA2a up-regulation. Complementing the gene expression data are an increase in SERCA2a protein levels and oxalate-supported Ca^{2+} uptake by isolated SR membranes following LVAD. Although the relationship between SERCA2a and FFR has been more extensively studied, properties of the RyR, which regulates Ca^{2+} release to the myofilaments, also play a pivotal role in the ability of the SR to store and rapidly release Ca^{2+} (22). Our data indicate up-regulated expression of the gene encoding for RyR following LVAD but little change in the protein content, a finding consistent with the fact that blockade of the RyR with an excess of ryanodine had the same effect on Ca^{2+} uptake by SR membranes isolated from both failing and failing/LVAD hearts. In a recent study, we showed that hyperphosphorylation of

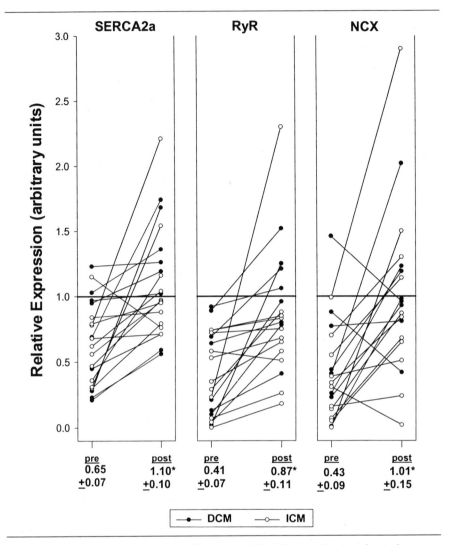

Figure 8. Individual mRNA values (normalized to non-failing) for sarcoplasmic endoreticular calcium ATPase subtype 2a (SERCA2a); the ryanodine receptor (RyR) and the sarcolemmal sodium: calcium exchanger (NCX) obtained from the same hearts before (pre) and after (post) LVAD support. Open circles represent ischemic cardiomyopathy (ICM) and closed circles dilated cardiomyopathy (DCM). Numerical data are mean ± SE with *representing a pre/post difference. (Adapted from reference 4, used by permission).

RyR in failing human myocardium disrupts the normal coupled gating of neighboring receptors resulting in abnormal ensemble gating patterns, less coordinated SR Ca^{2+} release during excitation, and Ca^{2+} leak during diastole (28). Post-LVAD, these abnormalities are reversed, possibly in response to normalization of the β-

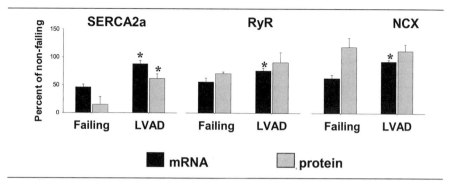

Figure 9. Comparison of mRNA and protein for sarcoplasmic endoreticular calcium ATPase subtype 2a (SERCA2a); the ryanodine receptor (RyR) and the sarcolemmal sodium : calcium exchanger (NCX) within the same myocardial samples obtained from failing or LVAD hearts and normalized to non-failing samples. *designates a failing/LVAD difference. Only SERCA2a exhibited significant increases in both mRNA and protein.

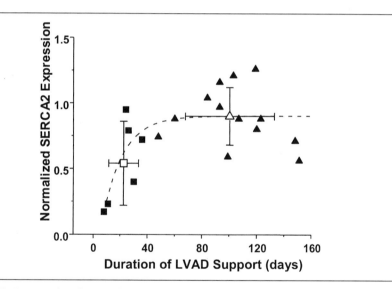

Figure 10. Protein values for sarcoplasmic endoreticular calcium ATPase subtype 2a (SERCA2a); normalized to non-failing and plotted as a function of LVAD duration. Squares depict <40 days and triangles >40 days; open symbols represent mean ± SE.). Adapted from reference 11, used by permission).

adrenergic signaling pathway. Thus, despite subtle changes in gene expression and/or protein content, it appears that channel or pump function may be more affected by post-translational events. Results of some studies have indicated that with decreased SERCA2a function in heart failure, a compensatory increase in the activity of the NCX occurs as this sarcolemmal protein assumes a greater role in extruding Ca^{2+} during diastole (20,29,30). Consistent with this process is data indicating up-

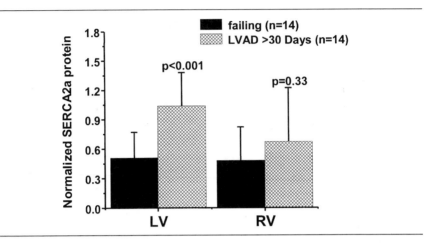

Figure 11. mRNA values for sarcoplasmic endoreticular calcium ATPase subtype 2a (SERCA2a) normalized to non-failing for left (LV) and right (RV) ventricular samples harvested from failing or LVAD hearts with >30 days of support. A marked increase in the LV but not RV of LVAD hearts is evident. (Adapted from reference 6, used by permission).

regulated myocardial expression of NCX mRNA in human heart failure (26). However, recent data indicate that levels of NCX exchanger protein are not necessarily changed in severe human heart failure (25), and animal studies have suggested that there can be decreased gene expression, and reduced Ca^{2+} flux through the NCX in the setting of cardiac failure (31–33). Our data showed that LVAD support lead to up-regulated gene expression but no change in NCX protein content. Thus, as for RyR, isolated measurement of gene expression may not fully clarify pathophysiologic or LVAD-induced changes of the NCX properties.

Regional heterogeneity

A potential limitation in the characterization of reverse molecular remodeling is the probability that changes are not uniform within a given chamber. To approach this issue we compared mRNA for SERCA2a, RyR and the NCX obtained from the left ventricular apex and free wall of the same failing heart (4). As shown in Figure 12, there was a trend for apical expression of all 3 genes to be higher although the difference was only significant for SERCA2a. This observation underscores a potential caveat in the study of pre-and post-LVAD tissue obtained from the same heart because the pre-LVAD sample is from the apex and the post-LVAD sample from the free wall. Compounding this caveat is the fact that not all processes producing end-stage failure are uniform (see below).

Underlying disease

Although the functional end-point of severe, refractory heart failure is uniform among LVAD recipients, the underlying disease leading to end-stage failure is not.

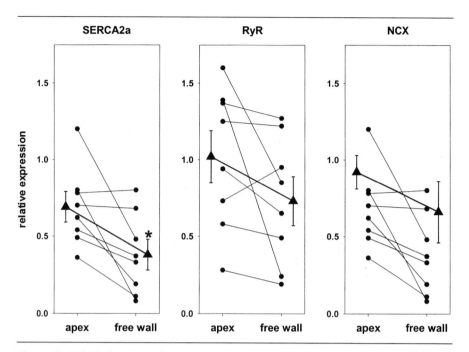

Figure 12. Individual mRNA values normalized to non-failing (circles) for sarcoplasmic endoreticular calcium ATPase subtype 2a (SERCA2a); the ryanodine receptor (RyR) and the sarcolemmal sodium: calcium exchanger (NCX) obtained from the left ventricular apex and free wall of the same hearts. Although the mean values (triangles) indicate a trend toward regional variation for all 3 genes, only SERCA2a exhibited a significant apical-free wall difference (designated by *). (From reference 4, used by permission).

For example, the patient with diffuse ischemic cardiomyopathy (ICM) may have a heterogenous process with areas of ischemia and infarction interspersed with relatively normal tissue. In contrast, idiopathic dilated cardiomyopathies (DCM) tend to be more homogeneous. Clarification of disease-dependent changes in gene expression is complicated by the fact the wide variability of mRNA values necessitates study of very large sample sizes. Nonetheless, as shown in Figure 13, application of nonparametric statistical analysis to mRNA data obtained from 80 samples in our laboratory have begun to suggest that LVAD-induced changes in RyR and NCX expression occur primarily in DCM hearts. In contrast, we have found that molecular remodeling of mitochondrial ultrastructure in heart failure, and its reversal by LVAD, occurs exclusively in ICM hearts (16).

Age, gender, pharmacotherapy

As with underlying disease, the impact of other factors such as age, gender and pharmacotherapy on reverse remodeling remain largely unexplored. In that aging alone has been shown to alter expression of calcium cycling genes (particularly SERCA2a)

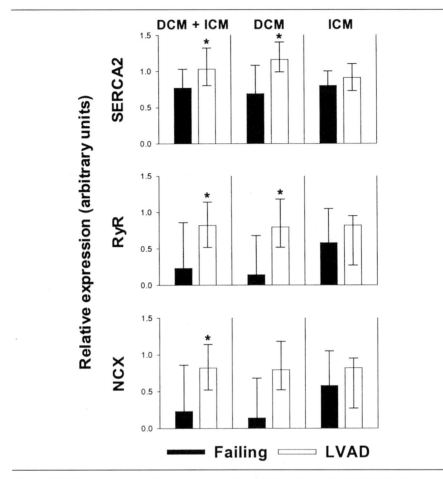

Figure 13. Values for sarcoplasmic endoreticular calcium ATPase subtype 2a (SERCA2a); the ryanodine receptor (RyR) and the sarcolemmal sodium : calcium exchanger (NCX) mRNA subdivided according to ischemic (ICM) or dilated (DCM) cardiomyopathy. Data are presented as median values with confidence limits, and demonstrate significant LVAD-induced change only for DCM hearts.

(34) and to dampen the process of forward remodeling in response to increased pressure and/or volume (35), there is a clear theoretical basis for a possible effect on reverse remodeling as well. Similarly, data demonstrating gender-related differences in SR calcium cycling in heart failure (36) indicate the possibility that the fundamental molecular abnormality may be influenced by gender with attendant effects on the nature of any LVAD-induced reversal. Finally, experimental and clinical studies have clearly indicated that drugs such as angiotensin converting enzyme inhibitors and β-blockers can prevent or reverse structural and perhaps molecular forward remodeling in the setting of heart failure (37,38). In that angiotensin

converting enzyme inhibitors exert direct effects on ventricular preload and after-load as well as effects on the neurohormonal system, it has been hypothesized that both hemodynamic and neurohormonal factors contribute to the beneficial effects on remodeling. However, whether the use of these drugs during LVAD-support alters the nature or time course of reverse remodeling remains unknown.

DISCUSSION

Work from our laboratory has demonstrated that LVAD-support reverses several aspects of ventricular pathophysiology including: 1) chamber enlargement and abnormal EDPVR; 2) globally increased LV mass and individual myocyte hyper-trophy; 3) diminished resting contractile properties and the inotropic response to β-adrenergic stimulation; 4) altered expression and/or function of proteins involved in calcium metabolism; and 5) altered mitochondrial ultrastructure. Other investigators have reported equally important findings, and it is likely that many more aspects of cardiac pathophysiology improved by LVAD support will be demonstrated in the future. As studies of this nature grow to include greater numbers of patients, it will also become increasingly important to analyze separately results from patients with different heart failure etiologies, age, gender and pharmacotherapy in order to characterize interdependent factors influencing heart failure in general and LVAD support in particular.

The precise mechanisms underlying the various aspects of reverse remodeling remain to be determined. Clearly the mechanisms involved with forward myocar-dial remodeling in response to pressure and volume load reflect intricately orches-trated up- and down-regulations of multiple intracellular signaling cascades. Indeed the complexities of these processes are evident in the fact that although having been investigated for over 20 years, these mechanisms are still not understood. It has been our working hypothesis that reverse remodeling involves the same mechanisms working in the opposite direction. However, in all probability additional mecha-nisms may also be in effect. By restoring cardiac output, blood pressure and renal perfusion, LVAD support leads to normalization of the neurohormonal and cytokine environment which may have profound effects in normalizing cellular properties.

Recent evidence suggests that in some patients, LVAD support may lead to improvement of global pump function of sufficient magnitude to permit removal of the device without subsequent transplantation (27,39). This has led to the concept of using LVADs as a bridge to recovery. The potential of this possibility is strength-ened by data demonstrating the global extent to which reverse remodeling occurs. However, current data indicate a very low incidence of sustained "full" recovery during LVAD support (40) thus weaning and device removal is not currently stan-dard of care. Nevertheless, the goal of using LVADs as a bridge to recovery is a worthy pursuit because of the severe imbalance between the number of patients requiring transplant and the number of available donor hearts. Better understand-ing of the process of reverse remodeling will aid the development of adjunctive therapies, better patient selection criteria and perhaps optimum LVAD use proto-cols to improve patient outcome following LVAD explantation.

REFERENCES

1. Levin HR, Oz MC, Chen JM, Packer M, Rose EA, Burkhoff D. 1995. Reversal of chronic ventricular dilation in patients with end-stage cardiomyopathy by prolonged mechanical unloading. Circulation 91:2717–2720.
2. McCarthy PM, Nakatani S, Vargo R, Kottke-Marchant K, Harasaki H, James KB, Savage RM, Thomas JD. 1995. Structural and left ventricular histologic changes after implantable LVAD insertion. Ann Thorac Surg 59:609–613.
3. Altemose GT, Gritsus V, Jeevanandam V, Goldman B, Margulies KB. 1997. Altered myocardial phenotype after mechanical support in human beings with advanced cardiomyopathy. J Heart Lung Transplant 16:765–773.
4. Heerdt PM, Holmes JW, Cai B, Barbone A, Madigan JD, Reiken S, Lee DL, Oz MC, Marks AR, Burkhoff D. 2000. Chronic unloading by left ventricular assist device reverses contractile dysfunction and alters gene expression in end-stage heart failure. Circulation 102:2713–2719.
5. Dipla K, Mattiello JA, Jeevanandam V, Houser SR, Margulies KB. 1998. Myocyte recovery after mechanical circulatory support in humans with end-stage heart failure. Circulation 97:2316–2322.
6. Barbone A, Holmes J, Heerdt PM et al. 2001. Comparison of right and left ventricular responses to left ventricular assist device support in patients with severe heart failure: A primary role of mechanical unloading underlying reverse remodeling. Circulation 104(6):670–675.
7. Lee SH, Doliba N, Osbakken M, Oz M, Mancini D. 1998. Improvement of myocardial mitochondrial function after hemodynamic support with left ventricular assist devices in patients with heart failure. J Thorac Cardiovasc Surg 116:344–349.
8. Calaghan SC, White E. 1999. The role of calcium in the response of cardiac muscle to stretch. Prog Biophys Molec Biol 71:59–90.
9. Swynghedauw B. 1999. Molecular mechanisms of myocardial remodeling. Pharmacological Reviews. 79:215–262.
10. Estrada-Quintero T, Uretsky BF, Murali S, Griffith BP, Kormos RL. 1995. Neurohormonal activation and exercise function in patients with severe heart failure and patients with left ventricular assist system. Chest 107:1499–1503.
11. Madigan JD, Barbone A, Choudhri AF, Morales DL, Cai B, Oz MC, Burkhoff D. 2001. Time course of reverse remodeling of the left ventricle during support with a left ventricular assist device. J Thorac Cardiovasc Surg 121(5):902–908.
12. Ogletree-Hughes ML, Stull LB, Sweet WE, Smedira NG, McCarthy PM, Moravec CS. 2001. Mechanical unloading restores beta-adrenergic responsiveness and reverses receptor downregulation in the failing human heart. Circulation 104(8):881–886.
13. Moravietz H, Szibor M, Goettsch W, Bartling B, Barton M, Shaw S, Koerfer R, Zerkowski HR, Holtz J. 2000. Deloading of the left ventricle by ventricualr assist device normalizes increased expression of endothelin ET_A receptors but not endothelin-converting enzyme-1 in patients with end-stage heart failure. Circulation 102(suppl III):III-188–III-193.
14. Bartling B, Milting H, Schumann H, Darmer D, Arusoglu L, Koerner MM, El-Babayosy A, Koerfer R, Holtz J, Zerkowski HR. 1999. Myocardial gene expression of regulators of myocyte apoptosis and myocyte calcium homeostasis during hemodynamic unloading by ventricular assist devices in patients with end-stage heart failure. Circulation 100(suppl II):216–223.
15. Grabellus F, Levkau B, Sokoll A, Welp H, Schmid C, Deng MC, Takeda A, Breithardt G, Baba HA. 2001. Reversible activation of nuclear factor-kappaB in human end-stage heart failure after left ventricular mechanical support. Cardiovasc Res 53(1):124–130.
16. Heerdt PM, Schlame M, Burkhoff D, Blanck TJJB. 2002. Disease-specific remodeling of mitochondrial membranes in failing human hearts following unloading by a left ventricular assist device. Ann Thorac Surg (in press).
17. Li YY, Feng Y, McTiernan CF, Pei W, Moravec CS, Wang P, Rosenblum W, Kormos RL, Feldman AM. 2001. Downregulation of matrix metalloproteinases and reduction in collagen damage in the failing human heart after support with left ventricular assist devices. Circulation 104(10):1147–1152.
18. Razeghi P, Mukhopadhyay M, Myers TJ, Williams JN, Moravec CS, Frazier OH, Taegtmeyer H. 2001. Myocardial tumor necrosis factor-alpha expression does not correlate with clinical indices of heart failure in patients on left ventricularassist device support. Ann Thorac Surg 72(6):2044–2050.
19. Aquila-Pastir LA, McCarthy PM, Smedira NG, Moravec CS. 2001. Mechanical unloading decreases the expression of beta-tubulin in the failing human heart. J Heart Lung Transplant 20(2):211.
20. Houser SR, Piacentino V 3rd, Weisser J. 2000. Abnormalities of calcium cycling in the hypertrophied and failing heart. J Mol Cell Cardiol 32(9):1595–1607.

21. Pieske B, Sutterlin M, Schmidt-Schweda S, Minami K, Meyer M, Olschewski M, Holubarch C, Just H, Hasenfuss G. 1996. Diminished post-rest potentiation of contractile force in human dilated cardiomyopathy. J Clin Invest 98:764–776.
22. Arai M, Alpert NR, MacLennan DH, Barton P, Periasamy M. 1993. Alterations in sarcoplamic reticulum gene experssion in human heart failure: a possible mechanism for alterations in systolic and diastolic properties of the failing myocardium. Circ Res 72:463–469.
23. Linck B, Boknik P, Eschenhagen T, Muller FU, Neumann J, Nose M, Jones LR, Schmitz W, Scholz H. 1995. Messenger RNA expression and immunological quantification of phospholamban and SR-Ca^{2+}-ATPase in failing and nonfailing human hearts. Cardiovasc Res 31:625–632.
24. Go LO, Moschella MC, Watras J, Handa KK, Fyfe BS, Marks AR. 1995. Differential regulation of two types of intracellular calcium release channels during end-stage heart failure. J Clin Invest 95:888–894.
25. Hasenfuss G, Reinecke H, Studer R, Meyer M, Pieske B, Holtz J, Holubarsch C, Posival H, Just H, Drexler H. 1994. Relation between myocardial function and expression of sarcoplasmic reticulum Ca2+-ATPase in failing and nonfailing human myocardium. Circ Res 75:434–442.
26. Studer R, Reinecke H, Bilger J, Eschenhagen T, Bohm M, Hasenfuss G, Just H, Holtz J, Drexler H. 1994. Gene expression of the cardiac Na+-Ca2+ exchanger in end-stage human heart failure. Circ Res 75:443–453.
27. Muller J, Wallukat G, Weng YG, Dandel M, Spiegelsberger S, Semrau S, Brandes K, Theodoridis V, Loebe M, Meyer R, Hetzer R. 1997. Weaning from mechanical cardiac support in patients with idiopathic dilated cardiomyopathy. Circulation 96:542–549.
28. Marx SO, Reiken S, Hisamatsu Y, Jayaraman T, Burkhoff D, Rosemblit N, Marks AR. 2000. PKA phosphorylation dissociates FKBP12.6 from the calcium release channel (ryanodine receptor): defective regulation in failing hearts. Cell 101(4):365–376.
29. Flesch M, Schwinger RH, Schiffer F, Frank K, Sudkamp M, Kuhn-Regnier F, Arnold G, Bohm M. 1996. Evidence for functional relevance of an enhanced expression of the Na(+)-Ca2+ exchanger in failing human myocardium. Circulation 94:992–1002.
30. Hasenfuss G, Schillinger W, Lehnart SE, Preuss M, Pieske B, Maier LS, Prestle J, Minami K, Just H. 1999. Relationship between Na+-Ca2+ exchanger protein levels and diastolic function of failing human ventricles. Circulation 99:641–648.
31. Yoshiyama M, Takeuchi K, Hanatani A, Kim S, Umura T, Toda I, Teragaki M, Akioka K, Iwao H, Yoshikawa J. 1997. Differences in expression of sarcoplasmic reticular Ca2+-ATPase and Na+-Ca2+ exchanger genes between adjacent and remote noninfarcted myocardium after myocardial infarction. J Mol Cell Cardiol 29:255–264.
32. Yao A, Su Z, Nonaka A, Zubair I, Spitzer KW, Bridge JH, Muelheims G, Ross J Jr, Barry WH. 1998. Abnormal myocyte Ca2+ homeostasis in rabbits with pacing-induced heart failure. Am J Physiol 275:H1441–H1448.
33. Dixon IMC, Hata T, Dhalla NS. 1992. Sarcolemmal calcium transport in congestive heart failure due to myocardial infarction in rats. Am J Physiol 262:H1387–H1394.
34. Lakatta EG. 1993. Myocardial adaptations in advanced age. Basic Res Cardiol 88(suppl 2)2:125–133.
35. Isoyama S, Grossman W, Wei JY. 1998. Effect of age on myocardial adaptation to volume overload in the rat. J Clin Invest 81(6):1850–1857.
36. Dash R, Frank KF, Carr AN, Moravec CS, Kranias EG. 2001. Gender influences on sarcoplasmic reticulum Ca2+-handling in failing human myocardium. J Mol Cell Cardiol 33(7):1345–1353.
37. Weber KT. 2001. Cardioreparation in hypertensive heart disease. Hypertension 38(3 Pt 2):588–591.
38. Sabbah HN. 1999. He cellular and physiologic effects of beta blockers in heart failure. Cardiol 22(Suppl 5):V16–V20.
39. Hetzer R, Mueller J, Weng Y, Wallukat G, Spiegelsberger S, Loebe M. 1999. Cardiac recovery in dilated cardiomyopathy by unloading with a left ventricular assist device. Ann Thorac Surg 68:742–749.
40. Mancini DM, Beniaminovitz A, Levin H, Catanese K, Flannery M, DiTullio M, Savin S, Cordisco M, Rose E, Oz M. 1998. Low incidence of myocardial recovery in patients with left ventricular assist devices. Circulation 98(22):2383–2389.

Signal Transduction and Cardiac Hypertrophy,
edited by N.S. Dhalla, L.V. Hryshko,
E. Kardami & P.K. Singal
Kluwer Academic Publishers, Boston, 2003

Stretch-Elicited Autocrine/Paracrine Mechanism in the Heart

Horacio E. Cingolani,★ Néstor G. Perez,★
and María C. Camilión de Hurtado★

Centro de Investigaciones Cardiovasculares
Facultad de Ciencias Médicas
Universidad Nacional de La Plata
Calle 60 y 120, 1900 La Plata
Argentina

Summary. An autocrine/paracrine mechanism is triggered by stretching the myocardium. This mechanism involves the release of angiotensin II (Ang II), the release/increased formation of endothelin (ET), the activation of the Na^+/H^+ exchanger (NHE), the increase in intracellular Na^+ concentration ($[Na^+]_i$), and the increase in the Ca^{2+} transient that underlies the so called slow force response (SFR) to stretch. This autocrine/paracrine mechanism could explain how a change in afterload alters cardiac contractility as was reported by Anrep in 1912.

Key words: myocardial stretch, Na^+/Ca^{2+} exchange, angiotensin II, endothelin hypertrophy.

INTRODUCTION

It is known that when the length of the cardiac muscle is increased, there is first a rapid and then a slow increase in twitch force. The first phase is thought to be due to an increase in myofilament responsiveness and is considered to be the basis of the Frank-Starling mechanism (1). The second phase that develops during the next 10 minutes or so is believed to be due to an increase in the Ca^{2+} transient (2–5) and its link with autocrine/paracrine mechanisms involving the tissue renin-angiotensin system has been recently suggested (5). We will discuss here the intra-

Address for Correspondence: Dr. Horacio E. Cingolani, Centro de Investigaciones Cardiovasculares, Facultad de Ciencias Médicas, UNLP, 60 y 120 (1900) La Plata, Argentina. Fax#: (54-221) 425-5861, Phone: (54-221) 483-4833, E-mail: cicme@atlas.med.unlp.edu.ar
★ Established Investigators of Consejo Nacional de Investigaciones Científicas y Técnicas (CONICET), Argentina.

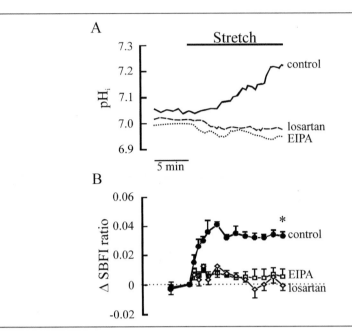

Figure 1. Stretch-induced NHE activation. Effects of EIPA and losartan. Activation of the NHE after stretching papillary muscles can be detected by both the increase in pH_i (typical experiment in panel A, "control") or in $[Na^+]_i$ (averaged experiments of panel B, "control", expressed as changes in the SBFI fluorescence ratio) in the absence of bicarbonate. When bicarbonate is present in the medium, the increase in $[Na^+]_i$ still occurs but pH_i changes are minimized. NHE blockade by EIPA as well as blockade of the Ang II AT_1 receptors by losartan abolished the changes promoted by the stretch (typical experiments in panel A and averaged data of panel B, "EIPA" and "losartan"). *indicates $p < 0.05$ vs EIPA and losartan. (Adapted from Cingolani et al. 1998 (8) and from Alvarez et al. 1999 (5) with permission).

cellular changes that follow the stretch of feline papillary muscles and the mechanical counterpart that results from the autocrine/paracrine mechanism triggered by myocardial stretch.

ACTIVATION OF THE NHE BY MYOCARDIAL STRETCH

Figure 1 shows the activation of the NHE that occurs after stretching papillary muscles from 92 to 98% of the length at which they developed the maximal twitch force (L_{max}). The activation of the NHE can be detected either by the increase in $[Na^+]_i$ (panel B) or by the increase in intracellular pH (pH_i) (panel A). When bicarbonate is present in the medium however, the changes in pH_i are minimized due to the activation of a bicarbonate acidifying mechanism (6,7) while the changes in $[Na^+]_i$ are still of similar magnitude. These changes can be abolished by NHE blockade with 5-(N-ethyl-N-isopropyl)-amiloride (EIPA) or by blockade of the Ang II AT_1 receptors with losartan (panels A and B) (8).

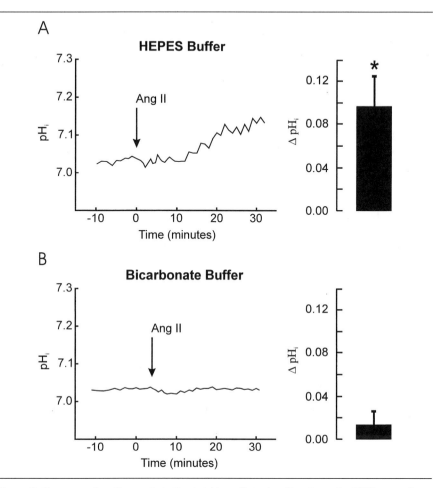

Figure 2. Exogenous Ang II can mimic the stretching effects. Ang II activates the NHE promoting an increase in pH_i that is prominent in the absence of bicarbonate (HEPES buffer) as shown in panel A (a typical experiment at left and the averaged pH_i value after 30 minutes in the column graph). In the presence of the physiological buffer (bicarbonate buffer) the changes in pH_i are minimized as shown in panel B (as in panel A, a typical experiment at left and the averaged pH_i value after 30 minutes in the column graph). *indicates $P < 0.05$ vs pre-Ang II control. (Adapted from Camilión de Hurtado et al. 1998 (6)).

ROLE OF ANG II IN THE ACTIVATION OF THE NHE

Since previous studies have shown that the stretch of isolated neonatal cardiomyocytes promotes the release of preformed Ang II (9), we were tempted to conclude that in our multicellular adult preparation the myocardial stretch releases preformed Ang II that, through the AT_1 receptors, stimulates the NHE in an autocrine or paracrine fashion (8–9). Figure 2 shows that in agreement with this, exogenous Ang II can mimic the effects of stretch. Ang II activates the NHE being reflected by an increase in pH_i (panel A). Note that the change in pH_i is minimized in the presence of bicarbonate (panel B), because of the already mentioned simultaneous activation of a bicarbonate acidifying mechanism by Ang II (6,7).

ROLE OF ET IN THE ANG II-INDUCED ACTIVATION OF THE NHE

Based in the experiments by Ito et al. (10) and considering that several effects previously attributed to Ang II are actually the result of the formation/release of ET (7,11,12), the possibility that Ang II-induced release/formation of ET mediates the effects of stretch was explored. Figure 3 shows that it was indeed the case, since the activation of the NHE by stretching papillary muscles was abolished by both nonselective and selective ET_A receptor blockade, and by inhibition of the endothelin-converting enzyme (ECE) activity with phosphoramidon. Similarly the activation of the NHE by exogenously applied Ang II was abolished by ET receptors blockade (8), as shown in Figure 4.

CROSS TALK BETWEEN ANG II AND ET

The fact that ET receptors blockade inhibits the activation of the NHE by Ang II, together with the notion that the NHE activation induced by ET is not abolished by AT_1 receptor blockade as previously reported by us (8), indicate that Ang II-induced release/formation of ET is the valid way of the cross talk between both peptides and not the opposite. These results suggest that it should be also the pathway for stretch, ruling out the possibility that myocardial stretch releases ET which in turn would release Ang II and cause the activation of the NHE. Figure 5 schematizes the complete sequence of events that are triggered by the stretch.

THE MECHANICAL COUNTERPART OF THE AUTOCRINE/PARACRINE EFFECTS

Figure 6 shows the typical changes in developed force that follows myocardial stretch (panel A) and the suppression of the second phase (the SFR) that causes the interference of the chain of the autocrine/paracrine events that follows myocardial stretch by NHE inhibition or the blockade of either Ang II AT_1 or ET receptors (panels B–D).

THE Na^+/Ca^{2+} EXCHANGER (NCX) AS THE CULPRIT OF THE INCREASE IN THE Ca^{2+} TRANSIENT

Since it was previously reported that the progressive increase in force during the SFR is due to an increase in the Ca^{2+} transient (2–5), we tested the hypothesis that the increase in the Ca^{2+} transient could be secondary to the increase in $[Na^+]_i$ that follows the NHE activation. It can be argued that the increase in pH_i after the NHE activation could mediate or contribute to the increase in contractility through an increase in the myofilament responsiveness to Ca^{2+}. However we should keep in mind that the changes in pH_i are minimized when bicarbonate is present in the medium and that previous studies have shown the absence of changes in myofilament Ca^{2+} responsiveness during the development of the SFR (4).

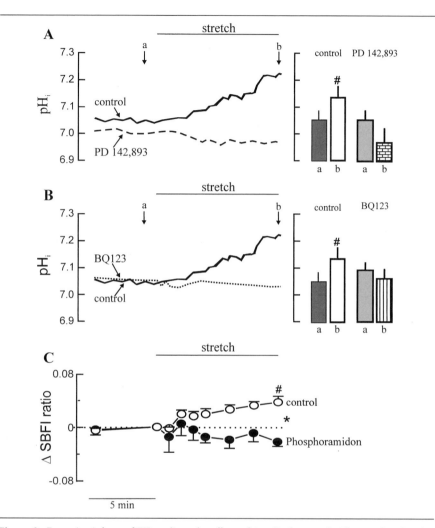

Figure 3. Formation/release of ET mediates the effects of Ang II after stretch. The stretch-induced NHE activation in isolated papillary muscles was abolished after non-selective ET receptor blockade (PD 142,893) and selective ET_A receptor blockade (BQ123), as detected by the lack of changes in pH_i after the stretch in both conditions (panels A and B, typical experiments and averaged data in the column graphs). Inhibition of the endothelin-converting enzyme activity by phosphoramidon gives further support to the hypothesis, as shown by the lack of changes in $[Na^+]_i$ (expressed as changes in the SBFI fluorescence ratio) after stretch under this condition (averaged data of panel C). "a" and "b" indicate the time at which the average for the column graphs were made. #indicates $p < 0.05$ vs pre-stretched control, ★indicates $P < 0.05$ between curves. (Adapted from Cingolani et al. 1998 (8) and from Pérez et al. 2001 (15) with permission).

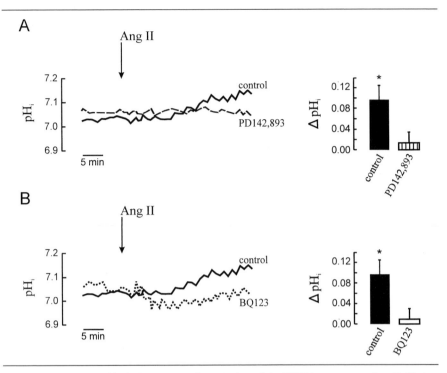

Figure 4. ET receptors blockade suppresses the activation of the NHE by exogenous Ang II. Similarly to the results for the stretch presented in Figure 3, pretreatment of the papillary muscles with a non-selective ET receptor blocker (PD 142,893, panel A) or with a selective ET_A receptor blocker (BQ123, panel B) prevented the expected increase in pH_i due to addition of Ang II. *indicates $p < 0.05$ vs pre-Ang II control. (Adapted from Cingolani et al. 1998 (8) with permission).

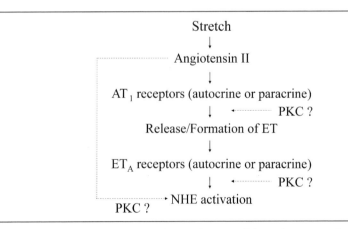

Figure 5. Chain of events triggered by the stretch. Myocardial stretch promotes the release of Ang II that will bind to the AT_1 receptors by an autocrine or paracrine mode and will stimulate the release/formation of ET probably by a protein kinase C (PKC)-mediated pathway. ET will bind to ET_A receptors (autocrine or paracrine) that will promote the activation of the NHE probably through another PKC dependent pathway. It is not possible to rule out a direct activation of the NHE by Ang II.

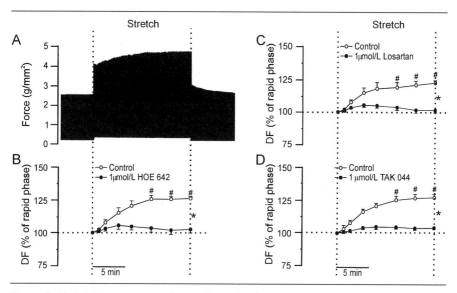

Figure 6. Typical force response to the stretch in isolated cat papillary muscle and effects of different interventions on the SFR. An original record showing the characteristic two-phase increase in force after the stretch is shown in panel A. The initial rapid phase is attributed to an increase in myofilament Ca^{2+} responsiveness, and the second one slowly developing (known as SFR) to an increase in Ca^{2+} transient. Panels B-D show the effect of three different interventions on the SFR, expressed as percent of the initial rapid phase. The SFR is abolished by NHE blockade (panel B), by Ang II AT_1 receptor blockade (panel C) and by non-selective ET receptors blockade (panel D). Taken together these results indicate that NHE activation is a key step for the development of the SFR, through a mechanism that needs the participation of Ang II and ET. #indicates $P < 0.05$ vs rapid phase, ★indicates $P < 0.05$ between curves. (Adapted from Pérez et al. 2001 (15) with permission).

It is interesting that in an ionic model of cardiac myocytes where the potential contribution of sarcolemmal ion fluxes to the SFR development was analyzed, Bluhm et al. (13) found that the SFR could be mimicked by an increase in $[Na^+]_i$ that concurred with an increase in Ca^{2+} entry through the NCX.

Figure 7 shows that when extracellular Na^+ was replaced either by equimolar amounts of choline chloride and N-methyl-D-glucamine (NMG) or by equimolar amounts of lithium chloride, the SFR was abolished. These experiments suggested that the NCX either by decreasing Ca^{2+} efflux (forward mode) or by increasing Ca^{2+} influx (reverse mode) could be responsible for the increase in the Ca^{2+} transient during the SFR. Experiments using KB-R7943, a blocker of the NCX preferentially in its reverse mode showed complete suppression of the SFR, as it can be appreciated in Figure 8A, indicating that Ca^{2+} increases by this way during the SFR. These results are in agreement with those predicted by the computerized model mentioned above. Interestingly, the compound also abolished the SFR either applied immediately or 15 minutes after the stretch (Figure 8B). However, since it has been reported a direct action of Ang II and ET on the NCX (14) we can not rule out the possibility that in addition to the increase in $[Na^+]_i$, a direct effect on the NCX could be necessary to drive the exchanger in reverse.

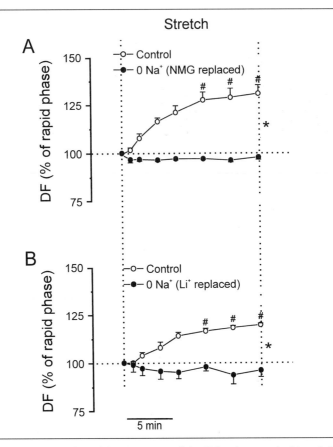

Figure 7. NCX in the generation of the SFR. Extracellular Na⁺ replacement by N–methyl-D-glucamine (NMG, panel A) or by lithium (Li^+, panel B) abolished the SFR. These results provide conclusive evidence that the NCX is involved in the development of the SFR, however they do not allow ascertaining whether the forward or the reverse mode of operation mediates the effect. #indicates $P < 0.05$ vs rapid phase, *indicates $P < 0.05$ between curves. (Adapted from Pérez et al. 2001 (15) with permission).

AUTOCRINE OR PARACRINE MECHANISM?

Since our experiments were performed in a multicellular preparation in which coexist myocytes, fibroblasts and endothelial cells, it is difficult to ascertain at present whether the elicited mechanism is autocrine or paracrine. To address whether endothelial cells were the source of ET, we performed experiments in which endocardial and vascular endothelial cells were functionally inactivated with triton X100 (15). After endothelial inactivation, the SFR and the increase in [Na⁺]$_i$ after the stretch both persisted and both were blocked by phosphoramidon. These data suggest that endothelial cells are not the source for ET. In the light of these results, Figure 9 summarizes two possible alternatives for the chain of events detected in a multicellular adult feline

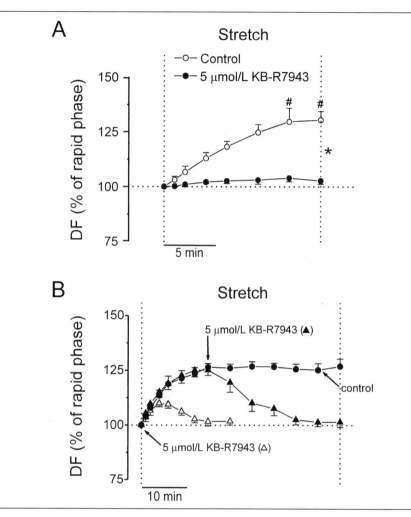

Figure 8. Effect of reverse mode NCX blockade by KB-R7943 on the development of the SFR. Panel A shows that pretreatment with KB-R7943 prevented the development of the SFR, giving strong support to the idea that Ca^{2+} influx through the NCX is the responsible for the increase in the Ca^{2+} transient that underlies the development of the SFR. Panel B shows that acute addition of the compound either at the beginning of the stretch or after 15 minutes also cancelled the SFR. #indicates $P < 0.05$ vs rapid phase, *indicates $P < 0.05$ between curves. (Adapted from Pérez et al. 2001 (15) with permission).

preparation that determines the development of the SFR. The upper panel schematizes the autocrine-signaling pathway to explain the SFR. In this alternative, stored Ang II is released from the myocyte and binds to its AT_1 receptors. The myocyte will form/release ET that, through the ET_A receptors, will stimulate the NHE activity by a PKC-dependent pathway. In the lower panel (paracrine) the mechanism is similar, but the source of ET would be the fibroblast instead of the myocyte. Ang II released

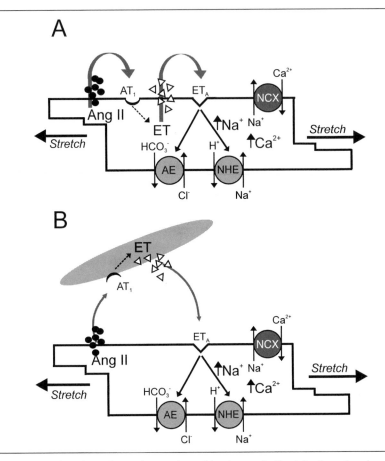

Figure 9. Hypothetical signaling pathways triggered by the stretch. Panel A schematizes the autocrine alternative in which the myocyte is the source and the target of Ang II. Ang II binds to AT_1 receptors and promotes the formation/release of ET, which, through the ET_A receptors, stimulates NHE activity by a PKC-dependent pathway. Simultaneous activation of the Na^+ independent Cl^-/HCO_3^- exchanger (AE) minimizes the increase in pH_i, but not in $[Na^+]_i$, which will activate the NCX in its reverse mode promoting the increase in the Ca^{2+} transient. Panel B schematizes the paracrine alternative in which the mechanism is essentially the same, but the source of ET is the fibroblast instead of the myocyte. Ang II released by the myocyte stimulates AT_1 receptors on fibroblasts, this promotes the formation/release of ET that will bind on the myocytes's ET_A receptors in a cross-talked paracrine loop. (Adapted from Pérez et al. 2001 (15) with permission).

by the myocyte will stimulate AT_1 receptors on fibroblasts in a paracrine fashion inducing the formation/release of ET and the ET released by fibroblasts will act on the myocytes's ET_A receptors in a cross-talked paracrine loop. Whatever the case, simultaneous activation of the acidifying mechanism Na^+ independent Cl^-/HCO_3^- exchanger (6,7) will preclude changes in pH_i, but not in $[Na^+]_i$ that will rise. The increase in $[Na^+]_i$ will favor the NCX in its reverse mode (Ca^{2+}_{in}–Na^+_{out}) and this will increase the $[Ca^{2+}]_i$ transient determining the development of the SFR.

CONCLUSIONS

The results presented herein are providing evidence of the autocrine/paracrine role played by the local myocardial renin-angiotensin system in the adult multicellular preparation.

The mechanical counterpart of this chain of events is an increase in contractility mediated by an increase in the Ca^{2+} transient through the NCX operating in reverse mode and can be the explanation for the Anrep effect (16) and the SFR.

The heart makes use of a dual mechanism for adapting its working output to changing hemodynamic conditions. First, there is a rapid increase in myofilament sensitivity, which depends on the stretch. This is followed by a slow increase in the Ca^{2+} transient, a response that results from a stretch-induced autocrine/paracrine loop involving the tissue renin-angiotensin system.

Although it is well known that myocardial stretch elicits an increase in protein synthesis leading to hypertrophy (9) and that the hypertrophic response is induced at least partly through an increase in secretion/synthesis of Ang II and ET (9,17), it still remains to be determined how the mechanical stretch is converted into biochemical signals that activate protein synthesis. Protein kinase cascades (18,19), calcium handling (20), calcineurin (21) and other mechanisms (22) have been extensively analyzed as possible mediators of the hypertrophic response. Whether or not the autocrine/paracrine system described here is linked to the development of myocardial hypertrophy is examined in another chapter of this book.

REFERENCES

1. Lakatta EG. 1992. Length modulation of muscle performance. Frank-Starling law of the heart. In: Fozzard HA, ed. The Heart and Cardiovascular System, 2nd ed. New York, NY: Raven;1325–1351.
2. Allen DG, Nichols CG, Smith GL. 1988. The effects of changes in muscle length during diastole on the calcium transient in ferret ventricular muscle. J Physiol (Lond) 406:359–370.
3. Parmley WW, Chuck L. 1973. Length-dependent changes in myocardial contractile store. Am J Physiol 224:1195–1199.
4. Kentish JC, Wrzosek A. 1998. Changes in force and cytosolic Ca^{2+} concentration after length changes in isolated rat ventricular trabeculae. J Physiol (Lond) 506:431–444.
5. Alvarez BV, Pérez NG, Ennis IL, Camilión de Hurtado MC, Cingolani HE. 1999. Mechanisms underlying the increase in force and Ca^{2+} transient that follow stretch of cardiac muscle. A possible explanation of the Anrep Effect. Circ Res 85:716–722.
6. Camilión de Hurtado MC, Alvarez BV, Pérez NG, Ennis IL, Cingolani HE. 1998. Angiotensin II Activates Na^+-independent Cl^--HCO_3^- Exchange in Ventricular Myocardium. Circ Res 82:473–481.
7. Camilión de Hurtado MC, Alvarez BV, Ennis IL, Cingolani HE. 2000. Stimulation of Myocardial Na^+-independent Cl^--HCO_3^- Exchanger by Angiotensin II is Mediated by Endogenous Endothelin. Circ Res 86:622–627.
8. Cingolani HE, Alvarez BV, Ennis IL, Camilión de Hurtado MC. 1998. Stretch-Induced Alkalinization of Feline Papillary Muscle. An autocrine-Paracrine System. Circ Res 83:775–780.
9. Sadoshima J, Xu Y, Sleiter HS, Izumo S. 1993. Autocrine release of angiotensin II mediates stretch-induced hypertrophy of cardiac myocytes in vitro. Cell 75:977–984.
10. Ito H, Hirata Y, Adachi S, Tanaka M, Tsujino M, Kioke A, Nogami A, Marumo F, Hiroe M. 1993. Endothelin-1 is an autocrine-paracrine factor in the mechanism of angiotensin II-induced hypertrophy in cultured rat cardiomyocytes. J Clin Invest 92:398–403.
11. Rajagopalan S, Laursen JB, Borthayre A, Kurz S, Keiser J, Haleen S, Glaid A, Harrison DG. 1997. Role for endothelin-1 in Angiotensin II-mediated hypertension. Hypertension 30:29–34.
12. Ortiz MC, Sanabria E, Manriquez MC, Romero JC, Juncos LA. 2001. Role of endothelin and isoprostanes in slow pressor responses to angiotensin II. Hypertension 37:505–510.

13. Bluhm WF, Lew WY, Garfinkel A, McCulloch AD. 1998. Mechanism of length history-dependent tension in an ionic model of the cardiac myocyte. Am J Physiol (Heart Circ Physiol) 274:H1032–H1040.
14. Ballard C, Schaffer S. 1996. Stimulation of the Na^+/Ca^{2+} exchanger by phenylephrine, angiotensin II and endothelin 1. J Mol Cell Cardiol 28:11–17.
15. Pérez NG, Camilión de Hurtado MC, Cingolani HE. 2001. Reverse mode of the Na^+/Ca^{2+} exchange following myocardial stretch. Underlying mechanism of the slow force response. Circ Res 88: 376–382.
16. von Anrep G. 1912. On the part played by the suprarenals in the normal vascular reactions on the body. J Physiol (Lond) 45:307–317.
17. Yamazaki T, Komuro I, Kudoh S, Zou Y, Shiojima I, Hiroi Y, Mizuno T, Maemura K, Kurihara M, Aikawa R, Takano H, Yazaki Y. 1996. Endothelin-1 is involved in mechanical stress-induced cardiomyocyte hypertrophy. J Biol Chem 271:3221–3228.
18. Komuro I, Yazaki Y. 1993. Control of cardiac gene expression by mechanical stress. Annu Rev Physiol 55:55–75.
19. Chien KR, Grace AA, Hunter JJ. 1998. Molecular biology of cardiac hypertrophy and heart failure. In: Molecular Basis of Cardiovascular Disease. Ed, KR Chien. Philadelphia, Pa: WB Saunders Co.
20. Marbán E, Koretsune Y. 1990. Cell calcium, oncogenes, and hypertrophy. Hypertension 15:652–658.
21. Zou Y, Hiroi Y, Uozumi H, Takimoto E, Toko H, Zhu W, Kudoh S, Mizukami M, Shimoyama M, Shibasaki F, Nagai R, Yazaki Y, Komuro I. 2001. Calcineurin plays a critical role in the development of pressure overload-induced cardiac hypertrophy. Circulation 104:97–101.
22. Molkentin JD. 2000. Calcineurin and beyond. Cardiac hypertrophic signaling. Circ Res 87:731–738.

Signal Transduction and Cardiac Hypertrophy,
edited by N.S. Dhalla, L.V. Hryshko,
E. Kardami & P.K. Singal
Kluwer Academic Publishers, Boston, 2003

L-Arginine at the Crossroads of Biochemical Pathways Involved in Myocardial Hypertrophy

Emanuele Giordano,[1,2] Lisa M. Shantz,[1] Rebecca A. Hillary,[1] Carlo Guarnieri,[2] Claudio M. Caldarera,[2] and Anthony E. Pegg[1]

[1] *Department of Cellular & Molecular Physiology H-166*
Penn State College of Medicine
The Milton S. Hershey Medical Center
Hershey, PA 17033-2390, USA
and [2] *Centro Studi e Ricerche sul Metabolismo Cardiaco*
Dipartimento di Biochimica "G. Moruzzi"
Università degli Studi di Bologna
40126 Bologna, Italia

Summary. Both ornithine decarboxylase (ODC) and nitric oxide synthase (NOS) activities rely on the availability of the common substrate L-arginine, which is directly processed by NOS to nitric oxide (NO) and L-citrulline. Alternatively, arginine is acted on by arginase in the urea cycle to produce ornithine, which then enters polyamine biosynthesis. Evidence in the literature points out that NO is able to inhibit ODC and polyamines can inhibit NOS. Both of these observations seem to indicate that the two metabolic pathways may crosstalk in regulating complex organic functions and the heart is a possible target organ for this interplay. It has been demonstrated that upregulation of ODC activity is critical in the hypertrophic myocardial response, which is also consistent with observations involving conditions of nitric oxide deficiency.

Key words: Arginase, Ornithine Decarboxylase, Nitric Oxide Synthase, Nitric Oxide, Polyamines.

Address for Correspondence: Emanuele Giordano MD PhD, Centro Studi e Ricerche sul Metabolismo Cardiaco, Dipartimento di Biochimica "G. Moruzzi", via Irnerio, 48, 40126 Bologna, Italia. Tel: +39 051 209 1207, Fax: +39 051 209 1224, E-mail giordano@biocfarm.unibo.it

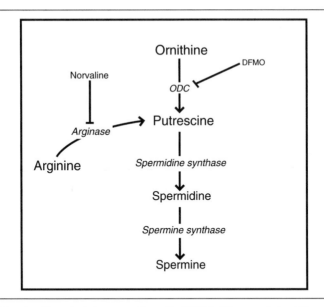

Figure 1. Polyamine biosynthesis in mammalian cells. *DFMO*, difluoromethylornithine; *ODC*, ornithine decarboxylase.

Muscle cell hypertrophy in the heart is part of an important adaptive response that results in an increase in the contractile power of the organ. This same hypertrophy, however, often is also an early stage in the clinical course of heart failure, a leading cause of death in Western countries (1). In hypertrophic cardiomyopathy the border between compensation and failure is not yet clear cut, and for this reason the molecular aspects of the pathophysiology of heart failure have been intensively studied in recent years, with the goal of designing more effective therapeutic strategies than those currently available (2).

At the cellular level, gene expression and protein synthesis activation are hallmarks of the hypertrophic phenotype, and it is known that both of these processes are promoted by the polyamines putrescine, spermidine and spermine, whose biosynthetic pathway is shown in Figure 1. These aliphatic amines, widely distributed in all cells, have been closely linked to cell growth, and a number of studies have pointed out that their synthesis and intracellular content are increased during cell proliferation and following growth stimuli (3–5).

Initial observations pointing out the relationship between polyamines and myocardial hypertrophy date back to the seventies. In these studies an increase in polyamine concentrations was found in the ventricular myocardium of animals that were either subjected to ascending aortic stenosis (6–7), undergoing stress (8) or intense muscular exercise (9), or treated with the β-adrenoceptor agonist isoprenaline (10), to induce cardiac hypertrophy. The rise in polyamine content was shown to be accompanied by increased histone acetylation (11), and increased rates of RNA

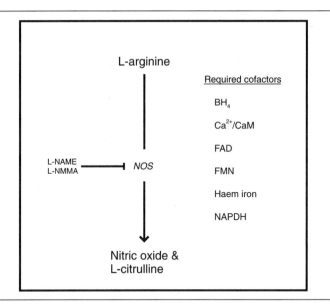

Figure 2. Nitric oxide biosynthesis in mammalian cells. BH_4, (6R)-5,6,7,8-tetrahydrobiopterin; *CaM*, calmodulin; *FAD*, flavinadenindinucleotide; *FMN*, flavinmononucleotide; *NADPH*, nicotinamide adeni-dinucleotide phosphate; *L-NAME*, L-N^ω-arginine-methyl ester; *L-NMMA*, N^G-monomethyl-L-arginine; *NOS*, nitric oxide synthase.

(9,11) and protein (12) synthesis. Moreover, the inhibition of polyamine synthesis decreased histone acetylation and RNA transcription, and this effect was reversed by spermine (13).

Many subsequent studies have confirmed and extended these early reports (14–30). New light was shed upon this field with the discovery of nitric oxide as a bioactive molecule (31,32). This nitrogen radical species is synthesized in virtually every cell type through an enzymatic pathway, sketched in Figure 2, that has been fully characterized (33). Three nitric oxide synthase (NOS) isoforms are known and all of them catalyze the synthesis of NO and L-citrulline from L-arginine (33,34). NO production is involved in a large number of physiological and patho-physiological functions in animal tissues, and the cardiovascular system is dramatically affected by its availability. NO is responsible for endothelium-mediated vasorelaxing tone, modulates platelet-vessel wall interactions, and regulates myocardial contractility as an inhibitor of the positive inotropic and chronotropic responses to β-adrenergic receptor stimulation (35–37). In addition, several recent reports have pointed out the antiproliferative effect of NO in smooth muscle cells (38) and its antihypertrophic potential in the myocardium (39–41). In light of their opposite effects on cell proliferation, the ability of polyamines to inhibit NOS activity and NO-mediated effects (42–47), coupled with the characterization of NO and its intermediate N^G-hydroxy-L-arginine as inhibitors of ODC and polyamine-mediated functions (48–52), suggest that the two metabolic pathways may crosstalk

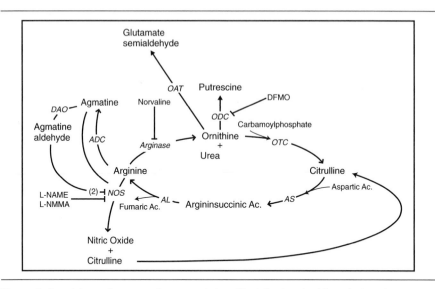

Figure 3. L-arginine at the crossroads among nitric oxide and polyamine biosynthetic pathways. *ADC*, arginine decarboxylase; *AL*, argininosuccinate lyase; *AS*, argininosuccinate synthase; *DAO*, diamino oxidase; *DFMO*, difluoromethylornithine; *L-NAME*, L-arginine-methyl ester; *L-NMMA*, N^{G}-monomethyl-L-arginine; *OAT*, ornithine aminotransferase; *ODC*, ornithine decarboxylase; *OTC*, ornithine transcarbamoylase.

in regulating complex organic functions and the heart is a possible target organ for this interplay. Evidence in support of this idea has been obtained in cardiomyocytes as well as in other cell systems (53–58).

Arginase converts L-arginine into L-ornithine (59,60), limiting the availability of L-arginine as a precursor of NO and shifting the equilibrium between NOS and ODC toward polyamine biosynthesis (61), as indicated in Figure 3. Indeed arginase activity has been shown to affect smooth muscle (62) and endothelial (63) cell proliferation in the vessel wall. Moreover, it has recently been demonstrated that the constitutive expression of arginase in microvascular endothelial cells counteracts nitric oxide-mediated vasodilatory function (64). This is entirely consistent with studies showing that the NO biosynthetic pathway intermediate N^{G}-hydroxy-L-arginine inhibits arginase activity (65–67) and limits cell proliferation (49). Taken together, these findings strongly support the differential regulation of NO and polyamine biosynthesis through the availability of arginine.

Catecholamines, which are classical myocardial hypertrophic stimuli, are able to increase ODC activity (10,25,26) and have recently been demonstrated to be responsible for stimulating arginase activity in macrophages (68). In this light, the role of NO as a mediator of parasympathetic inhibition of β-adrenergic autonomic tone in the myocardium may play a role not only as a modulator of muscle contractility, but also to limit such proliferative/hypertrophic cellular stimuli. All of this evidence suggests that L-arginine is a critical intermediate in the homeostasis of cardiomyocytes, and arginase, NOS and ODC all contribute to the maintenance of this homeostasis (Figure 3).

Recently the development of transgenic technology has proven useful as a new tool for gaining a deeper insight into this field. The targeted overexpression of ornithine decarboxylase to the heart has been shown to enhance β-adrenergic agonist-induced cardiac hypertrophy (28). This murine genotype is also more prone than wild type littermates to develop myocardial hypertrophy following pressure overload by aortic stenosis induced through abdominal aortic banding (unpublished observations). It is noteworthy that transgenic animals treated with isoproterenol develop a severe myocardial hypertrophy concomitantly with a dramatic increase of arginase activity as measured in total protein extracts from myocardial tissue (29). This is consistent with the increase in the expression of the endothelial constitutive isoform of NOS, which is presumably a compensatory adaptation to the reduced L-arginine availability (29).

The oral supplementation of L-arginine has been suggested as a tool to increase the activity of the NO/NOS biochemical pathway, expecially to ameliorate the endothelium-derived vasodilator tone (68–72). This intervention could possibly be relevant in the above described myocardial hypertrophic phenotype obtained in ODC-overexpressing mice. The exponential growth of the scientific work in this field indicates that this hypothesis deserves our attention.

ACKNOWLEDGEMENTS

Grants from CIRC (to EG), MIUR (to CG) and the American Heart Association (0040140N to LMS) are gratefully acknowledged.

REFERENCES

1. Levy D, Garrison RJ, Savage DD, Kannel WB, Castelli WP. 1990. Prognostic inplications of echocardiographically determined left ventricular mass in the Framingham heart study. N Engl J Med 322:1561–1566.
2. Hunter JJ, Chien KR. 1999. Signaling pathways for cardiac hypertrophy and failure. N Engl J Med 341:1276–1283.
3. Flamigni F, Rossoni C, Stefanelli C, Caldarera CM. 1986. Polyamine metabolism and function in the heart. J Mol Cell Cardiol 36:1297–1302.
4. Pegg AE. 1986. Recent advances in the biochemistry of polyamines in eukaryotes. Biochem J 234:249–262.
5. Shantz LM, Pegg AE. 1999. Translational regulation of ornithine decarboxylase and other enzymes of the polyamine pathway. Int J Biochem Cell Biol 31:107–122.
6. Caldarera CM, Casti A, Rossoni C, Visioli O. 1971. Polyamines and noradrenaline following myocardial hypertrophy. J Mol Cell Cardiol 3:121–126.
7. Feldman JM, Russel DH. 1972. Polyamine biogenesis in the left ventricle of the rat heart after aortic constriction. Am J Physiol 222:1199–1203.
8. Russel DH, Shiverick KT, Hamrell BB, Alpert NR. 1971. Polyamine synthesis during initial phases of stress-induced cardiac hypertrophy. Am J Physiol 221:1287–1291.
9. Caldarera CM, Orlandini G, Casti A, Moruzzi G. 1974. Polyamine and nucleic acid metabolism in myocardial hypertrophy of the overloaded heart. J Mol Cell Cardiol 6:95–104.
10. Warnica JW, Antony P, Gibson K, Harris P. 1975. The effect of isoprenaline and propranolol on rat myocardial ornithine decarboxylase. Cardiovasc Res 9:793–796.
11. Moruzzi G, Caldarera CM, Casti A. 1974. The biological effect of polyamines on heart RNA and histone metabolism. Mol Cell Biochem 3:153–161.

12. Gibson K, Harris P. 1974. The *in vitro* and *in vivo* effects of polyamines on cardiac protein biosynthesis. Cardiovasc Res 8:668–673.
13. Caldarera CM, Casti A, Guarnieri C, Moruzzi G. 1975. Regulation of ribonucleic acid synthesis by polyamines. Biochemical J 152:91–98.
14. Pegg AE, Hibasami H. 1980. Polyamine metabolism during cardiac hypertrophy. Am J Physiol 239:E372–E378.
15. Bartolome J, Huguenard J, Slotkin TA. 1980. Role of ornithine decarboxylase in cardiac growth and hypertrophy. Science 210:793–794.
16. Pegg AE. 1981. Effect of alpha-difluoromethylornithine on cardiac polyamine content and hypertrophy. J Mol Cell Cardiol 13:881–887.
17. Bartolome JV, Trepanier PA, Chait EA, Slotkin TA. 1982. Role of polyamines in isoproterenol-induced cardiac hypertrophy: effects of alpha-difluoromethylornithine, an irreversible inhibitor of ornithine decarboxylase. J Mol Cell Cardiol 14:461–466.
18. Harris P. 1982. Polyamine metabolism in myocardial hypertrophy. Eur Heart J 3(SA):73–74.
19. Flamigni F, Guarnieri C, Caldarera CM. 1986. Heart ornithine decarboxylase from control and isoproterenol-treated rats: kinetic properties, multiple forms and subcellular distribution. Gen Pharmacol 17:31–36.
20. Toraason M, Luken ME, Krueger JA. 1990. Cooperative action of insulin and catecholamines on stimulation of ornithine decarboxylase activity in neonatal rat heart cells. J Mol Cell Cardiol 22:637–644.
21. Lipke DW, Newman PS, Tofiq S, Guo H, Arcot SS, Aziz SM, Olson JW, Soltis EE. 1997. Multiple polyamine regulatory pathways control compensatory cardiovascular hypertrophy in coarctation hypertension. Clin Exp Hypertens 19:269–295.
22. Friberg P, Isgaard J, Wahlander A, Wickman A, Adams MA. 1998. Inhibited expression of insulin-like growth factor I mRNA and attenuated cardiac hypertrophy in volume overloaded hearts treated with difluoromethylornithine. Growth Horm IGF Res 8:159–165.
23. Cubria JC, Reguera RM, Balana-Fouce R, Ordonez C, Ordonez D. 1998. Polyamine-mediated heart hypertrophy induced by clenbuterol in the mouse. J Pharm Pharmacol 50:91–96.
24. Cubria JC, Ordonez C, Reguera RM, Tekwani BL, Balana-Fouce R, Ordonez D. 1999. Early alterations of polyamine metabolism induced after acute administration of clenbuterol in mouse heart. Life Sci 19:1739–1752.
25. Schafer M, Frischkopf K, Taimor G, Piper HM, Schluter K-D. 2000. Hypertrophic effect of selective β1-adrenoceptor stimulation on ventricular cardiomyocytes from adult rat. Am J Physiol 279:C495–C503.
26. Schluter K-D, Frischkopf K, Flesch M, Rosenkranz S, Taimor G, Piper HM. 2000. Central role for ornithine decarboxylase in β-adrenoceptor mediated hypertrophy. Cardiovasc Res 45:410–417.
27. Tipnis UR, He GY, Li S, Campbell G, Boor PJ. 2000. Attenuation of isoproterenol-mediated myocardial injury in rat by an inhibitor of polyamine synthesis. Cardiovasc Pathol 9:273–280.
28. Shantz LM, Feith DJ, Pegg AE. 2001. Targeted overexpression of ornithine decarboxylase enhances beta-adrenergic agonist-induced cardiac hypertrophy. Biochem J 358:25–32.
29. Giordano E, Shantz LM, Caldarera CM, Pegg AE. 2002. Ornithine decarboxylase overexpression and nitric oxide synthase activity in mouse heart: relationship to myocardial hypertrophy (*abs*). In: Molecular biology of the heart. Ed. LA Leinwand and MC Fishman, 54. Keystone, CO: Keystone Symposia 2002 Abstract Book.
30. Hillary RA, Shantz LM, Giordano E, Pegg AE. 2002. Role of calcineurin in the signal transduction pathway leading to cardiac hypertrophy induced by beta-adrenergic receptor stimulation in ornithine decarboxylase overexpressing mice (*abs*). In: Molecular biology of the heart. Ed. LA Leinwand and MC Fishman, 55. Keystone, CO: Keystone Symposia 2002 Abstract Book.
31. Ignarro LJ, Buga GM, Wood KS, Byrns RE, Chaudhuri G. 1987. Endothelium-derived relaxing factor produced and released from artery and vein is nitric oxide. Proc Natl Acad Sci USA 84:9265–9269.
32. Palmer RM, Ferrige AG, Moncada S. 1987. Nitric oxide release accounts for the biological activity of endothelium-derived relaxing factor. Nature 327:524–526.
33. Alderton WK, Cooper CE, Knowles RG. 2001. Nitric oxide synthases: structure, function and inhibition. Biochem J 357:593–615.
34. Palmer RM, Ashton DS, Moncada S. 1988. Vascular endothelial cells synthesize nitric oxide from L-arginine. Nature 333:664–666.
35. Ignarro LJ, Cirino G, Casini A, Napoli C. 1999. Nitric oxide as a signaling molecule in the vascular system: an overview. J Cardiovasc Pharmacol 34:879–886.

36. Paulus WJ. 2001. The role of nitric oxide in the failing heart. Heart Fail Rev 6:105–118.
37. Massion PB, Moniotte S, Balligand JL. 2001. Nitric oxide: does it play a role in the heart of the critically ill? Curr Opin Crit Care 7:323–336.
38. Ignarro LJ, Buga GM, Wei LH, Bauer PM, Wu G, del Soldato P. 2001. Role of the arginine-nitric oxide pathway in the regulation of vascular smooth muscle cell proliferation. Proc Natl Acad Sci USA 98:4202–4208.
39. Simko F, Simko J. 2000. The potential role of nitric oxide in the hypertrophic growth of the left ventricle. Physiol Res 49:37–46.
40. Grieve DJ, MacCarthy PA, Gall NP, Cave AC, Shah AM. 2001. Divergent biological actions of coronary endothelial nitric oxide during progression of cardiac hypertrophy. Hypertension 38:267–273.
41. Wollert KC, Fiedler B, Gambaryan S, Smolenski A, Heineke J, Butt E, Trautwein C, Lohmann SM, Drexler H. 2002. Gene transfer of cGMP-dependent protein kinase I enhances the antihypertrophic effects of nitric oxide in cardiomyocytes. Hypertension 39:87–92.
42. Hu J, Mahmoud MI, el-Fakahany EE. 1994. Polyamines inhibit nitric oxide synthase in rat cerebellum. Neurosci Lett 175:41–45.
43. Galea E, Regunathan S, Eliopulos V, Feinstein DL, Reis DJ. 1996. Inhibition of mammalian nitric oxide synthase by agmatine, an endogenous polyamine formed by decarboxylation of arginine. Biochem J 316:247–249.
44. Blachier F, Mignon A, Soubrane O. 1997. Polyamines inhibit lipopolysaccharide-induced nitric oxide synthase activity in rat liver cytosol. Nitric Oxide 1:268–272.
45. Blachier F, Briand D, Selamnia M, Robert V, Guihot G, Mayeur C. 1998. Differential inhibitory effects of three nitric oxide donors on ornithine decarboxylase activity in human colon carcinoma cells. Biochem Pharmacol 55:1235–1239.
46. Baydoun AR, Morgan DM. 1998. Inhibition of ornithine decarboxylase potentiates nitric oxide production in LPS-activated J774 cells. Br J Pharmacol 125:1511–1516.
47. ter Steege JC, Forget PP, Buurman WA. 1999. Oral spermine administration inhibits nitric oxide-mediated intestinal damage and levels of systemic inflammatory mediators in a mouse endotoxin model. Shock 11:115–199.
48. Blachier F, Robert V, Selamnia M, Mayeur C, Duee PH. 1996. Sodium nitroprusside inhibits proliferation and putrescine synthesis in human colon carcinoma cells. FEBS Lett 396:315–318.
49. Buga GM, Wei LH, Bauer PM, Fukuto JM, Ignarro LJ. 1998. N^G-hydroxy-L-arginine and nitric oxide inhibit Caco-2 tumor cell proliferation by distinct mechanisms. Am J Physiol 275:R1256–R1264.
50. Bauer PM, Fukuto JM, Buga GM, Pegg AE, Ignarro LJ. 1999. Nitric oxide inhibits ornithine decarboxylase by S-nitrosylation. Biochem Biophys Res Commun 262:355–358.
51. Satriano J, Ishizuka S, Archer DC, Blantz RC, Kelly CJ. 1999. Regulation of intracellular polyamine biosynthesis and transport by NO and cytokines TNF-alpha and IFN-gamma. Am J Physiol 276:C892–C899.
52. Bauer PM, Buga GM, Fukuto JM, Pegg AE, Ignarro LJ. 2001. Nitric oxide inhibits ornithine decarboxylase via S-nitrosylation of cysteine 360 in the active site of the enzyme. J Biol Chem 276:34458–34464.
53. Morgan DM. 1994. Polyamines, arginine and nitric oxide. Biochem Soc Trans 22:879–883.
54. Blachier F, Selamnia M, Robert V, M'Rabet-Touil H, Duee PH. Metabolism of L-arginine through polyamine and nitric oxide synthase pathways in proliferative or differentiated human colon carcinoma cells. Biochim Biophys Acta 1995 21:255–262.
55. Sooranna SR, Das I. 1995. The inter-relationship between polyamines and the L-arginine nitric oxide pathway in the human placenta. Biochem Biophys Res Commun 212:229–234.
56. Pignatti C, Tantini B, Stefanelli C, Giordano E, Bonavita F, Clô C, Caldarera CM. 1999. Nitric oxide mediates either proliferation or cell death in cardiomyocytes. Involvement of polyamines. Amino Acids 16:181–190.
57. Tantini B, Flamigni F, Pignatti C, Stefanelli C, Fattori M, Facchini A, Giordano E, Clô C, Caldarera CM. 2001. Polyamines, NO and cGMP mediate stimulation of DNA synthesis by tumor necrosis factor and lipopolysaccharide in chick embryo cardiomyocytes. Cardiovasc Res 49:408–416.
58. Tantini B, Pignatti C, Fattori M, Flamigni F, Stefanelli C, Giordano E, Menegazzi M, Clô C, Caldarera CM. 2002. NF-κB and ERK cooperate to stimulate DNA synthesis by inducing ornithine decarboxylase and nitric oxide synthase in cardiomyocytes treated with TNF and LPS. FEBS Lett 512:75–79.
59. Iyer R, Jenkinson CP, Vockley JG, Kern RM, Grody WW, Cederbaum S. 1998. The human arginases and arginase deficiency. J Inherit Metab Dis 21(Suppl 1):86–100.

60. Wu G, Morris SM Jr. 1998. Arginine metabolism: nitric oxide and beyond. Biochem J 336:1–17.
61. Li H, Meininger CJ, Hawker JR Jr, Haynes TE, Kepka-Lenhart D, Mistry SK, Morris SM Jr, Wu G. 2001. Regulatory role of arginase I and II in nitric oxide, polyamine, and proline syntheses in endothelial cells. Am J Physiol 280:E75–E82.
62. Wei LH, Wu G, Morris SM Jr, Ignarro LJ. 2001. Elevated arginase I expression in rat aortic smooth muscle cells increases cell proliferation. Proc Natl Acad Sci USA 98:9260–9264.
63. Li H, Meininger CJ, Kelly KA, Hawker JR Jr, Morris SM Jr, Wu G. 2002. Activities of arginase I and II are limiting for endothelial cell proliferation. Am J Physiol 282:R64–R69.
64. Zhang C, Hein TW, Wang W, Chang C, Kuo L. 2001. Constitutive expression of arginase in microvascular endothelial cells counteracts nitric oxide-mediated vasodilatory function. FASEB J 15:1264–1266.
65. Daghigh F, Fukuto JM, Ash DE. 1994. Inhibition of rat liver arginase by an intermediate in NO biosynthesis, N^G-hydroxy-L-arginine: implications for the regulation of nitric oxide biosynthesis by arginase. Biochem Biophys Res Commun 202:174–180.
66. Boucher JL, Custot J, Vadon S, Delaforge M, Lepoivre M, Tenu JP, Yapo A, Mansuy D. 1996. N-omega-hydroxyl-L-arginine, an intermediate in the L-arginine to nitric oxide pathway, is a strong inhibitor of liver and macrophage arginase. Biochem Biophys Res Commun 203:1614–1621.
67. Buga GM, Singh R, Pervin S, Rogers NE, Schmitz DA, Jenkinson CP, Cederbaum SD, Ignarro LJ. 1996. Arginase activity in endothelial cells: inhibition by N^G-hydroxy-L-arginine during high-output NO production. Am J Physiol 271:H1988–H1998.
68. Bernard AC, Fitzpatrick EA, Maley ME, Gellin GL, Tsuei BJ, Arden WA, Boulanger BR, Kearney PA, Ochoa JB. 2000. Beta adrenoceptor regulation of macrophage arginase activity. Surgery 127:412–418.
69. Sheridan BC, McIntyre RC Jr, Meldrum DR, Fullerton DA. 1998. L-arginine prevents lung neutrophil accumulation and preserves pulmonary endothelial function after endotoxin. Am J Physiol 274:L337–L342.
70. Hutchison SJ, Sudhir K, Sievers RE, Zhu BQ, Sun YP, Chou TM, Chatterjee K, Deedwania PC, Cooke JP, Glantz SA, Parmley WW. 1999. Effects of L-arginine on atherogenesis and endothelial dysfunction due to secondhand smoke. Hypertension 34:44–50.
71. Sheridan BC, McIntyre RC Jr, Meldrum DR, Fullerton DA. 1999. L-arginine attenuates endothelial dysfunction in endotoxin-induced lung injury. Surgery 125:33–40.
72. Siani A, Pagano E, Iacone R, Iacoviello L, Scopacasa F, Strazzullo P. 2000. Blood pressure and metabolic changes during dietary L-arginine supplementation in humans. Am J Hypertens 13:547–551.

Signal Transduction and Cardiac Hypertrophy,
edited by N.S. Dhalla, L.V. Hryshko,
E. Kardami & P.K. Singal
Kluwer Academic Publishers, Boston, 2003

Signal Transduction System in Human Aortic Smooth Muscle Cell Stimulated by Pure Pressure

Hideaki Kawaguchi, Noriteru Morita,
Takeshi Murakami, and Kenji Iizuka

Laboratory Medicine
Hokkaido University School of Medicine
N-15 W-7, Kita-Ku Sapporo 060-8638
Japan

Summary. Mechanical forces related to pressure and flow are important for cell hypertrophy and proliferation. We hypothesized the presence of mechanosensors that were solely sensitive to pure atmospheric pressure in the absence of shear and tensile stresses. A pressure-loading apparatus was set up to examine the effects of atmospheric pressure on human aortic smooth muscle cells (HASMC). Pressure application of 140 to 180 mmHg produced DNA synthesis in a pressure-dependent manner. In contrast, pressure of 120 mmHg or less produced no significant change. Pertussis toxin (PTx) completely inhibited the pressure-induced increase of DNA synthesis. Under the high pressure of 200 mmHg. Both extracellular signal-related kinase and c-Jun N-terminal kinase activities, but not p38 activity, were stimulated by pressure of more than 160 mmHg. ACE inhibitor inhibited cell proliferation under the pressure. But the addition of AII on ACE inhibitor under the pressure could not recover the cell proliferation.

These data suggest that HASMC have a mechanosensing cellular switch for DNA synthesis which is sensitive to pure atmospheric pressure, and that the molecular switch is activated by pressure of more than 140 mmHg. The mechanism of the inhibitory effect of ACE inhibitor on cell proliferation stimulated by pure pressure is under way.

Key words: mechanical stress, JUN, ERK, p38, ACE inhibitor.

Address for Correspondence: Hideaki Kawaguchi, Tel: +81-11-706-5154, Fax: +81-11-706-7877, E-mail: hideaki@med.hokudai.ac.jp

INTRODUCTION

Abnormal growth and proliferation of vascular smooth muscle cells have been implicated in the pathogenesis of atherosclerosis and hypertension (1). Mechanical stresses
are likely to be involved in this process since it has been demonstrated that they
regulate cell growth in many tissues (2). In arteries, for example, a mechanical stress
related to pressure and flow is crucial in promoting blood vessel wall remodeling.
Such vascular remodeling may have important clinical implications for the evolution of several vascular diseases, may alter vascular compliance in hypertension and
atherosclerosis, and may cause vascular fragility and compensatory changes in
atherosclerosis (3).

Various stresses have been studied, including cytokines, mitogens, ultraviolet light,
oxidant stress, hyperosmolarity, heat stress and mechanical stress (4). The vascular
endothelial and vascular smooth muscle cells covering the inner surface of blood
vessels are constantly exposed to such stress. The hemodynamic forces affecting
endothelial cells include shear stress due to the frictional force of blood flow,
and circumferential and pure pressure stress due to ransmural pressure. Recently, a
number of studies have shown that shear stress to the vessel wall, which is one of
the mechanical stresses generated by blood flow, modulates endothelial morphology
and function (5). However, in an *in vitro* cell culture model, it has been shown that
intracellular signalings produced by tensile and shear stresses may be influence not
only by pressure stress, but also by morphological and cytoskeletal changes of cells
(6). Vascular smooth muscle cells makeup the outer layer of the endothelium in
blood vessels and are thus indirectly exposed to blood flow. Therefore, mechanosensing intracellular signal transductions in vascular smooth cells are defined as a cellular response to transmural pure pressure and tensile stress in the absence of shear
stress. In previous studies, tensile stress was reported to accelerate DNA synthesis
and activate stretch-activated cation channels in vascular smooth muscle cells (7,8).
However, the molecular identities of these candidates for mechanosensitive receptors are currently unknown.

In this study, we hypothesized the presence of mechanosensors and intracellular
signal transductions acting under pure atmospheric pressure in the absence of tensile
and shear stresses. Based on this hypothesis, we evaluated the DNA synthesis and
intracellular signalings of human aortic smooth muscle cells using an original
pressure-loading apparatus that was capable of directly applying various levels of pure
pressure (maximum, 300 mmHg) on HASMC, in order to examine the effect of
pure pressure stress on mechanosensors without inducing morphological changes of
cells.

METHODS

Cell culture

HASMC (Clonetics) were cultured in smooth muscle cell basal medium (SmBM;
Clonetics) which was modified MCDB131 containing 5% fetal bovine serum,
gentacine (50 μg/ml), amphotericine (50 μg/ml) and several growth factors: human

epidermal growth factor (10 ng/ml), human fibroblast growth factor (2.0 ng/ml), and insulin (5.0 μg/ml). The cells were incubated at 37°C in a humidified, 5% CO2 atmosphere. The 4th through 8th passages of HASMC were plated on 6–well plates for further investigation.

Pure pressure-loading apparatus

An original pure pressure-loading apparatus was designed to exposed HASMC under pure atmosphere pressure stress. The chamber allows for pumping air or nitrogen gas to rise the internal pressure (maximum at 300 mmHg), and can be sealed tightly by placing several clamps at the edge. Internal pressure level were monitored with an aneroid barometer during the experiments. The compression chamber was established in the incubator and kept 37°C, and a digital thermometer was mounted in the incubator to monitor the exact internal temperature. In the following series of experiments, the chamber was kept at 37°C, and the partial pressure of pO2 and pCO2 were theoretically preserved as constants according to the Boyle-Gay-Lussac's law. The potential of hydrogen (pH) in the culture medium was supported at a constant level (7.41 ± 0.02) during the experiments. It was not possible to monitor the actual morphological changes of pressurizes cells in our system set-up. However, the light microscopic investigations failed to find any changes in cell size or morphology during and after pressurization.

HASMC were cultured on 6–well plates for 48 hours (hrs). In 3 wells of each plate, the medium was changed to a starving medium (Dulbecco's modified Eagle's medium without serum). In the other 3 wells, the medium was changed to the same starving medium but containing PTx (0.1 μg/ml; Seikagaku, Japan). After 8 hrs of incubation, the plates were placed in the pure pressure-loading apparatus in the medium containing 10 mM HEPES (N-2-hydroxyethyl-piperazine-N-2-ethane-sulfonic acid, pH 7.4), exposed to various levels of atmospheric pressure (0 through 240 mmHg), and then incubated in an incubator for 1 or 3 hrs at 37°C.

DNA synthesis

[^{3}H]-Thymidine (TdR) incorporation into DNA was studied as a marker for DNA synthesis acceleration by pure atmospheric pressure. [^{3}H]TdR (2 μCi/ml, Amersham) was added to the medium in all 6 wells of 6–well plate. After pressure-loading procedures, the plate was incubated in a 37°C CO2–incubator under normal pressure for 4 hrs. The cells were rinsed two times in ice-cold phosphate-buffered saline (PBS) followed by precipitation three times with ice-cold 10% trichloroacetic acid, and lysed in 0.5 N NaOH at 37°C by shaking for 30 min. The incorporation of [^{3}H]TdR into DNA was quantified by pipetting the DNA hydrolysate into counting vials containing 4 ml of liquid scintillation cocktail (Ready Gel, Beckman). The protein concentration of HASMC was normalized by Lowry's method with bovine serum albumin as a standard (9). The counting results were expressed as disintegrations per protein and were expressed as a percent-increase compared to controls at the basal level (0 mmHg) for 1 and 3 hrs. All the experiments for each pressure were performed in triplicate, and were repeated 2 to 3 times.

Immunoblotting

HASMC were incubated on 100-mm dishes until 80% confluent. The medium was replaced with a starving medium. After 8 hrs of incubation, the dishes were placed in the pure pressure-loading apparatus. In the medium containing 10 mM HEPES, and exposed to various levels of atomospheric pressure (0 mmHg, 120 through 180 mmHg, and 240 mmHg) for 3 hrs at 37°C. The cells were washed twice with ice-cold PBS, and harvested in a buffer containing 25 mM Tris-HCl (pH 6.8), 1% Triton X-100, 150 mM sodium chloride and protease inhibitors: benzamidine (100 μM), leupeptin (2 μM), aprotinin (0.15 μM), pepstatin A (1.5 μM), and phenylmethylsulfonyl fluoride (100 μM). The protein content of each sample was measured by Lowry's method. Samples (15 μg) were analyzed by SDS (sodium dodecyl sulfate)-polyacrylamide gel electrophoresis in a 12% gel using the Mini Gel Electrophoresis System (Marysol). Protein were transferred to a nitrocellulose membrane (Hybond ECL; Amersham) by Western Blotting apparatus (Semi dry type; Marysol) with a buffer containing 20% method, 48 mM Tris-base, 78 mM glycine, and 0.375% SDS for 2 hrs. The membranes were submerged for 1 hour in 4% non fat dry milk in TTBS (0.05% Tween-20, Tris-buffered saline, pH 7.4), followed by an incubation for 2 hrs in TTBS containing the appropriate primary antibodies (anti-active extracellular signal-regulated kinase (ERK), -active c-Jun N-terminal kinase (JUN), and -active p38 anti-rabbit polyclonal antibodies, Promega) in concentrations recommended by the manufacturer. The membranes were incubated in TTBS containing horseradish peroxidase-labeled donkey anti-rabbit Ig's (1 : 2500; Amersham), followed by washing three times in TTBS. The detection of the protein was performed using a chemiluminescence method (ECL; Amersham). Active phosphorylated forms of ERK, JNK and p38 were scanned with a digital image analyzing system and quantified NIH images.

Data analysis

All the results were expressed as means ± SEM, and statistical significance was assessed by Student's *t* test. Values of $p < 0.005$ were considered statistically significant.

RESULT

Pure pressure–dependent acceleration of DNA synthesis in HASMC

With the pure pressure-loading apparatus, an atomospheric pressure of 240 mmHg was applied on cultured HASMC. DNA synthesis was measured as [³H]-TdR incorporation into DNA. After one hour of pressure application, the pure pressure of 240 mmHg induced an approximately 20% increase in [³H]-TdR incorporation compared to the control HASMC. After more than 3 hrs, the degree of acceleration of DNA synthesis was similar.

Threshold of pure atmospheric pressure in acceleration of DNA synthesis

To determine the threshold of pure atmospheric pressure in acceleration of DNA synthesis, pure pressure was applied to HASMC for 1 or 3 hrs. Various levels of atmospheric pressure (0 mmHg, 100 through 200 mmHg increments, and 240 mmHg) were applied to analyze the threshold of pure pressure in acceleration of DNA synthesis. The atmospheric pressure of less than 120 mmHg produced no significant change in [^{3}H]-TdR incorporation at 1 and 3 hrs. However, pressure of 140 mmHg produced an approximately 20% increase in [^{3}H]-TdR incorporation (p < 0.005 vs. control) at 1 and 3 hrs. Pressure of more than 140 mmHg also produced an increase (14 ± 6% to 27 ± 4%; p < 0.005 vs. control). At 3 hr, the degree of increase of was dependent on pressure levels from 140 to 180 mmHg, with 180-mmHg pressure producing an increase of 49 ± 6% compared to control cells (p < 0.01 vs. control), 200 mmHg pressure significantly accelerated DNA synthesis at both 1 and 3 hrs. However, exposure to 200 mmHg pressure did not further increase the DNA synthesis.

PTx effect on pure pressure–dependent DNA synthesis

We examined whether Gi-proteins are involved in pure pressure-dependent acceleration of DNA synthesis in HASMC, DNA-synthesis in acceleration under 200-mmHg pressure was completely inhibited by PTx (0.1 µg/ml) at 3 hrs (increase of DNA synthesis vs. control: 18.8 ± 2.7 at 1 hr and 18.0 ± 1.4% at 3 hrs in the absence of PTx; 4.4 ± 2.7% at 1 hr and 2.3 ± 2.9% at 3 hrs in the presence of PTx). In contrast, an acceleration of DNA synthesis by 160-mmHg pressure was not significantly inhibited at this time point (increase of DNA synthesis vs. control: 21.6 ± 2.5% at 1 hr and 27.4 ± 5.5% at 3 hrs in the absence of PTx; 16.5 ± 6.9% at 1 hr and 32.5 ± 5.5% at 3 hrs in the presence of PTx), PTx also failed to significantly inhibit the acceleration produced by 180 mmHg pressure (increase of DNA synthesis vs. control: 24.6 ± 4.3%) at 1 hr and 40.1 ± 11.4% at 3 hrs in the absence of PTx; 24.2 ± 3.9% at 1 hr and 49.0 ± 6.0% at 3 hrs in the presence of PTx).

Signal transduction system under pure pressure

Pure atmospheric pressure stimulated ERK1/2 and JNK activities. Pressure of more than 160 mmHg induced an activation of ERK1 (p44), and ERK1 was activated to maximum level at pressure of 240 mmHg (increase in active form of ERK1 vs. control: 63.2 ± 12.1%). Pressures of more than 120 mmHg induced an activation of ERK2 (p42), and ERK2 was activated to maximum level at pressure of 180 mmHg (increase in active form of ERK2 vs. control: 49.5 ± 7.3%). JNK was activated at pressures of more than 160 mmHg in pressure-dependent manner and to a maximum level at pressure of 240 mmHg (increase in active form of JNK vs. control: 45.7 ± 6.9%). Application of pure atmospheric pressure induced no activation of p38.

Effect of ACE inhibitor on signal transduction system in HASMC stimulated by pressure

We studied the effect of ACE inhibitor on this system. ACE inhibitor perindoprilat is added to the culture medium, then determined DNA synthesis and ERK expression. Perindoprilat suppressed DNA synthesis under 160 mmHg. Perindpril,

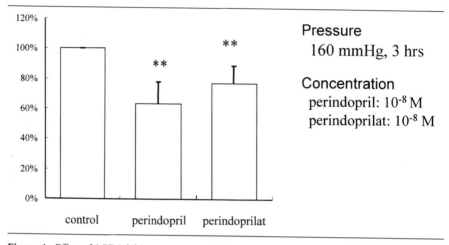

Figure 1. Effect of ACE inhibitor on pressure induced HASMC proliferation. Values are means ± SEM (n = 6–9). ★★p < 0.01 vs. controls.

inactive ACE inhibitor also suppressed DNA synthesis (Figure 1). AII was added on this incubation system. ACE inhibitor + AII do not recover DNA synthesis, which suppressed by ACE inhibitor (Figure 2). This result shows that AII do not effect on DNA synthesis under pressure, or ACE inhibitor directly inhibits the signal-pathway, which are activated by pure pressure. Perindoprilat and perindoril, inactive ACE inhibitor also suppressed ERK expression (Figure 3). We used other ACE inhibitors in this system, for example captopril. Captopril suppressed DNA synthesis (Figure 4).

DISCUSSION

Mechanical forces are important modulators of cellular functions, and particularly in the cardiovascular system. Mechanical stress has various components, such as well shear stress, tensile stress and pure pressure stress. In the case of shear stress, a fluid shear stress of 1.3–4.1 dynes/cm^2 affected endothelial cell DNA synthesis during regeneration (10). It is also reported that shear stress stimulated ERK and JNK activity in a force-dependent manner in endothelial cells (11). Shear stress is also known to activate phospholipase C and to generate inositol triphisphate (IP$_3$) and diacylglycerol. IP3 release Ca^{2+} from Ca^{2+} stores via IP3 receptor, and diacylglycerol activates protein kinase C (PKC) (12,13). Several PKC isoenzymes have been suggested to be involved in several downstream signalings, such as ERK activation, NF κ B-mediated gene transcription, erg-1 transcription and activation of c-Src families (14–16). Recently, It is reported that shear stress induced changes in the morphology and cytoskeltal organization of endothelial cells, and that these changes may be correlated to the functional change after exposure to shear stress (6). It is interesting to speculate role in shear stress-induced signalings, and that shear stress-induced signalings participate in intracellular cross-talk with integrine-coupled signal

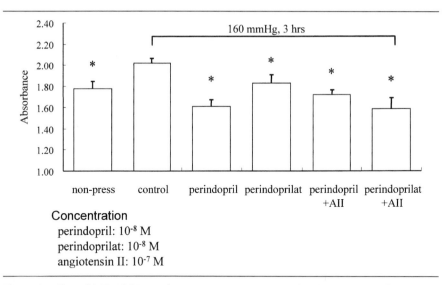

Figure 2. Effect of ACE inhibitor and angiotensin II on pressure-induced HASMC proliferation. Cells were incubated under an atmospheric pressure of 160 mmHg for 3 hours. Values are means ± SEM (n = 6–9). $\star p < 0.05$ vs. control.

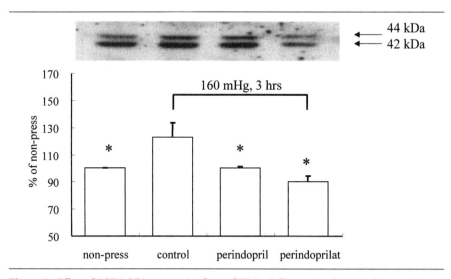

Figure 3. Effect of ACE inhibitor on active form of ERK. Cells were incubated under an atmospheric pressure of 160 mmHg for 3 hours. Values are means ± SEM (n = 3–5). $\star p < 0.05$ vs. controls.

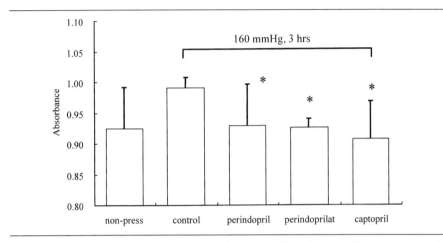

Figure 4. Effect of ACE inhibitors on pressure-induced HASMC proliferation. Cells were incubated under an atmospheric pressure of 160 mmHg for 3 hours.
Values are means ± SEM (n = 3–5). *p < 0.05 vs. controls.

transductions (17,18). In these studies, however, it is difficult to separate the direct effects of pure pressure from the indirect effects caused by the morphological change of cells. The pure stress is reported to promote DNA synthesis in rat cultured vascular smooth muscle cells in an original pressure-loading apparatus, as determined by immunocytochemical assay (19). This study suggests the possible presence of a mechanosensing cellular switch that is solely sensitive to pure pressure stress. However, in experiments with such apparatus, the threshold pressure for determining the on and off status of the mechanosensing cellular switch has not been clarified.

In this study, we demonstrated that pure pressure stress accelerated an increase of DNA synthesis in the absence of shear stress and tensile stress, and determined the threshold of pure pressure stress which presumably activates the mechanosensing cellular switch. Using an original pressure-loading apparatus, we investigated various pressure levels from 0 to 240 mmHg. Low atmospheric pressure of less than 120 mmHg had no significant effect on DNA synthesis, while pressures of more than 140 mmHg induced an acceleration of DNA synthesis. From these results, we conclude that a mechanosensing cellular switch for DNA synthesis that was solely sensitive to pure pressure was "on" or "off" at over or under 140 mmHg, respectively. Pressures of 140 to 180 mmHg promoted an increase of [³H]-TdR incorporation in a pressure-dependent manner at 1 and 3 hrs. Pressure of more than 200 mmHg also induced approximately 20% increase of DNA synthesis. However, degree of acceleration of DNA synthesis at pressure of more than 200 mmHg was similar and pressure-independent.

We also demonstrated the differential pathway in HASMC in response to pure atmospheric pressures. ERK1 was activated at pressures of more than 160 mmHg, and to a maximum level at pressure 2140 mmHg. ERK2 was activated at pressures of more than 120 mmHg, and to a maximum level at pressure of 180 mmHg. JNK was activated at pressures of more than 160 mmHg in a pressure-dependent manner. In contrast, p38 was not activated at pure atmospheric pressure. The mechanosensing mechanism stimulated by pure atmospheric pressure may consist of some differential pathways involving ERK and JNK signalings, and differential levels of pressure may activate each pathway. Moreover, differential activation of ERK and JNK in HASMC by pure atmospheric pressure may result in the selective phosphorylation and activation of transcription factors leading to selective gene regulatory events. It is not clear why the degrees of acceleration of DNA synthesis and activation of ERK2 were independent of pressure levels of more than 200 mmHg or why the pressure levels that accelerated DNA synthesis and activated ERK and JNK were different.

A role for heterotrimeric G-protein in mechanical stress-induced signal transductions in endothelial cells has recently emerged (20,21). It is known that both heterotrimeric G-proteins and small G-proteins are activated by shear stress. Shear stress-induced activation of G-proteins results in several flow-initiated endothelial responses that regulate vascular tone and that release such vasodilators as nitric oxide and prostaglandin I2, and such vasoconstrictors as endothelin (22–24). Therefore, we also investigated whether mechanosensing signaling pathways that are sensitive to pure pressure in HASMC were related to Gi-dependent pathways or Gi-independent pathways. At atmospheric pressures of 160 mmHg, PTx demonstrated no significant effect on [3H]TdR incorporation. However, at a high atmospheric pressure of 200 mmHg, PTx completely inhibited the increase of [3H]TdR incorporation. Pure pressure-induced DNA synthesis was produced through intracellular signaling pathways, including both Gi-dependent and -independent pathways. Although the molecular switch was "on" at an atmospheric pressure of more than 140 mmHg, an atmospheric pressure of below 180 mmHg may activate intracellular signalings predominantly through Gi-independent pathways, and a pressure of more than 200 mmHg may activate DNA synthesis predominantly through Gi-dependent pathways.

In summary, we demonstrated that HASMC had a mechanosensing molecular switch for DNA synthesis which was solely sensitive to pure atmospheric pressure, and the switch was "on" or "off" at over or under 140 mmHg, respectively. Moreover, mechanosensing cellular mechanisms may consist of some mechanosensors or intracellular pathways activated by different levels of pure atmospheric pressure. This study showed a change in dominance of Gi-dependent or Gi-independent intracellular signaling pathways in a pressure range from 160 to 200 mmHg. Recently, it has been reported that minimum risk for cardiovascular mortality was reached at 138.8 mmHg for a mean systolic arterial pressure in randomized clinical study of patients with hypertension (25). Activation of mechanosensing switches in HASMC at 140 mmHg may be involved in clinical cardiovascular events.

ACE inhibitor inhibited cell proliferation under the pressure. But the addition of AII on ACE inhibitor under the pressure could not recover the cell proliferation. ERKs and JNK are increased under pressure, and inhibited by ACE inhibitors. In

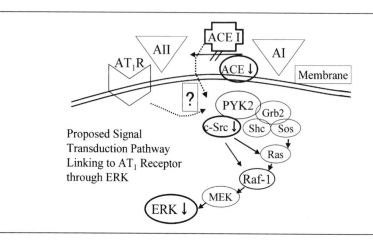

Figure 5. Proposed signal transduction pathway linking to AT1 receptor through ERK.

our recent studies, cSRC activated by pressure and suppressed ACE inhibitors. But Raf1 did not changed by pressure. Usually AII stimulates cell proliferation. But in our experiments, The addition of AII to incubation system do not recover the DNA synthesis suppressed by ACE inhibitor. At present time, we do not know how ACE inhibitor suppressed DNA synthesis by pressure (Figure 5). The mechanism of this inhibitory effect of ACE inhibitor on cell proliferation stimulated by pure pressure is under way in our laboratory.

REFERENCES

1. Safar ME, London G, Asmar R, Frohlich ED. 1998. Recent advances on large arteries in hypertension. Hypertension 32:156–161.
2. Vandenburgh HH. 1992. Mechanical forces and their second messengers in stimulating cell growth in vitro. Am J Physiol 262:R350-R355.
3. Cowan DB, Langill BL. 1996. Cellular and molecular biology of vascular remodeling. Curr Opi Lipidol 7:94–100.
4. Kyriakis JM, Avruch J. 1996. Sounding the alarm: protein kinase cascades activated by stress and inflammation. J Biol Chem 271:24313–24316.
5. Chien S, Li S, Shyy JYJ. 1998. Effects of mechanical forces on signal transduction and gene expression in endothelial cells. Hypertension 31:162–169.
6. Cucina A, Sterpetti AV, Pupelis G, Fragale A, Lpidi S, Cavallaro A, Giustiniani Q, D'Angelo LS. 1995. Shear stress induces changes in the morphology and cytoskeleton organization of arterial endothelial cells. Eur J Vas Endovasc Surg 9:86–92.
7. Weiser MC, Majack RA, Tucker A, Orton EC. 1995. Static tension is associated with increased smooth muscle cell DNA synthesis in rat pulmonary arteries. Am J Physiol 268:H1133–1138.
8. Setoguchi M, Ohya Y, Abe I, Fujishima M. 1997. Stretch activated whole-cell currents in smooth muscle cells from mesenteric resistance artery of guinea-pig. J Physiol 501:343–353.
9. Lowry OH, Rosenbrough NJ, Farr AL, Randall RJ. 1951. Protein measurement with the folin phenol reagent. J Biol Chem 193:265–275.
10. Ando J, Komatsuda T, Ishikawa C, Kamiya A. 1990. Fluid shear stress enhanced DNA synthesis in cultured endothelial cells during repair of mechanical denudation. Biorheology 27:675–684.
11. Jo H, Sipos K, Go YM, Law R, Rong J, McDonald JM. 1997. Differential effect of shear stress on extracellular signal-regulated kinase and N-terminal Jun kinase in endothelial cells. Gi2- and Gbeta/gamma-dependent signal pathways. J Biol Chem 272:1395–1401.

12. Helmlinger G, Berk BC, Nerem RM. 1995. Calcium responses of endothelial cell monolayers subjected to pulsatile and steady laminar flow differ. Am J Physiol 269:C367–375.
13. Tseng H, Peterson TE, Berk BC. 1995. Fluid shear stress stimulates mitogen-activated protein kinase in endothelial cells. Circ Res 77:869–878.
14. Mohan S, Mohan S, Sprague EA. 1997. Differential activation of NF-kappa B in human aortic endothelial cells conditioned to specific flow environments. Am J Physiol 273:C572–578.
15. Schwachtgen JL, Houston P, Campbell C, Sukhatme V, Braddock M. 1998. Fluid shear stress activation of erg-1 transcription in cultured human endothelial and epithelial cells is mediated via the extracellular signal-related kinase 1/2 mitogen-activated protein kinase pathway. J Clin Invest 101: 2540–2549.
16. Jalali S, Li YS, Sotoudeh M, Yuan S, Li S, Chien S, Shyy JYJ. 1998. Shear stress activates p60src-Ras-MAPK signaling pathways in vascular endothelial cells. Arterioscler Thromb Vas Biol 2:227–234.
17. Wang N, Butler JP, Ingber DE. 1993. Mechanotransduction across the cell surface and through the cytoskeleton. Science 260:1124–1127.
18. Miyamoto S, Teramoto H, Coso A, Gutkind JS, Burbelo PD, Akiyama SK, Yamada KM. 1995. Integrin function: molecular hierarchies of cytoskeletal signaling molecules. J Cell Biol 131:791–805.
19. Hishikawa K, Nakai T, Marumo T, Hayashi M, Suzuki H, Kato R, Saruta T. 1994. Pressure promotes DNA synthesis in rat cultured vascular smooth muscle cells. J Clin Invest 93:1975–1980.
20. Berthiaume F, Frangos JA. 1992. Flow-induced prostacyclin production is mediated by a pertussis toxin-sensitive G protein. FEBS Lett 308:277–279.
21. Gudi SRP, Clark CB, Frangos JA. 1996. Fluid flow rapidly activates G proteins in human endothelial cells. Involvement of G proteins in mechanochemical signal transduction. Circ Res 79:834–839.
22. Frangos JA, Eskin SG, McIntire LV, Ives CL. 1985. Flow effects prostacyclin production by cultured endothelial cells. Science 227:1477–1479.
23. Ranjan V, Xiao Z, Diamond SI. 1995. Constitutive NOS expression in cultured endothelial cells is elevated by fluid shear stress. Am J Physiol 269:H550–H555.
24. Kuchan MJ, Frangos JA. 1993. Shear stress regulates endothelin-1 release via protein kinase C and cGMP in cultured endothelial calls. Am J Physiol 264:H150–H156.
25. Hansson L, Zanchetti A, Carruthers SG, Dahlof B, Elmfeldt D, Julius S, Menard J, Rahn KH, Wedel H, Westerling S. 1998. Effect of intensive blood pressure lowering and low-dose aspirin in patients with hypertension: principal results of the hypertension optimal treatment (HOT) randomized trial. Lancet 351:1755–1762.

Signal Transduction and Cardiac Hypertrophy,
edited by N.S. Dhalla, L.V. Hryshko,
E. Kardami & P.K. Singal
Kluwer Academic Publishers, Boston, 2003

Role of Mitochondrial K$_{ATP}$ Channels in Improved Ischemic Tolerance of Chronically Hypoxic Adult and Immature Hearts

František Kolář, Ivana Ošťádalová, Bohuslav Ošťádal,
Jan Neckář, and Ondrej Szárszoi

Department of Developmental Cardiology
Institute of Physiology
Academy of Sciences of the Czech Republic and
Centre for Experimental Cardiovascular Research
Prague, Czech Republic

Summary. Adaptation to chronic hypoxia increases cardiac tolerance to acute ischemia/reperfusion injury, which manifests itself as a reduction of myocardial infarct size, improvement of post-ischemic contractile dysfunction and limitation of life-threatening ventricular arrhythmias. Hearts of chronically hypoxic adult animals can be further protected by classic ischemic preconditioning but the effects of these two phenomena are not additive. It appears that adaptation to hypoxia does not increase the total capacity of endogenous protective mechanisms. Moreover, the antiarrhythmic threshold of preconditioning is increased in chronically hypoxic animals.

Hearts of newborn animals which are "adapted" to hypoxic conditions *in utero* are more tolerant to ischemia/reperfusion injury than adults and can be further protected neither by preconditioning nor by prenatal exposure to chronic hypoxia. Decreasing cardiac ischemic tolerance after birth can be prevented by postnatal exposure to chronic hypoxia. In the rat, preconditioning develops only during the first postnatal week; unlike in adults, combination of chronic hypoxia and preconditioning provides better protection than each of the two conditions alone.

Address for Correspondence: Dr. František Kolář, Institute of Physiology AS CR, Vídeňská 1083, 142 20 Prague 4, Czech Republic. Tel.: +420-2-41062559, Fax: +420-2-41062125, E-mail address: kolar@biomed.cas.cz.

Although the detailed mechanism of cardioprotection induced by chronic hypoxia is unknown, several studies using selective pharmacological modulators of mitoK$_{ATP}$ suggest that activation of these channels plays an important role. Considering their involvement also in various forms of preconditioning, mitoK$_{ATP}$ may serve as the common component of both short-term and long-term cardioprotective mechanisms.

Key words: Chronic hypoxia, Myocardial ischemia, Protection, Preconditioning, K$_{ATP}$ channels.

INTRODUCTION: CARDIOPROTECTIVE EFFECTS OF CHRONIC HYPOXIA

The heart has the capability to cope with oxygen deprivation by activation of short-term and long-term adaptive mechanisms. Remarkable effort has been exerted to disclose the molecular signaling pathways, which underlie temporal protection of the heart against ischemic injury, afforded by prior brief periods of ischemia, the phenomenon widely known as preconditioning. Recent progress in understanding the two phases of protection, i.e. the classical preconditioning and the second window of protection, has been the subject of many reviews (e.g. 1–3). The detailed mechanism of this phenomenon remains, however, still unclear.

As compared with short-lived preconditioning, a more sustained improvement of cardiac ischemic tolerance can be achieved by prolonged exposure of animals to chronic hypoxia. Chronic myocardial hypoxia is the major pathophysiological feature of various cardiopulmonary diseases, such as chronic obstructive pulmonary disease and cyanotic congenital heart defects, and it is also naturally encountered in fetuses and in populations living at high altitude. Permanent or intermittent hypobaric hypoxia simulated in a low-pressure chamber (high altitude hypoxia, HAH) or normobaric hypoxia serve as relevant experimental models of chronic hypoxia. It is worth noting that Kopecky and Daum (4) first demonstrated the protection of the heart by HAH experimentally already in 1958. Their experiments were prompted by former clinical epidemiological studies demonstrating that the incidence of myocardial infarction and mortality from coronary heart disease is reduced in people living at high altitude (reviewed in 5). Kopecky and Daum found that cardiac muscle isolated from rats exposed every other day for six weeks to an altitude of 7000 m recovered its contractile function during reoxygenation following a period of acute anoxia to a higher level than that of control normoxic animals. Others, using various experimental models and adaptation protocols and various end points of injury have repeatedly confirmed this observation. The majority of these studies demonstrated that the hearts of adult chronically hypoxic animals develop smaller myocardial infarction (6–9) and exhibit better functional recovery (10–12) following ischemia/reperfusion insult than normoxic controls. These hearts are also less susceptible to toxic effects of isoprenaline, as indicated by the reduced size of necrotic lesions (13,14).

Of the three major end points of acute myocardial ischemia/reperfusion injury (ventricular arrhythmias, contractile dysfunction and lethal cell damage), the incidence and severity of arrhythmias have been the least studied and information on the effects

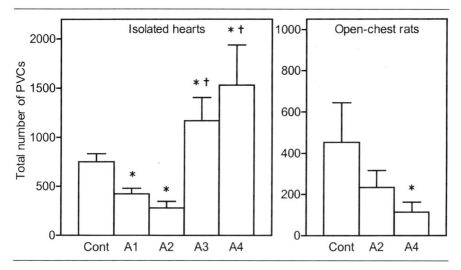

Figure 1. Total number of premature ventricular complexes (PVCs) over 30-min LAD coronary artery occlusion in isolated perfused hearts (left panel) and in anesthetized open-chest adult rats (right panel) adapted to intermittent HAH (groups A) and in normoxic animals (C). A1: adapted to 5000 m, 4 h/day, total of 10–14 exposures; A2: 5000 m, 4 h/day, 25–30 exposures; A3: 5000 m, 8 h/day, 25–30 exposures; A4: 7000 m, 8 h/day, 25–30 exposures.

Values are means ± SEM; *P < 0.05 vs normoxic controls; $^{\dagger}P$ < 0.05 vs group A2. Redrawn from (20) with permission.

of chronic high altitude hypoxia is less conclusive. Meerson et al. (15,16) observed a pronounced protection against ischemic arrhythmias in rats adapted to HAH (5000 m, 5–6 h/day, 40–45 exposures) using regional no-flow ischemia (coronary artery occlusion) in open-chest animals, but not in isolated perfused hearts. In another study (17), a similar protocol (4000 m, 5 h/day, 40 exposures) led to an antiarrhythmic effect that persisted in hearts even after their isolation. Chronic hypoxia protects the heart also against arrhythmias induced by adrenaline or high calcium (18). Recently we have shown that the effect of HAH on ischemic arrhythmias differs markedly when assessed on isolated perfused hearts or on open-chest animals (19,20). In isolated hearts the effect was strongly dependent on the degree (altitude) and duration of hypoxic exposure. Whereas the adaptation to 5000 m for 4 h/day decreased ectopic activity and severity of ischemic arrhythmias, extending the daily exposure to 8 h and/or increasing the degree of hypoxia to 7000 m led to a loss of protection and even a proarrhythmic effect of HAH was observed. In contrast, the open-chest rats adapted to HAH exhibited an antiarrhythmic protection, which was even more pronounced at the higher altitude (Figure 1). Hence, distinct effects occurred in the two experimental setups, in spite of the fact that both of them involved the same model of no-flow regional ischemia. The reason for this difference is unknown at present. Obviously, the presence of blood components and/or neurohumoral control mechanisms in open-chest animals may play a crucial role in maintaining the antiarrhythmic protection in rats adapted to a more severe hypoxia.

It is generally accepted that immature heart is less susceptible to ischemia/reperfusion injury as demonstrated in rabbits (21–23), dogs (24), pigs (25) as well as rats (26,27). We have shown, that cardiac tolerance decreases significantly already during the first postnatal week (28). The mechanism of the higher tolerance of newborn hearts to oxygen deprivation has not yet been satisfactorily clarified. As the fetus lives at very low oxygen partial pressure, the newborn heart is "adapted" to hypoxic conditions in utero. This view is supported by our observation that prenatal exposure (i.e. of pregnant mothers) to HAH fails to further increase ischemic tolerance in 1-day-old hearts (29). Newborn hearts exhibit a number of physiological features similar to those of adult hypoxia-tolerant animals, e.g. lower energy demand, greater anaerobic glycolytic capacity, altered ATP catabolic pathways, calcium handling and sensitivity to reactive oxygen species (reviewed in 30). Neonatal high tolerance to oxygen deprivation appears to be primarily based on the ability to maintain tissue aerobiosis as long as possible.

Normal postnatal decline of cardiac ischemic tolerance can be prevented by extension of hypoxic conditions beyond birth. Early postnatal exposure of rats to HAH maintains high resistance of their hearts, which better tolerate ischemia/reperfusion insult than age-matched normoxic controls even on day 10 of postnatal life. This effect has been demonstrated both in rats (29) and rabbits (23) in the form of better recovery of contractile function following ischemia. Perhaps for technical reasons, there are no data available as to whether similar effects would exist when the size of myocardial infarction or severity of ventricular arrhythmias are taken as the end points of ischemia/reperfusion injury.

CHRONIC HYPOXIA VERSUS PRECONDITIONING

The relationship between long-term cardioprotection by adaptation to chronic hypoxia and short-term protection by ischemic preconditioning is still poorly understood. Our experiments revealed that adaptation to HAH increases the antiarrhythmic threshold of ischemic preconditioning, as the single 3-min occlusion of the coronary artery, which was protective in normoxic hearts, was totally inefficient in the hypoxic group. Two occlusion periods of 5 min each were needed to precondition the chronically hypoxic hearts (Figure 2). It is conceivable that the stronger ischemic stimulus is needed to activate the signaling cascade leading to further short-term protection in a heart adapted to lack of oxygen.

The question arose whether a combination of chronic hypoxia and preconditioning may increase the total capacity of myocardial protective mechanisms, i.e. whether their effects are additive. Additive protective effects of these two phenomena were found when post-ischemic recovery of the contractile function was examined in isolated perfused hearts of adult rats (12). This observation led the authors to conclude that chronic hypoxia and preconditioning independently activate different protective mechanisms against ischemia. Recently, we analyzed the sole and combined protective effects of these phenomena on the size of myocardial infarction and the incidence and severity of ventricular arrhythmias in open-chest rat model (8). These experiments clearly demonstrated that chronically hypoxic hearts

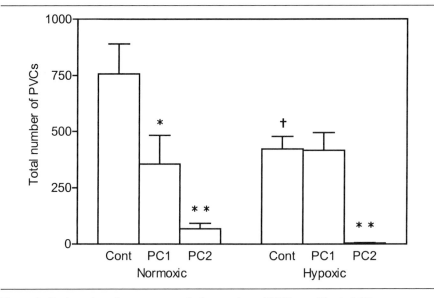

Figure 2. Total number of premature ventricular complexes (PVCs) over 30-min LAD coronary artery occlusion in preconditioned (PC) and non-preconditioned (Cont) isolated perfused hearts of adult rats adapted no intermittent HAH (5000 m, 4 h/day, 10–14 exposures) and of normoxic animals. Preconditioning was induced by either one 3-min (PC1) or two 5-min (PC2) occlusions of the same artery, each followed by 5-min reperfusion.
Values are means ± SEM; ⋆ $P < 0.05$ vs corresponding controls; ⋆⋆ $P < 0.05$ vs PC1; † $P < 0.05$ vs corresponding normoxic group. Redrawn from (19) with permission.

can be further preconditioned but the level of protection achieved by the combination of chronic hypoxia and preconditioning is the same as that provided by preconditioning alone in normoxic animals, indicating that these two protective phenomena are not additive and might share the same signalling pathway or element (Figures 3 and 4). It means that long-term adaptive processes do not increase the total capacity of endogenous protective mechanisms. In chronically hypoxic hearts, which are more tolerant to lethal cell injury and to arrhythmias, the efficiency of the short-term preconditioning is thereby reduced. This is unlikely to be explained by an increased threshold for preconditioning. These observations may be of potential clinical relevance in chronic ischemic/hypoxic states of the human heart; it seems likely that preconditioning or preconditioning-related pharmacological therapy will be less efficient in these situations than in the healthy heart. Moreover, various systemic diseases such as diabetes or hypercholesterolemia can further abrogate the myocardial response to preconditioning (reviewed in 31).

What is the relationship between chronic hypoxia and preconditioning in immature hearts? First of all it should be noted that the newborn rat heart could not be preconditioned. This endogenous protective mechanism is therefore absent at birth and it develops only at the end of the first postnatal week, counteracting the normally decreasing ischemic tolerance during this period (28). Surprisingly, when

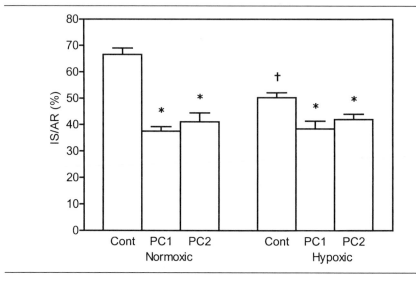

Figure 3. Myocardial infarct size expressed as percentage of the area at risk (IS/AR) in preconditioned (PC) and non-preconditioned (Cont) hearts of adult rats adapted to intermittent HAH (7000 m, 8 h/day, 24–30 exposures) and of normoxic animals. Infarct size (tetrazolium staining) was determined in anesthetized open-chest animals subjected to 30-min LAD coronary artery occlusion and 4-h reperfusion. Preconditioning was induced by either two (PC1) or five (PC2) occlusions of the same artery for 5 min, each followed by 5-min reperfusion.
Values are means ± SEM; ★$P < 0.05$ vs corresponding controls; †$P < 0.05$ vs corresponding normoxic group. Redrawn from (8) with permission.

prenatal exposure to HAH was combined with preconditioning in 1-day-old hearts, their ischemic tolerance was increased, despite the fact that each of the two sole phenomena failed to be protective. Moreover, unlike in adults, combination of chronic hypoxia and preconditioning in 10-day-old hearts provided better protection than each of the two phenomena alone (Figure 5). Similarly, Baker et al. (32) have observed that isolated perfused hearts of neonatal rabbits (7 to 10-day-old) normoxic from birth could be preconditioned; in contrast, age-matched hearts chronically hypoxic from birth could not, suggesting that these hearts are already fully protected by chronic hypoxia. This points to possible species and developmental differences in the interaction of the two protective phenomena.

CARDIOPROTECTIVE MECHANISM OF CHRONIC HYPOXIA: ROLE OF K$_{ATP}$

As compared with the temporal character of preconditioning, cardiac protection by adaptation to chronic hypoxia may persist long after the regression of other hypoxia-induced adaptive changes, such as polycythemia, pulmonary hypertension and right ventricular hypertrophy (reviewed in 33). This feature makes this phenomenon interesting for potential therapeutic exploitation. However, unlike preconditioning, chronic hypoxia has attracted much less attention and its cardioprotective

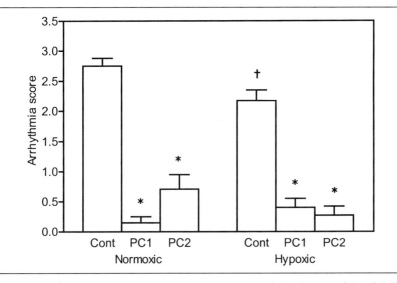

Figure 4. Arrhythmia score over 30-min LAD coronary artery occlusion in preconditioned (PC) and non-preconditioned (Cont) hearts of adult anesthetized open-chest rats adapted to intermittent HAH (7000 m, 8 h/day, 24–30 exposures) and of normoxic animals. Preconditioning was induced by either two (PC1) or five (PC2) occlusions of the same artery for 5 min, each followed by 5-min reperfusions. A 5-point arrhythmia score was determined in each individual heart and used for group analysis of severity of arrhythmias. Single PVCs were given a score of 1, salvos a score of 2, ventricular tachycardia a score of 3, reversible ventricular fibrillation a score of 4, and sustained fibrillation (lasting more than 2 min) a score of 5.
Values are means ± SEM; *$P < 0.05$ vs corresponding controls; $^{†}P < 0.05$ vs corresponding normoxic group. Redrawn from (8) with permission.

mechanism is far from clear. Though many potential factors have been proposed to play a role, direct evidence in favor of any of them is limited (reviewed in 34).

It has been shown that long-term adaptation to various metabolic stresses including chronic hypoxia results in activation of ATP-sensitive potassium channels (K_{ATP}) in various organs (35). An increasing body of evidence, based mostly on pharmacological experiments, indicates that these channels, in particular those that are localized in the inner mitochondrial membrane (mitoK_{ATP}) (36), play an important role in chronic hypoxia-induced protection of the heart against ischemia/reperfusion injury. We examined the effects of pharmacological modulators, that are considered to be selective for mitoK_{ATP}, on the size of myocardial infarction in open-chest adult rats and contractile dysfunction in isolated perfused hearts (9). Whereas the blocker, 5-hydroxydecanoate, completely abolished both the improvement of post-ischemic recovery of contractility and the reduction of infarct size in animals adapted to HAH, it had no appreciable influence in the normoxic group. In contrast, the opener, diazoxide, significantly reduced contractile dysfunction and infarct size in normoxic hearts to the same extent as achieved by chronic hypoxia, but it had no additive protective effect in the HAH-adapted group (Figures 6 and 7). These results are in accordance with our previous studies, which have shown that mitoK_{ATP} are

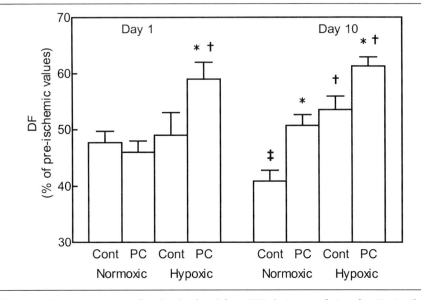

Figure 5. Maximum recovery of cardiac developed force (DF) during reperfusion after 40 min of global normothermic ischemia in preconditioned (PC) and non-preconditioned (Cont) isolated perfused hearts of 1-day-old (left panel) and 10-day-old (right panel) rats exposed to intermittent HAH (5000 m, 8 h/day) and of age-matched normoxic animals. In 1-day-old group, prenatal hypoxia was induced by exposure of mothers to HAH from day 15 to day 19 of pregnancy. The 10-day-old group was exposed to hypoxia between postnatal days 1 and 9. Preconditioning was elicited by three 3-min periods of global ischemia, each followed by 5-min reperfusion.
Values are means ± SEM; [*]$P < 0.05$ vs corresponding age-matched controls; [†]$P < 0.05$ vs corresponding age-matched normoxic group; [‡]$P < 0.05$ vs corresponding 1-day-old group. Data from (29) with permission.

involved in the antiarrhythmic mechanism of adaptation to chronic hypoxia. Likewise, pretreatment with 5-hydroxydecanoate prevented the decrease in both the number of premature ventricular complexes during ischemia and severity of reperfusion arrhythmias in animals adapted to HAH, while diazoxide was antiarrhythmic in the normoxic controls but not in the adapted group (19,37) (Figure 8). These effects cannot be attributed to hemodynamic actions of the drugs as they were demonstrated in both open-chest animals and in isolated hearts perfused under constant pressure or constant flow. Furthermore, BMS-191095, a novel highly selective mitoK$_{ATP}$ opener which is devoid of peripheral vasodilator activity (38,39), exhibited the same protective effect on myocardial infarction in the normoxic group (and its absence in the hypoxic group) as diazoxide (9) (Figure 7). This observation further supports our conclusion regarding the importance of mitoK$_{ATP}$ in cardioprotection by chronic hypoxia.

These channels also appear to play a role in increased cardiac ischemic tolerance of neonatal rats exposed to HAH for ten consecutive days starting at birth. Improved recovery of the contractile function of their isolated perfused hearts was blocked by

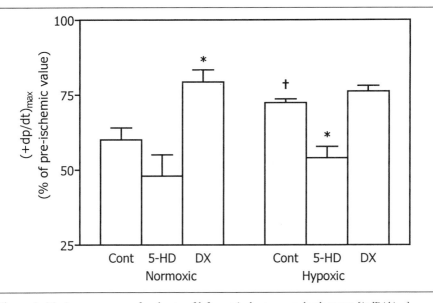

Figure 6. Maximum recovery of peak rate of left ventricular pressure development $[(+dP/dt)_{max}]$ during 45-min reperfusion after 20 min of global normothermic ischemia in control untreated (Cont), 5-hydroxydecanoate-treated (5-HD, 250 µmol/l) and diazoxide-treated (DX, 50 µmol/l) isolated perfused hearts of adult rats adapted to intermittent HAH (5000 m, 8 h/day, 24–32 exposures) and of normoxic animals.
Values are means ± SEM; $\star P < 0.05$ vs corresponding controls; $^\dagger P < 0.05$ vs corresponding normoxic group. Redrawn from (9) with permission.

5-hydroxydecanoate, which had no effect in the normoxic group. In fact, this substance reduced the ischemic tolerance of chronically hypoxic immature hearts even below the level observed in the untreated normoxic group (29) (Figure 9). A different situation was observed in hearts of neonatal rabbits: the non-selective K_{ATP} blocker, glibenclamide, completely abolished the protective effect of chronic hypoxia on post-ischemic contractile dysfunction in this species, whereas the opener, bimakalim, induced cardioprotection only in normoxic hearts (40,41). According to a recent study by the same group (42), both mitoK$_{ATP}$ and sarcolemmal K_{ATP} contribute to the cardioprotection in their model of chronic hypoxia. This protection was completely abolished by co-administration of selective sarcolemmal K_{ATP} (HMR 1098) and mitoK$_{ATP}$ blockers whereas 5-hydroxydecanoate alone exhibited only a partial inhibitory effect. Thus, our results obtained in adult and immature rats do not fully confirm the above conclusion, as mitoK$_{ATP}$ blockade led to a complete inhibition of protection, suggesting that species differences may play a role. Nevertheless, both our studies and those of Baker's group provide clear evidence that mitoK$_{ATP}$ are involved in the cardioprotective mechanism of chronic hypoxia, regardless of their quantitative importance.

MitoK$_{ATP}$ have also been implicated in the protection of the heart induced by preconditioning, as demonstrated in a number of reports. Their involvement was

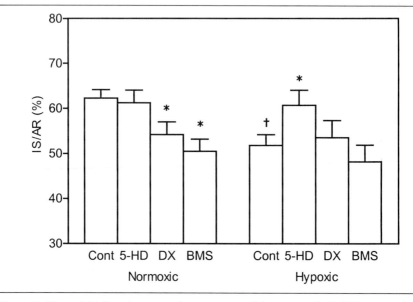

Figure 7. Myocardial infarct size expressed as percentage of the area at risk (IS/AR) in control untreated (Cont), 5-hydroxydecanoate-treated (5-HD, 5 mg/kg), diazoxide-treated (DX, 10 mg/kg) and BMS-191095-treated (BMS, 10 mg/kg) hearts of adult rats adapted to intermittent HAH (5000 m, 8 h/day, 24–32 exposures) and of normoxic animals. Infarct size (tetrazolium staining) was determined in anesthetized open-chest animals subjected to 20-min LAD coronary artery occlusion and 4-h reperfusion.
Values are means ± SEM; $\star P < 0.05$ vs corresponding controls; $^{\dagger} P < 0.05$ vs corresponding normoxic group. Data from (9) with permission.

demonstrated in various models and forms of preconditioning including acute (43–45) and delayed forms (3,46,47), pacing-induced protection (48), preconditioning on distance (49) and pharmacologically induced protection (1,50,51). It appears, therefore, that these channels may represent a common central component of both short-term and long-term cardioprotective mechanisms. The assumption that various protective phenomena may share the same molecular pathway or its element is further supported by the observation that protective effects of chronic hypoxia and classic ischemic preconditioning are not additive in adult rats (8,32) as discussed above. Moreover, the newborn rat heart, which is "adapted" to hypoxic conditions *in utero*, is also more tolerant to ischemic injury and cannot be preconditioned (28).

MITOK$_{ATP}$ AT CHRONIC HYPOXIA

It has been proposed that chronic hypoxia leads to sustained, tonic activation of cardiac mitoK$_{ATP}$ (19,41) that may explain the insensitivity of these hearts to diazoxide and BMS-191095. The mechanism by which mitoK$_{ATP}$ opening leads to improvement of ischemic tolerance of the heart remains obscure and little is known about factors that may maintain these channels in the active state under conditions

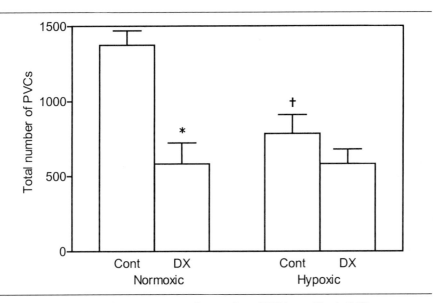

Figure 8. Total number of premature ventricular complexes (PVCs) over 30-min LAD coronary artery occlusion in control untreated (Cont) and diazoxide-treated (DX, 50 μmol/l) isolated perfused hearts of adult rats adapted to intermittent HAH (5000 m, 4 h/day, 10–14 exposures) and of normoxic animals.

Values are means ± SEM; *P < 0.05 vs corresponding controls; †P < 0.05 vs corresponding normoxic group. Redrawn from (19) with permission.

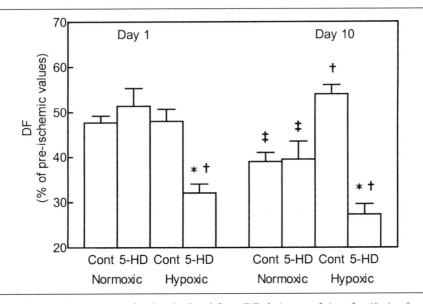

Figure 9. Maximum recovery of cardiac developed force (DF) during reperfusion after 40 min of global normothermic ischemia in control untreated (Cont) and 5-hydroxydecanoate-treated (5-HD, 300 μmol/l) isolated perfused hearts of 1-day-old (left panel) and 10-day-old (right panel) rats exposed to intermittent HAH (5000 m, 8 h/day) and of age-matched normoxic animals. In the 1-day-old group, prenatal hypoxia was induced by exposure of mothers to HAH from day 15 to day 19 of pregnancy. The 10-day-old group was exposed to hypoxia between postnatal days 1 and 9.

Values are means ± SEM; *P < 0.05 vs corresponding age-matched controls; †P < 0.05 vs corresponding age-matched normoxic group; ‡P < 0.05 vs corresponding 1-day-old group. Data from (29) with permission.

of chronic hypoxia and also following a restoration of normoxic conditions. Chronic hypoxia induces a large variety of adaptive changes in the myocardium, which may be protective (34) but their potential link to mitoK$_{ATP}$ has not yet been clearly established. Myocardial mitoK$_{ATP}$ can be activated, for instance, by protein kinase C (PKC) which appears to be a key player in signal transduction of various cardioprotective phenomena (47,52–54). It has been shown that PKC expression is modified by ischemic, hypoxic or pharmacological preconditioning with a translocation of individual isoforms to specific cellular structures (54–56). Limited information is available suggesting that PKC is up-regulated and permanently activated under conditions of chronic hypoxia (57). Our preliminary data also suggest that HAH leads to up-regulation of the PKC-δ isoform, particularly in the mitochondrial fraction (58). Chronic hypoxia also increases myocardial concentration of phosphatidylinositol, the substrate of PKC-activating signaling cascade (59). However, the involvement of PKC, or its particular isoform, in cardioprotection by HAH is questioned by the observation that the PKC inhibitor, chelerythrine, did not affect increased ischemic tolerance of these hearts (60).

Another potential candidate for endogenous mitoK$_{ATP}$ activator in chronic hypoxia is nitric oxide (NO) although its role is controversial. Rouet-Benzineb et al. (57) detected abundance and higher enzyme activity of inducible NO synthase (iNOS) in chronically hypoxic adult rat hearts due to hypoxia-inducible factor 1. Hypoxia increased this enzyme activity and gene expression also in atrial myocardium of children with cyanotic congenital heart defects, whereas constitutive NO synthase (eNOS) was down-regulated (61). In contrast, Baker et al. (62) showed that adaptation of neonatal rabbits to hypoxia increased NO production by up-regulation of eNOS; higher NO production in these hearts may activate K$_{ATP}$ by cGMP-dependent mechanism but other pathways cannot be excluded. Inhibition of NO synthase activity by L-NAME led to a complete abolition of protection by chronic hypoxia, whereas the NO donor, GSNO, was protective in normoxic but not in chronically hypoxic hearts (62). Similarly, NO synthase inhibition blocked completely the improved post-ischemic recovery of contractility of isolated perfused hearts of neonatal chronically hypoxic rats (29). In contrast to the above studies, L-NAME administration had no effect on improved recovery of the contractile function of chronically hypoxic adult rat hearts (60). Moreover, L-NAME efficiently reduced the severity of reperfusion arrhythmias in normoxic hearts but not in chronically hypoxic hearts, whereas GSNO abolished antiarrhythmic protection in the latter group, suggesting an adverse effect of NO on this manifestation of injury (63). The role of NO and its link to mitoK$_{ATP}$ in improved ischemic tolerance of chronically hypoxic hearts thus remain unclear. Future studies are necessary to disclose the complex mechanism of this long-term cardioprotective phenomenon.

ACKNOWLEDGEMENTS

This work was supported by the Grant Agency of the Czech Republic (grants No. 305/01/0279 to FK and 305/00/1659 to BO).

REFERENCES

1. Yellon DM, Baxter GF, Garcia-Dorado D, Heusch G, Sumeray MS. 1998. Ischaemic preconditioning: present position and future directions. Cardiovasc Res 37:21–33.
2. Cohen MV, Baines CP, Downey JM. 2000. Ischemic preconditioning: from adenosine receptor to K_{ATP} channel. Annu Rev Physiol 62:79–109.
3. Bolli R. 2000. The late phase of preconditioning. Circ Res 87:972–983.
4. Kopecky M, Daum S. 1958. Tissue adaptation to anoxia in rat myocardium (in Czech). Cs Fysiol 7:518–521.
5. Heath D, Williams DR. 1981. Man at High Altitude. Edinburgh: Churchil Livingstone.
6. Meerson FZ, Gomzakov OA, Shimkovich MV. 1973. Adaptation to high altitude hypoxia as a factor preventing development of myocardial ischemic necrosis. Am J Cardiol 31:30–34.
7. Turek Z, Kubat K, Ringnalda BEM, Kreuzer F. 1980. Experimental myocardial infarction in rats acclimated to simulated high altitude. Basic Res Cardiol 75:544–553.
8. Neckar J, Papousek F, Ostadal B, Novakova O, Kolar F. 2002. Cardioprotective effects of chronic hypoxia and preconditioning are not additive. Basic Res Cardiol 97:161–167.
9. Neckar J, Szarszoi O, Koten L, Papousek F, Ostadal B, Grover GJ, Kolar F. 2002. Effects of mitochondrial KATP modulators on cardioprotection induced by chronic high altitude hypoxia in rats. Cardiovasc Res 55:567–575.
10. McGrath JJ, Prochazka J, Pelouch V, Ostadal B. 1973. Physiological responses of rats to intermittent high altitude stress. Effects of age. J Appl Physiol 34:289–293.
11. Widimsky J, Urbanova D, Ressl J, Ostadal B, Pelouch V, Prochazka J. 1973. Effect of intermittent altitude hypoxia on the myocardium and lesser circulation in the rat. Cardiovasc Res 7:798–808.
12. Tajima M, Katayose D, Bessho M, Isoyama S. 1994. Acute ischemic preconditioning and chronic hypoxia independently increase myocardial tolerance to ischemia. Cardiovasc Res 28:312–319.
13. Poupa O, Krofta K, Prochazka J, Turek Z. 1966. Acclimatization to simulated high altitude and acute cardiac necrosis. Fed Proc 25:1243–1246.
14. Faltova E, Mraz M, Pelouch V, Prochazka J, Ostadal B. 1987. Increase and regression of the protective effect of high altitude acclimatization on the isoprenaline-induced necrotic lesions in the rat myocardium. Physiol Bohemoslov 36:43–52.
15. Meerson FZ, Ustinova EE, Orlova EH. 1987. Prevention and elimination of heart arrhythmias by adaptation to intermittent high altitude hypoxia. Clin Cardiol 10:783–789.
16. Meerson FZ, Ustinova EE, Manukhina EB. 1989. Prevention of cardiac arrhythmias by adaptation to hypoxia: regulatory mechanisms and cardiotropic effect. Biomed Biochim Acta 48:S83–S88.
17. Vovc E. 1998. The antiarrhythmic effect of adaptation to intermittent hypoxia. Folia Med (Plovdiv) 40(suppl 3):51–54.
18. Lishmanov YU, Uskina EV, Krylatov AV, Kondratiev BY, Ugdyzhekova DS, Maslov LN. 1998. A modulated effect of endogenous opioids on antiarrhythmic effect of hypoxic adaptation (in Russian). Russian J Physiol 84:363–372.
19. Asemu G, Papousek F, Ostadal B, Kolar F. 1999. Adaptation to high altitude hypoxia protects the heart agains ischemia-induced arrhythmias. Involvement of mitochondrial K_{ATP} channel. J Mol Cell Cardiol 31:1821–1831.
20. Asemu G, Neckar J, Szarszoi O, Papousek F, Ostadal B, Kolar F. 2000. Effects of adaptation to intermittent high altitude hypoxia on ischemic ventricular arrhythmias in rats. Physiol Res 49:597–606.
21. Nishioka K, Jarmakani J. 1982. Effect of ischemia on mechanical function and high-energy phosphates in rabbit myocardium. Am J Physiol 242:H1077–H1083.
22. Bove EL, Stammers AH. 1986. Recovery of left ventricular function after hypothermic global ischemia. J Thorac Cardiovasc Surg 91:115–122.
23. Baker EJ, Boerboom LE, Olinger GN, Baker JE. 1995. Tolerance of the developing heart to ischemia: impact of hypoxemia from birth. Am J Physiol 268:H1165–H1173.
24. Julia P, Young HH, Buckberg GD, Kofsky ER, Bugyi HI. 1990. Studies of myocardial protection in the immature heart. II. Evidence for importance of amino acid metabolism in tolerance to ischemia. J Thorac Cardiovasc Surg 100:888–895.
25. Baker JE, Boerboom LE, Olinger GN. 1990. Is protection of ischemic neonatal myocardium by cardioplegia species dependent? J Thorac Cardiovasc Surg 99:280–287.
26. Yano Y, Braimbridge MV, Hearse DJ. 1987. Protection of the pediatric myocardium: differential susceptibility to ischemic injury of the neonatal rat heart. J Thorac Cardiovasc Surg 94:887–896.

27. Riva E, Hearse DJ. 1993. Age-dependent changes in myocardial susceptibility to ischemic injury. Cardioscience 4:85–92.
28. Ostadalova I, Ostadal B, Kolar F, Parratt JR, Wilson S. 1998. Tolerance to ischaemia and ischaemic preconditioning in neonatal rat heart. J Mol Cell Cardiol 30:857–865.
29. Ostadalova I, Ostadal B, Jarkovska D, Kolar F. 2002. Combination of the protective effect of adaptation to chronic hypoxia and ischemic preconditioning in neonatal rat heart. Pediatr Res 52:561–567.
30. Ostadal B, Ostadalova I, Dhalla NS. 1999. Development of cardiac sensitivity to oxygen deficiency: comparative and ontogenetic aspects. Physiol Rev 73:635–659.
31. Ferdinandy P, Szilvassy Z, Baxter GF. 1998. Adaptation to myocardial stress in diseased states: is preconditioning a healthy heart phenomenon? Trends Pharmacol Sci 19:223–229.
32. Baker JE, Holman P, Gross GJ. 1999. Preconditioning in immature rabbit hearts: role of K_{ATP} channels. Circulation 99:1249–1254.
33. Ostadal B, Kolar F, Pelouch V, Prochazka J, Widimsky J. 1994. Intermittent high altitude and the cardiopulmonary system. In: The Adapted Heart. Ed. M Nagano, N Takeda, NS Dhalla, 173–182. New York: Raven Press.
34. Kolar F. 1996. Cardioprotective effects of chronic hypoxia: relation to preconditioning. In: Myocardial Preconditioning. Ed. Wainwright CL, Parratt JR, 261–275. Austin: RG Landes.
35. Cameron JS, Baghdady R. 1994. Role of ATP sensitive potassium channels in long term adaptation to metabolic stress. Cardiovasc Res 28:788–796.
36. Inoue I, Nagase H, Kishi K, Higuti T. 1991. ATP-sensitive K^+ channels in the mitochondrial inner membrane. Nature 352:244–247.
37. Neckar J, Papousek F, Ostadal B, Novakova O, Kolar F. 1999. Antiarrhythmic effect of adaptation to high altitude hypoxia is abolished by 5-hydroxydecanoate. J Mol Cell Cardiol 31:A51.
38. Grover GJ, D'Alonzo AJ, Garlid KD, Bajgar R, Lodge NJ, Sleph PG, Darbenzio RB, Hess TA, Smith MA, Paucek P, Atwal KS. 2001. Pharmacologic characterization of BMS-191095, a mitochondrial K_{ATP} opener with no peripheral vasodilator or action potential shortening activity. J Pharmacol Exp Therapeut 297:1184–1192.
39. Rovnyak GC, Ahmed SZ, Ding CZ et al. 1997. Cardioselective antiischemic ATP-sensitive potassium channel (K_{ATP}) openers. 5. Identification of 4-(N-aryl)-substituted benzopyran derivatives with high selectivity. J Med Chem 40:24–34.
40. Baker JE, Curry BD, Olinger GN, Gross GJ. 1997. Increased tolerance of the chronically hypoxic immature heart to ischemia. Contribution of the K_{ATP} channel. Circulation 95:1278–1285.
41. Eells JT, Henry MM, Gross GJ, Baker JE. 2000. Increased mitochondrial K_{ATP} channel activity during chronic myocardial hypoxia: is cardioprotection mediated by improved bioenergetics? Circ Res 87:915–921.
42. Kong X, Tweddell JS, Gross GJ, Baker JE. 2001. Sarcolemmal and mitochondrial K_{ATP} channels mediate cardioprotection in chronically hypoxic hearts. J Mol Cell Cardiol 33:1041–1045.
43. Garlid KD, Paucek P, Yarov-Yarovoy V, Murray HNM, Darbenzio RB, D'Alonzo AJ, Lodge NJ, Smith MA, Grover GJ. 1997. Cardioprotective effect of diazoxide and its interaction with mitochondrial ATP-sensitive K^+ channels. Possible mechanism of cardioprotection. Circ Res 81:1072–1082.
44. Ghosh S, Standen NB, Galinanes M. 2000. Evidence for mitochondrial K_{ATP} channels as effectors of human myocardial preconditioning. Cardiovasc Res 45:934–940.
45. Fryer RM, Ells JT, Hsu AK, Henry MM, Gross GJ. 2000. Ischemic preconditioning in rats: role of mitochondrial K_{ATP} channel in preservation of mitochondrial function. Am J Physiol 278: H305–H312.
46. Bernardo NL, D'Angelo M, Okubo S, Joy A, Kukreja RC. 1999. Delayed ischemic preconditioning is mediated by opening of ATP-sensitive potassium channels in the rabbit heart. Am J Physiol 276:H1323–H1330.
47. Takashi E, Wang Y, Ashraf M. 1999. Activation of mitochondrial K_{ATP} channel elicits late preconditioning against myocardial infarction via protein kinase C signaling pathway. Circ Res 85:1146–1153.
48. Macho P, Solis E, Sanchez G, Schwarze H, Domenech R. 2000. Mitochondrial ATP dependent potassium channels mediate non-ischemic preconditioning by tachycardia in dogs. Mol Cell Biochem 216:129–136.
49. Pell TJ, Baxter GF, Yellon DM, Drew GM. 1998. Renal ischemia preconditions myocardium: role of adenosine receptors and ATP-sensitive potassium channels. Am J Physiol 275:H1542–H1547.
50. Grover GJ, Garlid KD. 2000. ATP-sensitive potassium channels: A review of their cardioprotective pharmacology. J Mol Cell Cardiol 32:677–695.

51. O'Rourke B. 2000. Myocardial K_{ATP} channels in preconditioning. Circ Res 87:845–855.
52. Miura T, Liu Y, Kita H, Ogawa T, Shimamoto K. 2000. Roles of mitochondrial ATP-sensitive K channels and PKC in anti-infarct tolerance afforded by adenosine A1 receptor activation. J Am Coll Cardiol 35:238–245.
53. Sato T, O'Rourke B, Marban E. 1998. Modulation of mitochondrial ATP-dependent K^+ channels by protein kinase C. Circ Res 83:110–114.
54. Wang Y, Hirai K, Ashraf M. 1999. Activation of mitochondrial ATP-sensitive K^+ channel for cardiac protection against ischemic injury is dependent on protein kinase C activity. Circ Res 85:731–741.
55. Goldberg M, Zhang HL, Steinberg SF. 1997. Hypoxia alters the subcellular distribution of protein kinase C isoforms in neonatal rat ventricular myocytes. J Clin Invest 99:55–61.
56. Ping P, Zhang J, Qiu Y, Tang XL, Manchikalapudi S, Cao X, Bolli R. 1997. Ischemic preconditioning induces selective translocation of protein kinase C isoforms epsilon and eta in the heart of conscious rabbits without subcellular redistribution of total protein kinase C activity. Circ Res 81:404–414.
57. Rouet-Benzineb P, Eddahibi S, Raffestin B, Laplace M, Depond S, Adnot S, Crozatier B. 1999. Induction of cardiac nitric oxide synthase 2 in rats exposed to chronic hypoxia. J Mol Cell Cardiol 31:1697–1708.
58. Novak F, Markova I, Jezkova J, Kolar F, Neckar J, Novakova O. 2002. Effects of chronic hypoxia and acute ischemia on the expression of PKC isoforms in the rat myocardium. J Mol Cell Cardiol 34:A46.
59. Jezkova J, Novakova O, Kolar F, Tvrzicka E, Neckar J, Novak F. 2002. Chronic hypoxia alters fatty acid composition of phospholipids in right and left ventricular myocardium. Mol Cell Biochem 232:49–56.
60. Szarszoi O, Asemu G, Ostadal B, Kolar F. 2001. Role of mitochondrial K_{ATP} channels in increased ischemic tolerance of chronically hypoxic rat hearts. J Mol Cell Cardiol 33:A117.
61. Ferreiro CR, Chagas ACP, Carvalho MHC, Dantas AP, Jatene MB, de Souza LCB, da Luz PL. Influence of hypoxia on nitric oxide synthase activity and gene expression in children with congenital heart disease. A novel pathophysiological adaptive mechanism. Circulation 103:2272–2276.
62. Baker JE, Holman P, Kalyaranaman B, Griffith OW, Pritchard KA. 1999. Adaptation to chronic hypoxia confers tolerance to subsequent myocardial ischemia by increased nitric oxide production. Ann N Y Acad Sci 874:236–253.
63. Szarszoi O, Asemu G, Ostadal B, Kolar F. 2001. Role of nitric oxide in cardioprotection by chronic hypoxia. Physiol Res 50:P27.

Signal Transduction and Cardiac Hypertrophy,
edited by N.S. Dhalla, L.V. Hryshko,
E. Kardami & P.K. Singal
Kluwer Academic Publishers, Boston, 2003

Ca^{2+}-Dependent Signaling Pathways Through Calcineurin and Ca^{2+}/Calmodulin-Dependent Protein Kinase in Development of Cardiac Hypertrophy

Hiroyuki Takano, Yunzeng Zou, Hiroshi Akazawa, Toshio Nagai,
Miho Mizukami, Haruhiro Toko, and Issei Komuro★

Department of Cardiovascular Science and Medicine
Chiba University Graduate School of Medicine
1-8-1 Inohana, Chuo-ku
Chiba 260-8670, Japan

Summary. Cardiac hypertrophy is induced by a variety of cardiovascular diseases such as hypertension, valvular diseases, myocardial infarction, cardiomyopathy, and endocrine disorders. Although cardiac hypertrophy may be initially a beneficial response that normalizes wall stress and maintains normal cardiac function, prolonged hypertrophy becomes a leading cause of heart failure and sudden death. A number of studies have elucidated molecules responsible to the development of cardiac hypertrophy, including protein kinase C (PKC), protein kinase A (PKA), Raf-1 kinase, mitogen-activated protein (MAP) kinase family, and Janus kinase (JAK)/signal transducer and activator of transcription (STAT) family, Ras, and Rho family. It has been reported that Ca^{2+} regulates a number of cellular processes including cardiac hypertrophy. Since most hypertrophic signaling pathways are associated with an increase in intracellular Ca^{2+}, Ca^{2+}-dependent signaling pathways may be critical targets for therapies designed to prevent the progression of cardiac hypertrophy. Recently, a Ca^{2+}/calmodulin-dependent protein kinase, and a Ca^{2+}/calmodulin-dependent protein phosphatase, calcineurin, have attracted much attention as critical molecules that induce cardiac hypertrophy. In this review, we summarize the Ca^{2+}-dependent signaling pathways through Ca^{2+}/calmodulin-dependent protein kinase and calcineurin in cardiac hypertrophy.

★ Address for Correspondence: Issei Komuro, MD, PhD, Department of Cardiovascular Science and Medicine, Chiba University Graduate School of Medicine, 1-8-1 Inohana, Chuo-ku, Chiba 260-8670, Japan. Tel: 81-43-226-2097, Fax: 81-43-226-2557, E-mail: komuro-tky@umin.ac.jp

Key words: Ca^{2+}; calcineurin; CaMK; cardiac hypertrophy.

INTRODUCTION

Cardiac hypertrophy is recognized as an adaptive increase in heart size character-ized by a growth of cardiomyocyte rather than an increase in cell number. Cardiac hypertrophy is induced by a variety of cardiovascular diseases such as hypertension, valvular diseases, myocardial infarction, cardiomyopathy, and endocrine disorders (1,2). It has been well known that a variety of stimuli including mechanical stress, ischemia, and neurohumoral factors can activate multiple intracellular signaling pathways, leading to the development of cardiac hypertrophy (3). Although cardiac hypertrophy may be initially a beneficial response that normalizes wall stress and maintains normal cardiac function, epidemiological studies demonstrated that cardiac hypertrophy is a major risk factor of heart diseases and becomes a leading cause of heart failure and sudden death (4). Therefore, it is important to understand the pre-cise mechanisms and mediators of cardiac hypertrophy and to prevent it. Recently, a Ca^{2+}/calmodulin-dependent protein kinase (CaMK), and a Ca^{2+}/calmodulin-dependent protein phosphatase, calcineurin, have attracted much attention as criti-cal molecules that induce cardiac hypertrophy. Furthermore, the molecules related to CaMK and calcineurin, which include endogenous inhibitors of cardiac hyper-trophy, have been also elucidated. This article focuses on the Ca^{2+}-dependent sig-naling pathways through calcineurin and CaMK in cardiac hypertrophy.

Ca^{2+}/CALMODULIN

It has been known that Ca^{2+} regulates a number of cellular processes including cardiac hypertrophy (5). In response to external stimuli, cells increase their cytoso-lic Ca^{2+} levels (5). Because chelating of extracellular or intracellular Ca^{2+} abolishes hypertrophic responses by hypertrophic stimulators in cardiac myocytes, the increase in intracellular Ca^{2+} level and the activation of Ca^{2+}-dependent signaling pathway may be involved in cardiac hypertrophy (6–8). The elevation of cytosolic Ca^{2+} levels is accomplished by Ca^{2+} influx from external space and/or Ca^{2+} release from inter-nal stores such as sarcoplasmic reticulum (SR) (5). L-type Ca^{2+} channels, T-type Ca^{2+} channels, Na^+/Ca^{2+} exchanger, sarcolemmal Ca^{2+}-ATPase, SR Ca^{2+}-ATPase (SERCA), and ryanodine receptor are involved in Ca^{2+} transport in cardiac myocytes. Ca^{2+} influx through L-type Ca^{2+} channels induces a large Ca^{2+} release from SR through ryanodine receptor, which is called Ca^{2+}-induced Ca^{2+} release (CICR) (9,10). By using a Ca^{2+}-binding fluorescent dye (fluo3) and patch clamp technique, it has been shown that mechanical stress also induces Ca^{2+} influx through stretch-sensitive ion channels, leading to induction of CICR (11). The increase in intracellular Ca^{2+} levels usually evokes cellular events through its binding to Ca^{2+} binding proteins such as troponin C, calmodulin, calsequestrin, and calreticulin. Calmodulin has been well known as a major Ca^{2+} binding protein in all eukaryotic cells (12). It has been reported that the growth of cardiac myocytes is specifically regulated by calmodulin concentrations and that overexpression of calmodulin

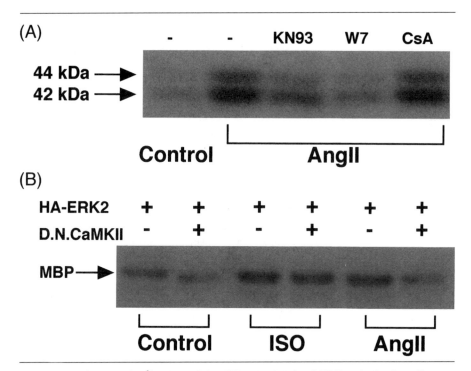

Figure 1. Involvement of Ca^{2+}, CaM, and CaMKII in AngII-induced ERKs activation in cardiomyocytes. (A) Cardiomyocytes were preincubated with KN93 (30 μM), W7 (30 μM) or cyclosporin A (CsA) (500 ng/ml) for 30 min. AngII were then added to the culture medium. ERKs activities were measured by "in-gel method". Bands corresponding to 44 kDa and 42 kDa ERKs are indicated. (B) cDNA encoding D.N.CaMKII was co-transfected with cDNA encoding HA-ERK2 into cultured cardiomyocytes. After stimulation with ISO or AngII, ERK2 activity was measured using MBP as the substrate. Representative autoradiograms from three independent experiments are shown.

induces cardiac hypertrophy in transgenic mice (13). Recently, we reported that endothelin-1 (ET-1)-, isoproterenol (ISO)-, or angiotensin II (Ang II)-induced hypertrophic responses were significantly suppressed by calmodulin inhibitor, W7, in cultured cardiomyocytes (14,15, Figure 1A). These findings suggest that calmodulin plays an important role in Ca^{2+}-dependent signals in cardiac myocytes.

CaMK-HDAC

Ca^{2+}/calmodulin modulates many molecules through activation of CaMKs (16). CaMKs are ubiquitous serine-threonine protein kinases involved in the regulation of diverse functions such as cell contraction, secretion, synaptic transmission, and gene expression (16). CaMKs are also implicated in the development of cardiac hypertrophy. CaMKII, a predominant isoform of CaMKs expressed in heart, increases the expression of atrial natriuretic peptide (ANP) gene in contraction- and phenylephrine (PE)-stimulated cardiac myocytes (17,18). We recently demonstrated that CaMKII plays an important role in ET-1-induced activation of β myosin heavy chain (βMHC) promoter and increases in protein synthesis, myofibrillar organization, and cell size in cardiac myocytes (14). In contrast, a CaMKII inhibitor, KN62, blocked ET-1-induced ANP secretion and βMHC promoter activation (19,20). We also demonstrated that another CaMKII inhibitor, KN93, inhibited Ang II-induced activation of ERKs (Figure 1A). CaMKI is expressed in a wide range of tissues including heart, while CaMKIV is expressed predominantly in brain (16,21). The level of CaMKIV expression is low in heart (21). Passier et al. reported that activated CaMKI and CaMKIV also induce cardiac hypertrophy in vitro and in vivo and that CaMKIV activates transcription factor myocyte enhancer factor-2 (MEF2) through a posttranslational mechanism in hypertrophic heart in vivo (22). A number of specific regulatory functions of MEF2 have been identified in immune, skeletal muscle, and cardiac muscle cells (23). MEF2 knockout mice have altered cardiac gene expression and die during embryonic development (24). And MEF2 has been shown to be activated by Ca^{2+} (25,26), calcineurin (27), and p38 MAPK (28). It is suggested that MEF2 plays important roles in both developmental and pathophysiological responses of cardiac myocytes and is a critical regulator of cardiac gene expression (29,30). However, the mechanism by which CaMKs activate MEF2 remains to be determined. Recently, it has been reported that MEF2 interacts with histone deacetylase (HDAC), resulting in repression of MEF2-dependent genes (31) and then the signaling pathway linking HDAC to CaMK and MEF2 has been extensively investigated.

Histone acetyltransferase (HAT) and HDAC play an important role in the regulation of transcription. Acetylation of histones and non-histone proteins is regulated by interaction of HATs and HDACs (32). HATs catalyze the acetylation of core histones of chromatin and relax nucleosomes, resulting in transcriptional activation. In contrast, HDACs deacetylate the N-terminal tails of core histones and repress transcription. HDACs are categorized into three classes, I, II, and III, based on size and sequence homology (32). Class I HDACs (HDAC1, 2, 3, and 8) are expressed ubiquitously, whereas class II HDACs (HDAC4, 5, 6, and 7) are observed primarily in heart, brain, and skeletal muscle. Class II HDACs interact with MADS/MEF2 domain of MEF2 through a unique 18-amino acid motif and repress the transcriptional activity of MEF2. Lu et al. recently reported that CaMKs stimulate MEF2 activity by dissociating class II HDACs from the DNA-binding domain and that the dissociation of HDACs by CaMKs signaling may let MAP kinases to maximally stimulate MEF2 activity by direct phosphorylation of the transcription activation domain (31). Subsequently, the same group demonstrated that CaMKs phosphorylate HDAC5 at serine-259 and −498 and that HDAC5 is subsequently transported from nucleus to cytoplasm through a C-terminal sequence (nuclear export sequence), resulting in dissociation of MEF2 from HDAC5 and activation of MEF2 (33). It was further demonstrated that 14-3-3 protein binds to phosphoserines of HDAC4/5 and masks nuclear localization signal of HDAC4/5 (34). As the result, 14-3-3 protein-HDAC4/5 complex is exported to cytoplasm (34,35). It has been well known that 14-3-3 protein family is expressed in all eukaryotic cells and is involved in numerous signal transduction pathways (36). Although localization of 14-3-3 in cytoplasm, nucleus, and membranes has been reported, the significance of such differential localization is still unclear. Furthermore, whether HDACs inhibit cardiac hypertrophy in vivo remains currently unknown.

CALCINEURIN-MCIP

Calcineurin, which is a serine-threonine phosphatase that is activated by $Ca^{2+}/$ calmodulin, has been shown to play an important role in neuronal functions and immune responses (37). Activated calcineurin dephosphorylates a family of transcription factors known as nuclear factor of activated T cells (NFAT), which subsequently translocates from cytoplasm to nucleus. NFAT may interact GATA4 or possibly transcription factors related to transcription of hypertrophic response genes in the nucleus. Molkentin et al. demonstrated that transgenic mice overexpressing activated calcineurin in the heart displayed significant cardiac hypertrophy and rapidly progressed to heart failure (38). Transgenic mice overexpressing constitutively active NFAT3 in the heart also showed pronounced cardiac hypertrophy. In vitro, adenoviral-mediated gene transfer of activated calcineurin also induced hypertrophy in cardiac myocytes (39). In contrast, calcineurin inhibitors cyclosporin A and FK506 suppressed PE-, angiotensin II (Ang II)-, or ET-1-induced hypertrophic responses in cardiac myocytes (38). These results suggest that calcineurin-mediated activation of NFAT plays a crucial role in cardiac hypertrophy. We examined the role of calcineurin in stretch-induced cardiac hypertrophy using the in vitro stretch device. Although mechanical stretch by 20% for 30 minutes induced hypertrophic responses, these responses were attenuated by calcineurin inhibitors (paper in preparation). Furthermore, cyclosporin A and FK506 blocked hypertrophic responses in some animal models of pressure overload-induced or genetic cardiac hypertrophy (40–48). However, several groups reported an opposite conclusion (49–52). Since many animals lost body weight and died possibly by severe side effects of the calcineurin inhibitors in these studies, it seemed to be difficult to reach a definite conclusion. To elucidate the precise roles of calcineurin in the development of pressure overload-induced cardiac hypertrophy without drug toxicity, we created transgenic mice overexpressing dominant negative forms of calcineurin in the heart and analyzed them. The transgenic mice had no detrimental effects under normal condition. Although wild type mice exhibited the increase in cardiac calcineurin activity by aortic banding, the increase in calcineurin activity was significantly reduced in the transgenic mice (53). Pressure overload-induced increases in left ventricular wall thickness, heart weight to body weight ratio, myocyte diameter, and interstitial fibrosis were significantly inhibited in the transgenic mice (53). The change of c-fos, ANP, brain natriuretic peptide (BNP), and SERCA2 mRNA levels induced by pressure overload was also attenuated in the transgenic mice but no change in skeletal α-actin and c-jun mRNAs were noted (53). Although it is suggested that calcineurin induces cardiac hypertrophy through the interaction between NFAT3 and GATA4, we have recently demonstrated that calcineurin is also involved in activation of extracellular signal-regulated kinases (ERKs), which are the most

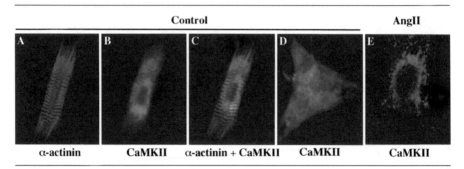

Figure 2. Localization of CaMKII in cultured cardiomyocytes. Cardiomyocytes of neonatal rats were cultured on glass cover slides in serum-free DMEM for 24 h before treatment. The cells were stained with anti α-actinin (rhodamine) (A, C) and CaMKII (FITC) (B–E) antibodies. A–D, control cells; E, AngII stimulation for 24 h.

extensively investigated members of MAP kinase family, in cardiac myocytes (15,53). Furthermore, our recent work elucidated that ISO and Ang II activate ERKs through two distinct Ca^{2+}-dependent pathways. Our results demonstrate that ISO translocates calcineurin from the Z-band to the perinuclear region and nucleus and activates ERKs through calcineurin by markedly elevating Ca^{2+} through CICR (15). While Ang II translocates CaMKII from the cytoplasm to the perinuclear region and activates ERKs through CaMKII in cardiac myocytes (Figure 1A, B and Figure 2). In contrast, ISO has no effect on the localization of CaMKII and Ang II has no effect on calcineurin (15, Figure 1A, B and Figure 2). These results suggest that CaMKII and calcineurin exist in different regions in cardiac myocytes and respond to the two agents in different manners.

Rex1p is a calcineurin-binding protein in Saccharomyces cerevisiae. A 30-amino acid segment of Rex1p shares homology to two different genes identified in the human gene sequence data base, DSCR1 and ZAKI-4. DSCR1 was designated because it resides within "Down syndrome critical region" of human chromosome 21 (54). ZAKI-4 was identified from cultured human skin fibroblasts by screening genes that are transcriptionally activated in response to thyroid hormone (55). It has been recently proposed that the protein products of the DSCR1 and ZAKI-4 are termed MCIP1 (myocyte-enriched calcineurin-interacting protein-1) and MCIP2, respectively (56). Rothermel et al. have identified a family of proteins, termed MCIP1 and MCIP2 that are highly expressed in striated muscles and that inhibit calcineurin activity by binding to catalytic subunit (CnA) of calcineurin (56). Expression of MCIP1, but not MCIP2, is induced by activated calcineurin in cardiac myocytes as well as skeletal myotubes (57). In contrast, expression of MCIP2 is upregulated by thyroid hormone. The region located between exons 3 and 4 of MCIP1 gene includes 15 consensus binding sites for NFAT and is mediated in the transcriptional regulation of MCIP1 gene by activated calcineurin. MCIP1 induced by activation of calcineurin inhibits the enzymatic activity of calcineurin and functions as a negative feedback regulation (57). Transgenic mice overexpressing MCIP1 in the heart were viable and exhibited no obvious abnormalities (58). However, heart weight to body weight ratio was slightly (5–10%) decreased in the transgenic mice than in wild type mice. Double transgenic mice (MCIP1 × CnA) displayed less cardiac hypertrophy and dilatation than transgenic mice overexpressing CnA alone (58). In the double transgenic mice, cardiac function was restored to the same as that of wild type mice. Moreover, ISO- and exercise-induced hypertrophy was also less in the double transgenic mice than in wild type mice (58). Because MCIP1 is abundantly expressed in cardiac myocytes and its expression is induced by activated calcineurin, it is expected to function as an endogenous inhibitor for cardiac hypertrophy.

CONCLUSION

It has been conceived that cardiac hypertrophy in response to pressure or volume overload is a necessary compensatory mechanism to normalize wall stress and maintain normal cardiac function. However, the results from Framingham Heart Study demonstrated that left ventricular hypertrophy is associated with increased cardiac mortality and is an independent risk factor for cardiac morbidity and mortality (4). Therefore, whether hypertrophic response to altered mechanical loading conditions is adaptive or maladaptive remains uncertain. Recently, Hill et al. reported that calcineurin inhibitor cyclosporin A maintains normal ventricular size and cardiac function despite inhibition of pressure overload-induced hypertrophy (44). Esposito et al. also demonstrated that the preventing the development of cardiac hypertrophy after aortic banding is not associated with deterioration in cardiac function using genetically engineered 2 model mice that have blunted hypertrophic responses to pressure overload (59). Indeed, cardiac function was better maintained in the genetic mice without hypertrophy than in wild type mice with hypertrophy. These results suggest that the development of cardiac hypertrophy and normalization of wall stress may not be necessary to preserve cardiac function. Further studies are needed to elucidate whether cardiac hypertrophy is good or bad at the different time from compensated hypertrophy to decompensated heart failure.

REFERENCES

1. Komuro I, Yazaki Y. 1993. Control of cardiac gene expression by mechanical stress. Annu Rev Physiol 55:55–75.
2. Chien KR. 1999. Stress pathways and heart failure. Cell 98:555–558.
3. Zou Y, Takano H, Akazawa H, Nagai T, Mizukami M, Komuro I. 2002. Molecular and cellular mechanisms of mechanical stress-induced cardiac hypertrophy. Endocr J 49:1–13.
4. Levy D, Garrison RJ, Savage DD, Kannel WB, Castelli WP. 1990. Prognostic implications of echocardiographically determined left ventricular mass in the Framingham Heart Study. N Engl J Med 322:1561–1566.
5. Berridge MJ, Bootman MD, Lipp P. 1998. Calcium-a life and death signal. Nature 395:645–648.
6. Bogoyevitch MA, Andersson MB, Gillespie-Brown J, Clerk A, Glennon PE, Fuller SJ, Sugden PH. 1996. Adrenergic receptor stimulation of the mitogen-activated protein kinase cascade and cardiac hypertrophy. Biochem J 314:115–121.
7. Yamazaki T, Komuro I, Zou Y, Kudoh S, Shiojima I, Hiroi Y, Mizuno T, Aikawa R, Takano H, Yazaki

Y. 1997. Norepinephrine induces the raf-1 kinase/MAP kinase cascade through both α1- and β-adrenoceptors. Circulation 95:1260–1268.

8. Yamazaki T, Komuro I, Zou Y, Kudoh S, Mizuno T, Hiroi Y, Shiojima I, Takano H, Kinugawa K, Kohmoto O, Takahashi T, Yazaki Y. 1997. Protein kinase A and protein kinase C synergistically activate the Raf-1 kinase/mitogen-activated protein kinase cascade in neonatal rat cardiomyocytes. J Mol Cell Cardiol 29:2491–2501.

9. Nabauer M, Morad M. 1990. Ca^{2+}-induced Ca^{2+} release as examined by photolysis of caged Ca^{2+} in single ventricular myocytes. Am J Physiol 258:C189–193.

10. Sham JS, Cleemann L, Morad M. 1995. Functional coupling of Ca^{2+} channels and ryanodine receptors in cardiac myocytes. Proc Natl Acad Sci USA 92:121–125.

11. Sigurdson W, Ruknudin A, Sachs F. 1992. Ca^{2+} imaging of mechanically induced fluxes in tissue-cultured chick heart: role of stretch-activated ion channels. Am J Physiol 262:H1110–1115.

12. Means AR, VanBerkum MF, Bagchi I, Lu KP, Rasmussen CD. 1991. Regulatory functions of calmodulin. Pharmacol Ther 50:255–270.

13. Gruver CL, DeMayo F, Goldstein MA, Means AR. 1993. Targeted developmental overexpression of calmodulin induces proliferative and hypertrophic growth of cardiomyocytes in transgenic mice. Endocrinology 133:376–388.

14. Zhu W, Zou Y, Shiojima I, Kudoh S, Aikawa R, Hayashi D, Mizukami M, Toko H, Shibasaki F, Yazaki Y, Nagai R, Komuro I. 2000. Ca^{2+}/calmodulin-dependent kinase II and calcineurin play critical roles in endothelin-1-induced cardiomyocyte hypertrophy. J Biol Chem 275:15239–15245.

15. Zou Y, Yao A, Zhu W, Kudoh S, Hiroi Y, Shimoyama M, Uozumi H, Kohmoto O, Takahashi T, Shibasaki F, Nagai R, Yazaki Y, Komuro I. 2001. Isoproterenol activates extracellular signal-regulated protein kinases in cardiomyocytes through calcineurin. Circulation 104:102–108.

16. Braun AP, Schulman H. 1995. The multifunctional calcium/calmodulin-dependent protein kinase: from form to function. Annu Rev Physiol 57:417–445.

17. McDonough PM, Glembotski CC. 1992. Induction of atrial natriuretic factor and myosin light chain-2 gene expression in cultured ventricular myocytes by electrical stimulation of contraction. J Biol Chem 267:11665–11668.

18. Ramirez MT, Zhao XL, Schulman H, Brown JH. 1997. The nuclear δB isoform of Ca^{2+}/calmodulin-dependent protein kinase II regulates atrial natriuretic factor gene expression in ventricular myocytes. J Biol Chem 272:31203–31208.

19. Irons CE, Sei CA, Hidaka H, Glembotski CC. 1992. Protein kinase C and calmodulin kinase are required for endothelin-stimulated atrial natriuretic factor secretion from primary atrial myocytes. J Biol Chem 267:5211–5216.

20. Zhu W, Zou Y, Shiojima I, Kudoh S, Aikawa R, Hayashi D, Mizukami M, Toko H, Shibasaki F, Yazaki Y, Nagai R, Komuro I. 2000. Ca^{2+}/calmodulin-dependent kinase II and calcineurin play critical roles in endothelin-1-induced cardiomyocyte hypertrophy. J Biol Chem 275:15239–15245.

21. Miyano O, Kameshita I, Fujisawa H. 1992. Purification and characterization of a brain-specific multifunctional calmodulin-dependent protein kinase from rat cerebellum. J Biol Chem 267:1198–1203.

22. Passier R, Zeng H, Frey N, Naya FJ, Nicol RL, McKinsey TA, Overbeek P, Richardson JA, Grant SR, Olson EN. 2000. CaM kinase signaling induces cardiac hypertrophy and activates the MEF2 transcription factor in vivo. J Clin Invest 105:1395–1406.

23. McKinsey TA, Zhang CL, Olson EN. 2002. MEF2: a calcium-dependent regulator of the cell division, differentiation and death. Trends Biochem Sci 27:40–47.

24. Lin Q, Schwarz J, Bucana C, Olson EN. 1997. Control of mouse cardiac morphogenesis and myogenesis by transcription factor MEF2C. Science 276:1404–1407.

25. Mao Z, Bonni A, Xia F, Nadal-Vicens M, Greenberg ME. 1999. Neuronal activity-dependent cell survival mediated by transcription factor MEF2. Science 286:785–790.

26. Youn HD, Sun L, Prywes R, Liu JO. 1999. Apoptosis of T cells mediated by Ca^{2+}-induced release of the transcription factor MEF2. Science 286:790–793.

27. Mao Z, Wiedmann M. 1999. Calcineurin enhances MEF2 DNA binding activity in calcium-dependent survival of cerebellar granule neurons. J Biol Chem 274:31102–31107.

28. Han J, Molkentin JD. 2000. Regulation of MEF2 by p38 MAPK and its implication in cardiomyocytes biology. Trends Cardiovasc Med 10:19–22.

29. Kolodziejczyk SM, Wang L, Balazsi K, DeRepentigny Y, Kothary R, Megeney LA. 1999. MEF2 is upregulated during cardiac hypertrophy and is required for normal post-natal growth of the myocardium. Curr Biol 9:1203–1206.

30. Molkentin JD, Markham BE. 1993. Myocyte-specific enhancer-binding factor (MEF-2) regulates

α-cardiac myosin heavy chain gene expression in vitro and in vivo. J Biol Chem 268:19512–19520.

31. Lu J, McKinsey TA, Nicol RL, Olson EN. 2000. Signal-dependent activation of the MEF2 transcription factor by dissociation from histone deacetylases. Proc Natl Acad Sci USA 97: 4070–4075.

32. Gray SG, Ekstrom TJ. 2001. The human histone deacetylase family. Exp Cell Res 262:75–83.

33. McKinsey TA, Zhang CL, Lu J, Olson EN. 2000. Signal-dependent nuclear export of a histone deacetylase regulates muscle differentiation. Nature 408:106–111.

34. Grozinger CM, Schreiber SL. 2000. Regulation of histone deacetylase 4 and 5 and transcriptional activity by 14-3-3-dependent cellular localization. Proc Natl Acad Sci USA 97:7835–7840.

35. McKinsey TA, Zhang CL, Olson EN. 2000. Activation of the myocyte enhancer factor-2 transcription factor by calcium/calmodulin-dependent protein kinase-stimulated binding of 14-3-3 to histone deacetylase 5. Proc Natl Acad Sci USA 97:14400–14405.

36. Tzivion G, Avruch J. 2002. 14-3-3 proteins: active cofactors in cellular regulation by serine/threonine phosphorylation. J Biol Chem 277:3061–3064.

37. Klee CB, Ren H, Wang X. 1998. Regulation of the calmodulin-stimulated protein phosphatase, calcineurin. J Biol Chem 273:13367–13370.

38. Molkentin JD, Lu JR, Antos CL, Markham B, Richardson J, Robbins J, Grant SR, Olson EN. 1998. A calcineurin-dependent transcriptional pathway for cardiac hypertrophy. Cell 93:215–228.

39. De Windt LJ, Lim HW, Taigen T, Wencker D, Condorelli G, Dorn GW II, Kitsis RN, Molkentin JD. 2000. Calcineurin-mediated hypertrophy protects cardiomyocytes from apoptosis in vitro and in vivo: an apoptosis-independent model of dilated heart failure. Circ Res 86:255–263.

40. Sussman MA, Lim HW, Gude N, Taigen T, Olson EN, Robbins J, Colbert MC, Gualberto A, Wieczorek DF, Molkentin JD. 1998. Prevention of cardiac hypertrophy in mice by calcineurin inhibition. Science 281:1690–1693.

41. Meguro T, Hong C, Asai K, Takagi G, McKinsey TA, Olson EN, Vatner SF. 1999. Cyclosporine attenuates pressure-overload hypertrophy in mice while enhancing susceptibility to decompensation and heart failure. Circ Res 84:735–740.

42. Shimoyama M, Hayashi D, Takimoto E, Zou Y, Oka T, Uozumi H, Kudoh S, Shibasaki F, Yazaki Y, Nagai R, Komuro I. 1999. Calcineurin plays a critical role in pressure overload-induced cardiac hypertrophy. Circulation 100:2449–2454.

43. Eto Y, Yonekura K, Sonoda M, Arai N, Sata M, Sugiura S, Takenaka K, Gualberto A, Hixon ML, Wagner MW, Aoyagi T. 2000. Calcineurin is activated in rat hearts with physiological left ventricular hypertrophy induced by voluntary exercise training. Circulation 101:2134–2137.

44. Hill JA, Karimi M, Kutschke W, Davisson RL, Zimmerman K, Wang Z, Kerber RE, Weiss RM. 2000. Cardiac hypertrophy is not a required compensatory response to short-term pressure overload. Circulation 101:2863–2869.

45. Lim HW, De Windt LJ, Steinberg L, Taigen T, Witt SA, Kimball TR, Molkentin JD. 2000. Calcineurin expression, activation, and function in cardiac pressure-overload hypertrophy. Circulation 101:2431–2437.

46. Murat A, Pellieux C, Brunner HR, Pedrazzini T. 2000. Calcineurin blockade prevents cardiac mitogen-activated protein kinase activation and hypertrophy in renovascular hypertension. J Biol Chem 275:40867–40873.

47. Oie E, Bjornerheim R, Clausen OP, Attramadal H. 2000. Cyclosporin A inhibits cardiac hypertrophy and enhances cardiac dysfunction during postinfarction failure in rats. Am J Physiol 278:H2115–2123.

48. Sakata Y, Masuyama T, Yamamoto K, Nishikawa N, Yamamoto H, Kondo H, Ono K, Otsu K, Kuzuya T, Miwa T, Takeda H, Miyamoto E, Hori M. 2000. Calcineurin inhibitor attenuates left ventricular hypertrophy, leading to prevention of heart failure in hypertensive rats. Circulation 102:2269–2275.

49. Luo Z, Shyu KG, Gualberto A, Walsh K. 1998. Calcineurin inhibitors and cardiac hypertrophy. Nat Med 4:1092–1093.

50. Ding B, Price RL, Borg TK, Weinberg EO, Halloran PF, Lorell BH. 1999. Pressure overload induces severe hypertrophy in mice treated with cyclosporin, an inhibitor of calcineurin. Circ Res 84: 729–734.

51. Zhang W, Kowal RC, Rusnak F, Sikkink RA, Olson EN, Victor RG. 1999. Failure of calcineurin inhibitors to prevent pressure-overload left ventricular hypertrophy in rats. Circ Res 84:722–728.

52. Hayashida W, Kihara Y, Yasaka A, Sasayama S. 2000. Cardiac calcineurin during transition from hypertrophy to heart failure in rats. Biochem Biophys Res Commun 273:347–351.

53. Zou Y, Hiroi Y, Uozumi H, Takimoto E, Toko H, Zhu W, Kudoh S, Mizukami M, Shimoyama M, Shibasaki F, Nagai R, Yazaki Y, Komuro I. 2001. Calcineurin plays a critical role in the development of pressure overload-induced cardiac hypertrophy. Circulation 104:97–101.
54. Fuentes JJ, Pritchard MA, Estivill X. 1997. Genomic organization, alternative splicing, and expression patterns of the DSCR1 (Down syndrome candidate region 1) gene. Genomics 44:358–361.
55. Miyazaki T, Kanou Y, Murata Y, Ohmori S, Niwa T, Maeda K, Yamamura H, Seo H. 1996. Molecular cloning of a novel thyroid hormone-responsive gene, ZAKI-4, in human skin fibroblasts. J Biol Chem 271:14567–14571.
56. Rothermel B, Vega RB, Yang J, Wu H, Bassel-Duby R, Williams RS. 2000. A protein encoded within the Down syndrome critical region is enriched in striated muscles and inhibits calcineurin signaling. J Biol Chem 275:8719–8725.
57. Yang J, Rothermel B, Vega RB, Frey N, McKinsey TA, Olson EN, Bassel-Duby R, Williams RS. 2000. Independent signals control expression of the calcineurin inhibitory proteins MCIP1 and MCIP2 in striated muscles. Circ Res 87:e61–e68.
58. Rothermel BA, McKinsey TA, Vega RB, Nicol RL, Mammen P, Yang J, Antos CL, Shelton JM, Bassel-Duby R, Olson EN, Williams RS. 2001. Myocyte-enriched calcineurin-interacting protein, MCIP1, inhibits cardiac hypertrophy in vivo. Proc Natl Acad Sci USA 98:3328–3333.
59. Esposito G, Rapacciuolo A, Naga Prasad SV, Prasad N, Takaoka H, Thomas SA, Koch WJ, Rockman HA. 2002. Genetic alterations that inhibit in vivo pressure-overload hypertrophy prevent cardiac dysfunction despite increased wall stress. Circulation 105:85–92.

Signal Transduction and Cardiac Hypertrophy,
edited by N.S. Dhalla, L.V. Hryshko,
E. Kardami & P.K. Singal
Kluwer Academic Publishers, Boston, 2003

Calreticulin, Cardiac Development and Congenital Complete Heart Block in Children

Barbara Knoblach,[1] Kimitoshi Nakamura,[2]
Murray Robertson,[3] and Marek Michalak[1]

*From the [1] Canadian Institutes of Health Research Membrane
Protein Research Group and the Department of Biochemistry
University of Alberta, Edmonton
Alberta, Canada T6G 2H7
the [2] Department of Pediatrics
Kumamoto University School of Medicine
Honjo 1-1-1, Kumamoto, Japan
[3] Department of Pediatrics
University of Alberta
Edmonton, Alberta, Canada T6G 2H7*

Summary. Calreticulin is a Ca^{2+} binding chaperone resident in the lumen of endoplasmic reticulum. The protein is highly expressed in developing heart and down-regulated after birth. In mice, calreticulin deficiency is lethal due to impaired cardiac development. Over-expression of calreticulin in developing and postnatal heart leads to bradycardia, complete heart block and sudden death. This indicates that calreticulin plays an important role in the development of the cardiac conduction system and in the pathology of congential heart block. These findings may have important implications on the molecular understanding of congenital heart block and may prove to be a target for future therapies.

Key words: cardiac development, congenital heart block, arrhythmias, calcium binding proteins, calreticulin, endoplasmic reticulum chaperones.

INTRODUCTION

Complete congenital heart block (CCHB), first described over a century ago (1), remains a poorly understood clinical entity in pediatric cardiac electrophysiology. It

Address for correspondence: Dr. M. Michalak, Department of Biochemistry, University of Alberta, Edmonton, Alberta, Canada T6G 2H7. Tel: 780-492-2256, Fax: 780-492-0886, E-mail: marek.michalak@ualberta.ca

is a disorder of cardiac electrical conduction characterized by marked bradycardia with clinical manifestations ranging from relatively asymptomatic individuals to patients with congestive cardiomyopathy and sudden death (2). The electrophysiological mechanism responsible for the bradycardia is a progressive disruption of the normal atrioventricular nodal (AVN) electrical conduction. Initial mild forms of AVN dysfunction (1st degree heart block) often develop into a complete interruption of AVN conduction (3rd degree heart block). It is a relatively uncommon disorder with an estimated frequency between $1:15,000$ to $1:20,000$ in live births. It has been diagnosed in fetuses as well as in newborns and older children. Symptomatic patients respond well to cardiac pacemaker implantation; however, despite adequate relief of the bradycardia, a significant number of patients go on to develop a severe form of dilated cardiomyopathy associated with sudden death (3). Currently the only effective therapy for these children is cardiac transplantation.

The cause of the AVN dysfunction remains poorly understood, although a relationship between CCHB and maternal connective tissue disorders has been recognized. Maternal IgG class antibodies anti-SSA/R_o and SSB/L_a freely cross the placenta and have been associated with fetal and neonatal CCHB (4). Candidate target antigens SSA/R_o and SSB/L_a have been extensively characterized at the molecular level as soluble tissue ribonucleoproteins (5). Maternal antibodies have also been shown to cross-react with human cardiac myosin heavy chain sarcomeric protein as well as sarcolemmal L-type Ca^{2+} channel, which important for cardiac excitation-contraction coupling (6). Studies with pregnant mice exposed to anti-SSA/R_o and anti-SSA/L_a antibodies have demonstrated fetal bradycardia and varying degrees of AVN block associated with impaired function of the L-type Ca^{2+} channel (7).

While the majority of infants with CCHB have been shown to be sero-positive for maternal antibodies, approximately 30–40% of affected children are sero-negative. In addition, the overall risk of an antibody-positive mother to have a child with CCHB is relatively small (8). Thus, AVN dysfunction involving this immune mechanism would not appear to account for all cases of CCHB. Recently, we have created transgenic mice over-expressing calreticulin, an endoplasmic reticulum (ER) Ca^{2+} binding chaperone, and discovered that these animals develop CCHB with clinical symptoms similar to those found in CCHB children (9).

CALRETICULIN

Calreticulin is a Ca^{2+} binding chaperone of the ER lumen (10). Several unique functions have been postulated for calreticulin, including modulation of gene expression (10), chaperone activity (11–13), regulation of cell adhesion (14–16), and of Ca^{2+} homeostasis (13,17–24). However, there are two principal cellular functions of the protein, which have been the most extensively studied: (i) molecular chaperone, and (ii) Ca^{2+} storage/signaling within the lumen of the ER.

Chaperone activity. Calreticulin functions as a molecular chaperone for many proteins and glycoproteins (11,12). The protein binds $Glc_1Man_9GlcNAc_2$ oligosaccharides, recognizing the terminal glucose and four internal mannose residues (25–27).

Calreticulin also binds to non-glycosylated proteins and therefore, is considered a true molecular chaperone (28). The N- and P-domains of the protein are likely responsible for its chaperone function (13). Many severe diseases including Alzheimer's, artherosclerosis, cystic fibrosis, α-1-antitrypsin deficiency, and defects in carbohydrate metabolism, result from deficiencies in protein folding (29–36). As yet protein conformational problems have not be attributed to any cardiovascular disorder.

Ca^{2+} binding and signaling. Calreticulin binds Ca^{2+} and plays an important role in the regulation of Ca^{2+} homeostasis (10,13,18–21,24,37,38). Over-expression of calreticulin results in an increased amount of intracellularly stored Ca^{2+} (18,20,22,24). Furthermore, the increased divalent cation permeability in response to Ca^{2+} store depletion is markedly diminished in calreticulin over-expressers suggesting that calreticulin affects the activation of Ca^{2+} influx in response to Ca^{2+} store depletion (18,20,22,24). Calreticulin was also implicated to play a role in integrin mediated Ca^{2+} signaling (39). Calreticulin knockout cells have impaired InsP$_3$-dependent Ca^{2+} release and reduced ER Ca^{2+} storage capacity (13,38). Ca^{2+} binding to calreticulin also affects its chaperone function and its abilities to interact with other components of the protein folding machinery (40–42). Therefore, calreticulin and normal intra-ER Ca^{2+} homeostasis are essential for quality control processes during protein synthesis and folding (12,41).

CALRETICULIN AND CARDIAC DEVELOPMENT

Since calreticulin is only a minor component of cardiac cells (38,43–47) it was initially surprising that calreticulin deficient mice die because of impaired heart development (38). However, we noticed that calreticulin gene expression is extremely high in the developing heart, indicating for the first time that an ER protein plays a critical role in cardiogenesis. Calreticulin may therefore be considered a novel cardiac embryonic gene (38). What is responsible for the observed cardiac pathology in calreticulin deficient embryos? *crt$^{-/-}$* cells exhibit impaired nuclear import of NF-AT transcription factor suggesting that calreticulin may control the availability of Ca^{2+} ions required for activation of calcineurin and NF-AT-dependent pathways during cardiac development (38). Therefore, the protein may be a regulator of Ca^{2+} homeostasis and of transcriptional pathways involved in cardiac development.

Cardiac development and growth are extremely complex processes under strict transcriptional control (48–51). A number of transcription factors are critical for specific stages of vertebrate cardiac morphogenesis and hypertrophy, including the homeobox protein Nkx-2.5 (52–55), the basic helix-loop-helix proteins dHAND and eHAND (49), MEF-2 (56–59), a member of the extended Sry family, Sox-4 (60) and GATA-4, a member of a family of zinc finger transcription factors (58,61). Nkx2.5 (*tinman*) transcription factor activates transcription of the calreticulin gene and COUP-TF1 binds to Nkx2.5 site in the calreticulin promoter and represses transactivation of the promoter (62). Nkx2.5 is essential for cardiac development (55) and is highly expressed during embryonic heart development. Disruption of the Nkx2.5 gene in mice leads to embryonic death due to cardiac morphogenetic

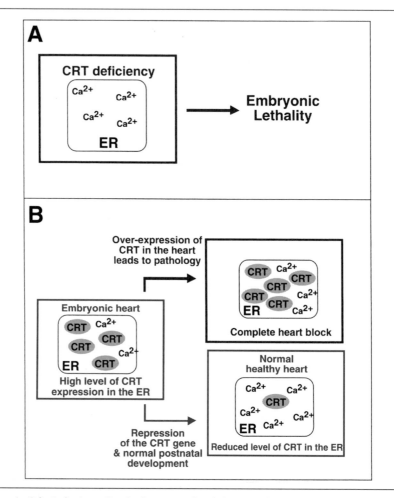

Figure 1. Calreticulin in cardiac development and pathology. A, calreticulin deficiency is embryonic lethal. B. Under normal physiological conditions calreticulin level is high in the embryonic heart. After birth calreticulin levels are reduced by transcriptional mechanisms. If calreticulin levels are maintained high after birth animals develop severe congenital arrhythmia and complete heart block followed by sudden death. CRT, calreticulin; ER, endoplasmic reticulum.

defects (63), reminiscent of the calreticulin deficiency (38). So far, the only reported cardiac specific targets of Nkx2.5 transcription factor had been ANF and α-cardiac actin gene (64–66), and now calreticulin is a newly identified target of this important cardiac specific transcription factor. The role of Ca^{2+} in cardiac specific Nkx2.5- and COUP-TF1-dependent transcriptional events has not been investigated.

Recent evidence indicates that intracellular, $InsP_3$-dependent Ca^{2+} stores play a role in cardiac development, growth and pathology including regulation and activation of the NF-AT/GATA-4/CaN transcriptional pathway (38,67–70). The activation of this Ca^{2+}-dependent pathway depends on a sustained Ca^{2+} release from ER stores (38,67–70) and, therefore, it would have to be independent of the SR Ca^{2+} store. Consequently, we proposed that cardiac muscle may contain two functionally different Ca^{2+} storage compartments (71). This idea is supported by recent reports indicating that InsP3 plays a role of a regulator of cardiac autonomic activity (71–73). Cardiomyocytes likely contain InsP3-sensitive, ER-like compartment that is functionally distinct from the SR (71–73).

CALRETICULIN OVER-EXPRESSING MICE—AN ANIMAL MODEL FOR CONGENITAL COMPLETE HEART BLOCK

Calreticulin expression is high in embryonic heart and declines sharply after birth likely due to activation of the gene by Nkx2.5 transcription factor and suppression by COUP-TF1 (62). Why is the expression of calreticulin so tightly regulated in the heart? We created transgenic mice over-expressing calreticulin in the heart and showed that these animals develop bradycardia associated with sinus node dysfunction, complete cardiac block, and death due to intractable heart failure indicating that calreticulin plays a role in the pathology of the conductive system (9). Histological analysis of transgenic hearts revealed dilated ventricular chambers, relatively thinner ventricular walls, and dilated atria with thrombosis and disarray of cardiomyocytes. Enlargement of the heart was not due to a hypertrophic response. Using M-mode echocardiography we established that transgenic animals exhibited a loss of systolic function. Electrocardiograms demonstrated that the P-R interval of transgenic mice was significantly prolonged in calreticulin over-expressers with subsequent development of complete AV nodal conduction block.

Calreticulin over-expresser hearts have very low levels of Connexin43 (Cx43) (9), a major component of gap junctions responsible for cell–cell communication (74,75). Phosphorylation of Cx43 is an important modulator of gap junction communication and affects conductance, metabolic coupling, growth and differentiation (75). Calreticulin transgenic animals exhibited significantly reduced phosphorylation of connexin further supporting a notion that gap junction function is impaired when levels of calreticulin are high in postnatal hearts. The current density of peak inward $I_{Ca,L}$ at 0 mV elicited in transgenic cardiomyocytes was also significantly smaller than the $I_{Ca,L}$ of in control animals under the same condition (9). The inactivation of $I_{Ca,L}$ in both groups could be fitted well to the bi-exponential decay. At 0 mV, the taus of fast and slow components were 16.8 ± 3.2 and 78.3 ± 9.2 ms in control (n = 5), 28.9 ± 8.9 and 92.6 ± 10.0 ms in transgenic cardiomyocytes (n = 5), respectively (9).

The phenotype of the calreticulin over-expresser mouse is very similar to that seen in children with complete heart block (9). The cause and molecular mechanism involved in the complete heart block is not known at present. However, calreticulin must be a part of a pathway responsible for the etiology of this disease (9). The protein may affect Ca^{2+} homeostasis in differentiating cardiomyocytes and it may play a critical role during synthesis, folding and targeting of Ca^{2+} channels, connexins and perhaps other cardiac specific proteins.

CONCLUSIONS

It is now evident that calreticulin is essential for development of the cardiac conductive system. These findings may have important implications on molecular understanding of congenital heart block and may prove to be a target for future therapies, particularly since it is now recognized that the elimination of the brady-cardia in congenital heart block does not prevent the late onset of heart failure. New therapeutic approaches to this potentially lethal disorder will have to be developed in the future.

ACKNOWLEDGEMENTS

Research in our laboratories is supported by grants from the Canadian Institutes of Health Research, from the Heart and Stroke Foundations of Alberta (to M.M.), and from the Northern Alberta Children Health Foundation and University of Alberta Hospital Foundation (to M.M. and M.R.). M.M. is a Canadian Institutes of Health Research Senior Investigator and a Medical Scientist of the Alberta Heritage Foundation for Medical Research.

REFERENCES

1. Morquio L. 1901. Sur une maladie infantile et familial characterisee par des modifications perma-nents du pouls des attaques syncopales et epileptiforms et la mort subite. Arch Med Inf 4:467–469.
2. Michaelsson M, Riesenfeld T, Jonzon A. 1997. Natural history of congenital complete atrioventric-ular block. Pacing Clin Electrophysiol 20:2098–2101.
3. Moak JP, Barron KS, Hougen TJ, Wiles HB, Balaji S, Sreeram N, Cohen MH, Nordenberg A, Van Hare GF, Friedman RA, Perez M, Cecchin F, Schneider DS, Nehgme RA, Buyon JP. 2001. Con-genital heart block: development of late-onset cardiomyopathy, a previously underappreciated sequela. J Am Coll Cardiol 37:238–242.
4. McCue CM, Mantakas ME, Tingelstad JB, Ruddy S. 1977. Congenital heart block in newborns of mothers with connective tissue disease. Circulation 56:82–90.
5. Scott JS, Maddison PJ, Taylor PV, Esscher E, Scott O, Skinner RP. 1983. Connective-tissue disease, antibodies to ribonucleoprotein, and congenital heart block. N Engl J Med 309:209–212.
6. Qu Y, Xiao GQ, Chen L, Boutjdir M. 2001. Autoantibodies from mothers of children with con-genital heart block downregulate cardiac L-type Ca^{2+} channels. J Mol Cell Cardiol 33:1153–1163.
7. Boutjdir M. 2000. Molecular and ionic basis of congenital complete heart block. Trends Cardiovasc Med 10:114–122.
8. Frohn-Mulder IM, Meilof JF, Szatmari A, Stewart PA, Swaak TJ, Hess J. 1994. Clinical significance of maternal anti-Ro/SS-A antibodies in children with isolated heart block. J Am Coll Cardiol 23:1677–1681.
9. Nakamura K, Robertson M, Liu G, Dickie P, Guo JQ, Duff HJ, Opas M, Kavanagh K, Michalak M. 2001. Complete heart block and sudden death in mouse over-expressing calreticulin. J Clin Invest 107:1245–1253.
10. Michalak M, Corbett EF, Mesaeli N, Nakamura K, Opas M. 1999. Calreticulin: one protein, one gene, many functions. Biochem J 344:281–292.
11. Bergeron JJM, Brenner MB, Thomas DY, Williams DB. 1994. Calnexin: a membrane-bound chap-erone of the endoplasmic reticulum. Trends Biochem Sci 19:124–128.
12. Helenius A, Trombetta ES, Hebert DN, Simons JF. 1997. Calnexin, calreticulin and the folding of glycoproteins. Trends Cell Biol 7:193–200.
13. Nakamura K, Zuppini A, Arnaudeau S, Lynch J, Ahsan I, Krause R, Papps S, De Smedt H, Parys, JB, Müller-Esterl W, Lew DP, Krause K-H, Demaurex N, Opas M, Michalak M. 2001. Functional specialization of calreticulin domains. J Cell Biol 154:961–972.
14. Opas M, Szewczenko-Pawlikowski M, Jass GK, Mesaeli N, Michalak M. 1996. Calreticulin modu-lates cell adhesiveness via regulation of vinculin expression. J Cell Biol 135:1913–1923.

15. Fadel MP, Dziak E, Lo CM, Ferrier J, Mesaeli N, Michalak M, Opas M. 1999. Calreticulin affects focal contact-dependent but not close contact-dependent cell-substratum adhesion. J Biol Chem 274:15085–15094.
16. Fadel MP, Szewczenko-Pawlikowski M, Leclerc P, Dziak E, Symonds JM, Blaschuk O, Michalak M, Opas M. 2001. Calreticulin affects β-catenin associated pathways. J Biol Chem 276:27083–27089.
17. Liu N, Fine RE, Simons E, Johnson RJ. 1994. Decreasing calreticulin expression lowers the Ca^{2+} response to bradykinin and increases sensitivity to ionomycin in NG-108-15 cells. J Biol Chem 269:28635–28639.
18. Bastianutto C, Clementi E, Codazzi F, Podini P, De Giorgi F, Rizzuto R, Meldolesi J, Pozzan T. 1995. Overexpression of calreticulin increases the Ca^{2+} capacity of rapidly exchanging Ca^{2+} stores and reveals aspects of their lumenal microenvironment and function. J Cell Biol 130:847–855.
19. Camacho P, Lechleiter JD. 1995. Calreticulin inhibits repetitive intracellular Ca^{2+} waves. Cell 82:765–771.
20. Mery L, Mesaeli N, Michalak M, Opas M, Lew DP, Krause K-H. 1996. Overexpression of calreticulin increases intracellular Ca^{2+} storage and decreases store-operated Ca^{2+} influx. J Biol Chem 271:9332–9339.
21. John LM, Lechleiter JD, Camacho P. 1998. Differential modulation of SERCA2 isoforms by calreticulin. J Cell Biol 142:963–973.
22. Fasolato C, Pizzo P, Pozzan T. 1998. Delayed activation of the store-operated calcium current induced by calreticulin overexpression in RBL-1 cells. Mol Biol Cell 9:1513–1522.
23. Roderick HL, Lechleiter JD, Camacho P. 2000. Cytosolic phosphorylation of calnexin controls intracellular Ca^{2+} oscillations via an interaction with SERCA2b. J Cell Biol 149:1235–1248.
24. Xu W, Longo FJ, Wintermantel MR, Jiang X, Clark RA, DeLisle S. 2000. Calreticulin modulates capacitative Ca^{2+} influx by controlling the extent of inositol 1,4,5-trisphophate-induced Ca^{2+} store depletion. J Biol Chem 275:36676–36682.
25. Spiro RG, Zhu Q, Bhoyroo V, Söling H-D. 1996. Definition of the lectin-like properties of the molecular chaperone, calreticulin, and demonstration of its copurification with endomannosidase from rat liver Golgi. J Biol Chem 271:11588–11594.
26. Zapun A, Petrescu SM, Rudd PM, Dwek RA, Thomas DY, Bergeron JJM. 1997. Conformation-independent binding of monoglucosylated ribonuclease B to calnexin. Cell 88:29–38.
27. Vassilakos A, Michalak M, Lehrman MA, Williams DB. 1998. Oligosaccharide binding characteristics of the molecular chaperones calnexin and calreticulin. Biochemistry 37:3480–3490.
28. Saito Y, Ihara Y, Leach MR, Cohen-Doyle MF, Williams DB. 1999. Calreticulin functions *in vitro* as a molecular chaperone for both glycosylated and non-glycosylated proteins. EMBO J 18:6718–6729.
29. Thomas PJ, Qu BH, Pedersen PL. 1995. Defective protein folding as a basis of human disease. Trends Biochem Sci 20:456–459.
30. Brooks DA. 1997. otein processing: a role in the pathophysiology of genetic disease. FEBS Lett 409:115–120.
31. Brooks DA. 1999. Introduction: molecular chaperones of the ER: their role in protein folding and genetic disease. Semin Cell Dev Biol 10:441–442.
32. Gething MJ. 1999. Role and regulation of the ER chaperone BiP. Sem Cell Dev Biol 10:465–472.
33. Halaban R, Svedine S, Cheng E, Smicun Y, Aron R, Hebert DN. 2000. Endoplasmic reticulum retention is a common defect associated with tyrosinase-negative albinism. Proc Natl Acad Sci USA 97:5889–5894.
34. Rudd PM, Wormald MR, Wing DR, Prusiner SB, Dwek RA. 2001. Prion glycoprotein: structure, dynamics, and roles for the sugars. Biochemistry 40:3759–3766.
35. Rudd PM, Elliott T, Cresswell P, Wilson IA, Dwek RA. 2001. Glycosylation and the immune system. Science 291:2370–2376.
36. Sherman MY, Goldberg AL. 2001. Cellular defenses against unfolded proteins: a cell biologist thinks about neurodegenerative diseases. Neuron 29:15–32.
37. Baksh S, Michalak M. 1991. Expression of calreticulin in *Escherichia coli* and identification of its Ca^{2+} binding domains. J Biol Chem 266:21458–21465.
38. Mesaeli N, Nakamura K, Zvaritch E, Dickie P, Dziak E, Krause K-H, Opas M, MacLennan DH, Michalak M. 1999. Calreticulin is essential for cardiac development. J Cell Biol 144:857–868.
39. Coppolino MG, Woodside MJ, Demaurex N, Grinstein S, St-Arnaud R, Dedhar S. 1997. Calreticulin is essential for integrin-mediated calcium signalling and cell adhesion. Nature 386:843–847.
40. Corbett EF, Oikawa K, Francois P, Tessier DC, Kay C, Bergeron JJM, Thomas DY, Krause K-H, Michalak M. 1999. Ca^{2+} regulation of interactions between endoplasmic reticulum chaperones. J Biol Chem 274:6203–6211.

41. Corbett EF, Michalak M. 2000. Calcium, a signaling molecule in the endoplasmic reticulum? Trends Biochem Sci 25:307–311.

42. Corbett EF, Michalak KM, Oikawa K, Johnson S, Campbell ID, Eggleton P, Kay C, Michalak M. 2000. The conformation of calreticulin is influenced by the endoplasmic reticulum lumenal environment. J Biol Chem 275:27177–27185.

43. Fliegel L, Burns K, MacLennan DH, Reithmeier RAF, Michalak M. 1989. Molecular cloning of the high affinity calcium-binding protein (calreticulin) of skeletal muscle sarcoplasmic reticulum. J Biol Chem 264:21522–21528.

44. Milner RE, Baksh S, Shemanko C, Carpenter MR, Smillie L, Vance JE, Opas M, Michalak M. 1991. Calreticulin, and not calsequestrin, is the major calcium binding protein of smooth muscle sarcoplasmic reticulum and liver endoplasmic reticulum. J Biol Chem 266:7155–7165.

45. Tharin S, Dziak E, Michalak M, Opas M. 1992. Widespread tissue distribution of rabbit calreticulin, a non-muscle functional analogue of calsequestrin. Cell Tissue Res 269:29–37.

46. Imanaka-Yoshida K, Amitani A, Ioshii SO, Koyabu S, Yamakado T, Yoshida T. 1996. Alterations of expression and distribution of the Ca^{2+}-storing proteins in endo/sarcoplasmic reticulum during differentiation of rat cardiomyocytes. J Mol Cell Cardiol 28:553–562.

47. Tsutsui H, Ishibashi Y, Imanaka-Yoshida K, Yamamoto S, Yoshida T, Urabe Y, Takeshita A. 1997. Alterations in sarcoplasmic reticulum calcium-storing proteins in pressure-overload cardiac hypertrophy. Am J Physiol 272:H168–H175.

48. Chien KR, Zhu H, Knowlton KU, Miller-Hance W, van-Bilsen M, O'Brien TX, Evans SM. 1993. Transcriptional regulation during cardiac growth and development. Annu Rev Physiol 55:77–95.

49. Srivastava D, Cserjesi P, Olson EN. 1995. A subclass of bHLH proteins required for cardiac morphogenesis. Science 270:1995–1999.

50. Olson EN, Srivastava D. 1996. Molecular pathways controlling heart development. Science 272:671–676.

51. Sucov HM. 1998. Molecular insights into cardiac development. Annu Rev Physiol 60:287–308.

52. Tonissen KF, Drysdale TA, Lints TJ, Harvey RP, Krieg PA. 1994. XNkx-2.5, a Xenopus gene related to Nkx-2.5 and tinman: evidence for a conserved role in cardiac development. Dev Biol 162:325–328.

53. Patterson KD, Cleaver O, Gerber WV, Grow MW, Newman CS, Krieg PA. 1998. Homeobox genes in cardiovascular development. Curr Top Dev Biol 40:1–44.

54. Schwartz RJ, Olson EN. 1999. Building the heart piece by piece: modularity of cis-elements regulating Nkx2–5 transcription. Development 126:4187–4192.

55. Evans SM. 1999. Vertebrate tinman homologues and cardiac differentiation. Semin Cell Dev Biol 10:73–83.

56. Edmondson DG, Lyons GE, Martin JF, Olson EN. 1994. Mef2 gene expression marks the cardiac and skeletal muscle lineages during mouse embryogenesis. Development 120:1251–1263.

57. Ross RS, Navankasattusas S, Harvey RP, Chien KR. 1996. An HF-1a/HF-1b/MEF-2 combinatorial element confers cardiac ventricular specificity and established an anterior-posterior gradient of expression. Development 122:1799–1809.

58. Fishman MC, Chien KR. 1997. Fashioning the vertebrate heart: earliest embryonic decisions. Development 124:2099–2117.

59. Christensen TH, Kedes L. 1999. The myogenic regulatory circuit that controls cardiac/slow twitch troponin C gene transcription in skeletal muscle involves E-box, MEF-2, and MEF-3 motifs. Gene Expr 8:247–261.

60. Schilham MW, Oosterwegel MA, Moerer P, Ya J, de Boer PA, van de Wetering M, Verbeek S, Lamers WH, Kruisbeek AM, Cumano A, Clevers, H. 1996. Defects in cardiac outflow tract formation and pro-B-lymphocyte expansion in mice lacking Sox-4. Nature 380:711–714.

61. Orkin SH. 1992. GATA-binding transcription factors in hematopoietic cells. Blood 80:575–581.

62. Guo L, Lynch J, Nakamura K, Fliegel L, Kasahara H, Izumo S, Komuro I, Agellon LB, Michalak M. 2001. COUP-TF1 antagonizes Nkx2.5-mediated activation of the calreticulin gene during cardiac development. J Biol Chem 276:2797–2801.

63. Lyons I, Parsons LM, Hartley L, Li R, Andrews JE, Robb L, Harvey RP. 1995. Myogenic and morphogenetic defects in the heart tubes of murine embryos lacking the homeo box gene Nkx2–5. Genes Dev 9:1654–1666.

64. Grepin C, Dagnino L, Robitaille L, Haberstroh L, Antakly T, Nemer MA 1994. hormone-encoding gene identifies a pathway for cardiac but not skeletal muscle gene transcription. Mol Cell Biol 14:3115–3129.

65. Durocher D, Charron F, Warren R, Schwartz RJ, Nemer M. 1997. The cardiac transcription factors Nkx2–5 and GATA-4 are mutual cofactors. EMBO J 16:5687–5696.
66. Sepulveda JL, Belaguli N, Nigam V, Chen CY, Nemer M, Schwartz RJ. 1998. GATA-4 and Nkx-2.5 coactivate Nkx-2 DNA binding targets: role for regulating early cardiac gene expression. Mol Cell Biol 18:3405–3415.
67. Timmerman LA, Clipstone NA, Ho SN, Northrop JP, Crabtree GR. 1996. Rapid shuttling of NF-AT in discrimination of Ca^{2+} signals and immunosuppression. Nature 383:837–840.
68. Dolmetsch RE, Lewis RS, Goodnow CC, Healy JI. 1997. Differential activation of transcription factors induced by Ca^{2+} response amplitude and duration. Nature 386:855–858.
69. Rao A, Luo C, Hogan PG. 1997. Transcription factors of the NFAT family: regulation and function. Annu Rev Immunol 15:707–747.
70. Molkentin JD, Lu JR, Antos CL, Markham B, Richardson J, Robbins J, Grant SR, Olson EN. 1998. A calcineurin-dependent transcriptional pathway for cardiac hypertrophy. Cell 93:215–228.
71. Mesaeli N, Nakamura K, Opas M, Michalak M. 2001. Endoplasmic reticulum in the heart, a forgotten organelle? Mol Cell Biochem 224:1–6.
72. Jaconi M, Bony C, Richards SM, Terzic A, Arnaudeau S, Vassort G, Puceat M. 2000. Inositol 1,4,5-trisphosphate directs Ca^{2+} flow between mitochondria and the endoplasmic/sarcoplasmic reticulum: A role in regulating cardiac autonomic Ca^{2+} spiking. Mol Biol Cell 11:1845–1858.
73. Lipp P, Laine M, Tovey SC, Burrell KM, Berridge MJ, Li W, Bootman MD. 2000. Functional $InsP_3$ receptors that may modulate excitation-contraction coupling in the heart. Curr Biol 10:939–942.
74. Gros DB, Jongsma HJ. 1996. Connexins in mammalian heart function. Bioessays 18:719–730.
75. Kardami E, Doble BW. 1998. Cardiomyocyte gap junctions: a target for growth factor signaling. Trends Cardiovasc Med 8:180–187.

Signal Transduction and Cardiac Hypertrophy,
edited by N.S. Dhalla, L.V. Hryshko,
E. Kardami & P.K. Singal
Kluwer Academic Publishers, Boston, 2003

Expression of Sodium-Calcium Exchanger Genes in Heart and Skeletal Muscle Development. Evidence for a Role of Adjacent Cells in Regulation of Transcription and Splicing

Marie Millour,[1] Laurent Lescaudron,[2] Alexander Kraev,[3]
and Dmitri O. Levitsky[1]

[1] *Faculté des Sciences et des Techniques*
Université de Nantes
CNRS UMR 6018, Nantes cedex 3
France
[2] *INSERM U-437, ITERT*
CHU Hôtel Dieu et Faculté des Sciences et des Techniques
Université de Nantes
[3] *Samuel Lunenfeld Research Institute*
Mt. Sinai Hospital, 600 University Avenue
Toronto, ON, Canada M5G 1X5

Summary. Sodium-calcium exchangers (NCX) are universal plasmalemma proteins regulating intracellular calcium concentration in animal tissues. While gene structure and regulation of the cardiac-specific isoform NCX1 are known in considerable detail, no data are available on the effect of extrinsic and/or extrinsic factors that govern tissue-specific transcription of all three isoforms (NCX1-NCX3) as well as their still hypothetical alternative splicing. We studied NCX gene expression in cardiac and skeletal muscles and in brain during rat development, as well as their expression in muscle cells grown in presence of neuron-conditioned medium. Our data demonstrate that NCX1 and NCX3 expression in cardiac and skeletal muscle is coordinately regulated and is sensitive to as yet unidentified factors apparently produced by the neighboring cells. Correct splicing of NCX3 transcript is rapidly disrupted within minutes of tissue dissection, consequently most of the previously reported splicing variants featuring exon skipping appear to be artefactual.

Address for Correspondence: Dmitri O. Levitsky, CNRS UMR 6018, Faculté des Sciences et des Techniques, Université de Nantes, 2, rue de la Houssinière, Nantes cedex 3, France. E-mail: *dmitri.levitsky@svt.univ-nantes.fr*; Phone: (33) 240-29-89-59; Fax: (33) 251-12-56-32.

Key words: sodium-calcium exchanger isoforms, alternative splicing, heart, brain, skeletal muscle, development.

INTRODUCTION

Plasma membrane Na^+-Ca^{2+}-exchanger (NCX) plays an important role in regulating intracellular free calcium levels in a variety of tissues (for a recent review, see ref. 1). Most of the studies have focused on molecular, structural and kinetic properties of a "cardiac" Na^+-Ca^{2+}-exchanger isoform (NCX1). However, its expression is not limited to the cardiac muscle and its role as major regulator of intracellular Ca^{2+} has been proven for a number of cellular systems. In brain, NCX1 provides lowering of intracellular calcium after neurotransmitter release (2). In kidney, NCX1 participates in Ca^{2+} reabsorption (3). In heart, acting in concert with the sarcoplasmic reticulum Ca^{2+} pump and Ca^{2+}-release channel, NCX1 regulates contraction-relaxation cycle (for ref., see 1,4).

The NCX1 gene is comprised of 14 exons (5). Its transcription is driven by a peculiar multipartite (6) promoter, in which "housekeeping" and "tissue-specific" components correspond to spatially distinct transcription sites. Each transcription site is identified by its specific 1st exon, spliced to the common transcript core, encoded by exons 2–14. In certain tissues basal transcription, driven by the relatively weak housekeeping promoter, is augmented by a more powerful regulatable promoter (6). Indeed, NCX1 transcript level in heart changes considerably during development (7,8) and under pathological conditions (1). Involvement of specific transcription factors in the function of the "cardiac" (synonyms, Ht, 1d) portion of the multipartite promoter has been studied in considerable detail (9–11).

Exons 2 to 14 encode the protein that is modeled to contain 9 transmembrane segments (12). A large intracellular loop between S5 and S6 comprises half of the exchanger molecule. It does not participate directly in Na^+-Ca^{2+} exchange but is essential for secondary regulation of the exchanger activity (13). In the middle portion of the loop two highly acidic sequences were identified (14). They form a high affinity calcium-binding domain (CBD) and mediate regulation of the Na^+/Ca^{2+} exchange by intracellular Ca^{2+} (15,16). The transition of the Ca^{2+}-free to Ca^{2+}-bound form of the CBD is associated with a change of conformation of the exchanger molecule, easily detectable as a mobility shift in SDS-PAGE (15,17).

Another intracellular loop region of particular interest is located downstream of the CBD (18,19). It is encoded by a series of alternatively spliced exons (A to B or 3 to 8). RT-PCR data suggest that splicing of these exons follows a tissue-specific pattern (10) which may result in translation of as many as 32 variants of the intracellular loop. Although on protein level these variants are difficult to identify, recent studies show that expressed alternatively spliced transcripts encode proteins with altered ion transport properties (20). However, precise purpose of this putative protein diversity remains obscure.

Proteins, encoded by two other NCX genes, NCX2 (21) and NCX3 (22) are studied in much less detail. According to Northern blotting (22) and RT-PCR (19) data, NCX3 expression is limited to skeletal muscle and brain. With regard to the

NCX2 transcript, the available data on its distribution in rat tissues (19,21) and even on the size of its transcripts (21,22) are contradictory. Since structural and functional properties of NCX1, NCX2, and NCX3 *in vitro* are quite similar (23), there is no apparent explanation for their co-expression in some tissues. This redundancy could be due to peculiarities of their plasmalemma localization. Otherwise it can be explained by increased options for regulation of NCX activity by transcriptional factors available at several distinct promoters.

While the excitation-contraction coupling in cardiac and skeletal muscle has many common features, particularly, both largely depend on interactions between a plasma membrane dihydropyridine receptor, a sarcoplasmic reticulum calcium channel (ryanodine receptor) and a SR calcium-transporting ATPase, the current role delegated to sodium-calcium exchange in the two tissues appears to be vastly different.

The role of intrinsic and extrinsic factors modulating developmental changes of NCX expression has not been addressed yet. We used two approaches to address this problem. The developmental approach allowed us to follow the profile of NCX isoform expression in different tissues (heart, skeletal muscle, brain). The model of isolated muscle satellite cells grown in presence of neuron-conditioned medium was used to assess influence of extrinsic factors on expression of different NCX transcripts. Muscle satellite cells are found between the basal lamina and the plasma membrane of muscle fibers and considered to be primary source of myogenic cells (24,25). Grown in culture, satellite cells isolated from adult muscle may proliferate and differentiate into myotubes in a sequence of events resembling muscle growth *in vivo* (26). In an attempt to elucidate influence of factors modulating NCX levels we also studied the expression of all three NCX genes in native muscles and cultivated muscle cells, as well as at different stages of muscle development.

We demonstrate that NCX1/NCX3 expression undergoes a reciprocal developmental switch in cardiac and skeletal muscle. We also demonstrate that alternative splicing of NCX transcripts appears to be extremely sensitive to the extracellular environment. Together, these data indicate that the true role of sodium-calcium exchange in muscle function may have been overlooked possibly due to the relative fragility of these proteins in experimental preparations as compared to other calcium transporters.

MATERIALS AND METHODS

Animals

Wistar-Kyoto and SHR rats, used at the Nantes laboratory, were obtained from R. Janver Breeding Center. Male and female rats born to pregnant 3-mo-old dams were used in this study. BALB/c × CD1 or C57BL/6 mice were purchased at the mouse facility of the Centre for Modeling of Human Disease, Mount Sinai Hospital, Toronto. For muscle biopsy, mouse was anesthetized by an intraperitoneal injection with lidocaine/phenobarbital and a small portion of tibialis muscle was dissected while the animal was immobilized by the anesthetic. Muscle biopsy was frozen in liquid nitrogen within 10 seconds of dissection. Portions of mouse brain were obtained as a by-product of a procedure to generate hippocampus slices for electrophysiological studies. Briefly, mouse was anesthetized by halothane inhalation and its dissected head was immediately submerged in partially frozen ACSF solution (27), previously saturated with oxygen. Portions of the brain were dissected under the buffer and frozen in liquid nitrogen typically within two minutes of decapitation.

Other experiments were carried out on 13 day old Swiss mice raised at the animal facility of the University of Nantes for satellite cell extraction and on E-11 days old Swiss embryos for neuronal cells isolation. Animals were sacrificed by cervical dislocation.

Conditioned medium production

Satellite cells were isolated as described previously (28,29). Pectoralis muscles (PM) were removed under sterile conditions and finely dissected to remove connective and fat tissues as well as blood vessels. After several washes in Dulbecco's phosphate-buffered saline, PM fragments were dissociated in a solution containing Pronase E (Sigma), Ham's F12/Hepes (Invitrogen) and 20% fetal calf serum (FCS, Gibco) for 60 minutes at 37°C. Then satellite cells were mechanically dissociated from myofibers and collected by centrifugation. This procedure was repeated 3 times and the final pellet was diluted in DMEM with 10% FCS. Satellite cells were plated alone or with neural cells at a density of 50,000 cells/ml in collagen pre-coated culture dishes (Iwaki). The media were removed and kept for further use after 3 days of culture.

Some satellite cells were allowed to grow with neuronal cells from Swiss mouse neural tube. E-11 days old embryos were dissected out and their neural tube was removed using microscalpel surgery. Only the ventral part of the neural tube (containing motor neurons) was transferred into DMEM with 10% FCS and mechanically dissociated by repeated pipetting through a syringe (30). Neuronal cells were collected by centrifugation, resuspended in DMEM and added at the density of 50,000 cells/ml to the Petri dish containing growing satellite cells. The culture media from both types of culture were collected after 3 days of culture and used for conditioned media experiments.

Satellite cells grown in conditioned media

Newly isolated satellite cells from PM were allowed to grow in conditioned medium with satellite cells alone or with satellite cells with neuronal cells. Both conditioned media were changed after 3 days of culture. The cultures were stopped and frozen either at day 3 or day 6 for further analysis.

RNA Isolation and Northern analysis

Total RNA was isolated by the guanidinium/phenol/chloroform solvent extraction method (RNA Plus, Bioprobe Systems, or Trizol, Life Technologies, Inc), dissolved in DEPC-treated water, or in 0.1 mM EDTA (Ambion) and stored at −80°C prior to use. Twenty micrograms of total RNA were applied per lane of formaldehyde-denatured 1% agarose gels with DIG-labeled RNA markers (Boehringer Mannheim). The electrode buffer was supplemented with 2.2% formaldehyde. After electrophoresis, the gels were soaked for 20 min in 50 mM NaOH, washed with DEPC-treated water and impregnated for 45 min with 10 × SSC (1 × SSC: 150 mM NaCl-15 mM sodium citrate, pH 7.0). The upward capillary transfer to nylon membranes (Boehringer Mannheim) was performed in 10 × SSC for 3 to 5 h. The RNA was fixed at 120°C for 30 min and the blots were prehybridized for 3 h at 68°C in the solution composed of 50% formamide, 5 × SSC, 0.2% SDS, 0.1% N-lauroylsarcosine and 4% of the blocking reagent (Boehringer Mannheim). Hybridization with digoxigenin-labeled riboprobes was performed overnight under the same conditions. The membranes were washed at room temperature with 2 × SSC, 0.1% SDS and twice for 15 min at 69°C with 0.1 × SSC, 0.1% SDS. The Northern blots were developed with alkaline phosphatase-coupled anti-DIG antibody (diluted 1 : 10000) and a chemiluminescent substrate (CSPD), and exposed to an X-ray film according to the manufacturer's recommendations (Boehringer Mannheim). The wet nitrocellulose membranes were sealed in plastic bags and stored at 4°C prior to rehybridization with 28S RNA and GAPDH DIG-labeled riboprobes.

Digoxigenin-UTP-labeled antisense RNA probes were synthesized as described previously (17). The plasmids containing inserts of rat brain NCX1 and NCX2 cDNA were a generous gift from K. D. Philipson (UCLA).

Reverse transcriptase assisted polymerase chain reaction

To disrupt DNA-RNA complexes, a sample of total RNA (2 to 4 µg in 25 µl) was heated for 10 min at 95°C and quickly chilled on ice. The contaminating DNA was eliminated using a "DNA-free" kit (Ambion). The DNAse I was removed by a resin, according to the manufacturer's protocol. The RNA from one third of the final volume was transcribed with Superscript II (Life Technologies, Inc.), using random hexamers. The cDNA was amplified using Goldstar Red DNA polymerase (Eurogentec). Following preheating of the samples at 95°C for 10 min, 1 U of the DNA polymerase was added at 75°C. Amplification was carried out for 34 to 36 cycles (30 s at 94°C, 45 s at 55°C, 30 s at 72°C) followed by 10 min incubation at 72°C. Two to 10 µl were applied per well of ethidium bromide-stained agarose gel and the bands were visualized under UV. Control RT-PCR experiments included a mock reverse transcription wherein the reverse transcriptase had been omitted from the incubation medium. These negative controls proved absence of a genomic DNA contamination after the "DNA-free" treatment.

NCX-specific primers

In most cases forward and reverse primers corresponded to distinct exons. The following pairs of primers used in PCR were synthesized (Cybergene). For NCX1, forward primers covering portions of exons 1 were coupled to an exon 2 reverse primer (306 to 325). These primer pairs are designated below as 1-Br, 1-Ht, and 1-Kc. The primer pairs were the following: forward 5′-1456 to 3′-1474 and reverse

5'-1964 to 3'-1944 (a-NCX2); forward 5'-1455 to 3'-1473 and reverse 5'-1984 to 3'-1964 (b-NCX2); forward 5'-979 to 3'-996 and reverse 5'-1295 to 3'-1276 (c-NCX2). For NCX3, the forward primer was between 1797 and 1816 bp while the reverse primers were between 5'-2829 and 3'-2809 (primer pair a-NCX3) or 5'-2128 and 3'-2109 (primer pair b-NCX3).

Immunodetection

100–200 milligrams of frozen rat tissues were homogenized using a Polytron in 1 to 2 ml of medium containing 20 mM HEPES (pH 7.0), 1 mM sodium azide, 1 mM phenylmethylsulfonyl fluoride, 1 µg aprotinin and 1 mM dithiothreitol. To remove cell debris, the tissue homogenates were centrifuged for 20 min at 700× g, frozen in liquid nitrogen and stored at −80°C. The dishes of cultured mouse cells were frozen and stored at −80°C. The cells were directly suspended in the above isolation medium.

Laemmli sodium dodecylsulfate-polyacrylamide gel electrophoresis and electrotransfer of the proteins to nitrocellulose membranes (Bio-Rad) were done as previously described (15). The membranes were treated for 1 h with a solution of 150 mM NaCl, 10 mM Tris-HCl, (pH 7.6), 5% skim milk powder and 0.1% Tween-20; preincubated for 1 h with polyclonal antibodies against rat brain NCX2 or NCX3 and treated with peroxidase-linked goat anti-rabbit IgG (Jackson ImmunoResearch Laboratories). The blots were developed with an enhanced chemiluminescence (ECL) detection kit (Amersham) and exposed to X-Omat film (Kodak).

RESULTS

NCX1 expression during rat development

Two rat strains (Wistar-Kyoto and SHR) differing in many functional aspects were chosen to generalize the changes in NCX1 expression in muscle. Whole hindlimb muscles were removed from 1- to 16-day-old animals. Slow (soleus) and fast (tibialis and extensor digitorum longus, EDL) muscles were excised from 26-day-old and 7-week-old rats. Hybridization of the total RNA isolated from skeletal muscle with a NCX1 DIG-riboprobe revealed a 7.5-kb band (Figure 1) corresponding to a major transcript of the cardiac exchanger. For both strains of rats, the level of NCX1 expression was stable from 1 day till 2 weeks, then it progressively declined. Its expression in a 7-week-old slow skeletal muscle (soleus) was lower than in fast skeletal muscles (tibialis and EDL).

Expression of NCX1 alternative first exons

Since alternative first exons of the NCX1 gene are linked to their specific promoter regions (6,31), changes the expression of each alternative exon 1 could be used as a measure of the relative activity of the promoters of "heart", "brain" or "kidney" type. In adult rat, the three alternative exons are easily detected by RT-PCR (Figure 2A). We confirmed previous data concerning more or less tissue-specific expression of the exons. In particular, in adult heart exon 1-Ht is predominant over 1-Br, while

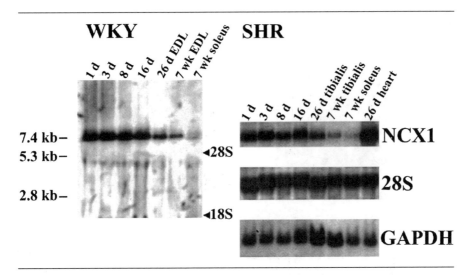

Figure 1. Developmental changes of NCX1 transcripts in skeletal muscles of two rat strains. Note that expression of the 7.5 kb NCX1 transcript is higher in fast muscles (EDL, tibialis) than in slow muscle (soleus).

in brain the 1-Br prevails (Figure 2B). No exon 1-Kc transcript was detected in adult skeletal muscle (Figure 3A) and adult heart (Figure 3B). We determined if the levels of the three transcript types vary during rat heart development. In embryonic heart, both 1-Ht and 1-Br-driven transcripts are expressed at higher levels than in adult heart (Figure 3B). Moreover, in embryonic heart 1-Kc-driven transcript is also expressed. We may thus suggest that during prenatal heart development multiple transcriptional factors are involved in NCX1 expression.

To obtain an insight into the mechanism of regulation of NCX transcription, we used a model of skeletal muscle satellite cells grown in the presence of neuron-conditioned medium, NCM (Figure 4). Analysis of RT-PCR products of the total RNA isolated from the growing satellite cells shows much weaker expression of 1-Br-driven transcript as compared to 1-Ht. The level of 1-Br-driven transcript does not change and that of 1-Ht increases only slightly under the influence of NCM. By contrast, the 1-Kc-driven transcript, not observed in the satellite cells grown in the absence of NCM, was detected when the cells had been exposed to factors presumably originating from neurons.

NCX2 expression during rat development and in mouse cell culture

Previous Northern data have shown that NCX2 expression is quite high in rat brain and skeletal muscle (21,22). A far more sensitive RT-PCR technique allowed to detect NCX2 transcript in a number of other rat tissues (19). Surprisingly, on Northern blots of rat skeletal muscle RNA from developing rat as well as on Western

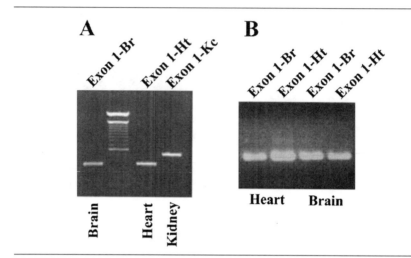

Figure 2. RT-PCR evidence of a relative tissue specificity of expression of the three exon 1 types of NCX1 gene. The sources of RNA isolated from adult rat were indicated below while the types of exons tested are shown above the figure.

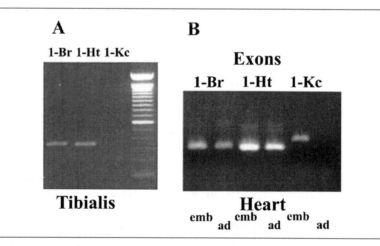

Figure 3. Expression of the three NCX1 exon 1 types in rat muscle. In fast skeletal muscle (A), and in adult heart (B) the levels of exon 1-Ht are higher than those of exon 1-Br, while exon 1-Kc is not expressed. All of the exon 1 types are expressed in embryonic heart at much higher levels as compared to adult heart.

blots of adult rat skeletal muscle we were not able to detect this transcript. As shown in Figure 5, in rat brain NCX2 transcript of 5 kb is quite low after birth and increases sharply on the 2nd postnatal day. In contrast to this result, no transcript of the same size was observed in the Northern of RNA from different muscle samples from rats of different age (Figure 5).

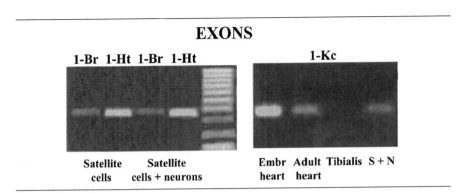

Figure 4. Absence of neuron-conditioned medium influence on expression of exons 1-Br and 1-Ht in skeletal muscle satellite cells (3 days in culture) and upregulation of exon 1-Kc expression in the cells grown in the presence of the NCM.

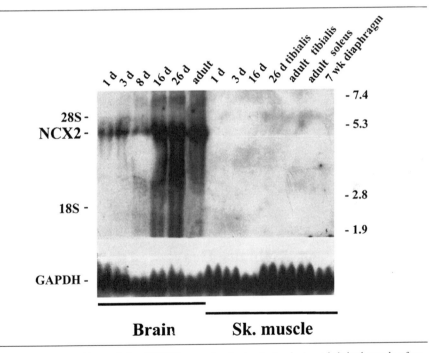

Figure 5. Northern blot analysis of NCX2 expression in developing brain and skeletal muscle of rat.

Western blots yielded similar results. Strong signals were observed for adult rat brain (Figures 6,7), aorta (Figure 6), stomach, uterus, colon, and intestine (not shown). In brain, the level of NCX2 polypeptide increased sharply between 5th and 10th postnatal day and stabilized after the 3rd week (Figure 6). It is worthwhile to mention that the immunoreactive bands revealed in brain and aorta homogenates

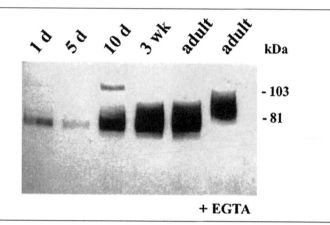

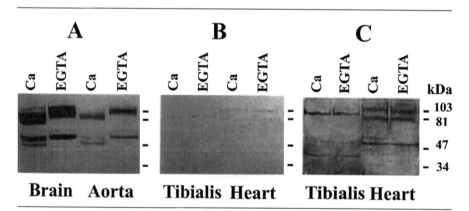

Figure 6. Western blotting experiment, demonstrating a dramatic increase in NCX2 expression in post-natal rat brain. Note that the major polypeptide revealed brain by the anti-NCX2 polyclonal antibody changed its electrophoretic mobility when a homogenate sample had been pretreated with EGTA. This indicates the presence in brain NCX2 of a high affinity Ca^{2+}-binding domain similar to that found in NCX1.

Figure 7. Western blotting analysis of NCX2 expression in adult rat tissues. A. NCX2 is expressed in brain and aorta. In both cases the major immunoreactive polypeptide and some of its proteolytic products were sensitive to EGTA pretreatment. The blot was exposed to X-ray film for 30 s. B. The blot corresponds to skeletal muscle and heart homogenates. Exposure for 30 s. C. The same blot as in panel B. Five minute exposure. Note that the immunoreactive bands of weak intensity do not change their electrophoretic mobility after EGTA pretreatment of tissue homogenates in sample buffer.

with a polyclonal antibody changed its electrophoretic mobility after the sample was pre-treated with EGTA (Figures 6,7). This strongly indicated that the observed signals correspond to a typical sodium-calcium exchanger. In contrast, these polypeptides were not found either in heart or in skeletal muscle homogenates (Figure 7). While a number of weakly immunoreactive bands was observed in these

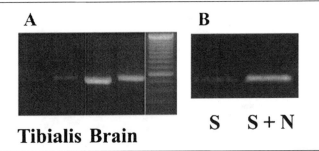

Figure 8. RT-PCR analysis of NCX2 expression. A. RNA was isolated from fast skeletal muscle and brain of adult rat. The primer pairs were a-NCX2 (1st and 3rd lanes) and b-NCX2 (2nd and 4th lanes). B. Influence of the NCM on mouse skeletal muscle satellite cells grown in culture for 3 days. c-NCX2 primer pair.

tissues, they were not sensitive to EGTA treatment. These signals are clearly due to nonspecific binding of the anti-NCX2 polyclonal antibody.

In summary, our data demonstrate that the levels of NCX2 expression in rat heart and skeletal muscle are too low to be detected by standard Northern and Western techniques. Only RT-PCR revealed a weak NCX2 expression in rat skeletal muscle (Figure 8A) and heart (not shown). In satellite cells the NCX2 expression level was also quite low but it increased considerably when the cells were grown in the presence of NCM (Figure 8B).

NCX3 expression

Our previous Northern and Western blotting data indicate that expression of this exchanger isoform in adult rat is limited to skeletal muscle and brain (17). In brain, NCX3 level does not change during the postnatal development, while in skeletal muscle it increases progressively during first postnatal weeks and eventually stabilizes by the 7th week. RT-PCR revealed no NCX3 transcript in either adult or embryonic heart but showed gradual increase of its concentration in skeletal muscle (Figure 9). Figure 10A shows that NCX3 level in muscle satellite cells is quite low as compared to that in brain. Once again, when the cells were grown in the presence of NCM, the expression of this exchanger isoform increased considerably.

NCX3 transcript splicing in live mouse muscle biopsy

The studies described in previous sections demonstrated that NCX gene expression is sensitive to as yet undefined set of extracellular factors that could be generally defined as "cellular environment". It was therefore logical to suggest that the process of tissue dissection and/or generation of a cultivated cell line from a tissue may have influence on NCX gene expression. Indeed, limited data of one of us briefly described in (6) indicate that NCX1 expression, although prominent in intact brain, is not detected in certain cell lines, such as PC-12. In an attempt to obtain a true

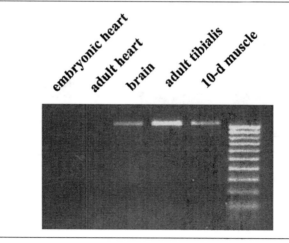

Figure 9. Comparison of NCX3 expression in rat heart, brain, and skeletal muscle. a-NCX3 primer pair.

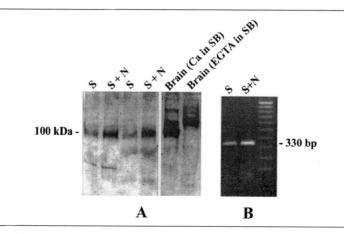

Figure 10. A. Western blot showing stimulating effect of NCM on satellite cells grown in culture for 3 days (lanes 1 and 2) and 6 days (lanes 3 and 4). The major immunoreactive polypeptide of the same molecular mass was revealed in brain and it changed the electrophoretic mobility under the influence of EGTA. B. RT-PCR of RNA isolated from the satellite cells (6 days of culture).

"snapshot" of the transcript structure in live tissue, a mouse was anesthetized and tibialis muscle biopsy was performed while the animal was alive. The sample was flash frozen in liquid nitrogen within 10 seconds of dissection and RNA was later extracted from it. In another case, mouse brain was isolated while the dissected head was submerged in partially frozen oxygenated ACSF solution to prevent neuronal death, the procedure used to prepare hippocampus slices for electrophysiological studies. In the latter case the dissected portions of the forebrain and cerebellum were frozen in liquid nitrogen within 2 minutes after decapitation. Transcript structure of NCX3 was examined by RT-PCR with primers flanking alternatively spliced areas.

The results of this analysis are shown on Figure 11. Along with the RT-PCR banding profile, schemes of splicing are shown to demonstrate the exon structure of the amplified product as deduced from direct sequencing of the PCR products. Our results show that in a muscle biopsy taken from a live animal essentially only one splicing variant is dominant, that containing exons BCD. The presence of a minor amount of another variant, skipping exon C, is inferred from the presence of secondary peaks on sequencing gels in the respective area. NCX3 transcripts from forebrain and cerebellum contain a similar pair of variants, except that exon A replaced exon B. Although in brain sample about half of the splicing products also appear to skip exon C, no significant amount of variants wherein both exons A and B were skipped (19) could be detected in either tissue.

DISCUSSION

Previous studies demonstrated elaborate regulation of transcription of the NCX1 gene (6,10,11). This work extends these observations and further demonstrates that all three isoforms of the sodium–calcium exchanger appear to be coordinately up- or down-regulated in skeletal muscle, brain and heart.

Most interestingly, NCX1 and NCX3 expression in developing rat skeletal muscle appear to be in a reciprocal relationship, i.e. up-regulation of one gene is accompanied by a down-regulation of the other. Consequently, while in skeletal muscle of newborn animals sodium–calcium exchange activity seems to be due largely to expression of NCX1 gene, in adult rats it is taken over by NCX3. In contrast, in rat brain the level of both NCX1 and NCX3 does not change appreciably during the post-natal development (our unpublished data). At odds with earlier data (19) no expression of NCX2 could be detected in skeletal muscle of any age by Northern or Western blotting techniques. However, RT-PCR analysis did allow us to detect trace levels of the NCX2 transcript in adult skeletal muscle that were much lower than those in adult brain. In brain of newborn rats, the NCX2 transcript level is also quite low but it increases dramatically between the 1st and the 2nd postnatal week. The latter data are in line with the observations on cerebellum granular cell culture maturation *in vitro* and on developing rat cerebellum (32,33). Overall, our data show that significant NCX2 expression is limited to brain and smooth muscle.

According to our data, the NCX1 level in heart, skeletal muscle, and brain is due to a more or less tissue-specific activity of 1-Ht and 1-Br-promoters. In adult muscle tissues exon 1-Ht predominates while in brain the expression of exon 1-Br is slightly higher than that of 1-Ht. In other words, in brain expression of NCX1 is largely driven by a GC-rich constitutive promoter, rather than by any of the two known regulatable promoters.

Previous observations indicate that NCX1 expression is especially high in perinatal heart (7). Moreover, Scheller et al. (6) demonstrated that splicing of the NCX1

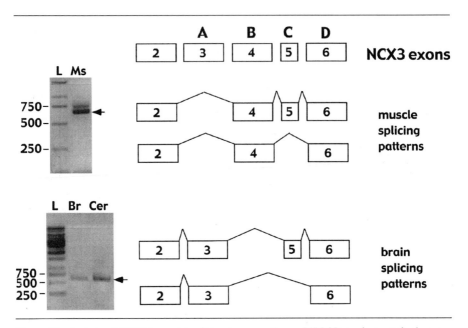

Figure 11. Analysis of NCX3 transcript splicing in mouse tissues. RT-PCR products resolved on a 1.2% agarose gels are shown on the left. Numbers at the left side of gel panels indicate marker fragment length in base pairs. Ms, muscle biopsy; Br, forebrain; Cer, cerebellum; L, length marker. NCX3 splicing variants, identified in each tissue by direct PCR product sequencing (marked by an arrow), are shown opposite of the corresponding gel panel. Exon designations for mouse NCX3 gene are assigned from 2 to 6 as in (5) for the human NCX3 gene and from A to D as in (19) for the rat NCX3 gene.

transcript in heart is going through an intermediate containing incomplete exon 1-Kc, although concentration of this intermediate in live adult rat tissues appeared to be extremely low. Our data lend further support to the existence of a regulatory circuit in developing cardiac muscle that selects between 1-Ht and 1-Kc promoters. Interestingly, concentration of a splicing product containing both exons 1-Ht and 1-Kc increases after death (6), which is in line with a hypothesis (see below) that a selection mechanism, switching between splicing of exon 1-Ht and 1-Kc is quickly disrupted *post mortem*.

The hypothetical selective mechanism appears to be strongly influenced by an as yet unknown component of the neuron-conditioned medium (NCM). While the levels of 1-Br- and 1-Ht-driven transcripts in the mouse satellite cells did not change in the presence of the NCM, expression of 1-Kc-driven transcript was markedly increased. A stimulating action of NCM was also observed in studies of NCX2 and NCX3 expression in muscle satellite cells. In particular, our RT-PCR data and Western blots analysis show an increase in NCX3 expression as early as 3 days of culture when the satellite cell are grown in presence of NCM as compared to satellite cells grown without it. In addition, NCX3 expression was not transient as it was also observed after 6 days of culture in newly formed myotubes. Similar influence of NCM on NCX2 expression was also observed.

The increase in NCX2 and NCX3 and of NCX1 exon 1-Kc-driven transcript in satellite cells grown in presence of NCM may be explained by trophic substances release from neuronal tissue that upregulate the NCX gene expression. A question raises as to the origin of the factor(s) influencing NCX1 level in satellite cells. It is worthwhile to mention that NCM was obtained from culture of neuronal cells isolated from the ventral part of neural tubes and grown with satellite cells for 3 days, while the other conditioned medium was obtained from 3 days old satellite cells grown alone. We used the ventral part of the neural tube as this region contains motor neurons, while the dorsal part of the neural tube does not.

The trophic effects of the innervation on muscle development and growth have been extensively studied (34,35). There is a large body of evidence that the ciliary neurotrophic factor (CNTF) plays an important role during skeletal muscle development, maturation and regeneration. CNTF levels are high in sciatic nerve and ventral spinal cord (36). CNTF can be found in motor neurons (37) and CNTF receptor alpha have been visualized on satellite cells (38) and on newly formed myotubes (38–40) by one of us. CNTF injection increases the number of mature myofibers (41) in intact rats and 4 days after a lesion, also the number of regenerating myofibers (42). In addition, the level of CNTF-receptor alpha mRNA is upregulated in newly formed myotubes after skeletal muscle injury (39).

Since the effects of CNTF on intact and denervated skeletal muscle are very pronounced, one could suggest that CNTF alone or in addition with others factors present in the NCM such as Sonic Hedgehog, Shh (43) or the neurotrophin 3 (NT-3) which are known to be present in a high concentration in the ventral part of the neural tube (44) could play a role on the effects we observed in the presence of NCM. However, no direct effects of those two molecules have been reported on satellite cells (as compared to CNTF). CNTF effects on other skeletal muscle proteins have already been reported and it has been found that protein turnover was time- and dose-dependent. A very small dose of CNTF (1 ng/ml) increased myofibrillar protein synthesis after 12 h indicating a rapid effect of CNTF on muscle protein synthesis (40). Although we cannot rule out that other molecules such as Shh or NT-3 could play a role in the effects of NCM on the expression of the three isoforms of the Na^+/Ca^{2+} exchanger in satellite cells, CNTF seems to be a plausible candidate.

Alternatively spliced variants of the three NCX genes were previously documented in rat tissues by Quednau et al. (19). These authors detected multiple splicing variants, resulting from combinations of the pair of mutually exclusive exons with various skipped cassette exons, which could together encode numerous protein variants. However, some of the variants previously detected in commercially available human tissues could not be confirmed in rat tissues (e.g. those containing "exon X" in ref. 5). In a previous work of one of us (6) it was shown that brief storage of rat corpses at room temperature before dissection disrupts tissue-specific transcription and associated alternative splicing of the rat NCX1 alternative first exons

1-Ht, 1-Kc and 1-Br. These data as well as the new data presented in this work together point to the existence of previously unknown modes of regulation of NCX gene transcription. The new observations prompted us to put forth a hypothesis that alternative splicing of NCX genes appears to be extremely sensitive to what could tentatively be defined as tissue homeostasis. Disruption of the homeostasis, which occurs during tissue dissection for RNA preparation, as well as during cell line generation from live tissues, induces aberrant splicing, which may or may not superimpose on the *bona fide* alternative splicing.

Since exon skipping on genomic scale indeed appears to be by far the most frequent event in alternative splicing (45), it seems plausible that inclusion of specific exons requires additional splicing factors only present in an intact tissue. As a first move to obtain support for this hypothesis, we sought to characterize NCX3 splicing variants in skeletal muscle, whereby a biopsy on a live anesthetized animal is possible. A similar, very rapid brain dissection was also performed. Our data suggest that NCX3 exons A and B are strictly tissue-specific and strictly mutually exclusive in muscle and brain. In other words, by "zero time" extrapolation to a live tissue brain contains only variant ACD, and muscle only BCD (Figure 11). Residual skipping of exon C, observed in this work, could be attributed to imperfections of the dissection procedure, since it appears to be slightly more pronounced in brain as compared to muscle, where instantaneous tissue removal and freezing was impossible. In contrast, previous studies have documented other splicing variants that lack one or more exons (19). Thus, it appears likely that all additional variants represent aberrations that rapidly accumulate during tissue dissection. Indeed, earlier data could be interpreted as imperfect selection of one exon from a pair of mutually exclusive exons (A/B), or exon skipping (exons A, B or C). A random combination of both aberrations was inevitably observed as a result of PCR amplification.

The results of our experiments do not question the essence of alternative splicing as a means of generating protein diversity, that appears to increase faster than genome complexity alone (46). Rather, they suggest that a significant portion of actually documented alternatively spliced variants, particularly featuring exon skipping, may represent aberrations resulting from tissue preparation procedures. Similarly, where tissue specific transcription is dependent on the use of alternative promoters, tissue preparation may induce apparent expression of an otherwise silent gene. Wide occurrence of possible splicing aberrations was already suggested by a large scale computer analysis of EST data (47). However, in the case of NCX genes, what previously was interpreted as a means of generating protein diversity, in view of our data may rather point to existence of as yet unknown mechanism, a sensor of tissue intactness, which serves to control transcript processing by specific exon inclusion or specific exon selection from a pair of mutually exclusive exons. This circuit appears to be rapidly disrupted after death, leading to accumulation of additional "alternatively spliced" transcripts. These aberrant transcripts cannot be easily distinguished from *bona fide* alternative splicing *in vivo* (such as tissue-specific selection between exons A and B in NCX genes) in cases where exon skipping does not disrupt the reading frame. From a widespread occurrence of exon skipping one may speculate that such "sensor exons" are found in many genes. A search for protein factors, mediating splicing of such exons, could now be initiated.

Observations, described in this paper, may gain a more general significance as more data on other calcium transporter expression accumulate. Current models of calcium handling are substantially based on electrophysiological experiments made 25–50 years ago. While it is generally accepted that various muscle/neuron preparations used for physiological studies have a limited lifetime for experimental measurements, they have never been checked for the intactness of their calcium transport system relative to the original tissue. Only recently, with the availability of complete genomic sequences of several model organisms, this problem can be approached in a systematic way. It is not unlikely that relative fragility of some calcium transporters had been overlooked and had led to their exclusion from current physiological models of calcium handling. Experimental models and approaches, described in this paper, will be instrumental in addressing this intriguing question.

ACKNOWLEDGMENTS

The authors are grateful to K.D. Philipson (UCLA) for generously supplying R3F1 and anti-NCX2 and NCX3 antibodies and plasmids. This work was supported by the University of Nantes, le Centre National de la Recherche Scientifique and l'Association Française contre les Myopathies. A.K. is grateful to John Georgiou for his expert assistance with mouse surgery and to John Roder for using his facilities for some of the experiments described in this work.

REFERENCES

1. Blaustein MP, Lederer WJ. 1999. Sodium/calcium exchange: Its physiological implications. Physiol Rev 79:763–854.
2. Sanches-Armass S, Blaustein MP. 1987. Role of Na/Ca exchange in regulation of intracellular Ca^{2+} in nerve terminals. Am J Physiol 252:C595–C603.
3. Lytton J, Lee SL, Lee WS, Van Baal J, Bindels RJM, Kilav R. 1996. The kidney sodium-calcium exchanger. Ann NY Acad Sci 779:58–72.
4. Philipson DK, Nicoll DA. 2000. Sodium-calcium exchange: A molecular perspective. Annu Rev Physiol 62:111–133.
5. Kraev A, Chumakov I, Carafoli E. 1996. The organization of human gene NCX1 encoding the sodium-calcium exchanger. Genomics 37:105–112.
6. Scheller T, Kraev A, Skinner S, Carafoli E. 1998. Cloning of the multipartite promoter of the sodium-calcium exchanger gene NCX1 and characterization of its activity in vascular smooth muscle cells. J Biol Chem 273:7643–7649.
7. Boerth SR, Zimmer DB, Artman M. 1994. Steady-state mRNA levels of the sarcolemmal Na^+-Ca^{2+} exchanger peak near birth in developing rabbit and rat hearts. Circ Res 74:354–359.
8. Vetter R, Studer R, Reinecke H, Kolar F, Ostadalova I, Drexler H. 1995. Reciprocal changes in the postnatal expresssion of the sarcolemmal Na^+-Ca^{2+} exchanger and SERCA2 in rat heart. J Mol Cell Cardiol 27:1689–1701.
9. Cheng G, Hagen TP, Dawson ML, Barnes KV, Menick DR. 1999. The role of GATA, CArG, E-box, and a novel element in the regulation of cardiac expression of the Na^+-Ca^{2+} exchanger gene. J Biol Chem 274:12819–12826.
10. Nicholas SB, Yang W, Lee SL, Zhu H, Philipson KD, Lytton J. 1998. Alternative promoters and cardiac muscle cell-specific expression of the Na^+/Ca^{2+} exchanger gene. Am J Physiol 274:H217–H232.

11. Muller JG, Isomatsu Y, Koushik SV, O'Quinn M, Xu L, Kappler CS, Hapke E, Zile MR, Conway SJ, Menick DR. 2002. Cardiac-specific expression and hypertrophic upregulation of the feline Na$^+$-Ca^{2+} exchanger gene H1-promoter in a transgenic mouse model. Circ Res 90:158–164.

12. Nicoll DA, Otolia M, Lu L, Lu Y, Philipson KD. 1999. A new topological model of the cardiac sarcolemmal Na$^+$-Ca^{2+} exchanger. J Biol Chem 274:910–917.

13. Matsuoka S, Nicoll DA, Railly RF, Hilgemann DW, Philipson KD. 1993. Initial localization of regulatory regions of the cardiac sarcolemmal Na$^+$-Ca^{2+} exchanger. Proc Natl Acad Sci USA 90:3870–3874.

14. Levitsky DO, Nicoll DA, Philipson KD. 1994. Identification of the high affinity Ca^{2+}-binding domain of the cardiac Na$^+$-Ca^{2+} exchanger. J Biol Chem 269:22847–22852.

15. Levitsky DO, Fraysse B, Léoty C, Nicoll DA, Philipson KD. 1996. Cooperative interaction between Ca^{2+} binding sites in the hydrophilic loop of the Na$^+$-Ca^{2+} exchanger. Mol Cell Biochem 160/161:27–32.

16. Matsuoka S, Nicoll DA, Hryshko LV, Levitsky DO, Weiss JN, Philipson KD. 1995. Regulation of the cardiac Na$^+$-Ca^{2+} exchanger by Ca^{2+}. J Gen Physiol 105:403–420.

17. Fraysse B, Rouaud T, Millour M, Fontaine-Pérus J, Gardahaut M-F, Levitsky DO. 2001. Expression of the Na$^+$/Ca^{2+} exchanger in skeletal muscle. Am J Physiol 280:C146–C154.

18. Kofuji P, Lederer WJ, Schulze DH. 1994. Mutually exclusive and cassette exons underlie alternatively spliced isoforms of the Na/Ca exchanger. J Biol Chem 269:5145–5149.

19. Quednau BD, Nicoll DA, Philipson KD. 1997. Tissue specificity and alternative splicing of the Na$^+$/Ca^{2+} exchanger isoforms NCX1, NCX2, and NCX3 in rat. Am J Physiol 272:C1250–C1261.

20. Dyck C, Omelchenko A, Elias CL, Quednau BD, Philipson KD, Hnatowich M, Hryshko LV. 1999. Ionic regulatory properties of brain and kidney splice variants of the NCX1 Na$^+$-Ca^{2+} exchanger. J Gen Physiol 114:701–711.

21. Li Z, Matsuoka S, Hryshko LV, Nicoll DA, Bersohn MM, Burke EP, Lifton RP, Philipson KD. 1994. Cloning of the NCX2 isoform of the plasma membrane Na$^+$-Ca^{2+} exchanger. J Biol Chem 269:17434–17439.

22. Nicoll DA, Quednau BD, Qui Z, Xia YR, Lusis AJ, Philipson KD. 1996. Cloning of a third mammalian Na$^+$-Ca^{2+} exchanger, NCX3. J Biol Chem 271:24914–24921.

23. Link B, Qui Z, He Z, Tong Q, Hilgemann DW, Philipson DK. 1998. Functional comparison of the three isoforms of the Na$^+$/Ca^{2+} exchanger (NCX1, NCX2, NCX3). Am J Physiol 274:C415–C423.

24. Mauro A. 1961. Satellite cells of skeletal muscle. J Biophys Biochem Cytol 9:493–495.

25. Campion DR. 1984. The muscle satellite cell; a review. Int Rev Cytol 87:225–251.

26. Jones, 1982. In vitro comparison of embryonic myoblasts and myogenic cells isolated from regenerating rat skeletal muscle. Exp Cell Res 139:401–403.

27. Henderson JT, Georgiou J, Jia Z, Robertson J, Elowe S, Roder JC, Pawson T. 2001. The receptor tyrosine kinase EphB2 regulates NMDA-dependent synaptic function. Neuron 32:1041–1056.

28. Creuzet S, Lescaudron L, Li Z, Fontaine-Pérus J. 1998. MyoD, myogenin, and desmin-nls-lacZ transgene emphasize the distinct patterns of satellite cell activation in growth and regeneration. Exp Cell Res 243:241–253.

29. Aubé AC, Barraud P, Fontaine-Pérus J, Lescaudron L. 1999. In vitro effects of neurons on satellite cell proliferation and differentiation: An in situ hybridization and immunocytochemical investigation. J Muscle Res Cell Motil 20:840.

30. Lefeuvre B, Crossin F, Fontaine-Pérus J, Bandman E, Gardahaut MF. 1996. Innervation regulates myosin heavy chain isoform expression in developing skeletal muscle fibers. Mech Dev 58:115–127.

31. Barnes KV, Cheng G, Dawson MM, Menick DR. 1997. Cloning of cardiac, kidney, and brain promoters of the feline ncx1 gene. J Biol Chem 272:11510–11517.

32. Carafoli E, Genazzani A, Guerini D. 1999. Calcium controls the transcription of its own transporters and channels in developing neurons. Biochem Biophys Res Commun 266:624–632.

33. Li L, Guerini D, Carafoli E. 2000. Calcineurin controls the transcription of Na$^+$/Ca^{2+} exchanger isoforms in developing cerebellar neurons. J Biol Chem 275:20903–20910.

34. Helgren ME, Squinto SP, Davis HL, Parry DJ, Boulton TG, Heck CS, Zhu Y, Yancopoulos GD, Lindsay RM, DiStefano PS. 1994. Trophic effect of ciliary neurotrophic factor on denervated skeletal muscle. Cell 76:493–504.

35. English AW, Schwartz G. 1995. Both basic fibroblast growth factor and ciliary neurotrophic factor promote the retention of polyneuronal innervation of developing skeletal muscle fibers. Dev Biol 169:57–64.

36. Ohta M, Ohi T, Nishimura M, Itoh N, Hayashi K, Ohta K. 1996. Distribution of and age-related changes in ciliary neurotrophic factor protein in rat tissues. Biochem Mol Biol Int 40:671–678.

37. Schorr M, Zhou L, Schwechheimer K. 1996. Expression of ciliary neurotrophic factor is maintained in spinal motor neurons of amyotrophic lateral sclerosis. J Neurol Sci 140:117–122.
38. Pelletier M, Caquineau C, Aubé AC, Barraud J, Fontaine-Pérus J, Zampieri M, Vallette F, Lescaudron L. 2000. Motor neurons stimulate adult muscle precursor cell behavior in vitro. Society for Neuroscience Abstract 514–511.
39. Kami K, Morikawa Y, Sekimoto M, Senba E. 2000. Gene expression of receptors for IL-6, LIF, and CNTF in regenerating skeletal muscles. J Histochem Cytochem 48:1203–1213.
40. Wang MC, Forsberg NE. 2000. Effects of ciliary neurotrophic factor (CNTF) on protein turnover in cultured muscle cells. Cytokine 12:41–48.
41. Peroulakis ME, Forger NG. 2000. Ciliary neurotrophic factor increases muscle fiber number in the developing levator ani muscle of female rats. Neurosci Lett 296:73–76.
42. Marques MJ, Neto HS. 1997. Ciliary neurotrophic factor stimulates in vivo myotube formation in mice. Neurosci Lett 234:43–46.
43. Litingtung Y, Chiang C. 2000. Control of Shh activity and signaling in the neural tube. Dev Dyn 219:143–154.
44. Dutton R, Yamada T, Turnley A, Bartlett PF, Murphy M. 1999. Regulation of spinal motoneuron differentiation by the combined action of Sonic hedgehog and neurotrophin 3. Clin Exp Pharmacol Physiol 26:746–748.
45. Nakai K, Sakamoto H. 1994. Construction of a novel database containing aberrant splicing mutations of mammalian genes. Gene 141:171–177.
46. Brett D, Pospisil H, Valcarcel H, Reich J, Bork P. 2002. Alternative splicing and genome complexity. Nature Genet 30:29–30.
47. Mironov AA, Fickett JW, Gelfandt MS. 1999. Frequent alternative splicing of human genes. Genome Research 9:1288–1293.

Signal Transduction and Cardiac Hypertrophy,
edited by N.S. Dhalla, L.V. Hryshko,
E. Kardami & P.K. Singal
Kluwer Academic Publishers, Boston, 2003

Na$^+$/H$^+$ Exchanger and Myocardial Hypertrophy

María C. Camilión de Hurtado,* Néstor G. Pérez,* Irene L. Ennis,
Bernardo V. Alvarez, and Horacio E. Cingolani*

Centro de Investigaciones Cardiovasculares
Facultad de Ciencias Médicas
Universidad Nacional de La Plata
60 y 120 (1900) La Plata
Argentina

Summary. Na$^+$/H$^+$ exchanger (NHE) is hyperactive in the hypertensive hypertrophied myocardium. Regression of cardiac hypertrophy (CH) induced by prolonged antihypertensive therapy with compounds of different pharmacological profiles (angiotensin converting enzyme inhibition, slow calcium channel and angiotensin II type 1 receptor blockade) normalizes the hyperactivity of myocardial NHE. Chronic treatment with selective NHE-1 inhibitors induced the regression of CH in SHR. Considered as a whole, these data support the notion of a causal link between the hyperactivity of the NHE-1 and the development of CH.

Key words: Na$^+$/H$^+$ exchanger; cardiac hypertrophy; hypertension.

INTRODUCTION

Cardiac hypertrophy (CH), generally considered as an adaptive response to increased hemodynamic load, is a major risk factor of morbidity and mortality in western societies. Although considerable progress has been made, the intracellular signaling pathways leading to the development of cardiac hypertrophy have not been completely defined yet. There is, however, growing evidence giving support to the notion that Na$^+$/H$^+$ exchanger (NHE) plays a primary role in the development of CH (1,2).

Address for Correspondence: María C. Camilión de Hurtado, Centro de Investigaciones Cardiovasculares, Facultad de Ciencias Médicas, Universidad Nacional de La Plata, 60 y 120 (1900) La Plata, Argentina. Phone: (54 221) 483 4833, Fax: (54 221) 425 5861, E-mail: mariacam@atlas.med.unlp.edu.ar
* Established Investigators of Consejo Nacional de Investigaciones Científicas y Técnicas (CONICET), Argentina.

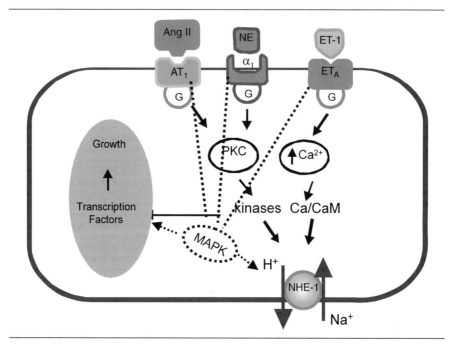

Figure 1. Intracellular signaling pathways involved in the activation of NHE-1 induced by agonists of G protein coupled receptors. Ang II: angiotensin II; NE: norepinephrine; ET-1: endothelin 1; PKC: protein kinase C; MAPK: mitogen activated protein kinase; NHE-1: Na^+/H^+ exchanger.

The sarcolemmal NHE is an integral membrane protein that pumps intracellular H^+ out of the cell in exchange for external Na^+. In this way, it is critical in the regulation of intracellular pH (pH_i) and Na^+ homeostasis as well as in the control of cell volume and growth (3–5). Among the various isoforms of the NHE family, isoform 1 is the predominant one in cardiac tissue. The activity of the antiporter is primarily regulated by pH_i by a H^+ sensor site on the membrane domain. The sensitivity of the H^+ sensor is greatly regulated by various extracellular stimuli at different regions of the C-terminal, both through phosphorylation-dependent and phosphorylation-independent mechanisms (6,7). Figure 1 schematizes possible signaling pathways leading to the activation of the NHE by agonists of G protein coupled receptors (GPCRs) with cell growth promoting actions like angiotensin II (Ang II), endothelin (ET) and norepinephrine (NE). The activation of these GPCRs stimulates phosphoinositide hydrolisis with a subsequent PKC activation and rise in intracellular Ca^{2+}, two well known signals promoting the activation of the antiporter and also of cellular growth (1,2,8,9). However, recent evidence suggests that NHE-1 activation by these agonists also involves a MAP kinase-dependent mechanism (1,10,11). Mechanical stretch of the myocardium, generally viewed as the trigger of CH in response to the elevation of arterial pressure, activates NHE through a

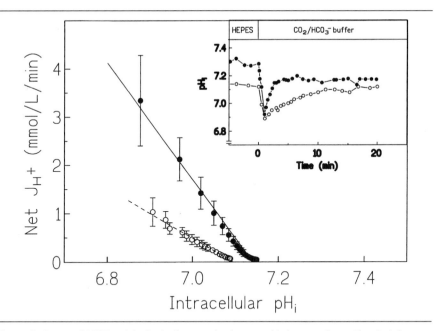

Figure 2. Increased NHE activity in the hypertensive hypertrophied myocardium. Closed circles: spontaneously hypertensive rats; open circles: normotensive rats; Net J_{H+}: net proton efflux during pH$_i$ recovery. Inset: representative recordings showing the faster pH$_i$ recovery from a CO_2-induced acid load in SHR compared to NT. (Modified with permission from Pérez et al. (13))

paracrine/autocrine mechanism with participation of Ang II and ET, as it is discussed in another chapter of this book (12).

This section will review results, mainly from our laboratory, about the activity of NHE in hypertrophied hypertensive myocardium and the effects of antihypertensive therapy or selective inhibition of the NHE-1, all of them providing evidence that NHE activity is an important determinant of CH.

1) NHE is hyperactive in hypertrophied hypertensive myocardium

Usually NHE activity is assessed by the rate of pH$_i$ recovery from an imposed acute intracellular load. The pH$_i$ tracings in Figure 2 (inset) shows that the rate of pH$_i$ recovery from an acid load is faster in the hypertrophied myocardium of spontaneously hypertensive rats (SHR) (13). The estimated rate of proton extrusion (J_{H+}) is increased at any given pH$_i$ value and the apparent "set-point" is shifted to a more alkaline pH$_i$ value in the hypertrophied myocardium (Figure 2). The increased pH$_i$ recovery from intracellular acidosis in the myocardium of SHR was also reported by another laboratory (14). Of interest, in essential hypertensive patients, a positive association was found between the amount of left ventricular hypertrophy and the level of NHE activity in erythrocytes (15).

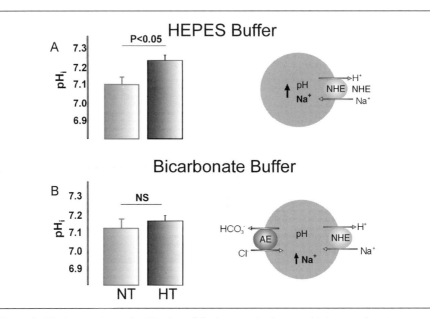

Figure 3. The increase in steady pH$_i$ value of the hypertensive hypertrophied myocardium is cancelled in the presence of bicarbonate. HT: spontaneously hypertensive rats; NT: normotensive rats; AE: Na$^+$-independent Cl$^-$/HCO$_3^-$ exchanger; NHE: Na$^+$/H$^+$ exchanger. (Modified with permission from Pérez et al. (13))

In view of the fact that tissue buffer capacity remains constant in hypertensive rats (13,16), the increase in proton extrusion should promote the rise of the resting pH$_i$ value in the hypertrophied hypertensive myocardium. However, this effect is evident only in the absence of bicarbonate (Figure 3A). When the bicarbonate-dependent mechanisms are also operative, the rise in pH$_i$ is cancelled by an increased extrusion of bicarbonate ions through the Na$^+$-independent Cl$^-$/HCO$_3^-$ exchanger (AE) (13) as it is schematized in Figure 3B. The increase in AE activity in the hypertrophied myocardium correlates with an increase in full length AE3 isoform mRNA expresion (17) and is also linked to PKC-dependent regulation of the exchanger activity (18). Even though the enhanced activity of the AE can compensate the rise in pH$_i$, it will not prevent the rise in Na^+_i caused by NHE-1 hyperactivity. The rise in Na^+_i might, through Na$^+$/Ca^{2+} exchange, cause the rise in Ca^{2+}. In this regard, the hypertrophied myocardium resembles the myocardial response to stretch, Ang II or ET in that all of them induce an increase in myocardial pH$_i$ due to the stimulation of NHE-1 activity only in the absence of bicarbonate (12,19–21).

The increase in NHE-1 activity in the hypertrophied myocardium may be due to an increase in the number of transport units and/or alterations of the intracellular signaling cascades converging on the NHE-1. Several pieces of evidence point to a change in intracellular signaling. In the first place, no difference at the level of

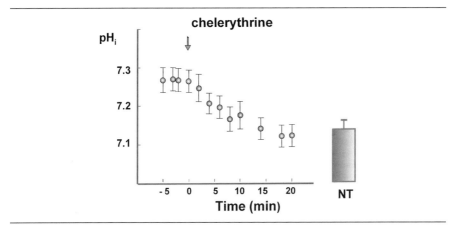

Figure 4. Inhibition of PKC activity normalizes the increase in steady pH_i value in hypertensive hypertrophied myocardium. NT: normotensive rats. (Modified with permission from Ennis et al. (18))

NHE-1 protein expression was detected in the myocardium of SHR (16). Secondly, the rise in myocardial pH_i found in hypertrophied myocardium in the absence of bicarbonate was cancelled after the inhibition of PKC activity (18). Figure 4 shows that myocardial pH_i of SHR decays after PKC inhibition approaching in ~20 minutes a similar value to that found in normotensive rats. Taken together, these data suggest the participation of a posttranslational PKC-dependent mechanism in the increase of NHE-1 activity in the hypertensive hypertrophied myocardium. These results would be in agreement with previous findings of a marked level of basal antiporter stimulation in vascular smooth muscle cells of SHR (22) and in platelets of hypertensive patients (23) as well as with reports about a higher phosphorylation level of NHE-1 in hypertensive compared to normotensive individuals (24,25).

2) Effect of antihypertensive therapy on NHE activity

It is well known that the reduction of arterial pressure induces the regression of CH in hypertensive individuals. It seemed interesting to explore the effect of reversing CH on the hyperactivity of the myocardial NHE-1. To this end, SHR were chronically treated with either one of the following frequently used antihypertensive drugs: nifedipine (slow calcium channel blocker), losartan (Ang II type 1 receptor blocker) or enalapril (angiotensin converting enzyme inhibitor). All the treatments decreased the systolic blood pressure to about the same value in the hypertensive rats, although arterial pressure remained elevated in comparison to normotensive rats (Figure 5A). As expected all three treatments induced the regression of CH (Figure 5B). The heart weight to body weight ratio, used as index of CH, decreased to values not different from that in normotensive rats with enalapril and nifedipine treatment whereas in the case of losartan the reduction in the cardiac index was even greater.

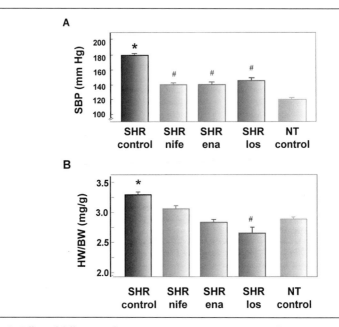

Figure 5. Effect of different antihypertensive treatments in SHR. A: Effect on systolic blood pressure (SBP). B: Effect on heart weight to body weight ratio (HW/BW). SHR control: untreated SHR; nife, ena and los indicate nifedipine, enalapril or losartan treatment respectively; NT control: untreated normotensive rats. *P < 0.05 vs. other groups; #P < 0.05 vs NT.

Myocardial NHE-1 activity was normalized after the antihypertensive treatment either when assessed in terms of steady values of pH_i in HEPES buffer (Figure 6A) or the rate of pH_i recovery from an acid load (Figure 6B–D). These data, therefore, indicate the existence of a close association between the level of NHE activity and of CH as it is illustrated in Figure 7. The plot of pH_i vs. HW/BW values shows that as pH_i decreases, so does the cardiac mass index, being the losartan treated group the one with greatest reduction in both pH_i and HW/BW ratio.

Interestingly, it has been recently reported that angiotensin converting enzyme inhibition reversed the increased NHE activity in blood cells of essential hypertensive patients (26,27) confirming our findings that the inhibition of the renin angiotensin system (RAS) promotes the normalization of NHE-1 hyperactivity. Whether it is the systemic in addition to local RAS involved still awaits to be clarified.

The fact that the three pharmacological interventions reduced CH as well as NHE-1 activity raised the question of whether there was a cause-effect relationship between these two effects or whether they were independent consequences of the therapy. The reduction in myocardial stretch subsequent to the decrease in afterload could had been a possible common factor. Although the notion of myocardial stretch as a cause of CH was long ago proposed, considerable progress in understanding

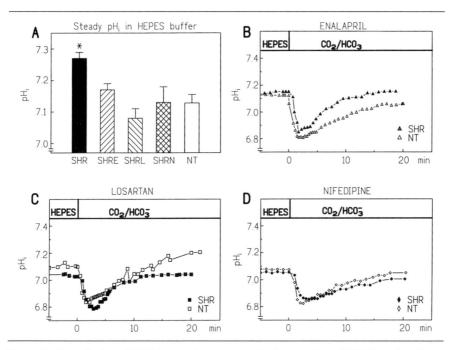

Figure 6. Normalization of NHE hyperactivity accompanies the regression of CH. A: steady pH_i values in Hepes buffer. SHR: untreated SHR; NT: untreated normotensive; SHR-E: enalapril-treated SHR; SHR-L: losartan-treated SHR; SHR-N: nifedipine treated SHR. B-D: Recovery of pH_i from a CO_2-induced acid load in SHR treated with enalapril, losatan or nifedipine respectively compared to untreated normotensive age-matched rats. Assessing NHE activity either by the steady pH_i value or the rate of pH_i recovery from intracellular acidosis revealed that the regression of CH was accompanied by normalization of the antiporter activity.

the process was made during the last decade. Most of the contribution derived from a series of elegant studies carried out on cultured neonatal rat cardiomyocytes, which proposed that stretch-induced CH involves NHE-1 activation and the autocrine-paracrine participation of ET and/or Ang II (28,29). Our own results in intact adult cardiac myocardium (12) allows us to propose that Ang II, ET and NHE are sequential steps of a single mechanism that begins with the stretch of the myocardium.

3) Effect of chronic inhibition of NHE-1 activity on CH

To further examine the relationship between NHE-1 activity and the regression of CH, SHR were treated with selective inhibitors of NHE-1 activity. Two compounds chemically related and manufactured by different companies were chosen. They were HOE642 (30) and BIIB 723, an orally active derivative of BIIB 513 (31). Figure 8 shows the reduction of CH observed in SHR after 1-month treatment with either of these compounds. Noticeably, NHE-1 inhibition induced the regression of CH in spite of the persistence of elevated hemodynamic afterload. By the end of

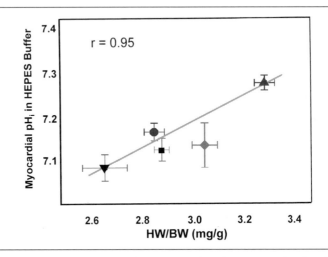

Figure 7. Relationship between myocardial pH$_i$ (as an index of NHE activity) and cardiac mass. Increased cardiac mass correlates with more alkaline pH$_i$ values. r: indicates correlation coefficient. ■ normotensive rats; ▲ untreated SHR; ▶ SHR treated with nifedipine; ● SHR treated with enalapril; ▼ SHR treated with losartan.

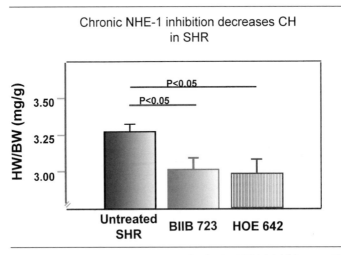

Figure 8. Effect of chronic treatment with selective NHE-1 inhibitors on CH. Significant reduction in CH was induced by one month of orally administration of either BIIB 723 or HOE 642.

the treatment, the decrease in arterial pressure (although statistically significant) amounted to no more than 6–8 mm Hg (32).

CONCLUSION

The present results unequivocally point to the existence of a causal link between the activity of the NHE-1 and the development of CH. Considered as a whole,

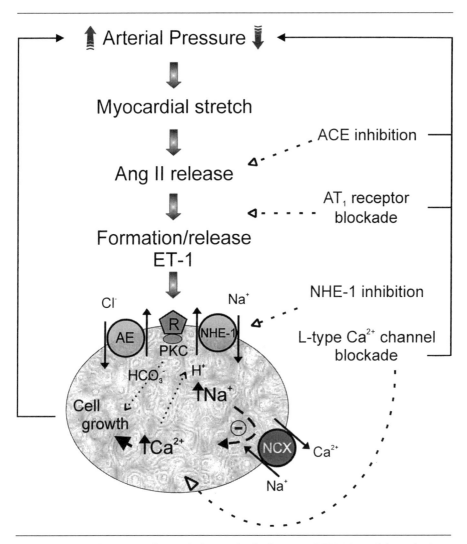

Figure 9. Proposed sequence of events leading to the development of CH. Myocardial stretch triggers an autocrine-paracrine mechanism initiated by the release of endogenous Ang II which in turn promotes the formation and release of ET. The latter peptide stimulates the activities of AE and NHE. The simultaneous activation of both pH$_i$ regulatory mechanisms while allows the maintenance of pH$_i$ within normal range causes the rise in Na^+_i that subsequently might lead to an increase in Ca$^{2+}_i$ through NCX, either by decreasing its extrussion or by promoting its influx (reverse mode of operation). This chain of events can be interrupted by various pharmacological interventions at different levels of the sequence, ultimately decreasing the stimulus for cellular growth.

these results and the previously mentioned data demonstrating the existence of a myocardial Ang II-ET mediated autocrine/paracrine mechanism triggered by stretch, allow us to propose that the mechanism schematized in Figure 9 is involved in the stimulation of NHE-1 and AE activities in the hypertensive hypertrophied myocardium. Interfering with the chain of events at any step will result in the interruption of the signaling cascades leading to myocardial growth.

ACKNOWLEDGEMENT

BIIB 723 was a kind gift of Dr. Randolph Seidler from Boehringer-Ingelheim, Pharma KG, Germany.

REFERENCES

1. Bianchini L, L'Allemain G, Pouysségur J. 1997. The p42/p44 mitogen-activated protein kinase cascade is determinant in mediating activation of the Na$^+$/H$^+$ exchanger (NHE1 isoform) in response to growth factors. J Biol Chem 272:271–279.
2. Yamazaki T, Komuro I, Yazaki Y. 1998. Signaling pathways for cardiac hypertrophy. Cell Signal 10:693–698.
3. Grinstein S, Rotin D, Mason M. 1989. Na$^+$/H$^+$ exchange and growth factor-induced cytosolic pH changes: role in cellular proliferation. Biochem Biophys Acta 988:73–97.
4. Counillon L, Pouysségur J. 1995. Structure-function studies and molecular regulation of the growth factor activatable sodium-hydrogen exchanger (NHE-1). Cardiov Res 29:147–154.
5. Takewaki S-I, Kuro-o M, Hiroi Y, Yamazaki T, Noguchi T, Miyagishi A, Nakahara K-I, Aikawa M, Manabe I, Yazaki Y, Nagai R. 1995. Activation of Na$^+$-H$^+$ antiporter (NHE-1) gene expression during growth, hypertrophy and proliferation of the rabbit cardiovascular system. J Mol Cell Cardiol 27:729–742.
6. Sardet C, Fafournoux P, Pouysségur J. 1991. α-Thrombin, epidermal growth factor, and okadaic acid activate the Na$^+$/H$^+$ exchanger, NHE-1, by phosphorylating a set of common sites. J Biol Chem 266:19166–19171.
7. Grinstein S, Woodside M, Sardet C, Pouyssegur J, Rodin D. 1992. Activation of the Na$^+$/H$^+$ antiporter during cell volume regulation: evidence for a phosphorylation-independent mechanism. J Biol Chem 267:23823–23828.
8. Marbán E, Koretsune Y. 1990. Cell calcium, oncogenes and hypertrophy. Hypertension 15:652–658.
9. Mende U, Kagen A, Cohen J, Aramburu J, Schoen FJ, Neer EJ. 1998. Transient cardiac expression of constitutively activated G$_q$ leads to cardiac hypertrophy and dilated cardiomyopaty by calcineurin-dependent and independent pathways. Proc Natl Acad Sci USA 95:13893–13898.
10. Moor AN, Fliegel L. 1999. Protein kinase-mediated regulation of the Na$^+$/H+ exchange in the rat myocardium by mitogen-activated protein kinase-dependent pathways. J Biol Chem 274: 22985–22992.
11. Snabaitis AK, Yokoyama H, Avkiran M. 2000. Roles of mitogen-activated protein kinases and protein kinase C in alpha (1A)-adrenoceptor-mediated stimulation of the sarcolemmal Na$^+$-H$^+$ exchanger. Circ Res 86:214–220.
12. Cingolani HE, Pérez NG, Camilión de Hurtado MC. Stretch-elicited autocrine/paracrine mechanism in the heart. This book.
13. Pérez NG, Alvarez BV, Camilión de Hurtado MC, Cingolani HE. 1995. pHi regulation in myocardium of the spontaneously hypertensive rat. Compensated enhanced activity of the Na$^+$-H$^+$ exchanger. Circ Res 77:1192–1200.
14. Schussheim AE, Radda GK. 1995. Altered Na$^+$-H$^+$ exchange activity in the spontaneously hypertensive perfused rat heart. J Mol Cell Cardiol 27:1475–1481.
15. de la Sierra A, Coca A, Paré JC, Sanitize M, Vas V, Urbano-Marquez A. 1993. Erythrocyte ion fluxes in essential hypertensive patients with left ventricular hypertrophy. Circulation 88:1628–1633.
16. Siczkowski M, Davies JE, Ng LL. 1994. Sodium-hydrogen antiporter protein in normotensive Wistar Kyoto and spontaneously hypertensive rats. J Hypert 12:775–781.
17. Chiappe de Cingolani G, Morgan P, Mundiña-Weilenmann C, Casey J, Fujinaga J, Camilión de

Hurtado M, Cingolani H. 2001. Hyperactivity and altered mRNA isoform expression of the Cl⁻/HCO$_3$⁻ anion exchanger in the hypertrophied myocardium. Cardiov Res 56:71–79.

18. Ennis IL, Alvarez BV, Camilión de Hurtado MC, Cingolani HE. 1998. Enalapril induces regression of cardiac hypertrophy and normalization of pH$_i$ regulatory mechanisms. Hypertension 31:961–967.

19. Cingolani HE, Alvarez BV, Ennis IL, Camilión de Hurtado MC. 1998. Stretch-induced alkanization of feline papillary muscle. An autocrine-paracrine system. Circ Res 83:775–779.

20. Camilión de Hurtado MC, Alvarez BV, Pérez NG, Ennis IL, Cingolani HE. 1998. Angiotensin II activates Na⁺-independent Cl⁻-HCO$_3$⁻ exchange in ventricular myocardium. Circ Res 82:473–481.

21. Camilión de Hurtado MC, Alvarez BV, Ennis IL, Cingolani HE. 2000. Stimulation of myocardial Na⁺-independent Cl⁻-HCO$_3$⁻ exchanger by endogenous endothelin. Circ Res 86:622–626.

22. Hoffman G, Ko Y, Sachinidis A, Gobel BO, Vetter H, Rosskopf D, Siffert W, Dussing R. 1995. Kinetics of Na⁺/H⁺ exchange in vascular smooth muscle cells from WKY and SHR: effects of phorbol ester. Am J Physiol 268:C14–20.

23. Livne AA, Aharonovitz O, Paran E. 1991. Higher Na⁺/H⁺ exchange rate and more alkaline intracellular pH set-point in essential hypertension: effects of protein kinase modulation in platelets. J Hypertens 9:1013–1019.

24. Siczkowski M, Ng LL. 1996. Phorbol ester activation of the rat vascular myocyte Na⁺/H⁺ exchange isoform 1. Hypertension 27:859–866.

25. Ng LL, Sweeney FP, Siczkowski M, Davies JE, Quinn PA, Krolwewski B, Krolwewski AS. 1995. Na⁺/H⁺ antiporter phenotype, abundance, and phosphorylation of immortalized lymphoblasts from humans with hypertension. Hypertension 25:971–977.

26. Fortuno A, Tisaire J, Lopez R, Bueno J, Diez J. 1997. Angiotensin converting enzyme inhibition corrects Na⁺/H⁺ exchanger overactivity in essential hypertension. Am J Hypertens 10:84–93.

27. Sánchez RA, Gimenez MI, Migliorini M, Giannone C, Ramirez AJ, Weder AB. 1997. Erythrocyte sodium-lithium countertransport in non-modulating offspring and essential hypertensive individuals: response to enalapril. Hypertension 30:99–105.

28. Sadoshima J, Xu Y, Slayter HS, Izumo S. 1993. Autocrine release of angiotensin II mediates stretch-induced hypertrophy of cardiac myocytes in vitro. Cell 75:977–984.

29. Yamazaki T, Komuro I, Kudoh S, Zou Y, Shiojima I, Hiroi Y, Mizuno T, Maemura K, Kurihara H, Aikawa R, Takano H, Yazaki Y. 1996. Endothelin-1 is involved in mechanical stress-induced cardiomyocyte hypertrophy. J Biol Chem 271:3221–3228.

30. Scholz W, Albus U, Counillon L, Gögelein H, Lang HJ, Linz W, Weichert A, Schölkens BA. 1995. Protective effects of HOE642, a selective sodium-hydrogen exchange subtype 1 inhibitor, on cardiac ischaemia and reperfusion. Cardiov Res 29:260–268.

31. Gumina RJ, Buerger E, Eickmeier C, Moore J, Daemmgen J, Gross JG. 1999. Inhibition of the Na⁺/H⁺ exchanger confers greater cardioprotection against 90 minutes of myocardial ischemia than ischemic preconditions in dogs. Circulation 100:2519–2526.

32. Camilión de Hurtado MC, Portiansky EL, Pérez NG, Rebolledo OR, Cingolani HE. 2002. Regression of cardiomyocyte hypertrophy in SIIR following chronic inhibition of the Na⁺/H⁺ exchanger. Cardiovasc Res 53(4):862–868.

II. Cardiac Signal Transduction

Signal Transduction and Cardiac Hypertrophy,
edited by N.S. Dhalla, L.V. Hryshko,
E. Kardami & P.K. Singal
Kluwer Academic Publishers, Boston, 2003

Role of the Electrogenic Na^+/HCO_3^- Symport in the Heart

Ernesto Alejandro Aiello

Centro de Investigaciones Cardiovasculares
Facultad de Ciencias Médicas
Universidad Nacional de La Plata
La Plata 1900, Argentina

Summary. The $Na^{+/}HCO_3^-$ cotransport (NBC) contributes to 40–50% of total acid extrusion in ventricular myocardium. There is, at least, one electrogenic isoform of the NBC in the heart, with a stoichiometry ratio of $2HCO_3^- : 1Na^+$. This cardiac electrogenic NBC abbreviates the action potential and hyperpolarizes the resting membrane potential, being these effects usually masked by the wide use of non-bicarbonate solutions in the electrophysiological recordings. The activation of the electrogenic NBC alkalinazes the cell after increases in heart rate, suggesting a role of this transporter in the compensation for the enhanced proton production induced by the acceleration of cell metabolism. The role of NBC in ischemic-reperfusion injury and heart failure remains to be determined. However, there is increasing evidence that involves this transporter as one of the Na^+-loading mechanisms during reperfusion.

Key words: cardiac myocytes, bicarbonate, cotransport.

INTRODUCTION

The maintenance of intracellular pH of heart cells in the physiological range requires mechanisms for H^+ extrusion, net OH^- (HCO_3^-) influx or both. The main mech-

Address for Correspondence and Reprints: Dr. Ernesto A. Aiello, Centro de Investigaciones Cardiovasculares, Facultad de Ciencias Médicas, 60 y 120, La Plata 1900, Argentina. Phone and Fax: (54-221) 483-4833, Email: aaiello@atlas.med.unlp.edu.ar
The author is an established investigator of the Consejo Nacional de Investigaciones Científicas y Técnicas (CONICET), Argentina.

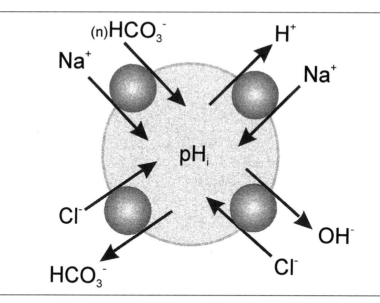

Figure 1. Mechanisms that modulate myocardial pH_i. Scheme showing the main mechanism that regulate cardiac pH_i. Two acid extruders (NBC and NHE) and two acid loaders (AE and CHE) are represented in the top and in the bottom of the figure, respectively.

anisms that regulate intracellular pH (pH_i) are shown in Figure 1. The best understood mechanism is the sarcolemmal sodium/hydrogen exchanger (NHE). This transporter is an acid extruder that is functional even in the absence of the physiological buffer bicarbonate. An acid loader, the chloride/hidroxile exchanger (CHE) is also functional in bicarbonate free solutions (1). In the last years it became apparent that the wide use of non-bicarbonate solutions was masking the existence of other mechanisms that play a role when the bicarbonate buffer is present. The main bicarbonate dependent mechanisms are the chloride/bicarbonate exchanger (anion exchanger, AE), which extrudes bicarbonate, and the bicarbonate loader, the Na^+/HCO_3^- cotransporter (NBC) (1). This mechanism mediates the co-influx of sodium and bicarbonate. The NBC was first described by Boron and Boulpaep (2) in renal proximal tubule of the salamander, with a HCO_3^-/Na^+ stoichiometry of 3:1, which generates a net flux of negative charge across the cell membrane. In the heart this mechanism was first reported to be present in sheep Purkinje fibers (3) and isolated guinea pig ventricular myocytes (4). In these studies the NBC was reported as electroneutral. However, the lack of electrogenicity of the symport in myocardium was challenged by experiments of our group performed in cat heart multicellular preparations (5,6) and rat ventricular myocytes (7). In these studies we proposed an NBC stoichiometry ratio of $2HCO_3^- : 1Na^+$. Recently, Choi et al. (8) reported the cloning of a human cardiac electrogenic isoform of the NBC (hhNBC) with a stochiometry of $2HCO_3^- : 1Na^+$. In addition, an electroneutral isoform of the NBC (NBCn1) has been shown to be also expressed in the heart (9,10). Thus, it seems likely that both isoforms coexist in the heart, the electrically silent and the electrogenic ones. However, whether both isoforms coexist in the plasma membrane of the same single myocyte or in different myocytes remains uncertain.

Contribution of the NBC to the maintenance of pH_i

Whereas in bicarbonate-free solutions, the regulation of pH_i could be entirely achieved by the NHE, in the presence of bicarbonate both mechanisms, the NHE and the NBC, contribute to pH_i modulation. Figure 2 shows experiments performed in cat papillary muscles in which the intracellular pH and the isometric force contraction were measured simultaneously. Extracellular solution was switched from a HEPES buffered solution, without bicarbonate, to a bicarbonate containing solution bubbled with CO_2. The initial transient acidification is due to rapid CO_2 permeation. The recovery of intracellular pH to control and even higher values is due to the activation of the mechanisms that expulse acid from the cell, the NHE and the NBC. Myocardial contractility assessed by developed tension showed parallel changes to intracellular pH. Figure 3 shows the recovery in intracellular pH after the acid load induced by CO_2 permeation in control conditions and in the presence of EIPA, a blocker of the NHE, or SITS, a non-specific blocker of the NBC. Both pharmacological interventions depressed the recovery in pH_i. Although EIPA inhibited the recovery in pH_i in the early phase to a larger extent, the pH reached after 25 minutes of superfusion with bicarbonate solution was the same, indicating that both acid extruders, the NHE and the NBC are contributing almost equally to the intracellular pH recovery. Thus, the NBC contributes to 40–50% of the total acid extrusion of the cardiac ventricular cell. Similar results were obtained by Lagadic-Gossman et al. in experiments performed in guinea-pig ventricular myocytes (4).

Contribution of the electrogenic NBC to the cardiac electrical properties

Measuring Na^+-dependent bicarbonate-sensitive currents with perforated-patch we were able to demonstrate the existence in the heart of an electrogenic NBC with a $HCO_3^-:Na^+$ stoichiometry ratio of 2:1 (7). This electrogenic NBC produces an anionic current which is outward (hyperpolarizing and repolarizing current) at potentials positive to the reversal potential of the NBC. Since the reversal potential for the NBC with a $HCO_3^-:Na^+$ stoichiometry ratio of 2:1 is close to $-95\,mV$, when rat or cat myocytes are exposed to a solution containing physiological concentration of bicarbonate a hyperpolarization of resting membrane potential (RMP) together with a shortening of action potential duration (APD) are observed. Figure 4, panel A, depicts a representative continuous recording of the RMP of a rat myocyte registered under current-clamp mode during the switch of a solution without bicarbonate to a bicarbonate containing solution. The exposure of the myocyte to bicarbonate induced a hyperpolarization of $4\,mV$ that was reversed upon bicarbonate washout (on average: $2.9 \pm 0.4\,mV$, n = 9). This hyperpolarization is

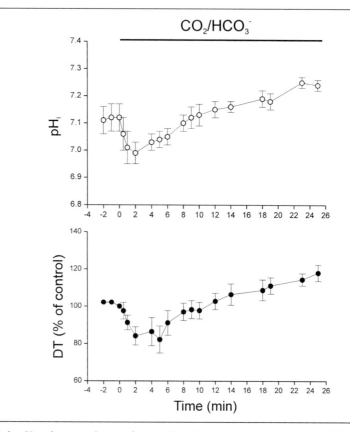

Figure 2. pH_i and tension changes after switching the extracellular solution from HEPES to HCO_3^- buffered solution. Upper panel: Average data of pH_i recorded with the fluorescent indicator BCECF/AM in 6 cat papillary muscles before and after changing the superfusate from a HEPES- to a HCO_3^--buffered solution. The change from HEPES to CO_2/HCO_3^--buffered superfusate (at constant pH_o) induced a transient acidification due to CO_2 permeation that was followed by a recovery to values slightly higher than control. Lower panel: Simultaneous recordings of contractility assessed by developed tension (DT) showed parallel changes to pH_i. Modified from Camilión de Hurtado et al. (5).

due to the influx bicarbonate. Consistent with the involvement of a Na-coupled mechanism, no bicarbonate induced hyperpolarization was observed in the absence of Na^+ (panel B). The effects of bicarbonate on the cat cardiac action potential (AP) waveform are shown in Figure 5. The presence of bicarbonate in the extracellular solution induced a gradual and marked shortening in the AP duration (APD) and a slight hyperpolarization of the RMP (panel A). The APD at 50% of repolarization time (APD_{50}) was $35 \pm 5\%$ (n = 6) shorter in the presence of bicarbonate than in its absence. This APD shortening was not observed when extracellular Na^+ was completely replaced with Li^+ (panel B), indicating the Na^+-dependence of these effects.

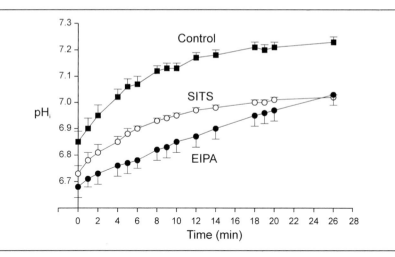

Figure 3. Relative contribution of the NBC to an acid load recovery. Time-course of recovery of pH$_i$ following the acid load induced by switching from HEPES to HCO$_3^-$ buffer under control conditions (n = 6), under 5 μM EIPA blockade of the Na$^+$/H$^+$ exchanger (n = 4) or under the blockade of HCO$_3^-$-dependent mechanisms by 0.1 mM SITS (n = 7). Both acid extruders, the NHE and NBC, contributed equally to the pH$_i$ recovery after the acid load. Modified from Camilión de Hurtado et al. (5).

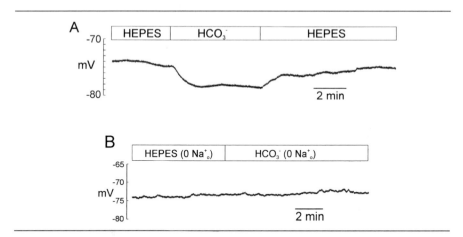

Figure 4. Hyperpolarization of RMP induced by external HCO$_3^-$. Perforated whole-cell configuration. Panel A: Continuous recording of RMP from a rat cardiac myocyte exposed successively to HEPES-, HCO$_3^-$- and HEPES-buffered solutions. Panel B: Representative recording of RMP of a myocyte during successive treatment with HEPES 0 Na^+_o and HCO$_3^-$ 0 Na^+_o. In the presence of HCO$_3^-$ a Na$^+$-dependent hyperpolarization of RMP was observed. Modified from Aiello et al. (7).

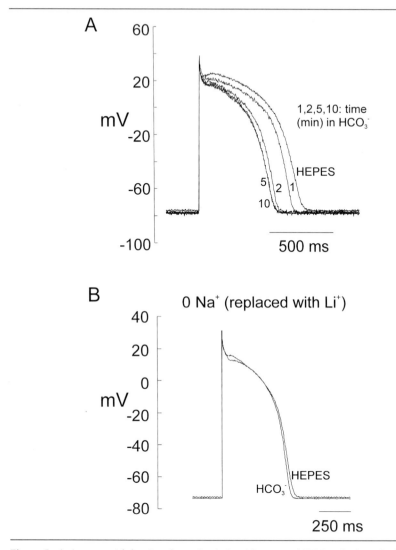

Figure 5. Action potential duration shortening induced by external HCO_3^-. Perforated whole-cell configuration. Panel A: AP recordings under current-clamp mode before (HEPES) and after 1, 2, 5 and 10 minutes of superfusion of a cat myocyte with external HCO_3^-. Panel B: AP recordings before and after exposure of a cat myocyte to HCO_3^- in the absence of extracellular Na^+. Na^+-dependent APD shortening was detected in the presence of HCO_3^- in the extracellular solution.

The bicarbonate-induced effects on RMP and APD were also prevented and reversed by SITS, a non-specific blocker of anionic transporters (7). These experiments demonstrate that rat and cat cardiac ventricular cells possess an electrogenic NBC that relevantly contributes to determine the shaping of the AP waveform.

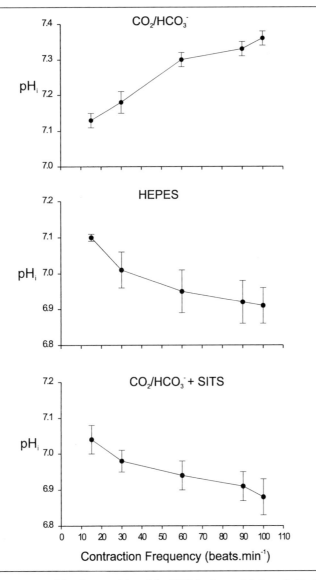

Figure 6. Consequences of the electrogenicity of the NBC in the modulation of pH$_i$. Changes in myocardial pH$_i$ induced by stepwise increments in the frequency of contractions of papillary muscles bathed in either bicarbonate-buffered solution (upper panel), bicarbonate-free medium (middle panel), or bicarbonate plus 0.1 mM SITS (lower panel). Increases in frequency induced a progressive elevation in pH$_i$ in papillary muscles bathed in a CO$_2$/bicarbonate medium (n = 5). In contrast, the same increments in frequency evoked a decrease in pH$_i$ in muscles either bathed in nominally bicarbonate-free medium (n = 5) or in bicarbonate-buffer solution plus SITS (n = 5). Modified from Camilión de Hurtado et al. (6).

Consequences of the electrogenicity of the NBC in the modulation of pH$_i$

Since there is an electrogenic NBC in the heart that regulates pH$_i$, voltage-sensitive changes in pH$_i$ should be present in this tissue. Consistently, when the frequency of stimulation of the heart increases, which also implies an increase in the total time that the myocardial cell spend in the depolarized state, an important alkalinization was observed in the presence of bicarbonate (Figure 6, upper panel). In contrast, when the same protocol was performed in the absence of bicarbonate (HEPES-buffered solution) an important acidification of the cell was observed (middle panel). In addition, in bicarbonate plus the NBC blocker SITS a similar acidification to the one seen in HEPES was observed (lower panel). From these experiments we can conclude that the availability of bicarbonate during an increase in heart rate would provide the myocardium with a mechanism that, by means of an elevated bicarbonate influx, substantially increase the ability of the cell to recover from the enhanced proton production produced by the accelerated metabolism.

Role of NBC in cardiac pathophysiology

After the acidification induced by ischemia, Na$^+$-coupled acid extrusion during ischemia and/or reperfusion contributes to net H$^+$ efflux. The associated Na$^+$ entry may contribute to a rise in [Na$^+$]$_i$ and therefore Ca^{2+} overload via Na$^+$/Ca^{2+} exchange. Vanderberg et al. (11) showed that the NBC contributes in about 20–30% to the total pH$_i$ recovery during reperfusion. Schafer et al. (12) demonstrated that during reoxygenation of rat myocytes exposed to 70 minutes of anoxia, the NBC also plays an important role in pH$_i$ recovery (approximately 30% of the total pH$_i$ recovery). Furthermore, these authors showed that the calcium oscillations that cause hypercontracture of the cells were diminished by DIDS, a blocker of the NBC (12). Recently, the group of Bril has shown in perfused rat hearts that the presence of a selective antibody against the electrogenic isoform of cardiac NBC (hhNBC) significantly improved the post-ischemic functional recovery (13). These authors also showed that the hhNBC protein expression in human myocardium from patients with heart failure was markedly increased in comparison to control hearts (13). Finally, Sandmann et al. (14) have recently shown that myocardial infarction induces up-regulation of NHE-1 and hhNBC. Accordingly, there is increasing evidence that involves the NBC as one of the Na$^+$-loading mechanisms during reperfusion. In addition the results described above suggest that the electrogenic isoform of NBC plays a pivotal role in ischemic heart diseases and congestive heart failure.

REFERENCES

1. Leem CH, Lagadic-Gossmann D, Vaughan-Jones RD. 1999. Characterization of intracellular pH regulation in the guinea-pig ventricular myocyte. J Physiol 517.1:159–180.
2. Boron WF, Boulpaep EL. 1983. Intracellular pH regulation in the renal proximal tubule of the salamander. J Gen Physiol 8:53–94.
3. Dart C, Vaughan-Jones RD. 1992. Na$^+$-HCO$_3^-$ symport in the sheep cardiac Purkinje fibre. J Physiol 451:365–385.
4. Lagadic-Gossman DK, Buckler J, Vaughan-Jones RD. 1992. Role of bicarbonate in pH recovery from intracellular acidosis in the guinea-pig ventricular myocyte. J Physiol 458:361–384.

5. Camilión de Hurtado MC, Pérez NG, Cingolani HE. 1995. An electrogenic sodium-bicarbonate cotransport in the regulation of myocardial intracellular pH. J Mol Cell Cardiol 27:231–242.

6. Camilión de Hurtado MC, Alvarez BV, Pérez NG, Cingolani HE. 1996. Role of an electrogenic Na$^+$/HCO$_3^-$ cotransport in determining myocardial pHi after an increase in heart rate. Circ Res 79:698–704.

7. Aiello EA, Vila Petroff MG, Mattiazzi A, Cingolani HE. 1998. Evidence for an electrogenic Na$^+$/HCO$_3^-$ symport in isolated rat cardiac myocytes. J Physiol 512.1:137–148.

8. Choi I, Romero MF, Khandoudi N, Bril A, Boron WF. 1999. Cloning and charactherization of a human electrogenic Na$^+$-HCO$_3^-$ cotransporter isoform (hhNBC). Am J Physiol 276:C576–C584.

9. Pushkin A, Abuladze N, Lee I, Newman D, Hwang J, Kurtz I. 1999. Cloning, tissue distribution, genomic organization, and funtional charactherization of NBC3, a new member of the sodium bicarbonate cotransporter family. J Biol Chem 274:16569–16575.

10. Choi I, Aalkjaer C, Boulpaep EL, Boron WF. 2000. An electroneutral sodium/bicarbonate cotransporter NBCn1 and associated sodium channel. Nature 405:571–575.

11. Vanderberg JI, Metcalfe JC, Grace AA. 1993. Mechanisms of pH$_i$ recovery after global ischemia in the perfused heart. Circ Res 72:993–1003.

12. Schafer C, Ladilov IV, Siegmund B, Piper HM. 2000. Importance of bicarbonate transport for protection of cardiomyocytes against reoxygenation injury. Am J Physiol 278: H1457–H1463.

13. Khandoudi N, Albadine J, Krief S, Berrebi-Bertrand I, Martin X, Bevensee MO, Boron WF, Bril A. 2001. Inhibition of the cardiac electrogenic sodium bicarbonate cotransporter reduces ischemic injury. Cardiovasc Res 52:387–396.

14. Sandmann S, Yu M, KaschiNaE, Blume A, Bouzinova E, Aalkjaer C, Unger T. 2001. Differential effects of angiotensin AT$_1$ and AT$_2$ receptors on the expression, translation and function of the Na$^+$-H$^+$ exchanger and Na$^+$-HCO$_3^-$ symporter in the rat heart after myocardial infarction. J Am Coll Cardiol 37:2154–2165.

Signal Transduction and Cardiac Hypertrophy,
edited by N.S. Dhalla, L.V. Hryshko,
E. Kardami & P.K. Singal
Kluwer Academic Publishers, Boston, 2003

Modulation of Atrial Natriuretic Peptide (ANP)-C Receptor and Associated Signaling by Vasoactive Peptides⋆

Madhu B. Anand-Srivastava and Malika Boumati

Department of Physiology and
Groupe de recherche sur le système nerveux central (GRSNA)
Faculty of Medicine
University of Montreal

Summary. We have previously shown that pretreatment of A10 smooth muscle cells (SMC) with angiotensin II (Ang II) attenuated atrial natriuretic peptide (ANP) receptor-C (ANP-C) mediated-inhibition of adenylyl cyclase without altering $[^{125}I]$-ANP binding. In the present studies, we have investigated the modulation of ANP-C receptor signaling by C-ANP_{4-23}, an analog of ANP that interacts specifically with ANP-C receptor and endothelin-1 (ET-1). Pretreatment of A10 SMC with C-ANP_{4-23} for 24 hrs resulted in the reduction in ANP receptor binding activity, whereas ET-1 treatment of the cells attenuated the expression of ANP-C receptor by about 60% as determined by immunoblotting. This decrease in receptor binding and receptor expression was reflected in attenuation of ANP-C receptor mediated-inhibition of adenylyl cyclase. C-ANP_{4-23} [des(Gln^{18},Ser^{19},Gln^{20},Leu^{21},Gly^{22}) $ANP_{4-23}NH_2$] a ring deleted peptide of ANP inhibited adenylyl cyclase activity in a concentration dependent manner with an apparent Ki of about 1 nM in control cells. The maximal inhibition observed was by about 30% which was almost completely attenuated by C-ANP_{4-23} and ET-1 treatments. In addition, Ang II-mediated inhibition of adenylyl cyclase was also attenuated by such treatments. The expression of $Gi\alpha$-2 and $Gi\alpha$-3 protein was decreased by C-ANP_{4-23} treatment, whereas it was augmented by ET-1 treatment. On the other hand, the expression of $Gs\alpha$ was augmented by C-ANP_{4-23} and not by ET-treatment, whereas the expression of $G\beta$ protein was unaltered by such treatments. The $Gs\alpha$-mediated effects of some agonists on adenylyl cyclase activity were significantly increased by C-ANP_{4-23} treatment and was decreased by ET-1 treatment. These results suggest that both the vasoac-

Address for Correspondence: Dr. Madhu B. Anand-Srivastava, Department of Physiology, Faculty of Medicine, University of Montreal, C.P. 6128, Succ. Centre-ville, Montreal, Quebec, Canada, H3C 3J7. Tel: (514) 343-2091, Fax: (514) 343-2111, E-mail: anandsrm@physio.umontreal.ca

tive peptides down regulate ANP-C receptor in A10 SMC. The C-ANP$_{4-23}$-induced down-regulation of ANP-C receptor and decreased expression of Giα proteins may be responsible for the attenuation of C-ANP$_{4-23}$-mediated inhibition of adenylyl cyclase activity, whereas ET-induced attenuation of C-ANP$_{4-23}$-mediated inhibition of adenylyl cyclase may be attributed to the decreased expression of ANP-C receptor and not to the overexpression of Giα proteins. From these studies it may be suggested that the desensitization of ANP-C receptors by ANP and endothelin *in vivo* may be one of the possible mechanisms for the pathophysiology of hypertension.

Key words: Adenylyl cyclase, ANP-C receptor, A10 smooth muscle cells, atrial natriuretic peptide, endothelin, G-proteins.

Atrial natriuretic peptide (ANP), a member of the family of natriuretic peptides, was discovered by de Bold et al. (1,2). ANP regulates a variety of physiological parameters, including the blood pressure, progesterone secretion, renin release, and vasopressin release (3,4), by interacting with receptors on the plasma membrane either to generate second messengers such as cyclic AMP (cAMP) (5–9) and cyclic GMP (cGMP) (10–12) or to affection channels (4).

ANP receptors are divided into two major categories, those that activate guanylyl cyclase (referred to as ANP-R$_1$) and those that do not (referred to as ANP-R$_2$) or (ANP-C). The ANP-R$_1$ are guanylyl cyclase-coupled receptors and have a relative molecular mass of 130–180 kDa, whereas ANP-R$_2$/ANP-C receptors exist as monomers (66 kDa) and dimmers (130 kDa). Molecular cloning techniques revealed three subtypes of natriuretic peptide receptor (NPR). These are NPR-A (13,14), NPR-B (15,16), and NPR-C (17,18). NPR-A and NPR-B are membrane guanylyl cyclases, whereas NPR-C (clearance receptors), also known as ANP-R$_2$ and ANP-C receptors, are coupled to adenylyl cyclase inhibition through inhibitory guanine nucleotide regulatory protein (17,19) or to activation of phospholipase C (20) and have been shown to mediate some of the physiological effects of ANP. The physiological role of ANP-C receptor and cAMP signal transduction includes inhibition of progesterone secretion from Leydig tumor cells, inhibition of thyroglobulin release from human thyroid cultured cells, inhibition of endothelial and vascular smooth muscle proliferation, inhibition of adrenergic and purinergic neurotransmission and *in vivo* translation of the endothelin message and the secretion of endothelin from cultured bovine endothelial cells (see review 4).

The ANP-C receptors have been reported to be regulated by various agents. Phorbol esters, calcium phospholipid-dependent protein kinase (PKC), and N-ethylmaleimide (NEM) attenuated the inhibitory effect of ANP on adenylyl cyclase (21) which may be due to the upcoupling of the ANP-C receptors from the catalytic subunit of the adenylyl cyclase. ANP receptors have also been shown to be regulated (down- or upregulated) in various pathophysiological conditions which are associated with increased levels of plasma ANP (4). ANP and angiotensin II (Ang II) appear to act as physiological antagonists in the regulation of blood pressure and fluid homeostasis through receptor-mediated actions in various target tissues (3,22–24). We have recently shown that Ang II attenuated the ANP-C receptor-mediated inhibition of adenylyl cyclase without affecting the ANP receptor binding sites in A10 vascular smooth muscle cells (VSMC) (25). In the present studies, we have examined the regulation of ANP-C receptor by C-ANP$_{4-23}$ and endothelial (ET-1) in A10 VSMC.

We have shown that both these peptides desensitize ANP-C receptor-mediated inhibition of adenylyl cyclase which may be attributed to the down regulation of ANP-C receptor alone or in combination with the inhibition of the levels of Gi protein which couple the ANP-C receptor to adenylyl cyclase signalling.

MATERIALS AND METHODS

Materials

Adenosine triphosphate, cyclic AMP, and other chemicals necessary for RNA extraction and Northern blot analysis were obtained from Sigma Chemical Co. (St. Louis, MO. Creatine kinase (EC 2.7.3.2), myokinase (EC 2.7.4.3), GTP, and GTPγS were purchased from Boehringer-Mannheim, Montreal, Quebec, Canada. 3-Isobutyl-1-methyl-xanthine (IBMX) was purchased from Aldrich Chemical Corporation (Milwaukee, WI)). [α-^{32}P]ATP, [α-^{32}]dCTP, and carrier-free [^{32}P]orthoposphate were purchased from Amersham Corp. (Oakville, Ontario, Canada). Angiotensin II and C-ANP4–23 were from Peninsula Laboratories Inc. (Belmont, CA), AS/7, EC/2, RM/1, and SW/1 antibodies directed against specific C-terminus sequences of Giα2, Giα3, Gsα, and Gβ respectively, were purchased from Dupont (Mississauga, Ontario).

Cell culture and incubation

The A10 cell line from embryonic thoracic aorta of rat was obtained from American Type Culture Collection, Rockville, MA. The cells were plated in 7.5 cm^2 flasks and incubated at 37°C in 95% air and 5% CO$_2$ humidified atmosphere in Dulbecco's modified Eagle's medium (DMEM) (with glucose, L-glutamine, and sodium bicarbonate) containing antibiotics and 10% heat-inactivated calf serum (FCS), as described previously (25). The cells were passaged upon reaching confluence with 0.5% trypsin containing 0.2% EDTA and utilized between passages 5 and 15. Confluent cell cultures were starved for 3 h in DMEM without FCS at 37°C. These cells were then incubated with C-ANP$_{4-23}$ or ET-1 for 24 h at 37°C. After incubation, cells were washed twice with ice-cold homogenization buffer (10 mM Tris-HCl, pH 7.5, containing 1 mM EDTA). The cells were scraped into ice-cold homogenization buffer using a rubber policeman and collected by centrifugation at 4°C for 10 min at 600 g. The cells were then homogenized in a Dounce homogenizer (10 strokes), and the homogenate was used for adenylyl cyclase assay and immunoblotting.

Adenylyl cyclase activity determination

Adenylyl cyclase activity was determined by measuring [^{32}P]cAMP formation from [α-^{32}P]ATP, as described previously (17,19). Typical assay medium contained 50 mM glycyglycine, pH 7.5, 0.5 mM Mg ATP, 5 mM MgCl$_2$ (in excess of the ATP concentration), 0.5 mM cAMP, 100 mM NaCl, 1 mM 3-isobutyl-1-methylxanthine (or as otherwise indicated), 0.1 mM EGTA, 10 μM GTP (or as otherwise indicated), [α-^{32}P]ATP (1–1.5 × 10^6 cpm), and an ATP-regenerating system consisting of 2 mM creatine phosphate. 0.1 mg/ml creatine kinase, and 0.1 mg/ml myokinase in a final volume of 200 μl. Incubations were started by the addition of the membrane preparations (20–30 μg) to the reaction mixture, which had been thermally equilibrated for 2 min at 37°C. The reactions conducted in triplicate for 10 min at 37°C were terminated by addition of 0.6 ml of 120 mM of zinc acetate containing 0.5 mM unlabeled cAMP. cAMP was purified by coprecipitation of other nucleotides with ZnCO$_3$ by addition of 0.5 ml of 144 mM Na$_2$CO$_3$ and subsequent chromatography by the double-column system as described by Salomon et al. (26). The unlabeled cAMP served to monitor the recovery of the [^{32}P]cAMP by measuring absorbance at 259 nm. Under the assay conditions used, adenylyl cycles activity was linear with respect to protein concentration and time of incubation. Protein concentration was determined by Lowry et al. (27) with crystalline bovine serum albumin (BSA) as standard.

Immunoblotting

Immunoblotting of G-proteins was performed as described previously (25). After SDS-PAGE, the separated proteins were electrophoretically transferred to nitrocellulose paper (Schleicher and Schuell) with a semidry transblot apparatus (Bio-Rad) at 15 V for 45 min. The proteins on the membranes were stained with Ponceau S to confirm that equivalent amount of proteins were loaded into each well. The membranes were then blocked with 5% BSA and washed twice in phosphate-buffered saline (PBS) and were incubated in PBS containing 3% dehydrated milk at room temperature for 2 h. The blots were then incubated with antisera against G-proteins (AS/7 against Giα-1 and Giα-2, EC/2 against Giα-3, RM/1 against Gsα and SW/1 against Gβ) and ANP-C receptor antibodies against ANP-C receptor in PBS containing 1.5% dehydrated milk and 0.1% Tween 20 at room temperature for 2 h. The antigen-antibody complexes were detected by incubating the blots with goat anti rabbit IgG (Bio-Rad) conjugated with horseradish peroxidase for 2 h at room temperature. The blots were washed three times with PBS before reacting with enhanced chemiluminescence (ECL) Western blotting detection reagents from Amersham. The autoradiograms were quantified by densitometric scanning using an enhanced laser densitometer (LKB Ultrason XL, Pharmacia, Quebec, Canada). The scanning was one dimensional and scanned the entire area of protein bands in autoradiograms.

ANP-C receptor binding determination. ANP receptor binding was determined as described previously (25,28). Briefly, [^{125}I]ANP binding was determined at 25°C by incubating 20 μl of membranes (~100 μg) for 60 min with 10 pM ^{125}I-ANP$_{99-126}$ peptide or as otherwise indicated (specificic radioactivity 1000 Ci/mmol) in 200 μl of a reaction mixture consisting of 50 mM Tris-HCl (pH 7.5), 5 mM MgCl$_2$, 1 mM aprotinin, bacitracin (1 mg/ml), BSA (4 mg/ml), 0,5 mM phenyl-methylsulfonyl fluoride, and various concentrations of the C-ANP$_{4-23}$ or as otherwise indicated. Binding reactions were initiated by the addition of membrane protein. The receptor [^{125}I]ANP complex was separated from free ^{125}I-ANP by filtration through GF/C filters pretreated with polyethyleneamine. The filters were washed three times with 4 ml of ice-cold Tris-HCl buffer (pH 7.5), and the associated radioactivity was determined in a LKB-Wallac 1277 Gamma Master counter.

Statistical analysis

Data are presented as mean ± SEM. Comparison between groups were made using Student's t test. The results were considered significantly different if P < 0.05.

RESULTS

Effect of C-ANP$_{4-23}$ and ET-1 treatment on C-ANP$_{4-23}$ mediated inhibition of adenylyl cyclase

We have recently shown that Ang II treatment of A10 SMC attenuated ANP-C and Ang II-receptor-mediated inhibition of adenylyl cyclase (25). To investigate if C-ANP$_{4-23}$ and ET-1 treatments also result in the modulation of ANP-C receptor, the effect of C-ANP$_{4-23}$ on adenylyl cyclase was examined in control and these vasoactive peptides-treated cells. Results shown in Figure 1 indicate that C-ANP$_{4-23}$ inhibited adenylyl cyclase in a concentration-dependent manner in control cells with an

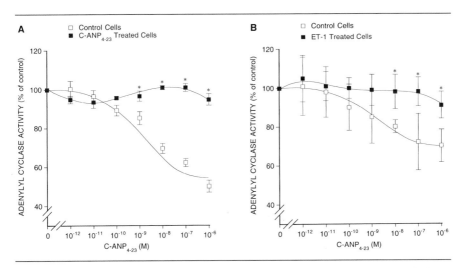

Figure 1. Effect of C-ANP$_{4-23}$ and ET-1 pre-treatment on C-ANP$_{4-23}$-mediated inhibition of adenylyl cyclase activity in A10 smooth muscle cells. A10 cells were incubated in the absence (control) or presence of 10^{-7} M C-ANP$_{4-23}$ or ET-1 (treated) for 24 h as described in "Materials and Methods". Membranes were prepared as described in "Materials and Methods". Adenylyl cyclase activity was determined in the membranes in the absence or presence of various concentrations of C-ANP$_{4-23}$ as described in "Materials and Methods". Values are means ± SEM of three separate experiments performed in triplicates. Basal enzyme activities in the presence of 10 μM GTPγS in control and C-ANP$_{4-23}$-treated membranes were 185.3 ± 9.0 and 161.5 ± 5 pmol (mg protein. 10 min)$^{-1}$, respectively and control and ET-1 treated cells were 288.6 ± 12.3 and 264.9 ± 7.9 pmol cAMP (mg protein. 10 min)$^{-1}$ respectively (⋆p < 0.05).

apparent Ki of about 1 nM. The maximal inhibition observed was about 30–40%, however, this inhibition was completely abolished in cells treated with C-ANP$_{4-23}$ (A) and ET-1 (B).

Effect of C-ANP$_{4-23}$ and ET-1 treatments on ANP receptors

To investigate if the attenuation of ANP-C receptor-mediated inhibition of adenylyl cyclase by C-ANP$_{4-23}$ or ET-1 treatment is attributed to the downregulation of ANP receptor, the receptor binding activity using [^{125}I]ANP$_{99-126}$ or expression of ANP-C receptor using antibodies against ANP-C receptor was determined.

[^{125}I]ANP binds to control and C-ANP$_{4-23}$ treated A10 smooth muscle cell membranes in a saturable manner, computer analysis of the saturation binding of labelled ANP over the concentration range studied in control and C-ANP$_{4-23}$-treated cells revealed a single class of saturable high affinity binding site with a dissociation constant (Kd) of 33.7 ± 6.0 and 35.0 ± 4.5 pM respectively, and a receptor density (Bmax) of 74.0 ± 5.0 and 57.0 ± 4.0 fmol/mg protein (n = 3) respectively. In addition, the specificity of [^{125}I]ANP binding to SMC membranes was also studied by competitive displacement of radiolabeled 10 pM [^{125}I]ANP by unlabeled C-ANP$_{4-23}$ peptide. As shown in Figure 2A, the total number of binding was significantly decreased in membranes prepared from C-ANP$_{4-23}$-treated cells as compared to control cells (3.7 ± 1.8 vs 5.6 ± 2.0 pmol/mg proteins, n = 3) without a significant change in the affinity (9.4 ± 1.0 vs 11.8 ± 1.5 nM, n = 3).

Figure 2B shows that ANP-C receptor antibody recognized ANP-C receptor of Mw of 66 kDa in control and ET-1 treated SMC membranes (top panel), however, the levels of the ANP-C receptor protein were significantly decreased in ET-1 treated cells by about 60 ± 4% (n = 3) as determined by densitometric scanning (lower panel).

Effect of C-ANP$_{4-23}$ and ET-1 treatments on Ang II-mediated inhibition of adenylyl cyclase

We have recently shown that Ang II pretreatment of A10 SMC for 24 hr resulted in the heterologous desensitization of Ang II and ANP-C receptor-mediated adenylyl cyclase inhibition (25). To investigate if C-ANP$_{4-23}$ and ET-1 pretreatments of A10 cells also result in an attenuation of Ang II-mediated inhibition of adenylyl cyclase, the effect of C-ANP$_{4-23}$ and ET-1 pretreatment of Ang II-mediated inhibition of adenylyl cyclase was examined and the results are shown in Figure 3. As reported earlier (25), Ang II at 10 μM inhibited adenylyl cyclase activity by about 30% in control cells, however, this inhibition was almost completely abolished in the cells treated with C-ANP$_{4-23}$ (A) and significantly attenuated by about 80% by ET-1 treatment (B).

Effect of C-ANP$_{4-23}$ and ET treatments on G-protein levels

A partial downregulation of ANP receptor and a complete attenuation of C-ANP$_{4-23}$-mediated inhibition of adenylyl cyclase by C-ANP$_{4-23}$ treatment for 24 h may suggest the involvement of postreceptor components in the desensitized

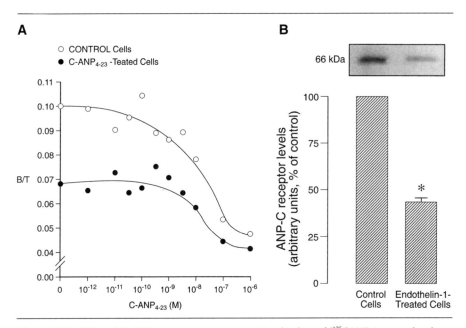

Figure 2(A). Effect of C-ANP$_{4-23}$ treatment on competition binding of [^{125}I]ANP in control and C-ANP$_{4-23}$ treated A10 smooth muscle cells. A10 cells were incubated in the absence (control) or presence (treated) of 10^{-7}M C-ANP$_{4-23}$ for 24 h as described in "Materials and Methods". Membranes were prepared as described in "Materials and Methods". A10 cell membranes were incubated at 25°C for 60 min with 10 pM [^{125}I]ANP and increasing concentrations of unlabeled peptide as described in "Materials and Methods". Each point represents the mean of triplicate determination from a single experiment. The binding curves are derived from the specific binding data analyzed by the ALLFIT program (multiple regression): control cells, Kd 12.4 nM, Bmax 4.2 pmol/mg of protein; C-ANP$_{4-23}$-treated cells, Kd 12.8 nM B$_{max}$ 2.8 pmol/mg of protein. Data from three separate experiments are given in the Results. **(B).** Quantification of ANP-C receptor protein by immunoblotting in control and ET-1-treated A-10 smooth muscle cells: A-10 smooth muscle cells (SMC) were incubated in the absence (control) or presence of 10^{-7} M endothelin-1 (ET-1 treated cells) for 24 h as described in "Materials and Methods". Membranes were prepared as described in "Materials and Methods". The membrane proteins (50 μg) from control and ET-1 treated cells were separated on sodium dodecyl sulfate-polyacrylamide gel electrophoresis (SDS-PAGE) and transferred to nitrocellulose which was then immunoblotted using antibody against ANP-C receptor (upper panel). The detection of ANP-C receptor protein was performed by using the chemiluminescence Western blotting detection reagents as described in "Materials and Methods". The immunoblots are representative of three separate experiments. Lower panel: densitometric scanning of ANP-C protein in control and ET-1-treated A-10 SMC. The results are expressed as percentage of control taken as 100%. Values are mean ± SEM of three separate experiments *p < 0.01.

response. To investigate this possibility, the levels of G-proteins that couple ANP-C receptor to adenylyl cyclase (17,19) were determined by immunoblotting technique using specific antibodies against Giα-2 and Giα-3 in control, C-ANP-$_{4-23}$ and ET-1-treated cells. As reported earlier, AS/7 antibodies that react with both Giα-1 and Giα-2 and EC/2 antibodies against Giα-3 recognized a single protein of 40 kDa (Giα-2) and 41 kDa (Giα-3) in control, C-ANP-$_{4-23}$ and ET-1-treated cells (Figure 4A and B) (25), however, the relative amounts of immunodetectable Giα-2 and Giα-

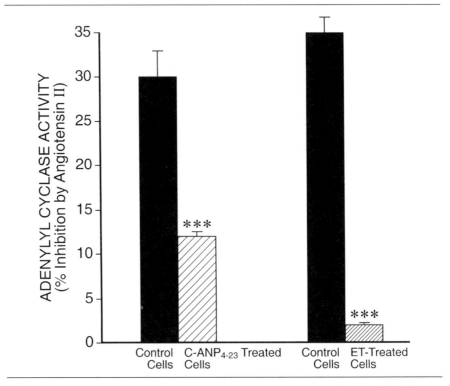

Figure 3. Effect of C-ANP$_{-4-23}$ and ET-1 treatments on Ang II-mediated inhibition of adenylyl cyclase activity in A10 smooth muscle cells. A10 smooth muscle cells (SMC) were incubated in the absence (control) or presence of 10^{-7}M C-ANP$_{4-23}$ or endothelin-1 for 24 h as described in "Material and Methods". Membranes were prepared as described in "Materials and Methods". Adenylyl cyclase activity was determined in the presence of 10 μM GTPγS alone (basal) or in the presence of 10 μM Ang II described in "Materials and Methods". Values are means ± SEM of four separate experiments performed in triplicates. Basal enzyme activities, in control and C-ANP$_{4-23}$-treated cells were 243.6 ± 5.8 and 210.4 ± 7.9 pmol cAMP (mg protein-10 min)$^{-1}$ respectively and in control and ET-1-treated cells, were 239.2 ± 8.8 and 249.7 ± 26.5 pmol cAMP (mg protein.10 min)$^{-1}$ respectively. ★★★ p < 0.001.

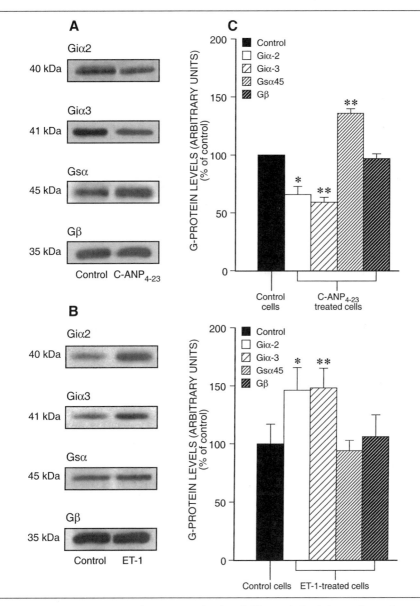

Figure 4(A,B). Determination of Gsα, Giα-2, Giα-3, and Gβ, protein levels in membranes from control, C-ANP$_{4-23}$ and ET-1-treated A-10 smooth muscle cells by immunoblotting: A10 smooth muscle cells (SMC) were incubated in the absence (control) or presence of 10^{-7}M C-ANP$_{4-23}$ (A) or endothelin (ET-1) (B) for 24 h as described in "Materials and Methods". Membranes were prepared as described in "Materials and Methods". The membrane proteins (50 μg) from control and treated cells were separated on sodium dodecyl sulfate-polyacrylamide gel electrophoresis (SDS-PAGE) and transferred to nitrocellulose which was then immunoblotted using AS/7 antibody for Giα-2, EC/2 antibody for Giα-3, RM/1 antibody for Gsα and SW/1 antibody for Gβ. The detection of G-proteins was performed by using ECL Western blotting technique as described in "Materials and Methods". The autoradiograms shown are representative of three separate experiments. **(C).** Summary of the quantification of immunoblots by densitometric scanning. Quantification of G-proteins was performed by densitometric scanning using an enhanced laser densitometer (LKB). The results are expressed as a percentage of the control taken as 100%. The values are means ± SEM of three separate experiments. *p < 0.05; **p < 0.01.

3 were significantly decreased in C-ANP$_{4-23}$-treated cells. At 10^{-7} M, the levels of Giα-2 and Giα-3 were decreased by about $35.0 \pm 3.5\%$ (n = 3) and $40.0 \pm 4.4\%$ (n = 3), respectively, as compared to control cells as determined by densitometric scanning (Figure 4C). On the other hand, the relative amounts of immunodetectable Giα-2 and Giα-3 were significantly increased by about 45 and 50% respectively in ET-treated cells as compared to control cells as determined by densitometric scanning (Figure 4C).

In addition, the levels of Gsα and Gβ, were also determined and the results are shown in Figure 4A and B. RM/1 antibodies against Gsα and SW/1 antibodies against Gβ recognized a single protein of 45 and 35 kDa, respectively, in control, C-ANP$_{4-23}$ and ET-1 treated cells; however, in contrast to Giα, the relative amounts of immunodetectable Gsα were increased by $35.6 \pm 4.0\%$ (n = 3) in C-ANP$_{4-23}$ treated cells and not in ET-1-treated cells as compared to control cells and the levels of Gβ, were not significantly different in control, C-ANP$_{4-23}$ and ET-1 treated cells as determined by densitometric scanning (Figure 4C).

Effect of C-ANP$_{4-23}$ and ET-1 treatments on agonist-stimulated adenylyl cyclase activity

Since C-ANP$_{4-23}$ treatments increased the levels of Gsα, it was of interest to also examine if the altered levels of Gsα could affect the responsiveness of adenylyl cyclase to guanine nucleotides, stimulatory hormones, and other agonists which activate adenylyl cyclase by receptor-independent mechanisms. Figure 5A shows the effect of C-ANP$_{4-23}$ treatment on GTPγS-stimulated adenylyl cyclase activity in control and C-ANP$_{4-23}$-treated cells. GTPγS stimulated adenylyl cyclase activity in a concentration-dependent manner in control and C-ANP$_{4-23}$-treated cells, but the stimulation was significantly enhanced in C-ANP$_{4-23}$-treated cells. For example, at $10\,\mu M$, GTPγS stimulated adenylyl cyclase activity by 100% in control and by 700% in C-ANP$_{4-23}$-treated cells. In addition, isoproterenol (ISO), sodium fluoride (NaF) and forskolin (FSK) stimulated adenylyl cyclase activity to various degrees in both control and C-ANP$_{4-23}$-treated cells; however, the extent of stimulation by these agonists was significantly augmented by about 2.3-, 2.8-, and 2.2 fold, respectively, in C-ANP$_{4-23}$-treated cells as compared to control cells (Table 1).

On the other hand, ET-1 treatment that increased the levels of Giα without affecting the levels of Gsα resulted in a significant decreased stimulation of adenylyl cyclase by GTPγS. GTPγS-stimulated adenylyl cyclase activity in a concentration-dependent manner in control as well as in ET-1-treated cells; however, the extent of stimulation was decreased in ET-1-treated cells (Figure 5B). GTPγS at $1\,\mu M$ stimulated the enzyme activity by about $600 \pm 75\%$ in control cells and about $300 \pm 24\%$ in ET-1-treated cells (n = 4). In addition, the stimulatory effects of isoproterenol, NaF and FSK on adenylyl cyclase activity were also significantly decreased in ET-1-treated cells compared to control cells (Table 1). Isoproterenol ($50\,\mu M$), FSK ($50\,\mu M$) and NaF ($10\,mM$) stimulated enzyme activity by about $480 \pm 24\%$, $6800 \pm 700\%$ and $950 \pm 49.9\%$ respectively, in control cells and by about $370 \pm 45\%$, $4200 \pm 632\%$ and $600 \pm 80\%$ in ET-1-treated cells.

Table 1. Effect of C-ANP$_{4-23}$ and ET-1 treatments on agonist-stimulated adenylyl cyclase activity in A10 smooth muscle cells

Adenylyl cyclase activity (pmol cAMP (mg protein 10 min)$^{-1}$)				
(A)				
Additions	Control cells	% stimulation	C-ANP$_{4-23}$-treated cells	% stimulation
None	63.6 ± 2.9		33.9 ± 1.6	
GTP (10 μM)	93.9 ± 3.3		37.2 ± 1.6	
GTP + ISO (50 μM)	469.5 ± 40.4	50%	427.8 ± 38.5	1150%
NaF (10 mM)	159.0 ± 12.9	250%	237.3 ± 25.2	700%
FSK (50 μM)	1150.2 ± 20.2	1800%	1356.8 ± 130.8	4200%
(B)				
Additions	Control cells	% stimulation	ET-1 treated cells	% stimulation
None	25.3 ± 1.6		34.0 ± 4.8	
GTP (10 μM)	65.8 ± 5.8		60.5 ± 3.5	
GTP + ISO (50 μM)	315.8 ± 19.7	480%	226.9 ± 27.1	375%
NaF (10 mM)	240.4 ± 12.6	950%	204.0 ± 20.2	600%
FSK (50 μM)	1720.4 ± 177.0	6800%	1428.0 ± 214.8	4002%

A10 cells were incubated in the absence (control) or presence (treated) of 10^{-7} M C-ANP$_{4-23}$ (A) or ET-1 (B) for 24 h as described in "Materials and Methods". Membranes were prepared as described in "Materials and Methods". Adenylyl cyclase activity in the membranes was determined in the absence (basal) or presence of 10 μM GTP, 50 μM isoproterenol (ISO) + 10 μM GTP, 10 mM sodium fluoride (NaF) or 50 μM forskolin (FSK), as described in "Materials and Methods". Values are mean ± SEM of three separate experiments performed in triplicate.

DISCUSSION

The present studies demonstrate that pretreatment of A10 smooth muscle cells by C-ANP$_{4-23}$ or ET-1 for 24 h results in a down regulation of ANP-C receptors which is reflected in an attenuation of ANP-C receptor-mediated inhibition of adenylyl cyclase. Our results are in agreement with the studies of other investigators (29–31) who have reported a significant decrease in ANP sites in vascular smooth muscle cells (VSMC) and A10 cells after 18 h exposure with ANP. In addition, a decreased responsiveness of guanylyl cyclase/cGMP system to ANP stimulation in VSMC exposed to ANP has also been demonstrated suggesting a down regulation of GC-coupled ANP receptor subtype by ANP treatment (29,30). However, these investigators have not performed any studies to examine the relationship between the changes in ANP sites and ANP receptor-adenylyl cyclase signal transduction but provided evidence suggesting that G-cyclase uncoupled sites are largely susceptible to a down regulation mechanism (29). On the other hand, our results are inconsistent with the previous studies (32), where 18 h exposure of VSMC from rat mesenteric arteries to ANP and ET-1 did not result in the down regulation of GC-coupled and uncoupled (ANP-C) ANP receptors. These apparent discrepancies may be due to the difference in the cell type (A10 cells versus cultured VSMC from mesenteric arteries) or to the method of treatment. We also demonstrate that C-ANP$_{4-23}$ and ET-1 treatments resulted in an attenuation of adenylyl cyclase inhibition in response to Ang II, which acts via a separate membrane-bound receptor, suggesting a

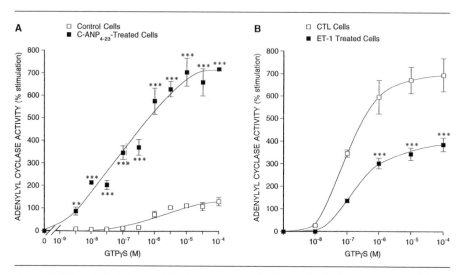

Figure 5. Effect of C-ANP$_{4-23}$ and ET-1 treatments on GTPγS-mediated stimulation of adenylyl cyclase activity in A10 smooth muscle cells: A10 smooth muscle cells (SMC) were incubated in the absence (control) or presence of 10^{-7} M C-ANP$_{4-23}$ (A) or endothelin-1 (B) (treated cells) for 24 h as described in "Materials and Methods". Membranes were prepared as described in "Materials and Methods". Adenylyl cyclase activity was determined in the absence or presence of various concentrations of GTPγS as described in "Materials and Methods". Values are means ± SEM of four separate experiments performed in triplicate. Basal enzyme activities in control and C-ANP$_{4-23}$-treated cells in the absence of GTPγS were 62.3 ± 2.7 and 47.1 ± 4.5 pmol of cAMP (mg of protein.10 min)$^{-1}$, respectively and in control and ET-1-treated cells were: 29.5 ± 3.5 and 32.1 ± 1.5 pmol cAMP (mg protein, 10 min)$^{-1}$, respectively. ★★p < 0.01,★★★p < 0.001.

heterologous desensitization. Our results are in agreement with previous studies showing a heterologous desensitization of inhibitory adenylyl cyclase-coupled receptors by adenosine and Ang II treatments (25,33). The mechanism by which C-ANP$_{4-23}$ and endothelin attenuates ANP-C expression is not known and needs to be investigated. However, endothelin receptors (ET$_A$) have been shown to be coupled to Gq/11, G12/13 and Gi heterotrimeric G-proteins leading to stimulation of phospholipase C/protein kinase C (PKC) pathway, small RhoA and inhibition of adenylyl cyclase respectively (34–37). Recently down regulation of ANP-C receptor by PKC activation has been reported (38). Taken together it may be possible that ET-1 induced-PKC activation may be responsible for the observed down regulation of ANP-C receptor expression in A10 SMC.

A complete attenuation of ANP-C receptor-mediated inhibition of adenylyl cyclase associated with partial down-regulation of ANP-C receptor by C-ANP$_{4-23}$ or ET treatments after 24 h is in agreement with our recent studies showing that the treatment of VSMC with ANP-C receptor antisense that inhibited the expression of ANP-C receptor protein by about 50% attenuated completely the ANP-C receptor-induced inhibition of adenylyl cyclase (39) and suggests that postreceptor modification such as an alteration in the levels of Giα proteins that couple ANP-C receptor to adenylyl cyclase system may also be responsible for the observed desensitization of adenylyl cyclase inhibition. In this regard, a relationship between the levels of Gi proteins and functions has been reported by several investigators (40–44). Thus, it may be possible that decreased expression of Gi protein by C-ANP$_{4-23}$ treatment may also contribute to the desensitization of ANP-C receptor-mediated inhibition of adenylyl cyclase. However, ET-1 treatment of the cells did not decrease the expression of Giα-2 and Giα-3 proteins, but resulted in the augmentation of the levels of Giα-2 and Giα-3 proteins. Taken together, it may be possible that about 60% reduction in ANP-C receptor expression by ET-1 treatment may be sufficient to completely attenuate the ANP-C receptor-mediated inhibition of adenylyl cyclase.

The ET-1–induced increased expression may be attributed to the enhanced RNA synthesis of Giα proteins, because of the fact that actinomycin D that inhibits RNA synthesis was also able to inhibit completely the ET-1–induced enhanced levels of Giα-2 and Giα-3 proteins (data not shown). However, the mechanism by which C-ANP$_{4-23}$ decreased and ET-1 increased the expression of Giα proteins respectively is not known and needs to be investigated. ET$_A$ receptor have been shown to be coupled to adenylyl cyclase and phospholipase C/PKC pathway (34). The implication of cAMP in the regulation of Giα protein expression has been reported (33,45,46). A chronic exposure of adipocytes with adenosine agonist N^6-phenylisopropyl adenosine that interacts with inhibitory adenosine receptor (A1) and inhibits adenylyl cyclase activity and cAMP levels has been shown to decrease the levels of Giα proteins (33). Similarly treatment of A10 SMC with C-ANP$_{4-23}$ that inhibits adenylyl cyclase activity also resulted in the attenuation of the expression of Gi proteins (45). In addition, isoprenaline that stimulates adenylyl cyclase activity and increase cAMP levels has been reported to increase the levels of Giα proteins (46). Taken together, it may be possible that the C-ANP$_{4-23}$-induced decreased levels of cAMP may be responsible for the decreased expression of Gi proteins. However, the fact that ET-1 increased and did not decrease the expression of Giα proteins in A10 SMC suggests the implication of other mechanisms or factors in ET-1–induced enhanced expression of Giα proteins. In this regard ET-1 behaves like Ang II that has also been shown to increase the expression of Giα proteins in A10 SMC (25).

We have also shown that C-ANP$_{4-23}$ treatment of A10 cells augmented the levels of Gsα proteins which was also reflected in increased functions of Gsα. An enhanced stimulation of adenylyl cyclase by GTPγS in C-ANP$_{4-23}$-treated cells as compared to control cells may be attributed to the increased levels and functions of Gsα, whereas decreased levels and functions of Giα, upregulation of β-adrenergic receptors, and increased levels and functions of Gsα may contribute to an increased responsiveness of adenylyl cyclase to isoproterenol stimulation. On the other hand, the decreased stimulation of adenylyl cyclase by GTPγS and isoproterenol in ET-1–treated cells may not be attributed to the decreased levels of Gsα, because the levels of Gsα were not altered by ET-1 treatment, and may be due to the enhanced expression of Giα proteins. In this regard, a relationship between decreased levels of Gi and augmented responsiveness of adenylyl cyclase to stimulatory hormones and increased levels of Giα and decreased responsiveness of adenylyl cyclase to GTPγS has been shown by previous studies (40,43,44). In addition, pertussis toxin (PT) and amiloride treatments that inactivate Giα proteins resulted in an augmentation of stimulatory responses of hormones on adenylyl cyclase (17,47). Furthermore, platelets from spontaneously hypertensive rats (43) and hypertensive patients (44) that exhibit decreased levels of Giα proteins elicited enhanced stimulation of adenylyl cyclase by N-ethylcarboxamide adenosine (NECA) and prostaglandins (PGE). Similarly the decreased stimulation of adenylyl cyclase by stimulatory hormones in different models of hypertensive rats that exhibit increased expression of Giα proteins has also been demonstrated (26,48,49).

An augmented stimulation of adenylyl cyclase by FSK in C-ANP$_{4-23}$-treated cells may be due to hypersensitivity of the catalytic subunit of adenylyl cyclase per se or to the decreased expression of Giα or to the enhanced expression of Gsα or to the alterations in all the components of adenylyl cyclase system. On the other hand, the decreased stimulation of adenylyl cyclase by FSK and NaF in ET-1-treated cells as compared to control cells may be attributed to the decreased sensitivity of the catalytic subunit of adenylyl cyclase per se or to the enhanced expression of Giα or to both. Our results are in agreement with the previous studies showing an increased stimulation of adenylyl cyclase by FSK in adipocytes exposed to adenosine inhibitory receptor agonist (33). The Gi-mediated regulation of FSK-stimulated enzyme activity can be further supported by the results of various studies showing an augmentation of FSK-stimulated adenylyl cyclase activity by PT treatment. In addition, the platelets from SHR (43) and hypertensive patients (44) that exhibited decreased levels of Giα showed an increased stimulation of adenylyl cyclase by FSK. Similarly, the overexpression of Giα has been shown to result in an attenuation of FSK-stimulated adenylyl cyclase activity (40). On the other hand, the requirement of Gsα and guanine nucleotides for the FSK activation of adenylyl cyclase has also been shown (50), which may suggest that C-ANP$_{4-23}$-induced enhanced levels of Gsα in A10 cells contribute to the enhanced sensitivity of adenylyl cyclase to FSK stimulation.

In conclusion, we have shown that exposure of A10 SMC to ET-1 and C-ANP$_{4-23}$ resulted in the down regulation of ANP-C receptor and associated adenylyl cyclase signaling. In addition, the levels of Giα proteins were augmented by ET-1 and attenuated by C-ANP$_{4-23}$ treatments, whereas the levels of Gsα were unaltered by ET-1 treatment and were augmented by C-ANP$_{4-23}$ treatments. The ET-1-induced enhanced levels of Giα may be responsible for the attenuation of Gsα-mediated functions, whereas C-ANP$_{4-23}$-induced attenuated levels of Giα proteins and enhanced levels of Gsα protein may be responsible for the augmentation of Gsα-mediated functions. From these results, it may be suggested that ANP and ET-1 by regulating the expression of ANP-C receptor and G-proteins and thereby cAMP levels may play an important role in the regulation of various physiological responses mediated by ANP-C receptor. The desensitization of ANP-C receptor by ANP and endothelin *in vivo* may be one of the possible mechanisms for the pathophysiology of hypertension.

This work was supported by the grants from Canadian Institute of Health Research.

ACKNOWLEDGEMENTS

We thank Christiane Laurier for her secretarial help.

REFERENCES

1. De Bold AJ, Borenstein HB, Veress AT, Sonenberg H. 1981. A rapid and potent natriuretic response to intravenous injection of atrial myocardial extracts in rats. Life Sci 288:289–294.
2. De Bold AJ. 1982. Atrial natriuretic factor of the rat heart, studies on isolation and properties. Proc Soc Exp Biol Med 170:193–198.
3. Cantin M, Genest J. 1985. The heart and the atrial natriuretic factor. Endocr Rev 6:107–127.
4. Anand-Srivastava MB, Trachte G. 1993. Atrial natriuretic factor receptors and signal transduction mechanisms. Pharmacol Rev 45:455–497.
5. Anand-Srivastava MB, Franks DJ, Cantin M, Genest J. 1984. Atrial natriuretic factor inhibits adenylyl cyclase activity. Biochem Ébiophys Commun 121:855–862.
6. Anand-Srivastava MB, Cantin M, Genest J. 1985. Inhibition of pituitary adenylyl cyclase by atrial natriuretic factor. Life Sci 36:1873–1879.
7. Anand-Srivastava MB, Cantin M. 1986. Atrial natriuretic factor receptors are negatively coupled to adenylyl cyclase activity in atrial and ventricular cardiocytes. Biochem Biophys Res Commun 138:427–436.
8. Anand-Srivastava, MB, Vinay P, Genest J, Cantin M. 1986. Effect of atrial natriuretic factor on adenylyl cyclase in various nephron segments. Am J Physiol 251:F417–F423.
9. Bianchi C, Anand-Srivastava MB, De Lean A, Gutkowska J, Genest J, Cantin M. 1986. Localisation and characterization of specific receptors for atrial natriuretic factor in the ciliary processes of the eye. Curr Eye Res 5:283–293.
10. Hamet P, Tremblay J, Pang SC, Garcia R, Thibault C, Gutrowska J. 1984. Effect of native and synthetic atrial natriuretic factor on cyclic GMP. Biochem Biophys Res Commun 123:515–527.
11. Waldman SA, Rapoport RM, Murad F. 1984. Atrial natriuretic factor selectively activates particulate guanylate cyclase and elevates cyclic GMP in rat tissues. J Biol Chem 259:15332–15334.
12. Winquist RJ, Farson EP, Waldman SA, Schwartz K, Murad F, Rapoport RM. 1984. Atrial natriuretic factor elicits an endothelium-independent relaxation and activates particulate guanylate cyclase in vascular smooth muscle. Proc. Natl Acad Sci USA 81:7661–7664.
13. Chinkers M, Garbers DL, Chang M, Lowe DG, Chin H, Goeddel DV, Shultz S. 1989. A membrane guanylate cyclase is an atrial natriuretic peptide receptor. Nature 338:78–83.
14. Lowe DG, Chang MS, Hellmiss R, Chen E, Singh S, Garbers DL, Goeddel DV. 1989. A membrane guanylate cyclase is an atrial natriuretic peptide receptor. Embo J 8:1377–1384.
15. Chang MS, Lowe DG, Lewis M, Hellaris R, Chen E, Goeddel DV. 1989. Differential activation of two different receptor guanylate cyclases. Nature 341:68–72.
16. Shultz S, Singh S, Bellet RA, Singh G, Tubb DJ, Chin H, Garbers DL. 1989. The primary structure of plasma membrane guanylate cyclase demonstrates diversity within this new receptor family. Cell 58:1155–1162.
17. Anand-Srivastava MB, Srivastava AK, Cantin M. 1987. Pertussis toxin attenuates atrial natriuretic factor mediated inhibition of adenylyl cyclase. Involvement of inhibitory guanine nucleotide regulatory protein. J Biol Chem 262:4913–4934.
18. Fuller F, Porter JG, Arfsten AE, Miller J, Schilling JW, Scarborough RM, Lewicki JA, Shenk DB. 1988. Atrial natriuretic peptide clearance receptor. Complete sequence and functional expression of cDNA clones. J Biol Chem 263:9395–9401.
19. Anand-Srivastava MB, Siram MR, Cantin M. 1990. Ring-deleted analogs of atrial natriuretic factor inhibit adenylyl/cAMP system. Possible coupling of clearance receptors (C-ANF) to adenylyl cyclase/cAMP signal transduction system. J Biol Chem 265:8566–8572.

20. Hirata M, Chang CH, Murad F. 1989. Stimulatory effects of atrial natriuretic factor on phosphoinositide hydrolysis in cultured bovine aortic smooth muscle cells. Biochim Biophys Acta 1010:346–351.

21. Anand-Srivastava MB. 1992. Characterization of ANF-R2-receptor-mediated inhibition of adenylyl cyclase. Mol Cell Biochem 6:83–92.

22. Burnett JC, Granger JP, Opgenosth TJ. 1984. Effect of synthetic atrial natriuretic factor on renal function and renin release. Am J Physiol 257:F863–F866.

23. De Léan A, Racz K, Gutkowska J, Nguyen TT, Cantin M, Genest J. 1984. Specific receptor-mediated inhibition by synthetic atrial natriuretic factor of hormone-stimulated steoidogenesis in cultured bovine adrenal cells. Endocrinology 115(4):1636–1638.

24. Chabrier PE, Roubert P, Lonchampt MO, Plas P, Braquet P. 1988. Regulation of atrial natriuretic factor by angiotensin II in rat vascular smooth muscle cells. J Biol Chem 263:13199–13202.

25. Palaparti A, Anand-Srivastava MB. 1998. Angiotensin II modulates ANP-R/ANP-C receptor-mediated inhibition of adenylyl cyclase in vascular smooth muscle cells. Role of protein kinase C. J Mol Cell Cardiol 30:1471–1482.

26. Salomon Y, Londos C, Rodbell MA. 1974. A highly sensitive adenylate cyclase assay. Annal Biochem 58:541–548.

27. Lowry OM, Rosebrough NJ, Farr AL, Randall RJ. 1951. Protein measurement with the folin phenol reagent. J Biol Chem 193:265–275.

28. Anand-Srivastava MB, Gutkowska J, Cantin M. 1991. The presence of atrial natriuretic factor receptors of ANF-R2 subtype in rat platelets. Coupling to adenylyl cyclase/cyclic AMP signal-transduction system. Biochem J 278:211–217.

29. Hirata Y, Hirose S, Takata S, Takagi Y, Natsubara. 1987. Down regulation of atrial natriuretic peptide receptor and cyclic GMP response in cultured rat vascular smooth msucle cells. Eur J Pharmacol 135:439–442.

30. Roubert P, Lonchampt MO, Chabrier PE, Plas P, Goulin J, Braquet P. 1987. Downregulation of atrial natriuretic factor receptors and correlation with cGMP accumulation in rat cultured vascular smooth msucle cells. Biochem Biophys Res Commun 148:61–67.

31. Neuser D, Bellemann P. 1986. Receptor binding, cGMP stimulation and receptor desensitization by atrial natriuretic peptides in cultured A10 vascular smooth muscle cells. FEBS Lett 209:347–351.

32. Schiffrin EL, Turgeon A, Tremblay J, Deslongchamps M. 1991. Effect of ANP, angiotensin, vasopressin and endothelin on ANP receptors in vascular cultured smooth msucle cells. Am J Physil 260:H58–H65.

33. Parson WJ, Stiles GL. 1987. Heterologous desensitization of the inhibitoty A1 adenosine receptor-adenylate cyclase system in rat epipolytes. Regulation of both Ns and Ni. J Biol Chem 262:841–847.

34. Vogelsang M, Broede-Sitz A, Schafer E, Zerkowski HR, Brodde OE. 1995. Endothelin ETA receptors couple to inositol phosphate formation and inhibition of adenylyl cyclase in human rat atrium. J Cardiovas Pharmacol 23:344–347.

35. Takagi Y, Ninomiya H, Sakamoto A, Miwa S, Masaki T. 1995. Structural basis of G protein specificity of human endothelin receptors. A study with endothelin A/B chimeras. J Biol Chem 270:10072–10078.

36. Wu Wong JR, Opgenorth TJ. 1998. Endothelin and isoproterenol counter-regulate cAMP and mitogen-activated protein. J Cardiovasc Pharmacol 31, Supp 1:185–191.

37. Mao J, Yuan H, Xie W, Simon MI, Wu D. 1998. Specific involvement of G proteins in regulation of serum response factor-mediated gene transcription by different receptors. J Biol Chem 273:27118–27123.

38. Yanaka N, Akatsuka H, Omari K. 1997. Protein kinase C activation down-regulates natriuretic peptide receptor C expression via transcriptional and post-translational pathway. FEBS Lett 418:333–336.

39. Palaparti A, Li Y, Anand-Srivastava MB. 2000. Inhibition of atrial natriuretic peptide (ANP)-C receptor expression by antisense oligodeoxynucleotides in A10 vascular smooth msucle cells is associated with attenuation of ANP-C receptor-mediated inhibition of adenylyl cyclase. Biochem J 346:313–320.

40. Anand-Srivastava MB. 1992. Enhanced expression of inhibitory guanine nucleotide regulatory protein in spontaneously hypertensive rats: relationship to adenylyl cyclase inhibition. Biochem J 288:79–85.

41. Marcil J, Thibault C, Anand-Srivastava MB. 1997. Enhanced expression of Gi protein precedes the development of blood pressure in spontaneously hypertensive rats. J Mol Cell Cardiol 29, 1009–1022.

42. Lynch CJ, Blakmore PF, Jonson EH, Wang RL, Krune PK, Exton JJ. 1989. Guanine nucleotide binding regulatory proteins and adenylate cyclase in livers of streptozotocin- and BB/w or diabetic rats. Immunodetection of Gs and Gi with antisera against synthetic peptides. J Clin Invest 83:2050–2062.

43. Anand-Srivastava MB. 1993. Rat platelets from spontaneously hypertensive rats exhibit decreased expression of inhibitory guanine nucleotide regulatory protein: relationship with adenylate cyclase activity. Circ Res 73:1032–1039.

44. Marcil J, Schiffrin EL, Anand-Srivastava MB. 1996. Aberrant adenylate cyclase/cAMP signal transduction and G protein levels in platelets from hypertensive patients: improve with antihypertensive drug therapy. Hypertension 28:83–90.

45. Anand-Srivastava MB. 2000. Dowregulation of atrial natriuretic peptide ANP-C receptor is associated with alterations in G-protein expresison in A10 smooth muscle cells. Biochemistry 39:6503–6513.

46. Reithman C, Geirschik P, Werdan K, Jakobs KH. 1990. Hormonal regulation of Gi alpha level and adenylyl cyclase responsiveness. Brit J Clin Pharmacol 30 suppl 1:118S-120S.

47. Anand-Srivastava MB. 1989. Amiloride interacts with guanine nucleotide regulatory proteins and attenuates hormonal inhibition of adenylate cylcase. J Biol Chem 264:9491–9496.

48. Marcil J, de Champlain J, Anand-Srivastava MB. 1998. Overexpression of Gi proteins precedes the development of DOCA-salt-induced hypertension: relationship with adenylyl cyclase. Cardiovas Res 39:492–505.

49. Di Fusco F, Anand-Srivastava MB. 2000. Enhanced expression of Gi proteins in non-hypertrophic hearts from rats with hypertension-induced by L-NAME treatment. J Hypertens 18:1081–1090.

50. Hildebrandt JD, Hanoune J, Birnbaumer J. 1982. Guanine nucleotide inhibition of cycS49 mouse lymphoma cell membrane adenylyl cyclase. J Biol chem 257:14723–14725.

Signal Transduction and Cardiac Hypertrophy,
edited by N.S. Dhalla, L.V. Hryshko,
E. Kardami & P.K. Singal
Kluwer Academic Publishers, Boston, 2003

Rab3 Small GTP-Binding Proteins: Regulation by Calcium/Calmodulin

Ranjinder S. Sidhu,[1] Richard R. Clough,[1] and
Rajinder P. Bhullar[1,2]

Departments of Oral Biology[1]
and Biochemistry & Medical Genetics[2]
University of Manitoba
780 Bannatyne Avenue
Winnipeg
Manitoba, Canada R3E 0W3

Summary. Rab proteins, forming a subfamily of 52 predominantly membrane-bound, low molecular weight GTP-binding proteins (G-proteins) of the Ras superfamily, are involved in vesicle traffic between intracellular organelles, endocytosis and exocytosis, and may be regulated by calcium (Ca^{2+}) and/or calmodulin (CaM). Rab3A and Rab3B bind CaM, and both RabGDP-dissociation inhibitor (RabGDI) and CaM cause dissociation of Rab3A from membranes, to form soluble cytoplasmic Rab/CaM or Rab/RabGDI complexes. This shuttling is intimately connected with the cycling of Rab between the active GTP-bound (at organelle membranes) and inactive GDP-bound (cytosolic) state, enabling Rab to function as molecular switches in the regulation of various cell functions. Rab3A inhibits, while Rab3B promotes, Ca^{2+}-dependent exocytosis. Recent work has demonstrated that Rab3's effects on exocytosis are regulated by CaM, in that CaM may enhance the dissociation of Rab by RabGDI in a Ca^{2+}-dependent manner. RabGDI binds only to inactive Rab, while CaM binds with much higher affinity to active Rab3A. Ca^{2+}/CaM can induce GDP to GTP exchange on Rab if RabGDI is not bound. It is proposed that increased intracellular Ca^{2+} concentration causes RabGDI to be replaced by CaM on Rab-GDP, allowing CaM to exert its effects through an activated Rab3. At high intracellular Ca^{2+} levels, the Rab3-GTP/CaM complex may predominate over the Rab3-GDP/RabGDI complex. Competitive rebinding of RabGDI to Rab-GDP, but not to Rab-GTP, would cause release of CaM and reversal of its effects. Thus, Ca^{2+} and CaM appear to be important regulators of Rab3 function. It is impor-

Address for Correspondence: Dr. R. P. Bhullar, Department of Oral Biology, University of Manitoba, 780 Bannatyne Avenue, Winnipeg, Manitoba, Canada R3E 0W3. Tel: 204-789-3703, Fax: 204-789-3913, E-mail: *BHULLAR@MS.UMANITOBA.CA*

tant to elucidate the exact mechanisms of such interactions, and which intracellular pathways are involved.

Key words: Rab, Rab3, RabGDI, calcium, calmodulin, exocytosis.

INTRODUCTION

The metabolism and function of a cell can be influenced by a wide variety of external factors. A signal from the extracellular environment impinging on the cell is initially detected at the surface by receptors and transferred onto other effectors inside the cell. It is here that the signals are further communicated, and often amplified, through the generation of second messengers (e.g. cyclic AMP, IP₃, diacylglycerol). These second messengers either participate in the cells' response by causing immediate alterations in the cell function or propagate the signal for further generation of long-term responses.

Signal transduction through the coupling of cell surface receptors to effectors inside the cell requires the participation of a group of proteins termed guanine nucleotide or GTP-binding proteins (G-proteins). There are two major families of G-proteins in the eukaryotic cell that participate in signal transduction pathways. The first family is made up of multisubunit heterotrimeric GTP-binding proteins, consisting of the α, β, and γ subunits (1). The α-subunit has molecular weight between 39–52 kDa, binds GTP/GDP, has intrinsic GTPase activity and 20 different mammalian α-subunits (coded for by 16 genes) have been identified (2). Five different β-subunits of molecular weight of ~35 kDa and eleven distinct γ-subunits of molecular weight between 7–10 kDa have been identified in mammalian cells (2). Upon occupation of the extracellular receptor, there is an exchange of GTP for GDP on the α-subunit, and the αβγ G-protein dissociates into α–GTP and βγ forms. The GTP-bound form of α-subunit links a wide variety of extracellular receptors to effectors (e.g. adenylyl cyclase, phospholipase C) inside the cell and the β-subunit has been shown to regulate ion channels (3). In addition, the βγ-subunit dimer complexes with GDP-bound form of the α-subunit upon inactivation of the G-protein through the conversion of bound GTP to GDP. This inactivation is achieved due to the intrinsic GTPase activity associated with the α-subunit and is facilitated by proteins termed regulators of G protein signalling or RGS proteins that stimulate the intrinsic GTPase activity (4–6).

The Ras-p21, and Ras-related proteins, make up the second family of GTP-binding proteins and are commonly referred to as the Ras superfamily of *small* or *low molecular weight GTP-binding proteins* (LMWG *proteins*) (7). The LMWG proteins have molecular weight between 20–30 kDa and consist of a single polypeptide chain that binds GTP/GDP. Based on their homology to Ras-p21, the LMWG proteins have been grouped into four subfamilies. These include, Ras-p21-related (~50% homology), Rho-related (30% homology), Rab-related (30% homology) and others (<30% homology). The Ras superfamily of GTP-binding proteins regulate a wide variety of cell functions including control of gene expression (Ras and Rho families), cytoskeletal reorganization (Rho family), vesicle trafficking and exocytosis (Rab family), vesicle budding (Sar1/Arf family), and nucleocytoplasmic transport and microtubule organization (Ran family). A recent review on the general properties and function of LMWG protein family has been published (8). The focus of this paper will be on the Ras-related Rab subfamily of small GTP-binding proteins with an emphasis on the role of calcium (Ca^{2+}) and calmodulin (CaM) in the regulation of the function of Rab3 proteins.

RAB LMWG PROTEINS

With the recent description of the Rab family motifs 1–5 conserved sequences, 52 members in the Rab subfamily have now been identified (9). Thus, Rab forms the largest branch of the Ras-related superfamily (8). Subcellular distribution analysis and functional studies have suggested a role for Rab proteins in vesicle traffic between intracellular organelles and in endocytosis and exocytosis (regulated and constitutive secretion) (10–12). Calmodulin, a ubiquitous calcium sensor involved in a multitude of signal transduction pathways, has been implicated in the process of regulated secretion from cells. The exact role of CaM in the process is still unknown but some information has emerged implicating CaM in the regulation of the Rab GTP-binding proteins (13). In this review, we will attempt to provide some insight into the role of calcium and/or calmodulin in the regulation of Rab-GTPase function. For more detailed information on the involvement of Ca^{2+} and/or CaM in other signaling pathways the reader is directed to other fine reviews (14–17).

REGULATION OF RAB-GTPASES

Like other members of the Ras superfamily, Rab proteins cycle between two states: an active GTP-bound state and an inactive GDP-bound state (18). The conversion of Rab-GDP to the GTP-bound form is facilitated by an upstream signal. This leads to a conformational change in the molecule, such that the Rab effector-binding region is now able to interact with downstream effector(s). As is the case with other GTP-binding proteins, Rab-GTP is converted back to the GDP state by the intrinsic GTPase activity associated with G-proteins, resulting in the termination of Rab-effector interaction. The intrinsic rate of GTP hydrolysis, which is the rate-limiting step, is an extremely slow reaction and would be little value to the cell without the aid of GTPase activating proteins (GAPs). Specific GAPs exist in the cell for each member or subfamily of LMWG proteins (8). This interconversion between the GTP- and GDP-bound form represents the conformational states equivalent to the active and inactive state of the G-protein. This cycling allows the G-proteins to act as molecular switches in the regulation of various cell functions.

LOCALIZATION OF RAB PROTEINS

Although Rab proteins are normally associated with the membrane, they are shuttled between the membrane bound and cytosol state, a process that is superimposed onto the GTP-GDP cycle. At any given time in a resting cell, about 10–50% of Rab proteins are present in the cytosol as a complex with Rab GDP-dissociation inhibitor (RabGDI) (19–21). As the name implies, RabGDI maintains the Rab protein in the GDP bound state while in the cytosol. Like most members of the LMWG protein family, Rab proteins contain a C-terminal post-translational lipid modification on cysteine residues called isoprenylation (22,23). The C-terminal iso-prenoid lipid moiety, which could be either a farnesyl group or a geranylgeranyl group, facilitates membrane anchoring. The binding of RabGDI masks the isoprenyl group and makes the G-protein more soluble. This partially explains how the GTP binding protein can shuttle between the cytosol and membrane compartments. In the case of Rab3, this lipid modification is believed to be necessary for the inter-action between Rab and either RabGDI or Ca^{2+}/CaM (24,25). The binding of RabGDI, and perhaps even CaM, to Rab3 masks the geranylgeranyl group through hydrophobic interactions, thus making the GTPase more soluble.

The mechanism by which Rab proteins are shuttled between the membrane and cytosol was elucidated with the finding that GDP-bound form of Rab is maintained in the cytosol by the binding of RabGDI (19). Once the Rab protein is ready to be delivered to the correct membrane compartment, a Rab escort protein (REP) facilitates targeting to the appropriate site (19,26). The GDI protein is then displaced from Rab by another factor called a GDI displacement stimulator (GDIGDS) or factor (GDIGDF) localized at specific organelle membranes (27–30). The mechanism by which this occurs is still unknown. The Rab protein is then converted to the GTP bound form by a GDP/GTP exchange protein (GEP, also called guanine nucleotide releasing factors or GEFs). The GTP-bound active form of Rab is then able to interact with downstream effector molecules such as, Rabphillin (31) and Rim (32). Shortly thereafter the GTP-bound form is converted back to the GDP-bound form by the action of the GTPase Activating Protein or GAP (33). The membrane bound Rab-GDP once again complexes with RabGDI and translocates back to the cytosol as a complex (20). *In vitro* studies have shown that CaM can also facilitate the dissociation of Rab3A protein from target mem-branes; however, less efficiently than RabGDI and with a less stringent requirement for the nucleotide state (25). RabGDI binds only to GDP-bound form of Rab pro-teins (19) while CaM binding to Rab3A has been reported to occur with a greater affinity to the GTP-bound form (34) than the GDP-bound state of Rab3A (25). Nevertheless, both RabGDI and CaM cause the dissociation of Rab3A from mem-brane, thus, forming a soluble complex in the cytosolic fraction (25).

RAB AND INTRACELLULAR VESICLE TRAFFIC

The Rab-GTPases are involved in the regulation of vesicle trafficking (35), a process found in many cell types, but especially in secretory cells such as neurons, exocrine cells, endocrine cells and platelets. Exocytosis proceeds by two distinct mechanisms, either by regulated secretion (biosynthetic pathway) or constitutive secretion (36). During regulated secretion, vesicles from the Golgi apparatus accumulate in the cytoplasm. Upon stimulation of the cells, the vesicles translocate near the periph-ery of the cell, fuse with the cell membrane, and then discharge their contents.

Some examples of regulated exocytosis include neurotransmitter release from synapses, hormone release from endocrine cells, and digestive enzyme release from exocrine cells. In contrast, cells with constitutive secretion do not accumulate vesicles that are supplied from the Golgi in the cytoplasm. Instead, during this process vesicles are continuously transported to the membrane and released extracellularly. Examples of constitutive secretion include plasma protein secretion from hepatocytes and immunoglobulin release from lymphocytes. The docking of vesicles to the membrane is dependent on GTP. Early evidence for this was obtained in studies using the non-hydrolyzable analogue GDPβS. This results in a decrease in the release of neurotransmitters and a selective loss of vesicle attachment to the presynaptic plasma membrane (37).

The first definitive evidence for a role of LMWG proteins in vesicle translocation was obtained from studies in yeast. The secretion of vesicles in yeast is mediated via the constitutive secretion pathway as the regulated mechanism for secretion is not operative in this unicellular organism. Mutations in genes that code for the two small G proteins, *Sec*4 and *Ypt*1, result in the accumulation of vesicles in the cell (38). Mammalian homologues of these yeast genes termed, *Rab*, have been discovered and localized to various regions of the cell. For instance, Rab7 protein is found in late endosomes and regulates the endocytic process (39). Rab4 and Rab5 are found in the early endosome and, mediate endosome-endosome fusion and receptor recycling, respectively (40). Rab1, Rab2, and Rab6 are localized at the endoplasmic reticulum and the Golgi apparatus, and regulate vesicle transport along the biosynthetic pathway (41). Rab3 is localized on secretory granules including synaptic vesicles and is involved in the regulation of the Ca^{2+}-dependent exocytosis. The involvement of CaM in the process of regulated exocytosis is now being intensely investigated.

REGULATION AND ACTIVATION OF CAM

Calmodulin is an intracellular calcium binding protein capable of regulating the biological activities of many cellular proteins and transmembrane ion transporters in a calcium-dependent manner. CaM is a 17 kDa dumbbell shaped acidic protein arranged in two globular domains connected with a long flexible linker α-helix (42). Each globular domain contains a pair of linked EF-hand motifs. When intracellular calcium levels rise to 10^{-5} M, four Ca^{2+} ions bind to CaM. This causes a conformational change in calmodulin such that a portion of the central linker α-helix unwinds allowing the binding of Ca^{2+}/CaM to target molecules (43). The bending of the central linker α-helix results in a conformational change into compact globular structure with two exposed hydrophobic surfaces surrounded by negative charges (44,45). The stability of this Ca^{2+}/CaM-target complex is contributed by electrostatic interactions (15). Although Ca^{2+}/CaM has been shown to activate a variety of molecules, the calcium free form apo-calmodulin (Apo-CaM) is often associated with a different set of target proteins (46). In addition, many target proteins bind CaM only within a narrow range of Ca^{2+} concentration and a low or high Ca^{2+} may inhibit binding.

One of the most intriguing properties of CaM is its ability to bind and activate numerous target proteins that share little similarity in amino acid sequence in their CaM binding regions (47). Pattern searches in sequences provide little help in predicting such sites in target proteins (http://calcium.oci.utoronto.ca/). As a result, CaM binding regions in target molecules must be empirically determined. Despite such obstacles in locating CaM binding partners some general properties can be ascribed to known CaM binding domains. Majority of the known CaM binding domains in partner proteins are composed of a stretch of 12–30 contiguous amino acids with positively charged amphiphilic characteristics that have a propensity to form an α-helix upon binding to CaM (48).

RAB3 AS CAM BINDING G-PROTEINS

Of the Rab proteins, the members of the Rab3 family have been shown to bind CaM in a calcium dependent manner (25,49). Four isoforms in the Rab3 (Rab3A, -3B, -3C and -3D) family have been identified (50). The different Rab3 proteins share considerable homology (73%) with majority of the differences clustered in the C-terminal region. Rab3A was the first member of the Rab3 family shown to bind CaM in a Ca^{2+}-dependent manner (25). The CaM binding domain in Rab3A has been localized to a region spanning amino acids 62–85 in this protein. Analysis of this region in Rab3B, Rab3C and Rab3D suggests that these proteins will also be able to bind CaM as there are only 6 conservative changes in the potential CaM binding region of Rab3B-Rab3D (Figure 1). Indeed, we have shown that Rab3B is a CaM binding protein (49) and one would expect that Rab3C and Rab3D will also be capable of binding CaM.

RAB3 IN CALCIUM-DEPENDENT EXOCYTOSIS

Although parallels have been drawn between pancreatic Rab3D and neuronal Rab3A, most of the research has focused on Rab3A. Thus, only Rab3A and Rab3B will be the focus of this review (see reference 51 for more information on Rab3D). Several lines of evidence suggest that Rab3 proteins participate in the control of storage granule content secretion in different cell types (10,52). Rab3 subfamily GTPases are localized to secretory granules in neuroendocrine cells (53,54) and on synaptic vesicles in neurons (55). Rab3A in the GTP-bound active state is believed to either inhibit calcium-dependent exocytosis or affect the cells sensitivity to calcium-dependent exocytosis (56–59). Evidence for a role of Rab3A in Ca^{2+}-dependent exocytosis has been obtained in studies using transient overexpression or microinjection of Rab3A and Rab3A mutants. Overexpression of wild type or the active Rab3A mutant (Rab3AQ81L) causes a marked inhibition of Ca^{2+}-dependent secretion from adrenal chromaffin cells and PC12 cells (57,58). While overexpression of Rab3AT36N, a dominant negative mutant homologous to the H-RasT17N mutant, was not able to inhibit Ca^{2+}-dependent exocytosis (58).

Gene knockout mice lacking Rab3A protein survive to maturity and remain fertile suggesting that perhaps Rab3A is not the essential element for synaptic vesicle

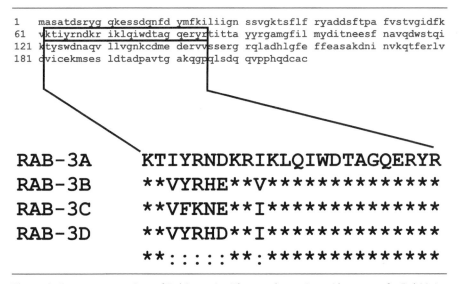

```
  1    masatdsryg qkessdqnfd ymfkiliign ssvgktsflf ryaddsftpa fvstvgidfk
 61    vktiyrndkr iklqiwdtag qeryrtitta yyrgamgfil myditneesf navqdwstqi
121    ktyswdnaqv llvgnkcdme dervvsserg rqladhlgfe ffeasakdni nvkqtferlv
181    dvicekmses ldtadpavtg akqgpqlsdq qvpphqdcac
```

RAB-3A   **KTIYRNDKRIKLQIWDTAGQERYR**
RAB-3B   ****VYRHE**V***************
RAB-3C   ****VFKNE**I***************
RAB-3D   ****VYRHD**I***************
              ::::::.*************

Figure 1. Sequence comparison of Rab3 proteins: The complete amino acid sequence for Rab3A is shown. Amino acids 62–85, which encompass the proposed CaM binding sequence in Rab3A, is highlighted and compared to the homologous regions in the Rab3B, 3C, and 3D proteins. Conservative amino acid changes are shown as dots underneath the sequences.

exocytosis (56). Instead, such transgenic animals have elevated levels of the Rab effector protein Rabphillin. The expression of this Rab3–interacting protein is specifically elevated while many other Rab3-effectors tested were unchanged (56). Based on these studies it was proposed that Rab3A plays a role in the recruitment of synaptic vesicles for exocytosis (56). Using cultured hippocampal cells deficient in Rab3A protein, it was shown that synaptic vesicles accumulate in the peripheral regions of these cells, thus, suggesting a role for Rab3A in a late step during vesicle fusion (60). Rab3A deficient mice also show a reduced development of postsynaptic long-term potentiation in the CA3 region of the hippocampus (61). In addition, intracellular injections of antisense oligonucleotides targeted to *rab3a* mRNA in adrenal chromaffin cells resulted in an increased potential to respond to repetitive stimulations while in control cells a desensitization occurs following repetitive stimulation (57). In short, Rab3A likely contributes to synaptic plasticity by modulating synaptic vesicle trafficking but is not essential for basal levels of synaptic transmission.

Some cells, such as platelet and endothelial cells do not express Rab3A protein; yet still have regulated secretion (62,63). Since other Rab family members, such as Rab3B, are present it is likely that they contribute to the regulated exocytosis in these cells (63,64). Though work on Rab3B is more limited, studies suggest that Rab3B may promote calcium-dependent exocytosis (65,66). Experiments using antisense oligonucleotides directed at *rab3B* mRNA have shown that anterior pituitary cells respond by a reduction in Ca^{2+}-dependent secretion (66). When domi-nant active Rab3B mutants are stably expressed in PC12 cells lacking endogenous Rab3B, Ca^{2+}-dependent secretion of norepinephrine was markedly stimulated (65). Thus, Rab3B apparently functions in opposition to Rab3A. However, since both Rab3A and Rab3B are able to bind CaM it is not likely that CaM functions as a GTPase activating protein and thus, promoting Rab inactivation.

The action of CaM on both Rab3A and -3B at first glance seems to be coun-terproductive due to the opposing functions of the two proteins. However, it is not unusual for CaM binding proteins with opposing functions to be activated by CaM. For example, CaM activates both CaM kinase (I and II), which phosphorylates target proteins, and the CaM-dependent phosphatase calcineurin, which dephosphorylates target proteins (48). In the case of Rab3, the inhibition or promotion of synaptic vesicle release may be determined by the action of the Rab3 protein on its effec-tor protein(s) and/or by changes in the intracellular Ca^{2+} concentration.

A MODEL FOR THE ROLE OF CALMODULIN IN RAB3 FUNCTION

The negative regulation of storage granule exocytosis by Rab3A has been linked to an interaction with CaM (13). Although the mechanism of calmodulin's involvement in the process is still unclear, it has been established that CaM can dissociate Rab3A from synaptic membranes (25). Recently, we have described that Rab3B can also bind calmodulin in cells lacking Rab3A in a guanine nucleotide-independent manner (49). As mentioned above CaM binds to a region between amino acids 62–85 in Rab3A. This region is very similar in all four Rab isoforms with only 6 conservative changes (Figure 1). Thus, not surprisingly CaM also binds to Rab3B, which is involved in promoting storage granule exocytosis. In addition, it seems plausible that calmodulin not only regulates Rab3A and Rab3B but likely also Rab3C and Rab3D. Although it cannot be ruled out, CaM's primary function may not be to promote activation or deactivation of the Rab protein by GTP-GDP exchange. Previous work on another Ras-related GTP-binding protein that binds CaM, called Ral, suggested regulation in this manner (67). Instead, CaM may facilitate the dissociation of Rab by RabGDI in the presence of increased levels of intracellular Ca^{2+} concentrations (25). A model depicting how this may function is shown (Figure 2).

It has been reported that CaM binds with higher affinity to GTP-Rab in pref-erence to the GDP-bound form (34), suggesting that nucleotide exchange may be facilitated by CaM. More recent work by Park et al. (68) has shown that Ca^{2+}/CaM can cause the exchange of GDP for GTP but not while Rab3 and RabGDI are in a complex. Thus, a signal (e.g. increase in intracellular Ca^{2+}) may cause a change in the Rab-GDI interaction and allow CaM to exert its effect(s) (Figure 3). This process will be reversed when CaM bound to GDP-Rab3 is replaced with Rab-GDI. Thus, CaM competes with RabGDI when Rab3 is in the GDP bound form, but Rab3-GTP bound to CaM is unimpeded when carrying out its physiological function. Though RabGDI has a greater affinity for Rab3-GDP than CaM, the Rab3-

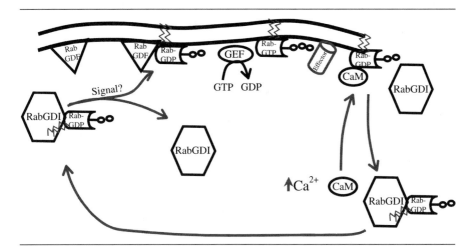

Figure 2. The Rab cycle and proposed role of calmodulin: Cytosolic Rab–GDP bound to RabGDI is targeted to the membrane by an upstream signal. A membrane bound RabGDI dissociation factor (Rab GDF) displaces RabGDI from the Rab complex. Removal of RabGDI allows the Rab protein to bind to the appropriate membrane while an initial targeting of *de novo* synthesized Rab proteins is facilitated by Rab Escort proteins (not shown). A guanine nucleotide exchange factor (GEF) allows the Rab protein to perform its function as a molecular switch by causing the exchange of GDP for GTP. The replacement of GDP causes a conformational change to occur on the Rab protein such that effector-binding region is exposed. The active-Rab protein is then able to bind to the appropriate effector and perform its function in the cell. Following this, a GTPase activating protein (GAP) enhances the hydrolysis of GTP to GDP thus recovering the inactive state. Recent *in vitro* evidence suggests that, like RabGDI, Ca^{2+}/CaM causes the dissociation of Rab from membranes. This is a generalized model that may be operative for other LMWG proteins that bind CaM.

GTP/CaM complex may predominate when Ca^{2+} levels are elevated. In such instances, CaM bound to Rab3-GTP may elicit other physiological responses by stimulating downstream effector molecules (Figure 3).

CONCLUSION

Calmodulin is an integral part of the signal transduction pathways operative in the cell. Now that role has expanded to the regulation of G˙protein function through a variety of mechanisms that are still being defined. However, it is clear that CaM plays a significant role in the function of Rab3 proteins by its ability to interact with these G proteins. Future research will be directed towards defining precisely the impact of Rab3-CaM interaction in controlling cell function.

ACKNOWLEDEGMENT

This work is supported by a grant from the Heart & Stroke Foundation of Manitoba to RPB and by a University of Manitoba Graduate Studies fellowship to R. Sidhu.

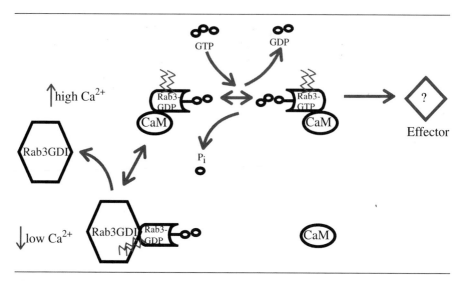

Figure 3. Rab GTP-GDP exchange cycle: In the inactive state RabGDI maintains the Rab protein in the cytosol as complex by masking the hydrophobic lipid tail. Upon removal of RabGDI from the complex by RabGDF and translocation to the membrane the Rab protein is then able to act on the appropriate effectors. As mentioned in the text, GTP is exchanged for GDP by the action of GEFs while the GTP is hydrolyzed to GDP with the aid of GAPs. In the figure, CaM is shown free and bound to both GDP- and GTP-Rab. Although CaM prefers GTP-bound Rab3, it is less selective than RabGDI for the nucleotide state. Thus, it is still unclear whether CaM causes dissociation prior to or following GTP hydrolysis. In the case of Rab3A, the GTP-bound form may interact with effectors in the cell that inhibit exocytosis while Rab3B-GTP may bind to effectors that promote exocytosis.

REFERENCES

1. Wieland T, Chen CK. 1999. Regulators of G-protein signaling: a novel protein family involved in timely deactivation and desensitization of signaling via heterotrimeric G proteins. Arch Pharmacol 360:14–26.
2. Offermanns S, Simon MI. 1996. Organization of transmembrane signalling by heterotrimeric G proteins. Cancer Surv 27:177–198.
3. Clapham DE, Neer EJ. 1997. G protein beta gamma subunits. Annu Rev Pharmacol Toxicol 37:167–203.
4. Berman DM, Gilman AG. 1998. Mammalian RGS proteins: barbarians at the gate. J Biol Chem 273:1269–1272.
5. Ross EM, Wilkie TM. 2000. GTPase-activating proteins for heterotrimeric G proteins: regulators of G protein signaling (RGS) and RGS-like proteins. Annu Rev Biochem 69:795–827.
6. Zerangue N, Jan LY. 1998. G-protein signaling: fine-tuning signaling kinetics. Curr Biol 8:R313–R316.
7. Bhullar RP. 1997. Small-molecular-weight G proteins. In: Neuromethods, Vol 31: G Protein methods and protocols. Ed RK Mishra, BG Baker and AA Boulton. New York: Humana Press. Inc.
8. Takai Y, Sasaki T, Matozaki T. 2001. Small GTP-binding proteins. Physiol Rev 81:153–208.
9. Pereira-Leal JB, Seabra MC. 2001. Evolution of the Rab family of small GTP-binding proteins. J Mol Biol 313:889–901.
10. Martinez O, Goud B. 1998. Rab proteins. Biochim Biophys Acta 1404:101–112.
11. Schimmoller F, Simon I, Pfeffer SR. 1998. Rab GTPases, directors of vesicle docking. J Biol Chem 273:22161–22164.

12. Stenmark H, Olkkonen VM. 2001. The Rab GTPase family. Genome Biol 2:Reviews3007.1–Reviews3007.7.
13. Coppola T, Perret-Menoud V, Luthi S, Farnsworth CC, Glomset JA, Regazzi R. 1999. Disruption of Rab3-calmodulin interaction, but not other effector interactions, prevents Rab3 inhibition of exocytosis. EMBO J 18:5885–5891.
14. Chin D, Means AR. 2000. Calmodulin: a prototypical calcium sensor. Trends Cell Biol 10:322–328.
15. Crivici A, Ikura M. 1995. Molecular and structural basis of target recognition by calmodulin. Annu Rev Biophys Biomol Struct 24:85–116.
16. Putney JW. 1998. Calcium signaling: Up, down, up, down . . . what's the point? Science 279:191–192.
17. Soderling TR. 1999. The Ca^{2+}-calmodulin-dependent protein kinase cascade. Trends Biochem Sci 24:232–236.
18. Sudhof TC. 1997. Function of Rab3 GDP-GTP exchange. Neuron 18:519–522.
19. Pfeffer SR, Dirac-Svejstrup AB, Soldati T. 1995. Rab GDP dissociation inhibitor: putting rab GTPases in the right place. J Biol Chem 270:17057–17059.
20. Regazzi R, Kikuchi A, Takai Y, Wollheim CB. 1992. The small GTP-binding proteins in the cytosol of insulin-secreting cells are complexed to GDP dissociation inhibitor proteins. J Biol Chem 267:17512–17519.
21. Ullrich O, Stenmark H, Alexandrov K, Huber LA, Kaibuchi K, Sasaki T, Takai Y, Zerial M. 1993. Rab GDP dissociation inhibitor as a general regulator for the membrane association of rab proteins. J Biol Chem 268:18143–18150.
22. Araki S, Kaibuchi K, Sasaki T, Hata Y, Takai Y. 1991. Role of the C-terminal region of smg p25A in its interaction with membranes and the GDP/GTP exchange protein. Mol Cell Biol 11:1438–1447.
23. Khosravi-Far R, Lutz RJ, Cox AD, Conroy L, Bourne JR, Sinensky M, Balch WE, Buss JE, Der CJ. 1991. Isoprenoid modification of rab proteins terminating in CC or CXC motifs. Proc Natl Acad Sci USA 88:6264–6268.
24. Musha T, Kawata M, Takai Y. 1992. The geranylgeranyl moiety but not the methyl moiety of the smg-25A/rab3A protein is essential for the interactions with membrane and its inhibitory GDP/GTP exchange protein. J Biol Chem 267:9821–9825.
25. Park JB, Farnsworth CC, Glomset JA. 1997. Ca^{2+}/calmodulin causes Rab3A to dissociate from synaptic membranes. J Biol Chem 272:20857–20865.
26. Alory C, Balch WE. 2000. Molecular basis for Rab prenylation. J Cell Biol 150:89–103.
27. Pfeffer SR. 1994. Rab GTPases: master regulators of membrane trafficking. Curr Opin Cell Biol 6:522–526.
28. Soldati T, Shapiro AD, Svejstrup AB, Pfeffer SR. 1994. Membrane targeting of the small GTPase Rab9 is accompanied by nucleotide exchange. Nature 369:76–78.
29. Dirac-Svejstrup AB, Sumizawa T, Pfeffer SR. 1997. Identification of a GDI displacement factor that releases endosomal Rab GTPases from Rab-GDI. EMBO J 16:465–472.
30. Ullrich O, Horiuchi H, Bucci C, Zerial M. 1994. Membrane association of Rab5 mediated by GDP-dissociation inhibitor and accompanied by GDP/GTP exchange. Nature 368:157–160.
31. Chung SH, Takai Y, Holz RW. 1995. Evidence that the Rab3a-binding protein, rabphilin3a, enhances regulated secretion. Studies in adrenal chromaffin cells. J Biol Chem 270:16714–16718.
32. Wang Y, Okamoto M, Schmitz F, Hofmann K, Sudhof TC. 1997. Rim is a putative Rab3 effector in regulating synaptic-vesicle fusion. Nature 388:593–598.
33. Clabecq A, Henry JP, Darchen F. 2000. Biochemical characterization of Rab3-GTPase-activating protein reveals a mechanism similar to that of Ras-GAP. J Biol Chem 275:31786–31791.
34. Kajio H, Olszewski S, Rosner PJ, Donelan MJ, Geoghegan KF, Rhodes CJ. 2001. A low-affinity Ca^{2+}-dependent association of calmodulin with the Rab3A effector domain inversely correlates with insulin exocytosis. Diabetes 50:2029–2039.
35. Pfeffer SR. 2001. Rab GTPases: specifying and deciphering organelle identity and function. Trends Cell Biol 11:487–491.
36. Augustine GJ, Burns ME, DeBello WM, Hilfiker S, Morgan JR, Schweizer FE, Tokumaru H, Umayahara K. 1999. Proteins involved in synaptic vesicle trafficking. J Physiol 520:33–41.
37. Hess SD, Doroshenko PA, Augustine GJ. 1993. A functional role for GTP-binding proteins in synaptic vesicle cycling. Science 259:1169–1172.
38. Novick P, Field C, Schekman R. 1980. Identification of 23 complementation groups required for post-translational events in the yeast secretory pathway. Cell 21:205–215.

39. Soldati T, Rancano C, Geissler H, Pfeffer SR. 1995. Rab7 and Rab9 are recruited onto late endosomes by biochemically distinguishable processes. J Biol Chem 270:25541–25548.

40. Ayad N, Hull M, Mellman I. 1997. Mitotic phosphorylation of rab4 prevents binding to a specific receptor on endosome membranes EMBO J 16:4497–4507.

41. Dorn GW 2nd, Mochly-Rosen D. 2002. Intracellular transport mechanisms of signal transducers. Ann Rev Physiol 64:407–429.

42. Chattopadhyaya R, Meador WE, Means AR, Quiocho FA. 1992. Calmodulin structure refined at 1.7 Å resolution. J Mol Biol 228:1177–1192.

43. Meador WE, Means AR, Quiocho FA. 1992. Target enzyme recognition by calmodulin: 2.4 Å structure of a calmodulin-peptide complex. Science 257:1251–1255.

44. Matsushima N, Hayashi N, Jinbo Y, Izumi Y. 2000. Ca^{2+}-bound calmodulin forms a compact globular structure on binding four trifluoperazine molecules in solution. Biochem J 347:211–215.

45. Wriggers W, Mehler E, Pitici F, Weinstein H, Schulten K. 1998. Structure and dynamics of calmodulin in solution. Biophys J 74:1622–1639.

46. Finn BE, Drakenberg T, Forsen S. 1993. The structure of apo-calmodulin. A ^1H NMR examination of the carboxy-terminal domain. FEBS Lett 336:368–374.

47. Rhoads AR, Friedberg F. 1997. Sequence motifs for calmodulin regulation. FASEB J 11:331–340.

48. James P, Vorherr T, Carafoli E. 1995. Calmodulin-binding domains: just two faced or multi-faceted? Trends Biochem Sci 20:38–42.

49. Sidhu RS, Bhullar RP. 2001. Rab3B in human platelet is membrane bound and interacts with Ca^{2+}/calmodulin. Biochem Biophys Res Commun 289:1039–1043.

50. Lin CG, Lin YC, Liu HW, Kao LS. 1997. Characterization of Rab3A, Rab3B and Rab3C: different biochemical properties and intracellular localization in bovine chromaffin cells. Biochem J 324:85–90.

51. Valentijn JA, Jamieson JD. 1998. On the role of rab GTPases: what can be learned from the developing pancreas. Biochem Biophys Res Commun 243:331–336.

52. Chung SH, Joberty G, Gelino EA, Macara IG, Holz RW. 1999. Comparison of the effects on secretion in chromaffin and PC12 cells of Rab3 family members and mutants. Evidence that inhibitory effects are independent of direct interaction with Rabphilin3. J Biol Chem 274:18113–18120.

53. Darchen F, Zahraoui A, Hammel F, Monteils MP, Tavitian A, Scherman D. 1990. Association of the GTP-binding protein Rab3A with bovine adrenal chromaffin granules. Proc Natl Acad Sci USA 87:5692–5696.

54. Darchen F, Senyshyn J, Brondyk WH, Taatjes DJ, Holz RW, Henry JP, Denizot JP, Macara IG. 1995. The GTPase Rab3a is associated with large dense core vesicles in bovine chromaffin cells and rat PC12 cells. J Cell Sci 108:1639–1649.

55. Fischer von Mollard G, Mignery GA, Baumert M, Perin MS, Hanson TJ, Burger PM, Jahn R, Sudhof TC. 1990. Rab3 is a small GTP-binding protein exclusively localized to synaptic vesicles. Proc Natl Acad Sci USA 87:1988–1992.

56. Geppert M, Bolshakov VY, Siegelbaum SA, Takei K, De Camilli P, Hammer RE, Sudhof TC. 1994. The role of Rab3A in neurotransmitter release. Nature 369:493–497.

57. Johannes L, Lledo PM, Roa M, Vincent JD, Henry JP, Darchen F. 1994. The GTPase Rab3a negatively controls calcium-dependent exocytosis in neuroendocrine cells. EMBO J 13:2029–2037.

58. Holz RW, Brondyk WH, Senter RA, Kuizon L, Macara IG. 1994. Evidence for the involvement of Rab3A in Ca^{2+}-dependent exocytosis from adrenal chromaffin cells. J Biol Chem 269:10229–10234.

59. Oishi H, Sasaki T, Nagano F, Ikeda W, Ohya T, Wada M, Ide N, Nakanishi H, Takai Y. 1998. Localization of the Rab3 small G protein regulators in nerve terminals and their involvement in Ca^{2+}-dependent exocytosis. J Biol Chem 273:34580–34585.

60. Geppert M, Goda Y, Stevens CF, Sudhof TC. 1997. The small GTP-binding protein Rab3A regulates a late step in synaptic vesicle fusion. Nature 387:810–814.

61. Castillo PE, Janz R, Sudhof TC, Tzounopoulos T, Malenka RC, Nicoll RA. 1997. Rab3A is essential for mossy fibre long-term potentiation in the hippocampus. Nature 388:590–593.

62. van der Meulen J, Bhullar RP, Chancellor-Maddison KA. 1991. Association of a 24-kDa GTP-binding protein, G_n24, with human platelet α-granule membranes. FEBS Lett 291:122–126.

63. Karniguian A, Zahraoui A, Tavitian A. 1993. Identification of small GTP-binding rab proteins in human platelets: thrombin-induced phosphorylation of rab3B, rab6, and rab8 proteins. Proc Natl Acad Sci USA 90:7647–7651.

64. Nagata K, Okano Y, Nozawa Y. 1997. Differential expression of low Mr GTP-binding proteins in human megakaryoblastic leukemia cell line, MEG-01, and their possible involvement in the differentiation process. Thromb Haemost 77:368–375.

65. Weber E, Jilling T, Kirk KL. 1996. Distinct functional properties of Rab3A and Rab3B in PC12 neuroendocrine cells. J Biol Chem 271:6963–6971.
66. Lledo PM, Vernier P, Vincent JD, Mason WT, Zorec R. 1993. Inhibition of Rab3B expression attenuates Ca^{2+}-dependent exocytosis in rat anterior pituitary cells. Nature 364:540–544.
67. Wang KL, Roufogalis BD. 1999. Ca^{2+}/calmodulin stimulates GTP binding to the ras-related protein ral-A. J Biol Chem 274:14525–14528.
68. Park JB, Kim JS, Lee JY, Kim J, Seo JY, Kim AR. 2002. GTP binds to Rab3A in a complex with Ca^{2+}/calmodulin. Biochem J 362:651–657.

Signal Transduction and Cardiac Hypertrophy,
edited by N.S. Dhalla, L.V. Hryshko,
E. Kardami & P.K. Singal
Kluwer Academic Publishers, Boston, 2003

Novel Aspects of Mechanical Signaling in Cardiac Tissue

Robert Denyer, Sandhya Sanghi,
Rajesh Kumar, and David E. Dostal

The Cardiovascular Research Institute
Division of Molecular Cardiology
The Texas A&M University System Health Science Center
Temple, TX 76504

Summary. Cardiac hypertrophy is a common outcome of hypertension or myocardial infarction and a major contributor to cardiovascular morbidity and mortality. Under increased hemodynamic load, the heart compensates by undergoing compensatory hypertrophy, a response that restores lost function and normalizes wall stress. Although initially beneficial, hypertrophy is an independent risk factor for heart failure since sustained cardiac hypertrophy can lead to decompensation and subsequent failure. Since cardiac myocytes are terminally differentiated and lose the ability to replicate soon after birth, these cells respond to increased work load by an increase in cell size. An intriguing and unresolved aspect of this process has been the ability of myocytes to sense mechanical stimuli and convert it into intracellular growth signals. Recent studies have focused on identifying the underlying mechanisms responsible for cardiac hypertrophy. A number of mechanosensors and signal transduction pathways have been identified as potential regulators of the hypertrophic response. Integrins and stretch-activated calcium channels have been shown to couple to low-molecular weight GTPases (Ras, Rac, RhoA), mitogen-activated protein kinases and protein kinase C. This review will discuss the key aspects of these signal transduction mechanisms.

Key words: Angiotensin II, Cardiac Myocytes, Fibroblasts, Heart Failure, Mechanical Stretch, Myocardium, Integrins, Stretch-Activated Cation Channels.

Address for Correspondence: David E. Dostal, Ph.D., The Cardiovascular Research Institute, Division of Molecular Cardiology, The Texas A&M University System HSC, 1901 South 1st Street, Bldg. 162, Temple, TX 76504. Phone: (254) 778-4811 (ext. 6619), Fax: (254) 899-6165, E-mail: ddostal@medicine.tamu.edu

INTRODUCTION

Cardiac hypertrophy, an important compensatory mechanism in response to chronic increases in hemodynamic load, is defined as an increase in heart size resulting from an increase in cardiac myocyte cell volume. The hypertrophic process is initially beneficial because of an increase in the number of contractile units and a reduction in ventricular wall stress. However, sustained hemodynamic overloading of the myocardium eventually results in heart failure, which is characterized by chamber dilatation, contractile dysfunction, and impaired survival. Considerable research efforts have focused on molecular mechanisms responsible for transducing hemodynamic load into myocardial growth and the transition to terminal heart failure. A growing number of intracellular signaling pathways have been identified as important transducers of the hypertrophic response in cardiac myocytes. The mitogen-activated protein (MAP) kinase and Janus kinase/signal transducers and activators of transcription (JAK/STAT) pathways (Figure 1) are the primary signal transduction pathways activated by mechanical stress in cardiac tissue. Calcineurin, an intracellular phosphatase has been implicated as a regulator of the hypertrophic response (Figure 2). Recently, integrins and stretch-activated cation channels have been shown to associate with signaling molecules and are thought to be responsible for sensing and transducing mechanical stimuli. We will present an overview of the growth-related mechanotransduction systems present in cardiac tissue.

THE MITOGEN-ACTIVATED PROTEIN KINASE PATHWAY

Mitogen-activated protein kinases are serine/threonine kinases that become activated by phosphorylation on tyrosine/threonine and in turn phosphorylate and activate nuclear substrates such as c-myc, c-jun, ATF-2 and $p62^{TCF}$ and other kinases such as $p90^{RSK}$ and MAPKAP kinase-2 [1,2] (Figure 1). Three subfamilies of MAP kinases have been characterized: (1) extracellular-regulated kinases (ERKs); (2) c-Jun N-terminal kinases (JNKs); and (3) p38-MAP kinases. The later two kinase families are referred to as stress-activated protein kinases (SAPK), which are preferentially activated by environmental stress.

The extracellular-regulated kinase pathway

The ERK family consists of six isoforms, ERK1–6, in which ERK1 is the most highly expressed form in the myocardium. Expression of ERK1–3 have been shown to decrease during cardiac development, in which ERK3 has very low expression in the adult heart [3]. In cultured cardiac myocytes, mechanical stretch has been shown to activate ERK1/2, Ras and $p90^{RSK}$ [4–10] and increase expression of c-fos and skeletal α-actin, suggesting a link between ERK1/2 activation and stretch-induced cardiac hypertrophy [4]. Although the precise mechanism of activation is unknown, the process appears to involve protein kinase C (PKC), tyrosine kinases and Ras [7–9]. The proximal mechanisms by which mechanical load induces activation of ERKs in the myocardium are currently being studied and remain to be elucidated.

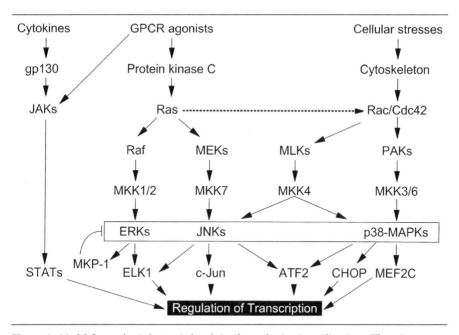

Figure 1. Model for mechanical stress-induced signal transduction in cardiac tissue. The mitogen-activated protein (MAP) kinase and Janus kinase and signal-transducers and activators of transcription (JAK/STAT) represent major pathways in cardiac tissue. G-protein-coupled receptors (GPCR) activate the MAP kinase pathways via Ras, which in turn stimulates Raf and MAP kinase kinase kinase (MEKs). MEKs lead to activation of MAP kinase kinase (MKK), which in turn lead to activation of three terminal MAP kinase effectors (extracellular-regulated kinases [ERKs]; c-Jun N-terminal kinases [JNKs], p38-MAP kinases), which regulate gene transcription. Mechanical stretch activates MAP kinase cascades via extracellular matrix and the cytoskeleton via the small G proteins Ras, Rac, Cdc42. Downstream targets of MAP kinases include nuclear transcription factors, such as ELK1, c-Jun, ATF2, CHOP and MEF2C. The JAK/STAT pathway is activated via gp 130 coupled mechanisms. Upon activation by JAKs, STATs dimerize and translocate to the nucleus resulting in induction of gene transcription. MAP kinase activation also results in activation and expression of MAP kinase phosphatases (e.g. MKP-1), which dephosphorylate and inactivate MAP kinases, leading to blockade of stretch-induced signaling.

The c-Jun N-terminal protein kinase pathway

JNK (c-Jun N-terminal protein kinase) was first reported to be activated in response to cellular stresses such as osmotic stress, UV irradiation, oxidative stress and heat shock. Although not activated by growth factors such as epidermal growth factor and basic fibroblast growth factor, JNK is activated by cytokines such as tumor necrosis factor-α and interleukin-1. Additionally, the JNK pathway has been demonstrated to have a role in mechanical stress-induced hypertrophy via phosphorylation of transcription factors c-Jun and ATF2. JNKs are encoded by three genes that all produce multiple products by alternative splicing yielding three isoforms: JNK1 (SAPK γ), JNK2 (SAPK α), and JNK3 (SAPK β), in which JNK1 and JNK2 are expressed in cardiac tissue (11). In cardiac myocytes, JNK isoforms are

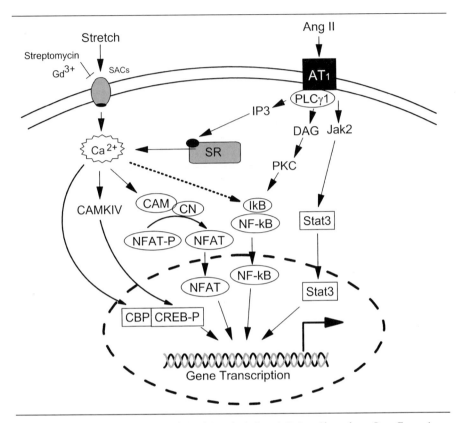

Figure 2. Schematic Depicting Coupling of Stretch-Activated Cation Channels to Gene Expression. Activation of stretch-activated cation channels (SACs) by mechanical stretch results in an influx of extracellular calcium ion (Ca^{2+}). Intracellular calcium can control gene expression by activating transcription factors in the cytoplasm (NFAT, NF-kb) or the nucleus (CREB). Intracellular calcium stimulates the Ca^{2+}-sensitive protein phosphatase calcineurin to dephosphorylate NFAT, which then enters the nucleus. When Ca^{2+} signaling stops, kinases in the nucleus rapidly phosphorylate NFAT, which then leaves the nucleus, and transcription of NF-AT-responsive genes ceases. The stimulatory action of calcium on the calmodulin (CAM)–calcineurin (CN) complex that dephosphorylates NFAT is inhibited by the immunosuppressants cyclosporin A (CsA) or FK506. An increase in Ca^{2+} can also trigger proteolysis of the inhibitory IKB subunit, allowing the active NF-kb subunit to enter the nucleus. CREB is a nuclear Ca^{2+}-responsive transcription factor phosphorylated by calmodulin kinases II and IV. Ca^{2+} acting within the nucleus is also responsible for activating the Ca^{2+} sensitive transcriptional co-activator CREB-binding protein (CBP). Cross-talk can occur with local factors, such as angiotensin II (Ang II) stimulates calcium mobilization and NF-kb activation. The AT_1 couples to phospholipase C1 (PLCγ1), which generates diacylglycerol (DAG) and inositol-1,4,5-trisphosphate (IP3). DAG activates Protein kinase C (PKC), which in turn phosphorylates IkB, thereby activating NF-kb. IP3 releases calcium ion (Ca^{2+}) from the sarcoplasmic reticulum (SR). The AT_1 receptor also activates JAK-STAT pathway, which leads to gene expression via Stat3 phosphorylation.

phosphorylated in response to mechanical stretch or G-protein-coupled receptor activation (12–14). JNK activation has been demonstrated in load-induced cardiac hypertrophy in rats, myocardial infarction and human heart failure (15–17). Mechanical stretch-induced activation of JNKs is poorly understood. In stretched myocytes, JNK activation has been shown to be independent of secreted angiotensin II (Ang II), extracellular calcium, and PKC activation (13). Although MEK4 and MEKK1 appear to activate JNKs (18,19), other proximal signaling mechanisms remain to be determined.

The p38-mitogen-activated protein kinase pathway

The p38 subfamily of MAP kinases have been shown to mediate stress-induced signaling in mammalian cells. The p38-MAP kinase family consists of six isoforms encoded by four genes (α, β, δ, γ) (20). The substrate for p38-MAP Kinase is MAP kinase-activated protein kinase-2 (MAPKAPK2). MAPKAPK2 can phosphorylate and activate the small heat-shock proteins Hsp 25 and Hsp 27 (21), which have cytoprotective effects in cardiac cells. Activation of the p38-MAP kinase cascade results in phosphorylation of ATF-2, which regulates gene expression. Upstream activators for p38-MAP kinases include MEK3, MEK4 and MEK6, and possibly MEK4 (20,22). Several reports suggest that the p38-MAP kinase pathway is involved in mechanical stretch-induced hypertrophy. For example, overexpression of activated MEK3 and MEK6 has been shown to induce hypertrophy and atrial natriuretic factor (ANP) expression in cultured neonatal rat cardiac myocytes (22,23). Pulsatile stretch has been shown to activate MAP kinase family members and focal-adhesion kinase (FAK) in cultured rat cardiac myocytes (7). In a mouse model, increased p38-MAP kinase activity was found during development of hypertrophy and heart failure in response to pressure-overload (23). Pharmacological inhibition of p38-MAP kinase activity with selective agonists has been shown to attenuate agonist-mediated hypertrophy in primary cultures of cardiac myocytes (22,24,25). In addition, pharmacologic or dominant-negative inhibition of p38-MAP kinase signaling significantly reduces agonist-induced ANP promoter activity in vitro (26,27). Further studies are required to determine whether p38-MAP kinase is a viable therapeutic target in the pressure-overloaded myocardium.

Mitogen-activated protein kinase phosphatases

In response to MAP kinase activation, a family of dual-specificity phosphatases becomes transcriptionally active and serve as counteracting factors, which directly regulate the magnitude and duration of ERK, JNK and p38-MAP kinase activation. These MAP kinase phosphatases (MKPs) dephosphorylate phospho-threonine and phospho-tyrosine residues in regulatory domains of MAP kinase family members (28,29). In cardiac tissue, MKP-1 has been demonstrated to have important regulatory effects on cardiac growth (30–32). Constitutive expression of MKP-1 in primary cultures of cardiac myocytes has been shown to block activation of MAP kinases, transcriptional responses and prevent agonist-induced hypertrophy (33,34). Transgenic mice expressing physiological levels of MKP-1 in the heart showed diminished developmental myocardial growth and attenuated hypertrophy in response to aortic banding and catecholamine infusion (34). These studies suggest that myocardium undergoing hypertrophy has decreased activation and expression of MKPs. However, the mechanisms by which mechanical and other hypertrophic stimuli regulate these phosphatases remain to be elucidated.

THE JANUS KINASE/SIGNAL TRANSDUCERS AND ACTIVATORS OF TRANSCRIPTION PATHWAY

The JAK/STAT pathway is a major signal transduction pathway of the cytokine superfamilies (35). JAK kinases were first identified as protein tyrosine kinases that associate with dimerized cytokine receptors activated by the ligands interferon-γ, interferon-α and interleukin-2. The JAK family consists of Jak1, Jak2, Jak3, Tyk2 and hopscotch. JAK kinases auto-phosphorylate on tyrosine and activate downstream proteins via tyrosine phosphorylation. The best characterized substrates of the JAK family are STAT proteins, which have a dual function, namely signal transduction in the cytoplasm and activation of transcription in the nucleus (36). Several STAT isoforms (STAT1–4, 5A, 5B, 6) have been identified in cardiac tissue (37–39). The JAK/STAT pathway has been shown to be activated in the pressure-overloaded rat heart (40). In this animal model, gp130, and cardiotrophin-1, leukemia inhibitory factor (LIF) and interleukin-6 were involved in activation of the JAK/STAT pathway (40). Both Ang II-dependent (Tyk2 and JAK2) and Ang II-independent (JAK1) mechanisms have been shown to contribute to load-induced activation of the JAK/STAT pathway (41). These observations are consistent with those observed in primary cultures of rat cardiac myocytes in which mechanical stretch stimulated phosphorylation of JAK1, JAK2, TYK2 and gp130 (42). Recent studies (37,38) have demonstrated that the promoter of the angiotensinogen (Ao) gene serves as a target for STAT proteins in cardiac myocytes, thereby linking the JAK/STAT pathway to autocrine regulation of Ang II. When subjected to ischemic injury, a significant increase in binding of activated STAT5A and STAT6 to the Ao promoter has been demonstrated in rat hearts (39). Inhibition of JAK2, which phosphorylates STAT5A and STAT 6, inhibited STAT-Ao promoter interactions and decreased Ao mRNA levels. Activation of STAT3 and STAT5A has also been demonstrated in myocardial hypertrophy. Adenovirus-mediated gene transfer of either wild type or dominant-negative STAT3 was shown to either stimulate or attenuate LIF-induced hypertrophy in cardiac myocytes (43); in the transgenic mouse, overexpression of STAT3 targeted to the heart has been shown to result in cardiac hypertrophy (44). Further studies are required to determine the relative role humoral factors and mechanosensors (e.g. integrins) in activation of the JAK/STAT pathway in the normal and pathological heart.

GUANINE NUCLEOTIDE-BINDING PROTEINS

Another candidate mechanism of mechanotransduction involves guanine nucleotide-binding proteins (G-proteins) that couple cell surface receptors to the appropriate effectors. There are two forms of signal transducing G-proteins: the "small G-proteins" and the "heterotrimeric G-proteins". In the inactive state, all G-proteins are bound to GDP. G-protein activation occurs by exchange of GDP to GTP, which is enhanced by guanine-nucleotide exchange factors. The small G-proteins are single polypeptides composed of approximately 200 amino acids and regulate a wide variety of cellular responses (45). Although five members of small G-proteins have been characterized (Ras, Rho, ADP-ribosylation factors, Rab, and Ran), only the Ras and Rho subfamilies have been studied in cardiac tissue. Classical Ras isoforms regulate cell survival, growth, and division and these effects are probably mediated through the ERK subfamily of MAP kinases. Several Ras family members are readily detected in primary cultures of rat ventricular myocytes. Transient transfection with a constitutively active Ras has been shown to induce hypertrophic gene expression (46–48). Ras binds to and activates several signaling proteins including c-Raf, the lipid kinase phosphatidylinositol 3-kinase (PI3K) and Ral-GDS, a GTPase exchange factor (49). The Rho subfamily includes RhoA, Rac1 and Cdc42, which regulate the actin/myosin cytoskeleton (50). RhoA and Rac1 have been implicated in cardiac myocyte hypertrophy. Transfection or infection of RhoA stimulates expression of ANF (51–53), and dominant-negative mutants of RhoA have been shown to prevent α-adrenergic-stimulated or Ras-induced hypertrophy (54). Transfection or adenoviral infection of cardiac myocytes with constitutively active Rac1 have been demonstrated to increase ANF expression and cause morphological changes associated with myocyte hypertrophy (22,55).

The heterotrimeric G-proteins mediate intracellular responses to extracellular stimuli during cardiac development. These transducing proteins are composed of separate α and βγ subunits. Agonist occupation of a membrane-bound receptor catalyzes the GDP to GTP exchange on the Gα subunit and subsequent dissociation of Gα from Gβγ. Both subunits are free to modulate activity of downstream signaling effectors, typically adenylyl cyclase or phospholipase C (PLC) (56). Most receptor-effector coupling pathways in the heart are mediated by Gα subunits. Four classes of subunits (Gs, Gi, Gq, and G12) are expressed in cardiac tissue (57). In cardiac fibroblasts, Gq and Gi are activated within 1 min of stretching and the responses are modulated by the rate and magnitude of the stimulus (58). Evidence that Gq may have an important role in mediating in vivo hypertrophy has been demonstrated in a transgenic mouse in which Gq overexpression was localized to the heart. Hearts from these animals displayed increased expression of cardiac hypertrophy marker genes, increased cardiac mass and an increase in cardiac myocyte size (59). Akhter and colleagues (60) have reported an attenuation of pressure overload-induced hypertrophy in transgenic mice that expressed an inhibitor peptide of the Gq subunit. However, the inability of the Gq knockout to completely prevent ventricular hypertrophy indicates that other pathways (e.g. other G-proteins, integrins, calcium channels, cytokines) are also important for the growth process.

MECHANORECEPTORS

The mechanisms responsible for converting mechanical stretch into biochemical signals are poorly understood. Integrins and stretch-activated cation channels (SACs) are the primary candidates for mediating mechanical transduction in cardiac tissue. Integrins, previously thought to function only as cell adhesive molecules, are transmembrane receptors that orchestrate essential functions between the extracellular matrix (ECM) and cells of the myocardium. These functions include cell proliferation and differentiation, organogenesis, regulation of gene expression, cell adhesion and migration, signal transduction and cell death (61).

Integrin structure and expression in cardiac tissue

Integrins are noncovalently associated heterodimeric receptors composed of α and β subunits with each subunit consisting of a large extracellular domain, a transmembrane region, and a short cytoplasmic signaling domain (62). The extracellular domain binds to proteins of the ECM or to counter receptors on other cell walls, whereas the intracellular domain couples to specific signal transduction cascades. Extracellular matrix-integrin interactions result in dynamic bidirectional signaling across cell membranes. Extracellular events, such as ligands binding to integrins, result in "outside-in" signaling. Conversely, intracellular signals can alter the binding affinity of integrins to the extracellular matrix causing "inside-out" signaling. These intracellular signals result from agonists binding to non-integrin cellular receptors. Different combinations of α/β heterodimers result in different signals for events such as cardiac development and cardiac disease. Extracellular ligands have different binding affinities for specific α/β combinations and individual ECM ligands bind to multiple integrins with different affinities.

In mammals, the integrin family consists of more than 18 α and 8 β subunits which dimerize (α/β heterodimers) to form over 24 pairs of non-tyrosine kinase receptors with distinct and often overlapping specificity for ECM proteins. Of this large number, only a few α- and β-chains are expressed in the myocardium. Cardiac myocytes express α_1, α_3, α_5, α_6, α_7, α_{10} subunits (61). The α_1 and α_5 integrin subunits are embryonic forms which are downregulated postnatal, but increase expression following pressure overload through aortic constriction. In cardiac myocytes, the α-subunits predominantly associate with splice variants of β_1, in which β_{1D} is the major isoform expressed in cardiac myocytes (63,64). Adult cardiac myocytes primarily express $\alpha_3\beta_1$ through binding to laminin and type IV collagen, but poorly adhere to other collagens and fibronectin (65,66). In neonatal rat cardiac myocytes and fibroblasts, β_3 and β_5 subunits also form heterodimers with α-subunits to evoke functional responses (67,68). Cardiac fibroblasts express many of the same α-subunits as myocytes, except α_6 or α_7, as cardiac fibroblasts lack a laminin containing basement membrane. Fibroblasts contain α_v and the collagen-specific α_2 subunits, both of which are not expressed by adult cardiac myocytes (61). However, it has been recently demonstrated that neonatal rat cardiac myocytes express $\alpha_v\beta_5$ based on functional studies in which $\alpha_v\beta_5$ blockade was found to prevent stretch-induced expression of brain natriuretic peptide (BNP) (68). Differential expression of integrins suggests that mechanical signaling changes during development of the myocardium and differs among cardiac cell types.

Integrins in cardiac disease

Disease models of cardiac hypertrophy, dilated cardiomyopathy and myocardial infarction have altered expression of collagens, fibronectin, and other ECM components (69–73). Integrin expression is also altered in these disease states. However, it remains to be determined whether these changes are a primary response to the disease or due to secondary alterations in the ECM. Previous studies have linked overexpression of β_1 integrin to the hypertrophic response in neonatal ventricular myocytes. The β_1 integrin has been shown to augment α_1 adrenergic-mediated hypertrophy in vivo and adrenergic stimulation of isolated neonatal ventricular myocytes increased β_{1D} integrin expression >350% (74,75). In hypertrophied hearts of aortic-constricted rats and mice, integrins β_{1A}, β_{1D}, α_3, and α_{7b} are increased and embryonic integrins, α_1 and α_5, are reexpressed (61). As the heart undergoes hypertrophy, dilation, and then failure, the cardiac myocyte changes its cell morphology significantly. During this process, the integrins change position on the cell surface and contacts with the ECM and cytoskeleton undergo changes as well. Extracellular matrix-integrin mismatches result in the release of cardiac myocytes from their ECM attachment sites and eventual apoptosis. Additionally, matrix-integrin-cytoskeleton alterations subject the cells to mechanical forces that are detrimental to survival. Shedding of integrins into the extracellular space has been reported during progression to heart failure, however the functional role of these free integrins remains to be determined (61). Mechanical stimulation and several growth factors, most notably platelet-derived growth factor, insulin-like growth factor, Ang II and transforming growth factor-β, upregulate expression of several integrins and specific ECM components (61). Although growth factors appear to modulate expression in a paracrine or autocrine manner, the precise signaling mechanisms responsible for this regulation remain to be elucidated (61,76). Although significant changes occur in the myocardium following myocardial infarction or injury, little is known regarding the role of integrins in this remodeling process. Additional work is required to determine the precise roles of integrins in the acute and recovery stages of myocardial infarction.

Integrin signaling in the myocardium

Integrin signaling in the myocardium is poorly understood. Since integrins lack enzymatic activity, these molecules must depend on association with other cellular proteins to initiate intracellular signals. The β-subunit links integrins with the cytoskeleton and the signal transduction apparatus of the cell. Cytoplasmic domains of β-subunits associate with non-receptor kinases (FAK, Src), cytoskeletal proteins (actin, α-actinin, talin, vinculin, paxillin, tensin, p130^{cas}), adapter proteins such as Shc, small G-proteins (RhoA, Rac1), signal-transducing molecules (JNK, PKC, MAP kinases) and transcription factors (nuclear factor-kB [NF-kB]) (61,77–80). In cardiac myocytes and fibroblasts, β-subunits have been shown to couple to FAK, MAP kinase cascades, gene expression, and hypertrophic growth (61,74,75,81–83). In neonatal rat myocytes, stretch-dependent gene expression of BNP is mediated via

ERK, JNK and p38-MAP kinase activation and inhibited when β_1, β_3 and $\alpha_v\beta_5$ are blocked. On-the-other-hand, overexpression of β_{1D}-integrin increases expression of atrial natriuretic peptide (68,75,84). These studies suggest that the integrin-MAP kinase pathway is an important regulator of hypertrophic-related genes in cardiac myocytes. Much less is known regarding β-integrin coupling mechanisms in cardiac fibroblasts. In adult rat cardiac fibroblasts, mechanical stretch has been demonstrated to activate ERK and JNK, but not p38-MAP kinase via β_1 integrin, suggesting that differences in integrin coupling exist between cardiac myocytes and fibroblasts (85). Disruption of integrin signaling in neonatal rat ventricular myocytes prevents adrenergic-mediated hypertrophic growth (74,75). FAK, a primary mediator of integrin signaling, has been shown to play a role in the hypertrophic and adhesive response of cardiac myocytes and is activated by vascular endothelial growth factor. Additionally, adrenergic agonist-mediated activation of ERK1/2 and other hypertrophic responses have been significantly blunted by dominant inhibition of FAK. This suggests that integrin signaling may converge with other hypertrophic agonists through ERK1/2 (61).

In summary, integrins are transmembrane receptors that orchestrate many essential functions between the ECM and the myocardium in order to maintain homeostasis and respond to different physiologic and pathophysiologic stimuli. Although changes in integrin expression have been identified in many disease states, including myocardial infarction, pressure overload, volume overload, and dilated cardiomyopathy, the role of specific integrins and their mechanisms of action remain to be determined.

Stretch-activated cation channels

Stretch-activated cation channels allow the passage of the major monovalent physiological cations, sodium and potassium, and the divalent cation, calcium (Ca^{2+}) across the plasma membrane. Calcium influx through SACs has been shown to lead to waves of calcium-induced calcium release in cardiac myocytes (86), indicating that SACs serve as initial responders to mechanical stress. These channels are primarily responsible for regulating the intracellular Ca^{2+} involved in modulating length-dependent contractility in the ventricular myocardium (87–89). The influx of extracellular Ca^{2+} through SACs is blocked when cardiac cells are pretreated with streptomycin or gadolinium ion (Gd^{3+}) (90). Recent evidence indicates a role for SACs in the regulation of gene expression (Figure 2). In isolated rabbit hearts, stretch-induced activation of heat-shock factor-1 (transcription factor) and the increase in heat-shock protein 72 mRNA were blocked by Gd^{3+}, but not diltiazem (L-type calcium channel blocker) (91), indicating that SAC activation mediates these processes. As shown in Figure 2, an increase in intracellular Ca^{2+} can control gene expression by activating transcription factors in the cytoplasm (NFAT, NF-kB) and nucleus (Cyclic AMP-Dependent Response Element Binding Protein [CREB]). When Ca^{2+} signaling stops, kinases in the nucleus rapidly phosphorylate NFAT, which then leave the nucleus, and transcription of NFAT-responsive genes ceases. A prolonged period of Ca^{2+} signaling is required to maintain NFAT in its active form. The stimulatory action of calcium on the calmodulin (CAM)–calcineurin (CN) complex that dephosphorylates NFAT is inhibited by the immunosuppressants cyclosporin A or FK506. Recently, a conserved role for calcineurin-NFAT signaling has been identified in the heart (92). Pharmacologic calcineurin inhibition has been shown to attenuate dilated and hypertrophic cardiomyopathy in three different mouse models of heart disease and pressure overload hypertrophy in aortic-banded rats (93). Increases in intracellular Ca^{2+} also triggers proteolysis of the inhibitory IkB subunit, allowing the active NF-kB subunit to enter the nucleus. The nuclear Ca^{2+}-responsive transcription factor CREB is phosphorylated by calmodulin kinases II and IV. Calcium acting within the nucleus is also responsible for activating the Ca^{2+}-sensitive transcriptional co-activator CREB-binding protein (CBP). Although SACs are primarily associated with calcium mobilization, these channels can also mediate activation of the focal-adhesion complex and MAP kinases. Treatment with Gd^{3+} or removal of extracellular calcium has been shown to prevent tyrosine phosphorylation of FAK, paxillin and morphological changes in endothelial cells exposed to uniaxial cyclical stretch (94). However, in stretched fibroblasts, these treatments blocked FAK-mediated activation of p38-MAP kinase (95). It is therefore possible that SACs work cooperatively with integrins to effect changes in gene expression and cellular function in the myocardium.

DIRECTIONAL STRETCH AND SIGNALING

Ventricular myocytes are subjected to a complex set of mechanical forces during the cardiac cycle. A selective increase in either preload or afterload has been shown to promote very different changes in ventricular and cellular architecture (96), protein metabolism (97) and mechanical indicators of cardiac performance (98,99). During the progression of concentric and eccentric hypertrophy, regional changes occur with regard to cardiac myocyte cell morphology (100,101). Pressure-overload conditions, such as aortic stenosis and hypertension, result in concentric hypertrophy characterized by an increase in ventricular wall thickness with little or no chamber dilation and parallel addition of sarcomeres. Conversely, volume-overload conditions, such as mitral regurgitation and aortic insufficiency, promote eccentric (dilated) hypertrophy characterized by a relatively little increase in wall thickness and a disproportionately large increase in chamber volume.

Recent in vivo studies have demonstrated that cardiac myocytes can "sense" the direction of mechanical stretch. The direction of mechanical stretch has been shown to be a determinant of gene expression, contractile protein turnover, and sarcomere structure in primary cultures of myocytes (102–104). When aligned cardiac myocytes were subjected to specific directions of uniaxial stretch, differential effects were observed with respect to cardiac gene expression and protein synthesis (104). Stretch across the short-axis of aligned myocytes promoted the accumulation of contractile proteins, branching myofibrils and other phenotypic characteristics observed in concentric hypertrophy (104). These changes did not occur when cells were exposed to stretch across the long-axis. In addition, these responses were not altered by manipulating the contractile state (i.e. isoproterenol treatment) of the cells (104).

This indicates that a detection/transduction system exists which enables cultured myocytes to discriminate between different directions of stretch and operate independent of the length-tension relationship. However, the mechanism(s) responsible for detecting the direction of mechanical stretch remain to be elucidated. Receptors capable of recognizing this information must have a unique and polarized distribution that allows for detection of a specific direction of stretch. This criteria appears to be met by matrix receptors of the integrin family. In neonatal rat cardiac myocytes, the $\alpha_1\beta_1$ integrin is preferentially distributed along the peripheral domains of the Z-discs (105). The concentration of $\alpha_1\beta_1$ integrins at the Z-discs could allow these molecules to serve as a discrimination and signal transduction system for converting physical information into the intracellular environment.

REGULATION OF THE RENIN-ANGIOTENSINSIN SYSTEM BY MECHANICAL STRETCH

The development of cardiac hypertrophy induced by hemodynamic load is very likely triggered by mechanical stress. However, there is considerable evidence that growth promoting factors, such as Ang II and endothelin-1 are involved. In neonate and adult myocytes, acute exposure (5–30 min) to mechanical stretch causes autocrine release of Ang II (106–110) and longer exposures (8–48 h) increase mRNA expression of angiotensin type I (AT_1) and type II (AT_2) receptors, angiotensinogen (Ao) and renin (108,111–113). A portion of the stretch induced increase in Ao gene expression occurs via AT_1 coupled mechanisms in neonatal and adult rat ventricular myocytes (112). In primary cultures of neonatal rat cardiac myocytes, the AT_1-dependent increase in Ao gene expression occurs primarily via activation of the JAK/STAT pathway (38,114–116). Acute pressure overload of the myocardium also activates the JAK-STAT system in the adult heart (41), suggesting that this pathway may be an important regulator of Ao gene expression in the pathological heart. In primary cultures of adult rat ventricular myocytes, mechanical stretch also increases p53 binding to the promoter regions of genes for Ao and AT_1 (117). The mechanosensor, proximal signaling mechanisms, and associated autocrine secretory pathways remain to be elucidated.

FUTURE DIRECTIONS

Myocardial stress is associated with alterations in gene expression that reflect the nature of the initial event, as well as in compensated and decompensated stages of cardiac failure. The development of cDNA microarray technology has allowed researchers to monitor expression of thousands of genes associated with the physiological status of the tissue. Characterization of gene expression under various cellular states has proved useful for identifying the underlying cellular pathophysiology. Microarray analysis has revealed that approximately 50 genes are differentially expressed in several models of cardiac hypertrophy, including transgenic and pressure-overload models (118–120). Additionally, more than 200 genes have been shown to be differentially expressed in response to myocardial infarction (121). Though these data look impressive, more comprehensive studies are required to identify genes responsible for initiation and progression of heart disease. Although cDNA microarray and other methods of gene expression profiling appear useful, the power of these technologies will not be fully established until they have been integrated with other biological information, such as biochemical pathways and biomedical literature for each associated gene. Expression data have limitations because mRNA levels do not necessarily reflect protein levels. Additionally, alternative splicing of hnRNA from a single gene can produce more than one protein. There are several post-transcriptional and post-translational events that can also affect the abundance and activity of proteins, some of which depend on the phenotype of the cell. For example, several proteins undergo chemical modifications essential for their biological activity, such as glycosylation and phosphorylation. All of these events make proteome diversity several orders of magnitude greater than genome diversity. Thus, both cDNA microarray analysis and proteinomics are essential for unraveling relationships between mechanical stress, gene expression, protein synthesis and cardiac function in the normal and diseased heart.

In conclusion, further study of the basic cellular mechanisms underlying load-induced mechanotransduction and gene expression will continue to provide insight into approaches to target cardiac hypertrophy. However, elucidation of the molecular basis of stress-induced hypertrophy remains a challenge due to the complex temporal and spatial interactions that occur between integrins, stretch-activated cation channels and signaling cascades activated by growth factors.

REFERENCES

1. Davis RJ. 1993. The mitogen-activated protein kinase signal transduction pathway. J Biol Chem 268:14553–14556.
2. Dalby KN, Morrice N, Caudwell FB, Avruch J, Cohen P. 1998. Identification of regulatory phosphorylation sites in mitogen-activated protein kinase (MAPK)-activated protein kinase-1a/p90rsk that are inducible by MAPK. J Biol Chem 273:1496–1505.
3. Boulton TG, Nye SH, Robbins DJ, Ip NY, Radziejewska E, Morgenbesser SD, DePinho RA, Panayotatos N, Cobb MH, Yancopoulos GD. 1991. ERKs: a family of protein-serine/threonine kinases that are activated and tyrosine phosphorylated in response to insulin and NGF. Cell 65: 663–675.
4. Sadoshima J, Izumo S. 1993. Mechanical stretch rapidly activates multiple signal transduction pathways in cardiac myocytes: potential involvement of an autocrine/paracrine mechanism. Embo J 12:1681–1692.
5. Yamazaki T, Tobe K, Hoh E, Maemura K, Kaida T, Komuro I, Tamemoto H, Kadowaki T, Nagai R, Yazaki Y. 1993. Mechanical loading activates mitogen-activated protein kinase and S6 peptide kinase in cultured rat cardiac myocytes. J Biol Chem 268:12069–12076.
6. Nyui N, Tamura K, Mizuno K, Ishigami T, Hibi K, Yabana M, Kihara M, Fukamizu A, Ochiai H, Umemura S, Murakami K, Ohno S, Ishii M. 1997. Stretch-induced MAP kinase activation in cardiomyocytes of angiotensinogen-deficient mice. Biochem Biophys Res Commun 235:36–41.
7. Seko Y, Takahashi N, Tobe K, Kadowaki T, Yazaki Y. 1999. Pulsatile stretch activates mitogen-activated protein kinase (MAPK) family members and focal adhesion kinase (p125(FAK)) in cultured rat cardiac myocytes. Biochem Biophys Res Commun 259:8–14.
8. Yamazaki T, Komuro I, Kudoh S, Zou Y, Shiojima I, Mizuno T, Takano H, Hiroi Y, Ueki K, Tobe K, et al. 1995. Mechanical stress activates protein kinase cascade of phosphorylation in neonatal rat cardiac myocytes. J Clin Invest 96:438–446.
9. Kashiwagi Y, Haneda T, Osaki J, Miyata S, Kikuchi K. 1998. Mechanical stretch activates a pathway linked to mevalonate metabolism in cultured neonatal rat heart cells. Hypertens Res 21:109–119.
10. Kudoh S, Komuro I, Hiroi Y, Zou Y, Harada K, Sugaya T, Takekoshi N, Murakami K, Kadowaki T,

Yazaki Y. 1998. Mechanical stretch induces hypertrophic responses in cardiac myocytes of angiotensin II type 1a receptor knockout mice. J Biol Chem 273:24037–24043.

11. Ito M, Yoshioka K, Akechi M, Yamashita S, Takamatsu N, Sugiyama K, Hibi M, Nakabeppu Y, Shiba T, Yamamoto KI. 1999. JSAP1, a novel jun N-terminal protein kinase (JNK)-binding protein that functions as a Scaffold factor in the JNK signaling pathway. Mol Cell Biol 19:7539–7548.

12. Choukroun G, Hajjar R, Kyriakis JM, Bonventre JV, Rosenzweig A, Force T. 1998. Role of the stress-activated protein kinases in endothelin-induced cardiomyocyte hypertrophy. J Clin Invest 102:1311–1320.

13. Komuro I, Kudo S, Yamazaki T, Zou Y, Shiojima I, Yazaki Y. 1996. Mechanical stretch activates the stress-activated protein kinases in cardiac myocytes. Faseb J 10:631–636.

14. Yano M, Kim S, Izumi Y, Yamanaka S, Iwao H. 1998. Differential activation of cardiac c-jun amino-terminal kinase and extracellular signal-regulated kinase in angiotensin II-mediated hypertension. Circ Res 83:752–760.

15. Cook SA, Sugden PH, Clerk A. 1999. Activation of c-Jun N-terminal kinases and p38-mitogen-activated protein kinases in human heart failure secondary to ischaemic heart disease. J Mol Cell Cardiol 31:1429–1434.

16. Li WG, Zaheer A, Coppey L, Oskarsson HJ. 1998. Activation of JNK in the remote myocardium after large myocardial infarction in rats. Biochem Biophys Res Commun 246:816–820.

17. Choukroun G, Hajjar R, Fry S, del Monte F, Haq S, Guerrero JL, Picard M, Rosenzweig A, Force T. 1999. Regulation of cardiac hypertrophy in vivo by the stress-activated protein kinases/c-Jun NH(2)-terminal kinases. J Clin Invest 104:391–398.

18. Cohen P. 1997. The search for physiological substrates of MAP and SAP kinases in mammalian cells. Trends in Cell Biology 7:353–361.

19. Tournier C, Whitmarsh AJ, Cavanagh J, Barrett T, Davis RJ. 1997. Mitogen-activated protein kinase kinase 7 is an activator of the c-Jun NH2-terminal kinase. Proc Natl Acad Sci USA 94:7337–7342.

20. New L, Han J. 1998. The p38 MAP Kinase Pathway and Its Biological Function. Trends in Cardiovascular Medicine 8:220–228.

21. Stokoe D, Engel K, Campbell DG, Cohen P, Gaestel M. 1992. Identification of MAPKAP kinase 2 as a major enzyme responsible for the phosphorylation of the small mammalian heat shock proteins. FEBS Letters 313:307–313.

22. Zechner D, Thuerauf DJ, Hanford DS, McDonough PM, Glembotski CC. 1997. A Role for the p38 Mitogen-activated Protein Kinase Pathway in Myocardial Cell Growth, Sarcomeric Organization, and Cardiac-specific Gene Expression. J. Cell Biol 139:115–127.

23. Wang Y, Huang S, Sah VP, Ross Jr. J, Brown JH, Han J, Chien KR. 1998. Cardiac Muscle Cell Hypertrophy and Apoptosis Induced by Distinct Members of the p38 Mitogen-activated Protein Kinase Family. J. Biol. Chem. 273:2161–2168.

24. Clerk A, Michael A, Sugden PH. 1998. Stimulation of the p38 mitogen-activated protein kinase pathway in neonatal rat ventricular myocytes by the G protein-coupled receptor agonists, endothelin-1 and phenylephrine: a role in cardiac myocyte hypertrophy? J Cell Biol 142:523–535.

25. Nemoto S, Sheng Z, Lin A. 1998. Opposing effects of Jun kinase and p38 mitogen-activated protein kinases on cardiomyocyte hypertrophy. Mol Cell Biol 18:3518–3526.

26. Liang F, Gardner DG. 1999. Mechanical strain activates BNP gene transcription through a p38/NF-kappaB-dependent mechanism. J Clin Invest 104:1603–1612.

27. Liang F, Lu S, Gardner DG. 2000. Endothelin-dependent and -independent components of strain-activated brain natriuretic peptide gene transcription require extracellular signal regulated kinase and p38 mitogen-activated protein kinase. Hypertension 35:188–192.

28. Guan KL. 1994. The mitogen activated protein kinase signal transduction pathway: from the cell surface to the nucleus. Cellular Signalling 6:581–589.

29. Keyse SM. 1995. An emerging family of dual specificity MAP kinase phosphatases. Biochimica et Biophysica Acta (BBA)—Molecular Cell Research 1265:152–160.

30. Chu Y, Solski PA, Khosravi-Far R, Der CJ, Kelly K. 1996. The mitogen-activated protein kinase phosphatases PAC1, MKP-1, and MKP-2 have unique substrate specificities and reduced activity in vivo toward the ERK2 sevenmaker mutation. J Biol Chem 271:6497–6501.

31. Franklin CC, Kraft AS. 1997. Conditional expression of the mitogen-activated protein kinase (MAPK) phosphatase MKP-1 preferentially inhibits p38 MAPK and stress-activated protein kinase in U937 cells. J Biol Chem 272:16917–16923.

32. Li C, Hu Y, Mayr M, Xu Q. 1999. Cyclic strain stress-induced mitogen-activated protein kinase (MAPK) phosphatase 1 expression in vascular smooth muscle cells is regulated by Ras/Rac-MAPK pathways. J Biol Chem 274:25273–25280.

33. Fuller SJ, Davies EL, Gillespie-Brown J, Sun H, Tonks NK. 1997. Mitogen-activated protein kinase phosphatase 1 inhibits the stimulation of gene expression by hypertrophic agonists in cardiac myocytes. Biochemical Journal 323:313–319.

34. Bueno OF, De Windt LJ, Lim HW, Tymitz KM, Witt SA, Kimball TR, Molkentin JD. 2001. The dual-specificity phosphatase MKP-1 limits the cardiac hypertrophic response in vitro and in vivo. Circ Res 88:88–96.

35. Ihle JN. 1995. Cytokine receptor signalling. Nature 377:591–594.

36. Schindler C, Darnell JE, Jr. 1995. Transcriptional responses to polypeptide ligands: the JAK-STAT pathway. Annu Rev Biochem 64:621–651.

37. Fukuzawa J, Booz GW, Hunt RA, Shimizu N, Karoor V, Baker KM, Dostal DE. 2000. Cardiotrophin-1 increases angiotensinogen mRNA in rat cardiac myocytes through STAT3: an autocrine loop for hypertrophy. Hypertension 35:1191–1196.

38. Mascareno E, Dhar M, Siddiqui MA. 1998. Signal transduction and activator of transcription (STAT) protein-dependent activation of angiotensinogen promoter: a cellular signal for hypertrophy in cardiac muscle. Proc Natl Acad Sci USA 95:5590–5594.

39. Mascareno E, El-Shafei M, Maulik N, Sato M, Guo Y, Das DK, Siddiqui MAQ. 2001. JAK/STAT Signaling Is Associated With Cardiac Dysfunction During Ischemia and Reperfusion. Circulation 104:325–329.

40. Pan J, Fukuda K, Kodama H, Sano M, Takahashi T, Makino S, Kato T, Manabe T, Hori S, Ogawa S. 1998. Involvement of gp130-mediated signaling in pressure overload-induced activation of the JAK/STAT pathway in rodent heart. Heart Vessels 13:199–208.

41. Pan J, Fukuda K, Kodama H, Makino S, Takahashi T, Sano M, Hori S, Ogawa S. 1997. Role of angiotensin II in activation of the JAK/STAT pathway induced by acute pressure overload in the rat heart. Circ Res 81:611–617.

42. Pan J, Fukuda K, Saito M, Matsuzaki J, Kodama H, Sano M, Takahashi T, Kato T, Ogawa S. 1999. Mechanical stretch activates the JAK/STAT pathway in rat cardiomyocytes. Circ Res 84:1127–1136.

43. Kunisada K, Tone E, Fujio Y, Matsui H, Yamauchi-Takihara K, Kishimoto T. 1998. Activation of gp130 transduces hypertrophic signals via STAT3 in cardiac myocytes. Circulation 98:346–352.

44. Kunisada K, Negoro S, Tone E, Funamoto M, Osugi T, Yamada S, Okabe M, Kishimoto T, Yamauchi-Takihara K. 2000. Signal transducer and activator of transcription 3 in the heart transduces not only a hypertrophic signal but a protective signal against doxorubicin-induced cardiomyopathy. Proc Natl Acad Sci USA 97:315–319.

45. Ruwhof C, van der Laarse A. 2000. Mechanical stress-induced cardiac hypertrophy: mechanisms and signal transduction pathways. Cardiovasc Res 47:23–37.

46. Thorburn A, Thorburn J, Chen SY, Powers S, Shubeita HE, Feramisco JR, Chien KR. 1993. HRas-dependent pathways can activate morphological and genetic markers of cardiac muscle cell hypertrophy. J Biol Chem 268:2244–2249.

47. Abdellatif M, Schneider MD. 1997. An effector-like function of Ras GTPase-activating protein predominates in cardiac muscle cells. J Biol Chem 272:525–533.

48. Fuller SJ, Finn SG, Downward J, Sugden PH. 1998. Stimulation of gene expression in neonatal rat ventricular myocytes by Ras is mediated by Ral guanine nucleotide dissociation stimulator (Ral.GDS) and phosphatidylinositol 3-kinase in addition to Raf. Biochem J 335 (Pt 2):241–246.

49. Sugden PH, Clerk A. 2000. Activation of the small GTP-binding protein Ras in the heart by hypertrophic agonists. Trends Cardiovasc Med 10:1–8.

50. Clerk A, Sugden PH. 2000. Small guanine nucleotide-binding proteins and myocardial hypertrophy. Circ Res 86:1019–1023.

51. Hoshijima M, Sah VP, Wang Y, Chien KR, Brown JH. 1998. The low molecular weight GTPase Rho regulates myofibril formation and organization in neonatal rat ventricular myocytes. Involvement of Rho kinase. J Biol Chem 273:7725–7730.

52. Fan WT, Koch CA, de Hoog CL, Fam NP, Moran MF. 1998. The exchange factor Ras-GRF2 activates Ras-dependent and Rac-dependent mitogen-activated protein kinase pathways. Curr Biol 8:935–938.

53. Sah VP, Hoshijima M, Chien KR, Brown JH. 1996. Rho is required for Galphaq and alpha1-adrenergic receptor signaling in cardiomyocytes. Dissociation of Ras and Rho pathways. J Biol Chem 271:31185–31190.

54. Hines WA, Thorburn A. 1998. Ras and rho are required for galphaq-induced hypertrophic gene expression in neonatal rat cardiac myocytes. J Mol Cell Cardiol 30:485–494.

55. Pracyk JB, Tanaka K, Hegland DD, Kim KS, Sethi R, Rovira, II, Blazina DR, Lee L, Bruder JT, Kovesdi I, Goldshmidt-Clermont PJ, Irani K, Finkel T. 1998. A requirement for the rac1 GTPase

in the signal transduction pathway leading to cardiac myocyte hypertrophy. J Clin Invest 102: 929–937.

56. Molkentin JD, Dorn IG, 2nd. 2001. Cytoplasmic signaling pathways that regulate cardiac hypertrophy. Annu Rev Physiol 63:391–426.

57. Sierra DA, Popov S, Wilkie TM. 2000. Regulators of G-protein signaling in receptor complexes. Trends Cardiovasc Med 10:263–268.

58. Gudi SR, Lee AA, Clark CB, Frangos JA. 1998. Equibiaxial strain and strain rate stimulate early activation of G proteins in cardiac fibroblasts. Am J Physiol 274:C1424–C1428.

59. D'Angelo DD, Sakata Y, Lorenz JN, Boivin GP, Walsh RA, Liggett SB, Dorn GW, 2nd. 1997. Transgenic Galphaq overexpression induces cardiac contractile failure in mice. Proc Natl Acad Sci USA 94:8121–8126.

60. Akhter SA, Luttrell LM, Rockman HA, Iaccarino G, Lefkowitz RJ, Koch WJ. 1998. Targeting the receptor-Gq interface to inhibit in vivo pressure overload myocardial hypertrophy. Science 280:574–577.

61. Ross RS, Borg TK. 2001. Integrins and the myocardium. Circ Res 88:1112–1119.

62. Humphries MJ. 2000. Integrin structure. Biochem Soc Trans 28:311–339.

63. Zhidkova NI, Belkin AM, Mayne R. 1995. Novel isoform of beta 1 integrin expressed in skeletal and cardiac muscle. Biochem Biophys Res Commun 214:279–285.

64. van der Flier A, Kuikman I, Baudoin C, van der Neut R, Sonnenberg A. 1995. A novel beta 1 integrin isoform produced by alternative splicing: unique expression in cardiac and skeletal muscle. FEBS Lett 369:340–344.

65. Terracio L, Rubin K, Gullberg D, Balog E, Carver W, Jyring R, Borg TK. 1991. Expression of collagen binding integrins during cardiac development and hypertrophy. Circ Res 68:734–744.

66. Borg TK, Rubin K, Lundgren E, Borg K, Obrink B. 1984. Recognition of extracellular matrix components by neonatal and adult cardiac myocytes. Dev Biol 104:86–96.

67. Nagai T, Laser M, Baicu CF, Zile MR, Cooper Gt, Kuppuswamy D. 1999. Beta3-integrin-mediated focal adhesion complex formation: adult cardiocytes embedded in three-dimensional polymer matrices. Am J Cardiol 83:38H–43H.

68. Liang F, Atakilit A, Gardner DG. 2000. Integrin dependence of brain natriuretic peptide gene promoter activation by mechanical strain. J Biol Chem 275:20355–20360.

69. Heling A, Zimmermann R, Kostin S, Maeno Y, Hein S, Devaux B, Bauer E, Klovekorn WP, Schlepper M, Schaper W, Schaper J. 2000. Increased expression of cytoskeletal, linkage, and extracellular proteins in failing human myocardium. Circ Res 86:846–853.

70. Kim HE, Dalal SS, Young E, Legato MJ, Weisfeldt ML, D'Armiento J. 2000. Disruption of the myocardial extracellular matrix leads to cardiac dysfunction. J Clin Invest 106:857–866.

71. Schaper J, Speiser B. 1992. The extracellular matrix in the failing human heart. Basic Res Cardiol 87 Suppl 1:303–309.

72. Tyagi SC. 2000. Physiology and homeostasis of extracellular matrix: cardiovascular adaptation and remodeling. Pathophysiology 7:177–182.

73. Farhadian F, Contard F, Corbier A, Barrieux A, Rappaport L, Samuel JL. 1995. Fibronectin expression during physiological and pathological cardiac growth. J Mol Cell Cardiol 27:981–990.

74. Pham CG, Harpf AE, Keller RS, Vu HT, Shai SY, Loftus JC, Ross RS. 2000. Striated muscle-specific beta(1D)-integrin and FAK are involved in cardiac myocyte hypertrophic response pathway. Am J Physiol Heart Circ Physiol 279:H2916–H2926.

75. Ross RS, Pham C, Shai SY, Goldhaber JI, Fenczik C, Glembotski CC, Ginsberg MH, Loftus JC. 1998. Beta1 integrins participate in the hypertrophic response of rat ventricular myocytes. Circ Res 82:1160–1172.

76. Hsueh WA, Law RE, Do YS. 1998. Integrins, adhesion, and cardiac remodeling. Hypertension 31:176–180.

77. Aplin AE, Howe A, Alahari SK, Juliano RL. 1998. Signal transduction and signal modulation by cell adhesion receptors: the role of integrins, cadherins, immunoglobulin-cell adhesion molecules, and selectins. Pharmacol Rev 50:197–263.

78. Ridley A. 2000. Rho GTPases. Integrating integrin signaling. J Cell Biol 150:F107–F109.

79. Ivaska J, Reunanen H, Westermarck J, Koivisto L, Kahari VM, Heino J. 1999. Integrin alpha2beta1 mediates isoform-specific activation of p38 and upregulation of collagen gene transcription by a mechanism involving the alpha2 cytoplasmic tail. J Cell Biol 147:401–416.

80. Kuppuswamy D, Kerr C, Narishige T, Kasi VS, Menick DR, Cooper Gt. 1997. Association of tyrosine-phosphorylated c-Src with the cytoskeleton of hypertrophying myocardium. J Biol Chem 272:4500–4508.

81. Matsushita T, Oyamada M, Fujimoto K, Yasuda Y, Masuda S, Wada Y, Oka T, Takamatsu T. 1999. Remodeling of cell-cell and cell-extracellular matrix interactions at the border zone of rat myocardial infarcts. Circ Res 85:1046–1055.
82. Fassler R, Rohwedel J, Maltsev V, Bloch W, Lentini S, Guan K, Gullberg D, Hescheler J, Addicks K, Wobus AM. 1996. Differentiation and integrity of cardiac muscle cells are impaired in the absence of beta 1 integrin. J Cell Sci 109(Pt 13):2989–2999.
83. Keller RS, Shai SY, Babbitt CJ, Pham CG, Solaro RJ, Valencik ML, Loftus JC, Ross RS. 2001. Disruption of integrin function in the murine myocardium leads to perinatal lethality, fibrosis, and abnormal cardiac performance. Am J Pathol 158:1079–1090.
84. Liang F, Wu J, Garami M, Gardner DG. 1997. Mechanical strain increases expression of the brain natriuretic peptide gene in rat cardiac myocytes. J Biol Chem 272:28050–28056.
85. MacKenna DA, Dolfi F, Vuori K, Ruoslahti E. 1998. Extracellular signal-regulated kinase and c-Jun NH2-terminal kinase activation by mechanical stretch is integrin-dependent and matrix-specific in rat cardiac fibroblasts. J Clin Invest 101:301–310.
86. Sigurdson W, Ruknudin A, Sachs F. 1992. Calcium imaging of mechanically induced fluxes in tissue-cultured chick heart: role of stretch-activated ion channels. Am J Physiol 262:H1110–H1115.
87. Gannier F, White E, Garnier, Le Guennec JY. 1996. A possible mechanism for large stretch-induced increase in $[Ca^{2+}]i$ in isolated guinea-pig ventricular myocytes. Cardiovasc Res 32:158–167.
88. Tatsukawa Y, Kiyosue T, Arita M. 1997. Mechanical stretch increases intracellular calcium concentration in cultured ventricular cells from neonatal rats. Heart Vessels 12:128–135.
89. Lab MJ, Zhou BY, Spencer CI, Horner SM, Seed WA. 1994. Effects of gadolinium on length-dependent force in guinea-pig papillary muscle. Exp Physiol 79:249–255.
90. Gannier F, White E, Lacampagne A, Garnier D, Le Guennec JY. 1994. Streptomycin reverses a large stretch induced increases in [Ca2+]i in isolated guinea pig ventricular myocytes. Cardiovasc Res 28:1193–1198.
91. Chang J, Wasser JS, Cornelussen RN, Knowlton AA. 2001. Activation of heat-shock factor by stretch-activated channels in rat hearts. Circulation 104:209–214.
92. Molkentin JD, Lu JR, Antos CL, Markham B, Richardson J, Robbins J, Grant SR, Olson EN. 1998. A calcineurin-dependent transcriptional pathway for cardiac hypertrophy. Cell 93:215–228.
93. Sussman MA, Lim HW, Gude N, Taigen T, Olson EN, Robbins J, Colbert MC, Gualberto A, Wieczorek DF, Molkentin JD. 1998. Prevention of cardiac hypertrophy in mice by calcineurin inhibition. Science 281:1690–1693.
94. Naruse K, Yamada T, Sai XR, Hamaguchi M, Sokabe M. 1998. Pp125FAK is required for stretch dependent morphological response of endothelial cells. Oncogene 17:455–463.
95. Wang JG, Miyazu M, Matsushita E, Sokabe M, Naruse K. 2001. Uniaxial cyclic stretch induces focal adhesion kinase (FAK) tyrosine phosphorylation followed by mitogen-activated protein kinase (MAPK) activation. Biochem Biophys Res Commun 288:356–361.
96. Cooper Gt. 1987. Cardiocyte adaptation to chronically altered load. Annu Rev Physiol 49:501–518.
97. Imamura T, McDermott PJ, Kent RL, Nagatsu M, Cooper Gt, Carabello BA. 1994. Acute changes in myosin heavy chain synthesis rate in pressure versus volume overload. Circ Res 75:418–425.
98. Cooper Gt, Satava RM, Jr., Harrison CE, Coleman HN, 3rd. 1973. Mechanisms for the abnormal energetics of pressure-induced hypertrophy of cat myocardium. Circ Res 33:213–223.
99. Cooper Gt, Puga FJ, Zujko KJ, Harrison CE, Coleman HN, 3rd. 1973. Normal myocardial function and energetics in volume-overload hypertrophy in the cat. Circ Res 32:140–148.
100. Hatt PY, Rakusan K, Gastineau P, Laplace M. 1979. Morphometry and ultrastructure of heart hypertrophy induced by chronic volume overload (aorto-caval fistula in the rat). J Mol Cell Cardiol 11:989–998.
101. Smith SH, Kramer MF, Reis I, Bishop SP, Ingwall JS. 1990. Regional changes in creatine kinase and myocyte size in hypertensive and nonhypertensive cardiac hypertrophy. Circ Res 67:1334–1344.
102. Komuro I, Katoh Y, Kaida T, Shibazaki Y, Kurabayashi M, Hoh E, Takaku F, Yazaki Y. 1991. Mechanical loading stimulates cell hypertrophy and specific gene expression in cultured rat cardiac myocytes. Possible role of protein kinase C activation. J Biol Chem 266:1265–1268.
103. Swynghedauw B. 1992. Biological adaptation of the myocardium to a permanent change in loading conditions. Basic Res Cardiol 87 Suppl 2:1–10.
104. Simpson DG, Majeski M, Borg TK, Terracio L. 1999. Regulation of cardiac myocyte protein turnover and myofibrillar structure in vitro by specific directions of stretch. Circ Res 85:e59–e69.
105. Terracio L, Simpson DG, Hilenski L, Carver W, Decker RS, Vinson N, Borg TK. 1990. Distribution of vinculin in the Z-disk of striated muscle: analysis by laser scanning confocal microscopy. J Cell Physiol 145:78–87.

106. Sadoshima J, Xu Y, Slayter HS, Izumo S. 1993. Autocrine release of angiotensin II mediates stretch-induced hypertrophy of cardiac myocytes in vitro. Cell 75:977–984.
107. Miyata S, Haneda T, Osaki J, Kikuchi K. 1996. Renin-angiotensin system in stretch-induced hypertrophy of cultured neonatal rat heart cells. Eur J Pharmacol 307:81–88.
108. Yamazaki T, Komuro I, Kudoh S, Zou Y, Shiojima I, Mizuno T, Takano H, Hiroi Y, Ueki K, Tobe K, et al. 1995. Angiotensin II partly mediates mechanical stress-induced cardiac hypertrophy. Circ Res 77:258–265.
109. Lin C, Baker KM, Thekkumkara TJ, Dostal DE. 1995. Sensitive bioassay for the detection and quantification of angiotensin II in tissue culture medium. Biotechniques 18:1014–1020.
110. Leri A, Claudio PP, Li Q, Wang X, Reiss K, Wang S, Malhotra A, Kajstura J, Anversa P. 1998. Stretch-mediated release of angiotensin II induces myocyte apoptosis by activating p53 that enhances the local renin-angiotensin system and decreases the Bcl-2-to-Bax protein ratio in the cell. J Clin Invest 101:1326–1342.
111. Malhotra R, Sadoshima J, Brosius FC, 3rd, Izumo S. 1999. Mechanical stretch and angiotensin II differentially upregulate the renin-angiotensin system in cardiac myocytes In vitro. Circ Res 85:137–146.
112. Tamura K, Umemura S, Nyui N, Hibi K, Ishigami T, Kihara M, Toya Y, Ishii M. 1998. Activation of angiotensinogen gene in cardiac myocytes by angiotensin II and mechanical stretch. Am J Physiol 275:R1–R9.
113. Kijima K, Matsubara H, Murasawa S, Maruyama K, Mori Y, Ohkubo N, Komuro I, Yazaki Y, Iwasaka T, Inada M. 1996. Mechanical stretch induces enhanced expression of angiotensin II receptor subtypes in neonatal rat cardiac myocytes. Circ Res 79:887–897.
114. McWhinney CD, Hunt RA, Conrad KM, Dostal DE, Baker KM. 1997. The type I angiotensin II receptor couples to Stat1 and Stat3 activation through Jak2 kinase in neonatal rat cardiac myocytes. J Mol Cell Cardiol 29:2513–2524.
115. McWhinney CD, Dostal D, Baker K. 1998. Angiotensin II activates Stat5 through Jak2 kinase in cardiac myocytes. J Mol Cell Cardiol 30:751–761.
116. Kodama H, Fukuda K, Pan J, Makino S, Sano M, Takahashi T, Hori S, Ogawa S. 1998. Biphasic activation of the JAK/STAT pathway by angiotensin II in rat cardiomyocytes. Circ Res 82:244–250.
117. Leri A, Fiordaliso F, Setoguchi M, Limana F, Bishopric NH, Kajstura J, Webster K, Anversa P. 2000. Inhibition of p53 function prevents renin-angiotensin system activation and stretch-mediated myocyte apoptosis. Am J Pathol 157:843–857.
118. Johnatty SE, Dyck JR, Michael LH, Olson EN, Abdellatif M. 2000. Identification of genes regulated during mechanical load-induced cardiac hypertrophy. J Mol Cell Cardiol 32:805–815.
119. Friddle CJ, Koga T, Rubin EM, Bristow J. 2000. Expression profiling reveals distinct sets of genes altered during induction and regression of cardiac hypertrophy. Proc Natl Acad Sci USA 97:6745–6750.
120. Aronow BJ, Toyokawa T, Canning A, Haghighi K, Delling U, Kranias E, Molkentin JD, Dorn GW 2nd. 2001. Divergent transcriptional responses to independent genetic causes of cardiac hypertrophy. Physiol Genomics 6:19–28.
121. Stanton LW, Garrard LJ, Damm D, Garrick BL, Lam A, Kapoun AM, Zheng Q, Protter AA, Schreiner GF, White RT. 2000. Altered patterns of gene expression in response to myocardial infarction. Circ Res 86:939–945.

Signal Transduction and Cardiac Hypertrophy,
edited by N.S. Dhalla, L.V. Hryshko,
E. Kardami & P.K. Singal
Kluwer Academic Publishers, Boston, 2003

Caspase Activation in a Cardiac Cell-Free Model of Apoptosis

Claudio Stefanelli, Carla Pignatti, Benedetta Tantini,
Emanuele D. Giordano Francesca Bonavita,
Maddalena Zini, Flavio Flamigni, Claudio Muscari,
Carlo Clo,[1] Claudio M. Caldarera, and Carlo Guarnieri

Department of Biochemistry "G. Moruzzi"
University of Bologna
Italy
[1] Institute of Biological Chemistry
University of Parma
Italy

Summary. The release of mitochondrial anapoptogenic factors, like cytochrome c, into the cytosol is a fundamental step for caspase activation and induction of apoptosis. In this report it is shown that the polyamine spermine causes the exit of cytochrome c from heart mitochondria. Polyamines are ubiquitous compounds necessary for growth processes, whose excessive accumulation can trigger apoptosis. The release of cytochrome c caused by spermine is a selective process that is independent of mitochondria damage. The cytochrome c-releasing power of spermine is not affected by cyclosporin A, differently from the effect of permeability transition inducers. Addition of cytochrome c to cytosol extracts from chick embryo heart cells (CEHC) or H9C2 ventricular cardiomyoblasts triggers the onset of caspase activity. In a cardiac cell-free model of apoptosis, the latent caspase activity of cytosolic extracts from CEHC can be activated by cytochrome c released from spermine-treated heart mitochondria. The activated caspase activity is inhibited by nitric oxide donor molecules. These data suggest that prolonged and sustained elevation of polyamines, characteristic of heart hypertrophy, could be involved in the development of apoptosis.

Key words: Apoptosis, Caspase, Cytochrome c, Polyamines, Spermine.

Address for Correspondence: Prof. Carlo Guarnieri, Dipartimento di Biochimica "G. Moruzzi", Via Irnerio, 48. 40126, Bologna, Italy. Fax: +39-51-2091224, E-mail: cguarn@biocfarm.unibo.it

INTRODUCTION

Much is known about the biosynthesis, degradation, and transport of polyamines (1) but despite several decades of extensive research, their function in cellular physiology remains unsettled, and the only established function of polyamines is their absolute requirement for cell growth. In the heart, polyamine metabolism is strongly affected by several factors both physiological and pathological that influence cardiac function and growth (2). An increase in heart polyamines is linked to hypertension and cardiac hypertrophy (2,3).

Even if polyamines are necessary for growth processes, their excessive accumulation can trigger apoptosis (4–6). Furthermore, in some cases, polyamine depletion can protect the cells from induction of apoptosis (7). Apoptosis consists in a cell death process whose deregulation is thought to be involved in several pathologies. Activation of the caspase proteases represents a fundamental step in apoptosis (8). Mitochondria can play a central role in this process because the release of apoptogenic factors, like cytochrome c, into the cytosol is a crucial step for caspase activation (9,10). Spermine causes caspase activation and the leakage of cytochrome c into the cytosol both in whole cells (6) and cell extracts containing mitochondria along with cytosol (11). To explore the mechanism of the proapoptotic action of spermine, we studied the ability of the polyamine to directly affect the translocation of cytochrome c out from the mitochondrion (12). In this report it is shown that caspase activity can be triggered in cytosolic extracts from heart cells by cytochrome c released from spermine-treated mitochondria. This caspase activity can be inhibited by nitric oxide.

MATERIALS AND METHODS

Preparation of cardiac mitochondria

Mitochondria were prepared from the hearts of female Wistar rats (13). Briefly, the hearts were homogenized in 3 vols (w/v) of 0.5% bsa containing 180 mM KCl and 10 mM EDTA (pH 7.2). The homogenate was centrifuged for 5 min at 1000 g, and the supernatant was filtered and centrifugated for 10 min at 8000 g. The pellet was resuspended in 0.5% bonine serum albumine containing 180 mM KCl and 1 mM EDTA (pH 7.2) and centrifugated at 5000 g for 5 min. The final pellet was gently resuspended in 0.5 ml of mitochondria incubation buffer (MIB) consisting of 0.25 M sucrose, 1 mM KH$_2$PO$_4$ and 10 mM Hepes (pH 7.4). This crude mitochondria suspension (0.5 ml) was layered on top of 15 ml of a solution consisting of 30% Percoll, 0.25 M sucrose, 1 mM EDTA, and 10 mM Hepes (pH 7.4). Self-generating Percoll gradient was developed by centrifugation at 35,000 g for 30 min at 4°C. The mitochondrial band was separated from less dense contaminants and broken mitochondria, collected with a Pasteur pipette, and washed twice in 5 ml of MIB by centrifugating 5 min at 8000 g. The final pellet was suspended in MIB at 10 mg protein/ml. Mitochondrial function was assayed with standard oxymetric tests (13). Oxygen consumption was monitored in an oxygen-electrode chamber (IC-Oxy, Gilson, France) at 25°C in a final volume of 1.5 ml containing 0.5 mg of mitochondrial protein in MIB. Succinate (10 mM) was the oxidable substrate (in the presence of 2 μM rotenone).

Release of cytochrome c from isolated mitochondria

An aliquot of 10 μl of the mitochondria preparation (0.1 mg of protein) was incubated for 15 min at 25°C in a final volume of 50 μl of MIB containing 10 mM succinate and 2 μM rotenone (to give a final mitochondrial protein concentration of 2 mg/ml). At the end of the incubation, mitochondria were pelleted for 20 s in a benchtop centrifuge at 12,000 rpm. Fourty μl of the clear supernatant were added with 10 μl of fivefold-concentrated loading buffer and boiled for 3 min. Aliquots of 20 μl were subject to SDS-PAGE and Western blotting analysis of cytochrome c (12). Depletion of cytochrome c from supernatant of spermine-treated mitochondria was achieved by immunoprecipitation of cytochrome c as described by Chauhan et al. (14).

Cytosolic extracts and caspase activation

Cytosolic extracts for *in vitro* caspase activation were prepared from confluent cultures of chick embryo heart cells (CEHC), obtained and maintained as described (15) or from H9C2 cardiomyoblasts. To prepare these extracts, the cells from 10–15 plates (10 cm diameter) were collected and washed in phosphate-buffered saline. The cell pellet was then suspended in 0.4 ml of CFS buffer (16), left 10 min in ice and then gently lysed in a glass-teflon Potter-Elvehjem homogenizer with 70 strokes at medium speed. Cell lysis was confirmed by microscopic examination. The homogenate was centrifugated for 5 min at 1000 g to remove whole cells and nuclei. The supernatant was recentrifuged for 15 min at 16,000 g and the resulting supernatant finally centrifuged for 30 min at 100,000 g. Generally, these extracts contained about 5 mg of protein/ml. For the detection of caspase activation, 10 μl of cytosol were incubated for 1 h at 30°C in a final volume of 40 μl along with (when added) 1 mM MgCl$_2$/1 mM dATP, 100 ng of cytochrome c, or 20 μl of supernatant obtained from incubations of mitochondria. At the end of the incubation, an aliquot of 10 μl in duplicate was used for the caspase assay. The activity of caspase enzymes was measured by the cleavage of the fluorogenic peptide substrate Ac-DEVD-AMC in a final volume of 30 μl during a 15 min incubation at 37°C as previously described (17).

RESULTS

Polyamines are able to cause the release of cytochrome c from heart mitochondria (Figure 1A). Spermine was the most effective, and the increase in cytochrome c was maximal at 100 μM (Figure 1B). Higher polyamine concentrations did not further increase the leakage of cytochrome c. Spermidine was somewhat less effective than spermine, while putrescine had effect only at concentrations higher than 2 mM (not shown). The release of cytochrome c was specific and was not accompanied by a generalized leakage of mitochondrial proteins or adenylate kinase activity.

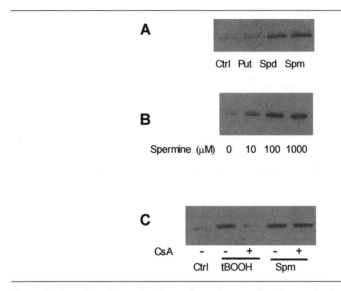

Figure 1. Spermine triggers the release of cytochrome c from heart mitochondria. (**A**) Mitochondria (2 mg/ml) were incubated for 15 min in the absence (Ctrl) or presence of a 100 μM concentration of polyamines. After centrifugation, cytochrome c was detected in the supernatants by Western blotting. (**B**) Rat heart mitochondria were fractionated on a self-generating Percoll gradient. Then aliquots of 0.1 mg of protein were incubated 15 min without any treatment (C, control), or in the presence of the indicated concentration (μM) of spermine (Spm). After centrifugation, cytochrome c was detected in supernatants by Western blotting. (**C**) Percoll-purified mitochondria (2 mg/ml) were incubated 15 min without any treatment (Ctrl) or in the presence of 100 μM spermine (Spm), or 100 μM *ter*-butyl hydroperoxide (tBOOH). Cyclosporin A (CsA, 1 μM) was added, when indicated. Following centrifugation, cytochrome c was determined by Western blotting in the supernatants.

Mitochondria were further purified by Percoll fractionation, that separate intact mitochondria from lighter damaged ones (13). Centrifugation on a self-generating Percoll gradient separated heavier mitochondria from lighter contaminants, consisting of membrane fragments and damaged mitochondria. Intact mitochondria accounted for more than one half of the protein content of crude preparations (49 to 60%) and were functional in standard oxymetric tests. They were strictly coupled and exhibited a RCR of 3.8 ± 0.2 using succinate (+ rotenone) as substrate and a P/O ratio of 1.59 ± 0.02, that are normal values for cardiac mitochondria (13). Spermine, but not polylysine (at a 100 μg/ml concentration, not shown), was able to trigger cytochrome c exit from purified mitochondria indicating that the effect of spermine is specific and is not caused by a displacement of cytochrome c electrostatically bound to membrane fragments.

Several data have shown that the release of cytochrome c from the intermembrane space of the mitochondrion can be triggered by the mitochondrial permeability transition (MPT) (9,10,16). MPT can be induced by oxidative stress obtained, for example, by treatment with *ter*-butyl hydroperoxide. We compared the effects of cyclosporine A (CsA), a MPT inhibitor, on the release of cytochrome c caused

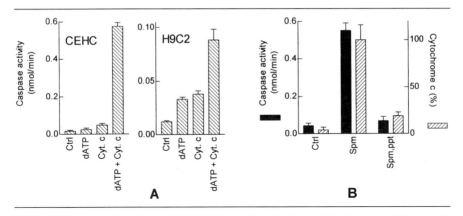

Figure 2. Spermine triggers caspase activation in a cardiac cell-free model of apoptosis. (**A**) Cytosolic extracts from CEHC or H9C2 cells were incubated 1h without any treatment (Ctrl), or in the presence of 1mM dATP, or with 100ng of cytochrome c (Cyt.c), then caspase activity was assayed. (**B**) Percoll-purified mitochondria (5mg/ml) were incubated 15min with or without 100μM spermine. After centrifugation, 20μl of the supernatants obtained from control (Ctrl) or spermine-treated (Spm) mitochondria were incubated 1h in the presence of 10μl of cytosolic extract from CEHC and 1mM dATP. An aliquot of the supernatant from spermine-treated mitochondria was also subject to immunoprecipitation of cytochrome c (Spm,ppt) prior to incubation with cytosol. At the end of the incubation, samples were assayed for caspase activity. Cytochrome c was assayed in an aliquot of 10μl of each of the supernatants by Western blotting followed by densitometry. The figure also shows the relative amount of cytochrome c, with respect to the content in supernatant obtained from spermine-treated mitochondria (100%).

by spermine or *ter*-butyl hydroperoxide. Oxidative stress caused the release of cytochrome c to an extent similar to spermine (Figure 1C). However, the leakage of cytochrome c triggered by *ter*-butyl hydroperoxide was inhibited by CsA, a classical inhibitor of MPT (18), whereas CsA did not block the effect of spermine. This finding is in agreement with reports showing that the polyamine has a protective effect in heart mitochondria (19). The experiments shown in Figure 1 show that spermine triggers the leakage of cytochrome c from intact mitochondria, without causing any apparent damage.

In further experiments we wanted to establish a cardiac cell-free model of apoptosis. A cytosolic extracts was obtained from chick embryo heart cells (CEHC). These non-transformed heart cells express a high caspase activity, albeit usually latent (15). Figure 2A shows that caspase activation can be achieved in these extract, as well as in extracts from H9C2 cells, by addition of dATP along with cytochrome c. Incubation of these cytosolic extracts with supernatants from spermine-treated mitochondria, that contain cytochrome c, resulted in caspase activation (Figure 2B). These supernatants were not able to cause caspase activation when depleted of cytochrome c by immunoprecipitation.

Caspase activity from staurosporine-treated CEHC undergoing apoptosis is inhibited both *in vitro* and *in vivo* by NO donor molecules (15). Actually, NO donors inhibited in a dose-dependent manner also caspase activity triggered in cytosol from

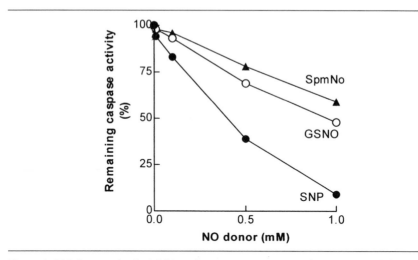

Figure 3. NO donor molecules inhibit cardiac caspase activity. Cytosolic extracts (10 μl) from CEHC were incubated 1 h in the presence of 1 mM dATP and 20 μl of the supernatants obtained from spermine-treated (Spm) mitochondria, similarly to experiment in Figure 2B. At the end of the incubation, samples were assayed for caspase activity cleaving the substrate sequence DEVD. Caspase activity was assayed in the absence or presence of the indicated concentration of NO donors. The activated caspase activity in the absence of any NO donor is indicated as 100% of remaining caspase activity. SpmNo, spermine-NO; GSNO, Glutathione-NO; SNP, sodium nitroprusside.

CEHC incubated with dATP and cytochrome *c*-containing supernatants from spermine-treated heart mitochondria (Figure 3).

DISCUSSION

The interaction of polyamines with mitochondria is known by many years. Polyamines are specifically transported into heart mitochondria (19) where appear to exert several functions, generally protective. We firstly described an unexpected mitochondrial effect of polyamines: the release of cytochrome *c* (12). This finding has been confirmed and extended by others (20,21). The exit of cytochrome *c* is not caused by the MPT and the mechanism remains to be determined, even if some data suggest the involvement of oxidative mechanism (21). Spermine is known to influence the movement of proteins across the external membrane of mitochondria (22), but one intriguing question may be why only a small fraction of cytochrome *c* is released. Even if the physiological relevance of our findings remains to be determined, it should be kept in mind that the translocation of cytochrome *c* into the cytosol represents a central step in many forms of apoptosis, since cytochrome *c* is a necessary component of the apoptosome, responsible for caspase activation (8).

We have described here a cardiac cell-free model of apoptosis: caspase activity in cytosol of embryonal cardiomyocytes is triggered by the cytochrome *c* released from mitochondria by spermine. The activated caspase activity is inhibited by NO donors, suggesting a possible antiapoptotic effect of NO in heart cells, observed in whole-cell models (15,23).

Our data also suggest a possible involvement of polyamines in some pathological forms of apoptosis. Actually, it is well established that the polyamines spermine and spermidine are present in high amounts within the cells bound to anionic structures, leaving only low concentrations of free polyamines (24). Cardiac hypertrophy, either pharmacologically-induced or consequent to hypertension, is characterized by a large and prolonged increase in polyamine level (2,3), and is coupled to excessive apoptosis (25). The abnormal accumulation of polyamines in cells stimulated to growth, but that cannot divide, may contribute to induction of apoptosis.

ACKNOWLEDGEMENTS

This work was supported by Compagnia di S. Paolo (Torino, Italy), "Fondi pluriennali di Dipartimento", and italian MIUR (fondi ex 60% and 40%).

REFERENCES

1. Pegg AE. 1988. Polyamine metabolism and its importance in neoplastic growth and as a target for chemotherapy. Cancer Res 48:759–774.
2. Flamigni F, Rossoni C, Stefanelli C, Caldarera CM. 1986. Polyamine metabolism and function in the heart. J Mol Cell Cardiol 18:3–11.
3. Pegg AE, Hibasami H. 1980. Polyamine metabolism during cardiac hypertrophy. Am J Physiol 239:E372–E378.
4. Poulin R, Pelletier G, Pegg AE. 1995. Induction of apoptosis by excessive polyamine accumulation in ornithine decarboxylase-overproducing L1210 cells. Biochem J 311:723–727.
5. Xie X, Tome ME, Gerner EW. 1997. Loss of intracellular putrescine pool-size regulation induces apoptosis. Exp Cell Res 230:386–392.
6. Stefanelli C, Bonavita F, Stanic I, Mignani M, Facchini A, Pignatti C, Flamigni F, Caldarera CM. 1998. Spermine causes caspase activation in leukaemia cells. FEBS Lett 437:233–236.
7. Stefanelli C, Pignatti C, Tantini B, Fattori M, Stanic I, Mackintosh CA, Flamigni F, Guarnieri C, Caldarera CM, Pegg AE. 2001. Effect of polyamine depletion on caspase activation: a study with spermine synthase-deficient cells. Biochem J 355:199–206.
8. Thornberry NA, Lazebnik J. 1998. Caspases: enemies within. Science 281:1312–1316.
9. Finkel E. 2001. The mitochondrion: is it central to apoptosis? Science 292:624–626.
10. Green DR, Reed JC. 1998. Mitochondria and apoptosis. Science 281:1309–1318.
11. Stefanelli C, Bonavita F, Stanic' I, Pignatti C, Flamigni F, Guarnieri C, Caldarera CM. 1999. Spermine triggers the activation of caspase-3 in a cell-free model of apoptosis. FEBS Lett 451:95–98.
12. Stefanelli C, Stanic' I, Zini M, Bonavita F, Flamigni F, Zambonin L, Landi L, Pignatti C, Guarnieri C, Caldarera CM. 2000. Polyamines directly induce release of cytochrome C from heart mitochondria. Biochem J 347:875–880.
13. Rickwood D, Wilson MT, Darley-Usmar VM. 1987. Isolation and characteristics of intact mitochondria. In: Mitochondria a pratical approach. Ed. VM Darley-Usmar, D Rickwood and MT Wilson, 1–16, Oxford: IRL Press.
14. Chauhan D, Pandey P, Ogata A, Teoh G, Krett N, Halgren R, Rosen S, Kufe D, Kharbanda S, Anderson K. 1997. Cytochrome *c*-dependent and -independent induction of apoptosis in multiple myeloma cells. J Biol Chem 272:29995–29997.
15. Stefanelli C, Pignatti C, Tantini B, Stanic' I, Bonavita F, Muscari C, Guarnieri C, Clo C, Caldarera CM. 1999. Nitric oxide can function as either a killer molecule or an antiapoptotic effector in cardiomyocytes. Biochim Biophys Acta 1450:406–413.
16. Ellerby HM, Martin SJ, Ellerby LM, Naiem SS, Rabizadeh S, Salvesen GS, Casiano CA, Cashman NR, Green DR, Bredesen DE. 1997. Establishment of a cell-free system of neuronal apoptosis: comparison of premitochondrial, mitochondrial, and postmitochondrial phases. J Neurosci 17:6165–6178.

17. Stefanelli C, Bonavita F, Stanic' I, Pignatti C, Farruggia G, Masotti L, Guarnieri C, Caldarera CM. 1998. Inhibition of etoposide-induced apoptosis with peptide aldehyde inhibitors of proteasome. Biochem J 332:661–665.
18. Fontaine E, Bernardi P. 1999. Progress on the mitochondrial permeability transition pore: regulation by complex I and ubiquinone analogs. J Bioenerg Biomembr 31:335–345.
19. Toninello A, Dalla Via L, Testa S, Siliprandi D, Siliprandi N. 1990. Transport and action of spermine in rat heart mitochondria. Cardioscience 1:287–294.
20. Mather M, Rottemberg H. 2001. Polycations induce the release of soluble intermembrane mitochondrial proteins. Biochim Biophys Acta 1503:357–358.
21. Maccarone M, Bari M, Battista N, Di Rienzo M, Falciglia K, Finazzi Agrò A. 2001. Oxidation products of polyamines induce mitochondrial uncoupling and cytochrome c release. FEBS Lett 507:30–34.
22. Bordin L, Cattapan F, Clari G, Toninello A, Siliprandi N, Moret V. 1994. Spermine-mediated casein kinase II-uptake by rat liver mitochondria. Biochim Biophys Acta 1199:266–270.
23. Weiland U, Haendler J, Ihling C, Albus U, Scholz W, Ruetten H, Zeiher AM, Dimmeler S. 2000. Inhibition of endogeneous nitric oxide synthase potentiates ischemia-reperfusion-induced myocardial apoptosis via a caspase-3 dependent pathway. Cardiovasc Res 45:671–678.
24. Davis R, Morris RD, Coffino P. 1992. Sequestered end products and enzyme regulation: the case of ornithine decarboxylase. Microbiol Rev 56:280–290.
25. Teiger E, Than, VD, Richard L, Wisnewsky C, Tea BS, Galboury L, Tremblay J, Schwartz K, Hamet P. 1996. Apoptosis in pressure overload-induced heart hypertrophy in the rat. J Clin Invest 97:2891–2897.

Signal Transduction and Cardiac Hypertrophy,
edited by N.S. Dhalla, L.V. Hryshko,
E. Kardami & P.K. Singal
Kluwer Academic Publishers, Boston, 2003

The Role of the Voltage-Sensitive Release Mechanism in Contraction of Normal and Diseased Heart

Susan E. Howlett and Gregory R. Ferrier

Cardiovascular Research Laboratories
Department of Pharmacology
Dalhousie University
Halifax, Nova Scotia
Canada B3H 4H7

Summary. The series of events which couple depolarisation of the cardiac cell membrane to initiation of contraction are known as excitation-contraction coupling (EC-coupling). A key event in EC-coupling is the release of Ca^{2+} from stores in the sarcoplasmic reticulum (SR). Until recently, it was believed that release of SR Ca^{2+} in heart could be triggered only by a process called Ca^{2+}-induced Ca^{2+} release (CICR). However, recent studies have demonstrated an additional separate mechanism which initiates release of SR Ca^{2+} independently of conventional CICR. This new mechanism, called the voltage-sensitive release mechanism (VSRM), contributes substantially to initiation of contraction and to changes in magnitude of contraction with changes in heart rate. Furthermore, the VSRM is a target for several major signalling pathways, which indicates that it may play a major role in regulation of the strength of cardiac contraction. The VSRM also may play an important role in contractile dysfunction accompanying heart disease, as the VSRM is selectively depressed in at least two models of heart failure. The mechanism by which the VSRM releases Ca^{2+} from the SR is currently the subject of experimental research, which may provide new targets for therapeutic actions to improve contractile function in heart disease.

Key words: voltage-sensitive release mechanism; calcium-induced calcium release; heart failure; phosphorylation; sarcoplasmic reticulum.

Address for Correspondence: S.E. Howlett, Ph.D. and G.R. Ferrier, Ph.D., Department of Pharmacology, Sir Charles Tupper Medical Building, Dalhousie University, Halifax, Nova Scotia, Canada B3H 4H7. Telephone: (902) 494-3552; (902) 494-2550, Fax: (902) 494-1388, E-mail: Susan.Howlett@dal.ca, Gregory.Ferrier@dal.ca

INTRODUCTION

In cardiac muscle, contraction is initiated by excitation of the cell membrane by an action potential. Excitation of the cell membrane triggers a rapid rise in intracellular free Ca^{2+}, which activates intracellular myofilaments. The rapid rise in intracellular free Ca^{2+} is derived largely through release of Ca^{2+} from the sarcoplasmic reticulum (SR). The process by which excitation of the sarcolemma is coupled to release of SR Ca^{2+} and contraction is called excitation-contraction coupling (EC-coupling). The mechanisms by which excitation causes SR Ca^{2+} release in heart have been the subject of intense research over the past several decades. This paper reviews recent developments in our concepts of cardiac EC-coupling.

MECHANISMS OF EC-COUPLING

Early studies demonstrated that release of SR Ca^{2+} could be initiated by Ca^{2+}-induced Ca^{2+} release (CICR). CICR was first demonstrated in heart by Fabiato (1–3). He showed that rapid application of Ca^{2+} to cardiac myocytes from which the sarcolemma had been removed, triggered release of Ca^{2+} from stores within the SR (1–3). CICR also is believed to occur in intact myocytes, where SR Ca^{2+} release is initiated primarily by L-type Ca^{2+} current (I_{Ca-L}) (4–8). The role of I_{Ca-L} in triggering Ca^{2+} SR release is supported by experiments which show that extracellular Ca^{2+} is required for CICR (9). Furthermore, blockade of I_{Ca-L} with Ca^{2+} channel blockers abolishes CICR (10,11). Under some conditions, Ca^{2+} entering cells by other routes also may play a role in triggering CICR (12).

Not only is Ca^{2+} release initiated by CICR, but Ca^{2+} release also is graded by this process. Thus, in voltage clamp experiments, CICR is directly proportional to the magnitude of peak inward I_{Ca-L} (4–8,12). Because the current-voltage (IV) relationship for I_{Ca-L} is bell-shaped, CICR also shows a bell-shaped voltage dependence, which is reflected in the amplitudes of both contractions (Figure 1A,B) and Ca^{2+} transients (4–8,12).

Although CICR is clearly proportional to I_{Ca-L}, cardiac contractions which are not proportional to I_{Ca-L} also can be initiated under appropriate experimental conditions (10,11,13–18). These contractions persist in the presence of Ca^{2+} channel blockade (10,11,14,16,17). Furthermore, these contractions are not proportional to the magnitude of I_{Ca-L}, and exhibit a sigmoidal dependence on membrane potential (Figure 1A,B). Because these contractions are graded by membrane voltage, rather than inward I_{Ca-L}, they have been attributed to a mechanism which has been named the voltage-sensitive release mechanism (VSRM) (11,15,18).

The VSRM and CICR can be differentiated from each other experimentally. This is possible because these two mechanisms exhibit distinctly different physiological and pharmacological characteristics. For example the VSRM and CICR are activated over different ranges of membrane potential (11). The activation curve for the VSRM begins near −60 mV, while CICR is first activated along with I_{Ca-L} near −30 mV (Figure 1A). The VSRM becomes maximal near −20 mV and remains maximal at membrane potentials as positive as +100 mV. In contrast, CICR exhibits

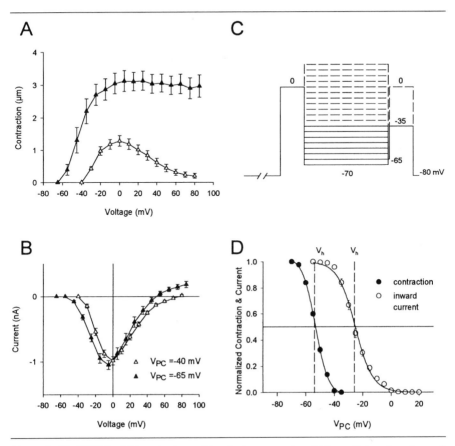

Figure 1. The VSRM exhibits activation and inactivation properties which are distinct from those of CICR and I_{Ca-L}. **Panels A, B.** Mean contraction-voltage (A) and current-voltage relations (B). Contractions and currents were activated by 200 ms steps to various membrane potentials from a post-conditioning potential of either −40 (open symbols) or −65 mV (filled symbols). When steps were made from a post-conditioning potential of −40 mV to inactivate the VSRM, the contraction-voltage relationship was bell-shaped as characteristic of CICR. When steps were made from −65 mV and both CICR and the VSRM were available, the contraction-voltage relationship was sigmoidal and activation was shifted to more negative potentials. The change in post-conditioning potential had little effect on current-voltage relations. **Panel C.** Voltage clamp protocol used to examine steady-state inactivation of currents or contractions. Following the last conditioning pulse, the membrane was clamped to different post-conditioning voltages (V_{PC}). The test step to −35 mV was used to activate the VSRM and the test step to 0 mV was used to examine I_{Ca-L}. **Panel D.** Mean steady-state inactivation curves for contractions initiated by the VSRM (filled symbols) and inward I_{Ca-L} (open symbols). The mean half-inactivation voltage for the VSRM was −53.2 ± 0.4 mV, which is significantly more negative than the half-inactivation voltage for I_{Ca-L} (−25.3 ± 0.9 mV, p < 0.001). Data were recorded from rat ventricular myocytes voltage clamped with high resistance microelectrodes (n = 9–12 cells per group). Reprinted with permission from Ferrier et al., 1998 and Ferrier & Howlett, 2001.

its characteristic bell-shaped contraction-voltage curve. Thus, CICR contractions are maximal near 0 mV and become minimal at membrane potentials near the reversal potential for I_{Ca-L} (+60 mV).

Phasic contractions initiated by the VSRM and CICR both exhibit steady-state inactivation. Thus, when activation steps are preceded by prolonged depolarisation, initiation of contraction by a subsequent activation step is inhibited. The degree of inhibition or inactivation is determined by the voltage of the preceding depolarisation. However, steady-state inactivation of the VSRM and CICR occurs over different distinct ranges of membrane potentials. The VSRM is approximately half inactivated at −50 mV (half-inactivation voltage), whereas the half-inactivation voltage of I_{Ca-L}/CICR is approximately −25 mV (11; Figure 1C,D). Thus, the inactivation curve for the VSRM lies about 25 mV negative to the curve for CICR (Figure 1C,D). Because of this difference, CICR is available while the VSRM is inactivated by a holding potential of −40 mV.

Although phasic VSRM contractions exhibit inactivation, the VSRM also is characterized by a non-inactivating sustained component (10,19). Both phasic and sustained components can be activated by depolarisation (Figure 2A). The phasic component rises to a maximum and then spontaneously declines, whereas the sustained component persists until the cell is repolarized. In contrast, CICR elicits only phasic contractions, which terminate spontaneously even when depolarization or Ca^{2+} influx are prolonged (20). The sustained component exhibits a sigmoidal voltage dependence similar to the phasic component, and is maximal at potentials positive to −20 mV (10). Relaxation (deactivation) of the sustained component in response to repolarization occurs over the same range of membrane potentials as the activation curve of the VSRM (10). Thus sustained VSRM contractions and transients exhibit activation and deactivation which follow the same voltage dependence. Because voltage can grade sustained Ca^{2+} release continuously, the sustained component may play an active role in controlling relaxation during repolarization. Thus, changes in resting membrane potential and action potential duration could affect the time course of relaxation through modulation of the VSRM.

The differences in activation and inactivation properties of phasic VSRM and CICR responses allow separation of the VSRM and CICR with voltage clamp protocols (e.g. 10,11). VSRM contractions can be activated selectively with voltage clamp steps from −65 to −40 mV (Figure 2A). However, voltage clamp steps from −40 to 0 mV activate phasic contractions that are almost exclusively initiated by CICR (Figure 2). This protocol for separation of the two mechanisms is useful for demonstrating differential effects of pharmacological agents on the VSRM and CICR in the same cell. However, under physiological conditions the cardiac action potential would activate both the VSRM and CICR together.

A number of pharmacological agents have differential effects on VSRM and CICR responses. The VSRM can initiate SR Ca^{2+} release and contraction when CICR coupled to Ca^{2+} entry by various routes is inhibited (10,11,13,14,16,17). For example, L-type Ca^{2+} channel blockers consistently inhibit contractions and Ca^{2+} transients initiated by CICR coupled to I_{Ca-L} (10,11,13,16,17,21,22). In contrast,

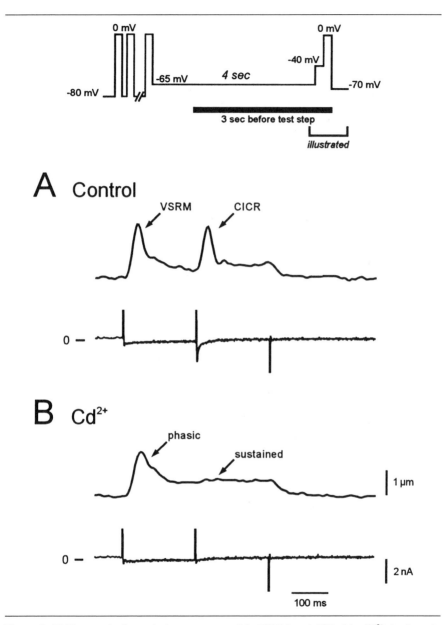

Figure 2. Neither sustained nor phasic components of the VSRM are inhibited by Cd^{2+}. A schematic of the voltage clamp protocol is shown at the top. Ten conditioning pulses were followed by a 4 sec step to −65 mV, and then by two sequential test steps to −40 and 0 mV. Drugs were applied with a computer controlled rapid solution switching device during the period indicated by the thick bar. **Panel A.** Test steps to −40 and 0 mV elicited phasic contractions (top trace) initiated by the VSRM and CICR, respectively. The VSRM was accompanied by a sustained component. I_{Ca-L} was observed with the step to 0 mV (bottom trace). **Panel B.** Both the CICR contraction and I_{Ca-L} were abolished by rapid application of 100 μM Cd^{2+}. Phasic and the sustained components of the VSRM were unaffected by Cd^{2+}. Reprinted with permission from Ferrier et al., 2000.

VSRM contractions and/or Ca^{2+} transients still can be elicited under these conditions. This differential blockade has been demonstrated when CICR is blocked by Cd^{2+}, Ni^{2+}, or low concentrations of the 1,4-dihydropyridine, nifedipine (Figure 2A,B) (10,11,13,16,17,19,21–23). Cd^{2+} and Ni^{2+} block permeation of the Ca^{2+} channel pore by Ca^{2+} (24). Brief application of low concentrations of nifedipine blocks opening of Ca^{2+} channels but does not eliminate Ca^{2+} channel gating charge movement (25). Thus, Ca^{2+} channel blockers which block permeation but not gating inhibit CICR but not the VSRM.

The VSRM also can be inhibited selectively by tetracaine or by low concentrations of ryanodine (22). Rapid application of tetracaine, a local anesthetic, selectively abolishes VSRM contractions without affecting SR Ca^{2+} load. The site of action mediating this effect is not clear. Tetracaine has actions on a variety of channels including Na channels and SR Ca^{2+} release channels (ryanodine receptors) (26–28). At high concentrations, or with prolonged exposure, tetracaine also affects CICR and SR Ca^{2+} load by additional actions (22,27,28). As inhibition of the VSRM by tetracaine can be observed when Na^+ current has been inhibited previously with lidocaine and/or tetrodotoxin (10,17,22), it is unlikely that the effect of tetracaine on the VSRM is related to blockade of Na^+ channels. However, it is possible that tetracaine may inhibit the VSRM through interactions with ryanodine receptors (27,28).

The VSRM can be inhibited selectively by very low concentrations of ryanodine (14). At micromolar concentrations, ryanodine partially opens SR Ca^{2+} release channels and causes depletion of SR Ca^{2+} stores (29–31). However, block of the VSRM occurs at nanomolar concentrations of ryanodine which do not deplete the SR of Ca^{2+}, and which have virtually no effect on contractions initiated by CICR (32). Higher concentrations of ryanodine that deplete SR Ca^{2+}, also block CICR in addition to the VSRM (32). These observations suggest that a high affinity binding site for ryanodine may modulate the VSRM.

The preceding discussion focuses on characteristics of phasic VSRM contractions and Ca^{2+} transients. The pharmacological responses of sustained transients and contractions initiated by the VSRM are essentially the same as described for phasic VSRM responses (10).

REGULATION OF THE VSRM BY SIGNALLING PATHWAYS

Cardiac contraction is regulated by a number of major signalling pathways. These include the Ca^{2+}-calmodulin dependent kinase (CamK), and the adenylyl cyclase-protein kinase A (AC-PKA) pathways. These pathways may be linked to different cell surface receptors such as β_1- and β_2-adrenergic receptors and muscarinic cholinergic receptors as well as ionic messengers such as Ca^{2+}. Studies of EC-coupling regulation have focussed mainly on signalling pathways impacting on CICR. However, several lines of evidence suggest that the VSRM is an important target for regulatory signalling pathways as well.

Regulation of the VSRM was first recognized through experiments that inadvertently disrupted intracellular signalling pathways (16,17). The VSRM was originally observed in discontinuous voltage–clamp experiments conducted with high resistance microelectrodes, which cause only limited dialysis of myocytes (11,14). However, when experiments were attempted with patch pipettes which readily exchange pipette solution with the cell interior, CICR was intact but the VSRM could not be detected (16,17). These initial experiments with patch pipettes utilized conventional intracellular solutions, and therefore had the potential to remove small diffusible second messengers through dialysis. When either calmodulin or 8-bromo-cAMP (8-br-cAMP) are added to the pipette solution, the VSRM becomes available for activation and VSRM contractions and Ca^{2+} transients are restored (16,17). The ability of calmodulin to rescue the VSRM is inhibited by KN-62, a specific inhibitor of CamK (17). Similarly, restoration of the VSRM by 8-br-cAMP is prevented or reversed by H-89, a specific inhibitor of PKA (16). These results indicate that disruption of the VSRM by conventional patch pipette solutions is most likely related to disruption of the CamK and AC-PKA pathways by dialysis with patch pipettes.

When addition of 8-br-cAMP to pipette solutions is used to restore activation of the VSRM, the amplitude of peak I_{Ca-L} also is moderately increased (16). This increase in I_{Ca-L} is accompanied by a parallel increase in CICR. Although I_{Ca-L} and CICR are increased by 8-br-cAMP, the gain of CICR (contraction per unit current) is not affected (16,18). Thus, the appearance of VSRM contractions with addition of 8-br-cAMP cannot be explained by induction of a high-gain CICR by 8-br-cAMP. Furthermore, when calmodulin, rather than 8-br-cAMP, is used to restore activation of the VSRM, neither CICR nor I_{Ca-L} are increased in amplitude.

In the absence of either calmodulin or 8-br-cAMP in the patch pipettes, contraction-voltage relations are bell-shaped as expected for CICR, even when test steps are made from very negative potentials to ensure that the VSRM is not inactivated by voltage. Inclusion of either calmodulin or 8-br-cAMP in the pipette solution restores sigmoidal contraction-voltage or Ca^{2+} transient-voltage relations typical of the VSRM (16,17). These contractions and transients also show steady-state inactivation characteristic of the VSRM. VSRM contractions or Ca^{2+} transients supported by either calmodulin or 8-br-cAMP exhibit characteristic resistance to block of I_{Ca-L} with Cd^{2+}, whereas CICR is still inhibited by Ca^{2+} channel blockers in the same cells (16,17). Furthermore, Mackiewicz et al. (23) showed that contractions supported by 8-br-cAMP also were resistant to block of I_{Ca-L} by 5 or 10 mM Ni^{2+}. Ca^{2+} transients supported by 8-br-cAMP also persist in the presence of block of I_{Ca-L} with Ni^{2+} (13). In addition, VSRM responses supported by calmodulin can be selectively blocked by rapid application of tetracaine (17). Thus, both the pharmacological and physiological characteristics of the VSRM in patch pipette experiments with calmodulin or 8-br-cAMP are identical to those in undialyzed myocytes.

These pathways also may play an important role in maintaining the VSRM in undialyzed myocytes. Application of either H-89 or KN-62 reduces the amplitudes of VSRM contractions in undialyzed myocytes (17). This suggests that both CamK and AC-PKA pathways regulate the VSRM in the absence of exogenous calmodulin or 8-br-cAMP. Further, simultaneous superfusion of undialyzed myocytes with both H-89 and KN-62 virtually abolishes the VSRM (17). In all cases CICR is affected much less than the VSRM by these inhibitors. These observations suggest that these phosphorylation pathways play a critical role in regulation of the VSRM in intact cardiac muscle.

The observation that the VSRM can be restored by addition of 8-br-cAMP to patch pipette solutions suggests that agents which increase intracellular levels of cAMP should also stimulate the VSRM. One can increase cAMP levels either by stimulating synthesis by AC or by inhibiting degradation by phosphodiesterases (PDE). Indeed, stimulation of AC with forskolin increases VSRM contractions but also increases CICR, I_{Ca-L}, and SR Ca^{2+} load (33). A similar non-selective response is observed with the PDE inhibitor isobutyl-methylxanthine (IBMX) (33). Both forskolin and IBMX are non-selective agents. Forskolin stimulates all AC isoforms, and IBMX inhibits all four major isoforms of PDE expressed in heart. When myocytes are exposed to the selective PDE-3 inhibitor amrinone, VSRM contractions are strongly stimulated with virtually no effect on I_{Ca-L} or CICR (Figure 3A–D), and only a small increase in SR Ca^{2+} stores (33). In contrast, rolipram, a selective inhibitor of PDE-4, has no effect on the VSRM (34). These observations suggest that regulation of the VSRM is highly targeted through compartmentalization. There is increasing evidence that phosphorylation of specific targets can be selectively regulated by PKA or PDE's anchored in the vicinity of specific proteins (35,36). Thus, in the case of the VSRM, it is likely that phosphorylation of a key site by PKA is regulated by PDE-3.

Evidence for an important role of PDE's in regulation of the VSRM also comes from experiments with patch pipettes in which different analogues of cAMP were added to the intracellular solutions. The VSRM is clearly supported by 8-br-cAMP, which is resistant to hydrolysis by PDE's (37). The VSRM also is supported by another PDE resistant analogue, dibutyryl-cAMP (38). In contrast, addition of either Na-cAMP or tris-cAMP to patch pipettes does not activate the VSRM (38). As Na-cAMP and tris-cAMP are readily hydrolysed by PDE's (37), it is likely that they are degraded before they can reach the phosphorylation site associated with the VSRM. This explanation likely accounts for the absence of the VSRM in other studies in which hydrolysable analogues of cAMP have been utilized in patch pipette solutions (39).

Recent evidence suggests that muscarinic agonists also selectively target the VSRM (40). Carbachol, a non-selective muscarinic agonist, selectively decreases the amplitudes of VSRM contractions with virtually no effect on I_{Ca-L} or CICR (40). Addition of the non-selective muscarinic antagonist atropine in the continued presence of carbachol results in a marked increase in VSRM contractions, again with little or no effect on I_{Ca-L} or CICR (40). Atropine by itself has no effect on EC-coupling. Although the specific muscarinic receptor subtypes which mediate these effects are not known, these observations suggest that the VSRM is highly targeted by signalling pathways, and imply that the VSRM represents an important regulatory site for cardiac contraction.

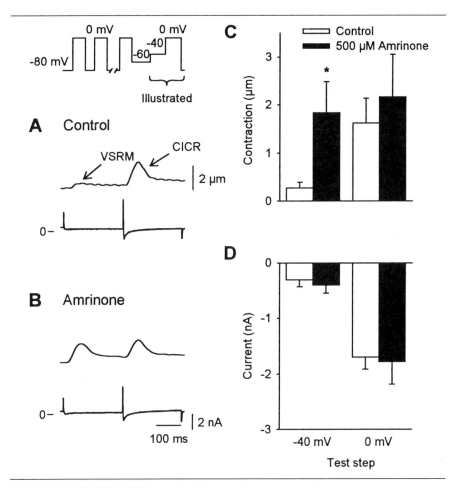

Figure 3. The PDE III inhibitor amrinone, increases the magnitude of VSRM contractions with no effect on CICR. Voltage clamp protocol shown at top. **Panel A.** VSRM and CICR contractions (top) and currents (bottom) were activated selectively by two sequential voltage clamp steps from −60 to −40 and 0 mV. **Panel B.** The magnitude of the VSRM contraction was increased by 500 μM amrinone. In contrast, amrinone had no effect on the CICR contraction or inward currents. **Panel C.** Mean data demonstrate that the effect of amrinone on VSRM contractions was significant (p < 0.05; n = 5 cells per group). **Panel D.** Amrinone had no significant effect on inward currents. Reprinted with permission from Xiong et al., 2001.

ROLE OF THE VSRM IN THE PHYSIOLOGY OF CONTRACTION

Under experimental conditions where the VSRM and CICR are activated separately, both mechanisms can trigger contractions with similar amplitudes. However, under physiological conditions the VSRM and CICR would be activated together by the cardiac action potential. It is not entirely clear whether these two mechanisms operate additively. However, when the VSRM is available for activation, contractions elicited by steps to membrane potentials corresponding to the overshoot and plateau of the action potential are substantially larger than when the VSRM is inactivated (11). Furthermore, in experiments utilizing single activation steps to activate both mechanisms simultaneously, 5 mM Ni^{2+}, which would strongly inhibit CICR, reduces the amplitudes of Ca^{2+} transients by only 20% (13). These observations suggest that the VSRM contributes substantially to the total contraction when both mechanisms are activated together.

The relative contribution of the VSRM to contraction may vary with experimental or physiological conditions. Several key factors which may influence the contribution of the VSRM are predicted by the conditions necessary to detect the presence of this mechanism. For example, depression of phosphorylation pathways by dialysis of diffusible intermediates can virtually abolish the VSRM. In contrast, CICR is still present under these conditions. Similarly, when EC-coupling is studied at room temperature, the VSRM also is inactivated although CICR persists (41). This may reflect effects of temperature on phosphorylation levels (e.g. 42). Thus, the degree to which the VSRM is phosphorylated likely will play a critical role in modulating the contribution of the VSRM to total contraction.

The amplitude of VSRM contractions and transients is extremely sensitive to activation history (11,43). The contribution of the VSRM is minimal in quiescent myocytes, but increases steeply with increasing rate and number of preceding activation steps, even when SR Ca^{2+} load is kept relatively constant (43). On the other hand, CICR shows much more modest changes in amplitude in response to activation history (43). The physiological correlate of activation history relates to the classic contraction-frequency and staircase phenomena (44,45). Our studies of these phenomena suggest that the VSRM contributes minimally to contraction at very low heart rates, but contributes progressively more as heart rate increases. The marked change in the contribution of the VSRM to contraction with changes in heart rate suggest that the VSRM is an important determinant of contraction-frequency relations and staircases.

Attention to phosphorylation levels and activation history is essential to activation of the VSRM in experimental studies of EC-coupling. Many studies have failed to detect the VSRM in isolated myocytes because of the particular experimental conditions utilized. Clearly experiments which utilized patch pipettes with conventional filling solutions, room temperature, or depolarised holding or conditioning potentials which would inactivate the VSRM, would detect only CICR. The use of conditioning pulses and specific additions to patch pipettes also are critical. For example, a recent study, conducted with appropriate temperature and membrane potentials, still failed to detect the VSRM. This study explored whether the VSRM could be elicited by addition of tris-cAMP to patch pipettes or by stimulation of cells with isoproterenol (39). However, in this study activation steps were preceded by only two conditioning pulses at an extremely slow repetition rate (0.2 to 0.5 Hz). There are at least two factors which would make it highly unlikely that these experiments would elicit the VSRM: the use of a PDE degradable analogue of cAMP (tris-cAMP), and an inadequate activation history. Indeed, two recent studies which utilized adequate conditioning pulse trains and the non-hydrolyzable analogue 8-br-cAMP in patch pipette solutions reported that contractions persisted in ventricular myocytes in the presence of 5–10 mM Ni^{2+} (19,23). These considerations show that physiological conditions which enhance the contribution of the VSRM to contraction also correspond to the conditions which optimise this mechanism experimentally.

ROLE OF THE VSRM IN HEART DISEASE

As the VSRM makes a major contribution to contraction in cardiac myocytes from normal heart, it is important to consider whether it plays a role in contractile dysfunction in heart disease. In fact, recent studies have demonstrated that the ability of the VSRM to initiate contraction is markedly decreased in cardiomyopathic hamsters and in rats with congestive heart failure secondary to myocardial infarction.

The cardiomyopathic hamster develops a genetic cardiomyopathy that leads to heart failure. Isolated myocytes from these animals exhibit a defect in contractile function that is attributable entirely to a reduction in contractions initiated by the VSRM, with no depression of CICR or I_{Ca-L} (21). This defect in the VSRM develops even before overt heart failure appears. In the rat model, congestive heart failure was confirmed by echocardiography and elevated left ventricular end-diastolic pressure (46). *In situ* hearts, isolated tissues and isolated ventricular myocytes from these animals all exhibit contractile dysfunction. Voltage clamp experiments in ventricular myocytes from these animals show that the contractile defect is due to a selective decrease in contraction initiated by the VSRM (46). CICR and I_{Ca-L} were unchanged. Many components of phosphorylation pathways have been found to be down-regulated in different models of heart failure (47,48). Therefore, it is possible that changes in phosphorylation levels may underlie depression of the VSRM in this disease state.

MECHANISM OF EC-COUPLING FOR THE VSRM

The mechanism by which release of SR Ca^{2+} by the VSRM is triggered by depolarisation of the sarcolemma is not clear. The hallmark of conventional CICR is that SR Ca^{2+} release and contraction are proportional to macroscopic Ca^{2+} current. Thus, gradation of CICR occurs with relatively large changes in Ca^{2+} current which are easily visualized and measured. However, the VSRM continues to operate when Ca^{2+} entry through L- and T-type Ca^{2+} channels, or the Na^+-Ca^{2+} exchanger are inhibited (18). Thus, conventional CICR cannot account for large contractions elicited by the VSRM during blockade of Ca^{2+} influx by inhibitors.

Despite the observation that the VSRM can initiate large contractions when Ca^{2+} influx is inhibited, the VSRM is inhibited when Ca^{2+} is omitted from the extracellular solution (14). The explanation for this requirement for extracellular Ca^{2+} is not clear. Two possibilities have been suggested (18): 1) the VSRM may represent an ultra-high gain form of CICR in which full sized contractions or transients are elicited by entry of minimal amounts of Ca^{2+}; 2) the VSRM may be activated by depolarisation of a voltage sensor in the sarcolemma without Ca^{2+} entry. In the latter case, extracellular Ca^{2+} might be required to occupy a binding site as an essential step in activation of the VSRM.

Conventional CICR can be shown to be proportional to macroscopic Ca^{2+} current in cells which also exhibit the VSRM with little or no accompanying current. Thus, if the VSRM represents ultra-high gain CICR, this mechanism must co-exist along with conventional CICR in the same cells. If, on the other hand, the VSRM represents a voltage-sensor coupled mechanism, it is not necessary to postulate that both ultra-high and low gain CICR co-exist in the same cell. Because the VSRM requires extracellular Ca^{2+}, it is more difficult to provide definitive evidence that distinguishes between these two mechanisms. Nonetheless, Mackiewicz et al. (23) demonstrated that block of Ca^{2+} permeation of L-type Ca^{2+} channels with 5 or 10 mM Ni^{2+} did not inhibit initiation of contraction by depolarisation. However, high concentrations of 1,4-dihydropyridines, which are expected to block gating charge in L-type Ca^{2+} channels (25), inhibit all contractions (23). This led Mackiewicz et al. (23) to suggest that dihydropyridine receptors/L-type Ca^{2+} channels could serve as voltage sensors which couple SR Ca^{2+} release to gating charge movement in the heart. The idea that L-channels can communicate directly with ryanodine receptors is supported by experiments which document modulation of ryanodine receptor function by BAY K8644, which binds to L-channels (49). In addition, there is evidence that the II–III intracellular loop of the cardiac L-channel can affect SR Ca^{2+} release visualized as Ca^{2+} sparks (50). However, it is not clear whether these putative interactions are related to a role for dihydropyridines in activation of the VSRM.

Regardless of the mechanism by which the VSRM is activated by depolarisation, it is clear that the VSRM represents a separate mechanism for Ca^{2+} release which has distinctly different characteristics from conventional CICR. Furthermore, the VSRM likely represents a central target in regulation of cardiac contractile function, and may play a role in heart diseases involving contractile dysfunction. Compelling evidence that the VSRM represents a new entity which is separate from conventional CICR raises the prospect that agents which target the VSRM may provide new therapeutic avenues for treatment of contractile dysfunction.

AKNOWLEDGEMENTS

This work was supported in part by grants from the Heart and Stroke Foundation of Nova Scotia and from The Canadian Institutes for Health Research. The authors wish to thank Peter Nicholl for assistance in preparation of illustrations.

REFERENCES

1. Fabiato A. 1985. Rapid ionic modifications during the aequorin-detected calcium transient in a skinned canine cardiac Purkinje cell. J Gen Physiol 85:189–246.
2. Fabiato A. 1985. Time and calcium dependence of activation and inactivation of calcium-induced release of calcium from the sarcoplasmic reticulum of a skinned canine cardiac Purkinje cell. J Gen Physiol 85:247–290.
3. Fabiato A. 1985. Simulated calcium current can both cause calcium loading in and trigger calcium

release from the sarcoplasmic reticulum of a skinned canine cardiac Purkinje cell. J Gen Physiol 85:291–320.

4. Barcenas-Ruiz L, Wier WG. 1987. Voltage dependence of intracellular $[Ca^{2+}]_i$ transients in guinea pig ventricular myocytes. Circ Res 61:148–154.

5. Beuckelmann DJ, Wier WG. 1988. Mechanism of release of calcium from sarcoplasmic reticulum of guinea-pig cardiac cells. J Physiol (Lond) 405:233–255.

6. Cleemann L, Morad M. 1991. Role of Ca^{2+} channel in cardiac excitation-contraction coupling in the rat: evidence from Ca^{2+} transients and contraction. J Physiol (Lond) 432:283–312.

7. duBell WH, Houser SR. 1989. Voltage and beat dependence of the Ca^{2+} transient in feline ventricular myocytes. Am J Physiol 257:H746–H759.

8. London B, Krueger JW. 1986. Contraction in voltage-clamped, internally perfused single heart cells. J Gen Physiol 88:475–505.

9. Nabauer M, Callewaert G, Cleemann L, Morad M. 1989. Regulation of calcium release is gated by calcium current, not gating charge, in cardiac myocytes. Science 244:800–803.

10. Ferrier GR, Redondo IM, Mason CA, Mapplebeck CL, Howlett SE. 2000. Regulation of contraction and relaxation by membrane potential in cardiac ventricular myocytes. Am J Physiol 278: H1618–H1626.

11. Howlett SE, Zhu JQ, Ferrier GR. 1998. Contribution of a voltage-sensitive calcium release mechanism to contraction in cardiac ventricular myocytes. Am J Physiol 274:H155–H170.

12. Bers DM. 2001. Excitation-Contraction Coupling and Cardiac Contractile Force, 2nd Edition. Dordrecht, The Netherlands: Kluwer Academic Publishers, 2001.

13. Hobai IA, Howarth FC, Pabbathi VK, Dalton GR, Hancox JC, Zhu JQ, Howlett SE, Ferrier GR, Levi AJ. 1997. "Voltage-activated Ca release" in rabbit, rat and guinea-pig cardiac myocytes, and modulation by internal cAMP. Pflugers Arch 435:164–173.

14. Ferrier GR, Howlett SE. 1995. Contractions in guinea-pig ventricular myocytes triggered by a calcium-release mechanism separate from Na^+ and L-currents. J Physiol (Lond) 484:107–122.

15. Howlett SE, Ferrier GR. 1997. The voltage-sensitive release mechanism: a new trigger for cardiac contraction. Can J Physiol 75:1044–1057.

16. Ferrier GR, Zhu JQ, Redondo IM, Howlett SE. 1998. A role for cAMP dependent kinase A in activation of the voltage-sensitive release mechanism for cardiac contraction. J Physiol (Lond) 513:185–201.

17. Zhu JQ, Ferrier GR. 2000. Regulation of a voltage-sensitive release mechanism by Ca^{2+}-calmodulin dependent kinase in cardiac myocytes. Am J Physiol 279:H2104–H2115.

18. Howlett SE, Ferrier GR. 2001. Cardiac excitation-contraction coupling: role of membrane potential in regulation of contraction. Am J Physiol 280:H1928–H1944.

19. Emanuel K, Mackiewicz U, Lewartowski B. 2001. On the source of Ca^{2+} activating the tonic component of contraction of myocytes of guinea pig heart. Cardiovasc Res 52:76–83.

20. Sham JS, Song LS, Chen Y, Deng LH, Stern MD, Lakatta EG, Cheng H. 1998. Termination of Ca^{2+} release by a local inactivation of ryanodine receptors in cardiac myocytes. Proc Natl Acad Sci USA 95:15096–15101.

21. Howlett SE, Xiong W, Mapplebeck C, Ferrier GR. 1999. Role of the voltage-sensitive release mechanism in depression of cardiac contraction in myopathic hamsters. Am J Physiol 277:H1690–H1700.

22. Mason CA, Ferrier GR. 1999. Tetracaine can inhibit contractions initiated by a voltage-sensitive release mechanism in guinea pig ventricular myocytes. J Physiol (Lond) 519:851–865.

23. Mackiewicz U, Emanuel K, Lewartowski B. 2000. Dihydropyridine receptors functioning as voltage sensors in cardiac myocytes. J Physiol Pharmacol 51:777–798.

24. McDonald TF, Pelzer S, Trautwein W, Pelzer DJ. 1994. Regulation and modulation of calcium channels in cardiac, skeletal, and smooth muscle cells. Physiol Rev 74:365–507.

25. Hadley RW, Lederer WJ. 1995. Nifedipine inhibits movement of cardiac calcium channels through late, but not early, gating transitions. Am J Physiol 269:H1784–H1790.

26. Katzung B. 2001. Basic and Clinical Pharmacology, 8th edition. New York: McGraw-Hill.

27. Overend CL, Eisner DA, O'Neill SC. 1997. The effect of tetracaine on spontaneous Ca^{2+} release and sarcoplasmic reticulum Ca^{2+} content in rat ventricular myocytes. J Physiol (Lond) 502:471–479.

28. Overend CL, O'Neill SC, Eisner DA. 1998. The effect of tetracaine on stimulated contractions, sarcoplasmic reticulum Ca^{2+} content and membrane current in isolated rat ventricular myocytes. J Physiol (Lond) 507:759–769.

29. Meissner G. 1986. Ryanodine activation and inhibition of the Ca^{2+} release channel of sarcoplasmic reticulum. J Biol Chem 261:6300–6306.

30. Rousseau E, Smith JS, Meissner G. 1987. Ryanodine modifies conductance and gating behavior of single Ca^{++} release channel. Am J Physiol 253:C364–C368.
31. Shattock JM, Bers DM. 1987. Inotropic response to hypothermia and the temperature-dependence of ryanodine action in isolated rabbit and rat ventricular muscle: implications for excitation-contraction coupling. Circ Res 61:761–771.
32. Mason CA, Howlett SE, Ferrier GR. 1998. Ryanodine selectively inhibits the voltage-sensitive release mechanism for SR Ca in guinea-pig ventricular myocytes. Biophys J 74:A55.
33. Xiong W, Moore HM, Howlett SE, Ferrier GR. 2001. In contrast to forskolin and 3-isobutylmethylxanthine, amrinone stimulates the cardiac voltage sensitive release mechanism without increasing calcium-induced calcium release. J Pharmacol Exp Ther 298:1–10.
34. Howlett SE, Ferrier GR. 2002. Differential effects of specific phosphodiesterase (PDE) III and IV inhibition on contraction in cardiac myocytes. Biophys J 82:67a.
35. Housley MD, Milligan G. 1997. Tailoring cAMP signalling responses through isoform multiplicity. Trends Biol Sci 22:217–224.
36. McCartney S, Little BM, Langeberg LK, Scott JD. 1995. Cloning and characterization of A-kinase anchor protein 100 (AKAP100). A protein that targets A-kinase to the sarcoplasmic reticulum. J Biol Chem 270:9327–9333.
37. Meyer RB, Miller JP. 1974. Analogs of cyclic AMP and cyclic GMP: general methods of synthesis and the relationship of structure to enzymic activity. Life Sci 14:1019–1040.
38. Ferrier GR, Redondo IM, Zhu JQ, Howlett SE. 2000. A critical role for phosphodiesterase in regulation of the cardiac voltage-sensitive release mechanism (VSRM) by cAMP analogs in whole cell voltage clamp investigations. Biophys J 78:371A.
39. Piacentino V, Dipla K, Gaughan JP, Houser SR. 2000. Voltage-dependent Ca^{2+} release from the SR of feline ventricular myocytes is explained by Ca^{2+}-induced Ca^{2+} release. J Physiol (Lond) 523:533–548.
40. Felix CA, Howlett SE, Ferrier GR. 2002. Muscarinic agonists modulate the cardiac voltage-sensitive release mechanism (VSRM) in the absence of adrenergic stimulation. Biophys J 82:67a.
41. Ferrier GR, Redondo IM. 1996. Low temperature inhibits cardiac contractions initiated by the voltage-sensitive release mechanism. J Mol Cell Cardiol 28:A180.
42. Miyamoto S, Hori M, Izumi M, Ozaki H, Karaki H. 2001. Species- and temperature-dependency of the decrease in myofilament Ca^{2+} sensitivity induced by beta-adrenergic stimulation. Jpn J Pharmacol 85:75–83.
43. Zhu JQ, Ferrier GR. 1999. Role of the voltage-sensitive release mechanism in force-interval relations and staircases in cardiac ventricular myocytes. Biophys J 76:A458.
44. Bowditch HP. 1871. Über die Eigenthümlichkeiten der Reizbarkeit, welche die Muskelfasern des Herzens zeigen. Ber. Sächs. Akad. Wiss. 23:652–689.
45. Koch-Weser J, Blinks JR. 1963. The influence of the interval between beats on myocardial contractility. Pharmacol Rev 15:601–651.
46. Sjaastad I, Birkeland JA, Ferrier GR, Howlett SE, Wasserstrom JA, Sejersted OM. 2000. Rats with congestive heart failure exhibit a defect in excitation-contraction coupling caused by suppression of the voltage sensitive release mechanism. Circ 102:II-297.
47. Frank K, Kranias EG. 2000. Phospholamban and cardiac contractility. Ann Med 32:572–578.
48. Wang X, Dhalla NS. 2000. Modification of beta-adrenoceptor signal transduction pathway by genetic manipulation and heart failure. Mol Cell Biochem 214:131–155.
49. Katoh H, Schlotthauer K, Bers DM. 2000. Transmission of information from cardiac dihydropyridine receptor to ryanodine receptor: evidence from Bay K 8644 effects on resting Ca^{2+} sparks. Circ Res 87:106–111.
50. Li Y, Bers DM. 2001. A cardiac dihydropyridine receptor II–III loop peptide inhibits resting Ca^{2+} sparks in ferret ventricular myocytes. J Physiol (Lond) 537:17–26.

Signal Transduction and Cardiac Hypertrophy,
edited by N.S. Dhalla, L.V. Hryshko,
E. Kardami & P.K. Singal
Kluwer Academic Publishers, Boston, 2003

Role of AT₁ Receptor Blockade in Reperfused Myocardial Infarction

Bodh I. Jugdutt

From the Division of Cardiology
Department of Medicine
and Cardiovascular Research Group
Faculty of Medicine, University of Alberta
Edmonton, Alberta, Canada

Summary. Angiotensin II (AngII) type 1 (AT₁) receptor blockade is an attractive therapeutic strategy for blocking the effects of AngII mediated through the AT₁ receptor after ischemia-reperfusion (IR) or reperfused myocardial infarction (MI). Cumulative evidence indicates that blocking the effects of excessive AngII might produce benefits beyond those of lowering of blood pressure. Although early coronary artery reperfusion is becoming established for the initial management of patients with acute MI, it results in reperfusion injury, with myocardial stunning and persistent left ventricular (LV) dysfunction. Since AngII is released during IR and MI, and exerts several effects that enhance IR injury, AT₁ receptor blockade might be beneficial as adjunctive therapy after IR and reperfused MI. Recent studies suggest that the AngII type 2 (AT₂) receptor and downstream signaling via PKCε (protein kinase Cε) and nitric oxide (NO) might contribute to the cardioprotection induced by AT₁ receptor blockade during IR.

Key words: Angiotensin receptors; ischemia-reperfusion; ventricular function; apoptosis; angiotensin receptor antagonists.

INTRODUCTION

Angiotensin II (AngII) type 1 (AT₁) receptor blockade has become an attractive therapeutic strategy for blocking the effects of AngII mediated through the AT₁

Address for Correspondence: Dr. Bodh I. Jugdutt, 2C2.43 Walter Mackenzie Health Sciences Center, Division of Cardiology, Department of Medicine, University of Alberta, Edmonton, Alberta, Canada T6G 2R7. Tel: (780) 407-7729, Fax: (780) 437-3546, E-mail: bjugdutt@ualberta.ca

receptor (1). Cumulative evidence indicates that blocking the effects of excessive AngII might produce benefits beyond the lowering of blood pressure in cardio-vascular disease (1–4). Early coronary artery reperfusion is now widely used for the management of patients with acute myocardial infarction (MI) (5), and every effort is being made to restore flow as rapidly and completely as possible (6). However, even early reperfusion results in reperfusion injury, with myocardial stunning and persistent left ventricular (LV) dysfunction (7–9). The role of oxygen free radicals and oxidative stress in reperfusion injury have been reviewed (8–12). The release of AngII during ischemia-reperfusion (IR) (13–15), MI (16) and heart failure (17,18) appears to contribute to the pathophysiology of these states. Several of the physio-logic effects of AngII enhance IR injury (14). In fact, the renin-angiotensin system (RAS), of which AngII is the primary effector peptide, is upregulated during IR and MI (17–21). AT_1 receptor blockade might therefore be beneficial as adjunctive therapy after IR and reperfused MI. Some recent studies that provide insight into the mechanisms of cardioprotection by AT_1R blockade during IR and involving AngII type 2 (AT_2) receptor are discussed.

THE AT_2 RECEPTOR DURING IR AND AT_1 RECEPTOR BLOCKADE

In the normal adult heart, most of the cardiovascular physiological effects of Ang II are mediated through the AT_1 receptor and the AT_2 receptor is mostly inactive (20,21). The AT_2 receptor is abundant and active in the fetus and its levels normally decline after birth (22). However, the AT_2 receptor is re-expressed in the adult heart following IR injury (23–29), MI (30), heart failure (19) and hypertension (19,20) as part of the re-expression of the fetal gene programs under stress. Accumulating evidence show that the AT_2 receptor is counter-regulatory and antagonizes the effects of the AT_1 receptor, thereby exerting antigrowth, antihypertrophic and pro-apoptotic effects (21). The increase in AT_2 receptor levels after injury may also oppose other effects of AngII such as vasoconstriction (20). In the presence of AT_1 receptor blockade and injury-induced increase in AT_2 receptor levels, unopposed AT_2 receptor stimulation, activation and signaling may therefore augment and/or contribute to the beneficial effects of AT_1 receptor blockade (1). As shown in Figure 1, AT_2 receptor activation may lead to increased bradykinin (BK), nitric oxide (NO) and cGMP (24,31–33), or increased protein kinase Cε (PKCε) activation (24,34).

AT_2 RECEPTOR ACTIVATION AND PKCε/cGMP SIGNALING DURING AT_1 RECEPTOR BLOCKADE AND IR

The hypothesis that AT_2 receptor activation and signaling via PKCε and cGMP might contribute to cardioprotection during AT_1 receptor blockade was tested in the in vivo dog model of IR (28). Briefly, anesthetized, opened chest dogs were instrumented with arterial and left atrial catheters for monitoring hemodynamics. Left ventricular (LV) function was measured by two-dimensional echocardiograms and Doppler (2-Echo/Doppler). AT_1 receptor blockade was produced by candesartan (CV-11974, 1 mg/kg over 30 min i.v.) before IR and confirmed by inhibition of AngII pressor responses (0.25 μg/kg I.V.) at baseline and after drug infusions.

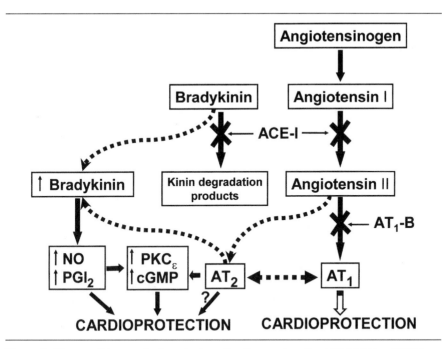

Figure 1. Diagram of the postulated mechanism of cardioprotection after ACE inhibition (ACE-I) and AT$_1$ receptor blockade (AT$_1$-B). PGI$_2$ = prostacyclin. See text for other abbreviations.

The animals were randomized to 7 groups: sham (no IR, saline or CN); controls (IR, saline i.v. infusion); AT$_1$ receptor blockade (candesartan, 1 mg/kg over 30 min i.v. + IR; AT$_2$ inhibitor (PD123319, 3 mg/kg/min i.c. for 30 min) + candesartan i.v. + IR; PKC inhibitor (chelerythrine, 17 µg/kg/min i.c. for 30 min) + candesartan i.v. + IR; NO synthase (NOS) inhibition (N^6-monomethyl-L-arginine [L-NMMA], 75 mg/kg/min i.c. for 30 min) + candesartan i.v. + IR; BK inhibition (HOE-140, 10 ng/kg/min i.c. for 30 min) + candesartan i.v. + IR. The intracoronary (i.c.) injections were made (via a PE-50 catheter) into the occluded bed distal to the site of the occlusion site of the left anterior descending (LAD) coronary artery. Ischemia for 90 minutes was then produced by LAD coronary occlusion made by a snare device around the middle region of the LAD coronary artery. This was followed by reperfusion for 120 minutes, achieved by releasing the occluding snare.

In vivo hemodynamic and functional recordings were made at baseline, post-drug pre-occlusion, 90 minutes post-occlusion, and 120 minutes post-reperfusion. The hearts were arrested in diastole (with 1 M potassium chloride) and processed for ex vivo measurements of infarct size using the triphephyl tetrazolium chloride (TTC) method and computerized planimetry. As described previously (27,28), the AT$_1$ receptor, AT$_2$ receptor and PKCε proteins were measured by Western immunoblots and cGMP by enzyme immunoassay on fresh frozen (liquid nitrogen) samples taken from the ischemic and non-ischemic zones. The 2D-Echo/Doppler recordings were

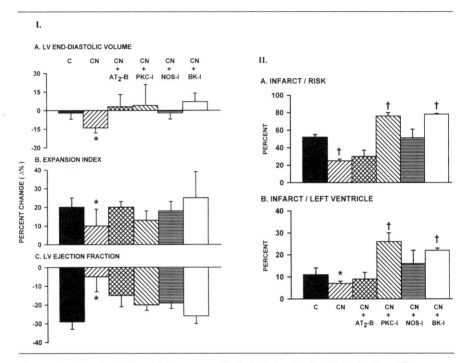

Figure 2. I. Beneficial effects of AT$_1$ receptor blockade during in vivo IR in the dog. Effect on diastolic volume **(A.)**, expansion index **(B.)** and LV ejection fraction **(C.)**. Percent changes are shown. *P ≤ 0.05 versus control. **II.** Effects on infarct size as percent risk region **(A.)** or left ventricle **(B.)**. AT$_2$-B = AT$_2$ receptor blockade with PD123319; BK-I = bradykinin inhibition with HOE-140; C = control; CN = candesartan; NOS-I = nitric oxide synthase inhibition with L-NMMA; PKC-I = protein kinase C inhibition with chelerythrine; LV = left ventricular. *P < 0.05, †P < 0.001 versus control.

analyzed for parameters of LV systolic and diastolic function and remodeling, as described previously (27,28).

As reported previously (27,28), the results showed that candesartan alone improves global systolic and diastolic function, limits acute LV remodeling (Figure 2), decreases infarct size (Figure 2) and regionally increases AT$_2$ receptor and PKCε proteins (Figure 3) as well as cGMP (not shown) in the ischemic zone. Importantly, the AT$_2$ receptor antagonist and the inhibitors of BK, PKCε and NOS attenuated these beneficial effects of candesartan and the regional increase in AT$_2$ receptor and PKCε proteins. The AT$_1$ receptor protein did not change in this model.

The findings of these studies (27,28) indicate that AT$_1$ receptor blockade induces cardioprotection during IR in the dog vivo model. This beneficial effect is abolished by AT$_2$R blockade and inhibition of PKC, NO synthesis and BK. The overall findings support the hypothesis that AT$_2$ receptor activation and downstream signaling through BK, PKCε, NO and cGMP play a significant role in the cardioprotective effect of AT$_1$ receptor blockade during IR. AngII has been shown to be

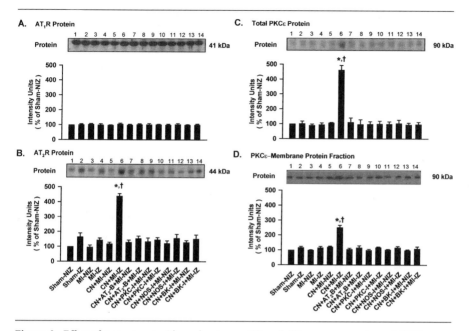

Figure 3. Effect of pretreatment with candesartan on AT₁ and AT₂ receptor proteins and PKCε proteins in acutely reperfused myocardial infarction in the dog. The effects of the AT₁ receptor blocker candesartan (CN, 1 mg/kg 30 min pre-ischemia) alone intravenously or after intracoronary (into the occluded zone) AT₂ receptor blockade (AT₂-B, PD123319), PKC inhibition (PKC-I, chelerythrine), NOS inhibition (NOS-I, L-NMMA) and bradykinin inhibition (BK-I, HOE-140) on ex vivo AT₁/AT₂ receptor and PKCε proteins. Representative gels with bar graphs of mean ± SD (n = 5). AT₁ receptor protein did not change **(A)**. Increase in AT₂ receptor protein **(B)** and PKCε proteins **(C, D)** were abolished by AT₂ receptor, PKC, NO and BK inhibition. IZ, infarct size; NIZ, non-infarct zone; MI, myocardial infarction.

harmful during IR (35) while AT₁ receptor blockade induces cardioprotection during IR (36–39). AT₁ receptor blockade has also been shown to reduce infarct size, improve LV function and limit LV remodeling after MI in the in vivo dog model (40). AT₁ receptor blockade was also cardioprotective in chronic heart failure after MI in the rat model (32). The findings support previous observations that AT₂ receptor activation is involved in the cardioprotective effect of AT₁ receptor blockade after myocardial injury (24–26,31–33). It is pertinent that the dog model of IR is associated with necrosis (41) and often low flow ischemia (42) and candesartan induces cardioprotection in both this model (42) and the mini-pig model (33) of in vivo IR.

CARDIOPROTECTION AND AT₂R UPREGULATION DURING AT₁ RECEPTOR BLOCKADE IN DOG AND RAT IN VIVO MODELS OF REPERFUSED MI

Although AT₁ receptor blockade has been shown to be cardioprotective during MI and IR in dog in vivo models, whether AT₁ receptor blockade produces similar

Table 1. Summary of the effects of AT_1 receptor blockade on cardioprotection

Author	Reference	AT_1 Blocker	Series	Model	Effect
Liu	48	Losartan	Rat	IR, in vivo	$\leftrightarrow$ TTC infarct size; $\downarrow$ with ramiprilat
Liu	32	L158809	Rat	Remote HF, in vivo	$\uparrow$ LV function / $\downarrow$ remodeling (– by HOE-140, PD123319)
Sladek	49	Losartan	Rat	Acute MI, in vivo	$\leftrightarrow$ infarct size; $\downarrow$ LVEDP, τ, RVSP; less $\downarrow$ capillary density
Stauss	50	Losartan	Rat	MI, in vivo	$\leftrightarrow$ TTC infarct size
Milavetz	51	Losartan	Rat	MI, in vivo	$\uparrow$ survival
Ford	43, 44	Losartan	Rat	IR, in vitro, WH	$\downarrow$ function
Yang	39	Losartan	Rat	NWH, in vitro	$\uparrow$ function ($\uparrow AT_1R$)
Yang	47	Losartan	Rat	NWH, in vitro	$\uparrow$ function (as AS-ODNs to AT_1R mRNA
Xu	23	PD123319	Rat	IR, in vitro, WH	LV function $\uparrow$ with PD123319; $\uparrow AT_2R$
Xu	46	Losartan	Rat	IR, in vitro, WH	LV function $\downarrow$ with Losartan ($\leftrightarrow AT_2R$); $\uparrow$ with PD123319 ($\uparrow AT_2R$)
Moudgil	26	Losartan UP269-6	Rat	IR, in vitro, WH	$\uparrow AT_2R$; LV function $\leftrightarrow$ with losartan; $\downarrow$ with UP269-6
Richer	52	Irbesartan	Rat	MI, in vivo	$\uparrow$ survival
Hartman	54	Losartan	Rabbit	Acute MI, in vivo	$\uparrow$ TTC infarct size ($\downarrow$ with AngII, ramiprilat)
Liu	55	Losartan	Rabbit	IR, in vitro	$\leftrightarrow$ TTC infarct size
Diaz	56	Losartan	Rabbit	IPC, NWH, in vitro	Abolish infarct-limiting (TTC) effect of IPC (not PD123319)
Bastien	53	Losartan	Hamster	Cardiomyopathy, in vivo	$\uparrow$ contractility
Schwarz	59	EXP3174	Pig	IR, in vivo	$\downarrow$ infarct size (as enalaprilat); $\uparrow$ IPC

cardioprotection in rodents is controversial. Table 1 summarizes the effects of AT_1 receptor blockade on cardioprotection in several studies using different models (23–26,32,33,39,40,42–64). Thus, AT_1 receptor blockade has been reported to: have no effect on myocardial blood flow during IR in dogs (42); impair (43,44) or enhance (36–39,47) functional recovery after IR in rats; decrease infarct size in dogs (40), pigs (59) and mini-pigs (33); have no effect on infarct size in rats (48–50), rabbits (55,56), or dogs (57,58); increase infarct size in rabbits (54); limit remodeling after MI in rats (32,65) and dogs (40); improve survival in rats after MI (51,52) and patients after heart failure (61); and increase LV contractile function in

Table 1. Cont.

Author	Reference	AT$_1$ Blocker	Series	Model	Effect
Jalowy	33	Candesartan	Pig	IR; low flow ischemia; in vivo	↓ TTC infarct size
Spinale	60	Valsartan	Pig	Pacing HF, in vivo	↔ LV function; ↑ with benazaprilat ± valsartan (− by HOE-140)
Richard	57	EXP3174	Dog	Acute MI, in vivo	↔ infarct size (↓ with enalaprilat)
Dörge	42	Candesartan	Dog	IR, in vivo	↔ flow
McDonald	58	DuP532	Dog	DC shock, necrosis, in vivo	↔ necrosis; ↓ LV remodeling
Ford	40	L-158809	Dog	MI, in vivo	↓ infarct size; ↓ LV remodeling; ↑ LV function
Xu	24	Losartan, UP269-6	Dog	IR, in vivo	↑AT$_2$R; LV function ↑ with losaratan and UP269-6
Jugdutt	25	Candesartan	Dog	IR, in vivo	↑AT$_2$R; ↑ LV function with candesartan
O'Brien	45	Losartan, UP269-6	Dog	IR, in vivo	UP269-6 ↓ LV volume more than losartan
ELITE I	61	Losartan	Human	HF	↓ mortality vs. captopril
ELITE II	62	Losartan	Human	Elderly HF	↔ survival
RESOLVD	63	Candesartan	Human	HF	↑ contractility
Val-HeFT	64	Valsartan	Human	HF	↑ survival with ACE inhibitor

Abbreviations: AS-ODN, antisense oligodeoxynucleotides; EDP, end-diastolic pressure; HF, heart failure; IR, ischemia-reperfusion; IPC, ischemic preconditioning; LV, left ventricular; MI, myocardial infarction; NWH, non-working heart; R, receptor; RVSP, right ventricular systolic pressure; τ, tau as index of diastolic function; TTC, triphephyl tetrazolium chloride; WH, working hearts; ↑, increase; ↔, no change; ↓, decrease; −, inhibited. See text for other abbreviations.

cardiomyopathic hamsters (53) and heart failure patients (63). AT$_1$ receptor blockade was also shown to decrease post-ischemic arrhythmias in rats (65,66).

The finding that the protective effect of AT$_1$ receptor blockade in dogs was associated with blockers that displayed characteristic insurmountable inhibition of vascular contractile responses to AngII (67), such as candesartan (33) and UP269-6 (24), as well as those that show surmountable inhibition, such as losartan (24), challenges the idea that the property of insurmountability, reflecting tight receptor binding, might translate into a therapeutic advantage.

Whether AT$_1$ receptor blockade with valsartan (surmountable inhibitor) and irbesartan (insurmountable inhibitor) would be equally protective in rodents was therefore studied. The effects of the AT_1 receptor blockers, valsartan and irbesartan on in vivo LV function (Echo/Doppler) and infarct size (TTC) and regional AT_2 receptor expression (immunoblots) after reperfused anterior MI were therefore determined in rats and dogs (68). The animals (38 rats and 25 dogs) were randomized to intravenous valsartan (10 mg/kg), irbesartan (10 mg/kg) and vehicle control over 30 minutes before IR, or to sham groups. AT_1 receptor blockade was confirmed by inhibition of AngII-induced pressor responses.

The overall results of that study (68) indicated that AT_1 receptor blockade induces cardioprotection after IR in both the dog and rat hearts after IR with improved global LV systolic and diastolic function, and infarct size. In addition, this cardioprotective effect involves enhanced AT_2 receptor expression in both animal models. The findings with valsartan and irbesartan also suggest that differences in "surmountability" of inhibition might not always translate into more protection, at least in the acute setting.

POSTISCHEMIC APOPTOSIS AND FUNCTIONAL RECOVERY AFTER AT_1 RECEPTOR BLOCKADE IN WORKING RAT HEARTS IN VITRO

Apoptosis (programmed cell death) has been suggested to play a critical role in the pathophysiology of cardiovascular disease (69,70). Apoptosis has been suggested to contribute to LV dysfunction after IR, MI and post MI remodeling (69,70). Cardiomyocyte (CM) apoptosis has been detected during IR injury (71–74) and acute MI (75–80), especially in the border zones (75), and has been suggested to precede CM necrosis (81). CM apoptosis was suggested to contribute to IR injury (71). Reperfusion of ischemic myocardium reduces the number of apoptotic CMs but also accelerates apoptosis in non-salvageable CMs (71). Inhibition of CM apoptosis has been suggested to attenuate LV dysfunction after IR (82,83). Cardiac AngII increases after acute MI (16,84) and IR (15), and AngII is involved in CM (84–87) and smooth muscle cell apoptosis (88,89). Thus, AngII induces apoptosis in cultured adult rat CMs and this effect is blocked by an AT_1 receptor blocker (losartan) but not by an AT_2 receptor blocker (PD123319) (87). Inhibition of AngII formation by enalapril in dogs with heart failure (90) and captopril in spontaneously hypertensive rats (SHRs) limited CM apoptosis (91). Inhibition of the effffects of AngII at the AT_1 receptor level with losartan also attenuates smooth muscle cell apoptosis (89).

Although chronic pretreatment with the AT_1 receptor blocker TCV-116 attenuates LV dysfunction after IR in rats (36), whether chronic AT_1 receptor blockade applied after acute IR or acutely reperfused MI might decrease apoptosis found after IR (71–74) has not been addressed. This is a pertinent issue because evidence indicates that AT_1 receptor blockade after IR results in AT_2 receptor activation (27,28) and AT_2 receptor receptors are believed to be pro-apoptotic (21). AT_2 receptor stimulation inhibits responses to AT_1 receptor activation (92) and this effect would be especially enhanced when the AT_2 receptor is over-expressed after injury. While candesartan decreases infarct size in the in vivo mini-pig model of IR, the AT_2 receptor blocker PD123319 only produced a non-significant decrease from 22% to 17% in that model (33). However, during AT_1 receptor blockade with candesartan in the in vivo dog model of IR, PD123319 abrogated its beneficial effect on infarct size (28).

The possibility that enhanced AT_2 receptor protein during AT_1 receptor blockade might not increase CM apoptosis was therefore examined. Whether chronic AT_1 receptor blockade inhibits apoptosis and attenuates LV dysfunction after ischemia-reperfusion (IR) was studied in the isolated working rat heart (29). The results indicated that LV dysfunction after IR is associated with apoptosis in the working rat heart and chronic AT_1 receptor blockade inhibited CM apoptosis after acute IR without improving functional recovery in that model (29). These results suggested that decrease in CM apoptosis does not necessarily translate into decreased LV dysfunction after acute IR. In addition, the results indicated that AT_1 receptor blockade can improve LV function after IR independent of a decrease in CM apoptosis.

Although i) the AT_2 receptor is upregulated in cardiac hypertrophy, MI and heart failure (21,93), ii) AngII activity is enhanced in heart failure, and iii) AT_2 receptors are upregulated and AT_1 receptors are downregulated in heart failure (19), the idea that the AT_2 receptor might play a significant functional role has been questioned by other researchers (94). Moreover, AT_2 receptor gene (+1675 G/A) polymorphism was recently implicated in LV structure in humans with arterial hypertension (95). Also, apoptosis was recently found not to be increased in myocardium overexpressing the AT_2 receptor in transgenic mice (96). The results of the recent study (29) suggest that this might also be true in the presence of AT_1 receptor blockade.

MYOCARDIAL PROTECTION THROUGH AT₁ RECEPTOR BLOCKADE AND IMPLICATIONS

There is considerable experimental evidence indicating that AT_1 receptor blockade is cardioprotective during in vivo IR, by improving recovery of mechanical function, improving LV systolic and diastolic function and limiting acute infarct expansion. Other mechanisms remain to be defined. Cumulative experimental evidence also indicates that the AT_2 receptor plays a significant role in the cardioprotective effects of AT_1 receptor blockade (24,25,27,28,33). The findings on the effects of pretreatment with AT_1 receptor blockers on IR are especially pertinent for the large population of hypertensive patients who might develop acute coronary syndromes while receiving these drugs. Further long-term studies on the effect of chronic AT_1 receptor blockade after reperfused MI and heart failure are needed. It is important to note that the ratio of AT_1 to AT_2 receptor is 1:1 in rat hearts and 1:2 in human hearts (97), and this ratio increases further in human heart failure (19). It is also important to note that AngII levels are elevated during angiotensin-converting-enzyme (ACE) inhibition (98–101), providing the rationale for AT_1 receptor blockade (102). This increase in AngII during ACE inhibition appears to be related to production via non-ACE pathways, especially chymase which is dominant in human hearts (103).

New advances in the clinical use of AT_1 receptor blockers (or ARBs) have been reviewed elsewhere (1) and the results of several ongoing clinical trials are eagerly awaited. A major drawback of clinical trials is that ARBs have to be tested on top of a background therapy, including ACE inhibitors, reperfusion therapies and other agents. A placebo group is currently considered to be unethical. The ELITE [Evaluation of Losartan in the Elderly] (62) and RESOLVD [Randomized Evaluation of Strategies for Left Ventricular Dysfunction], using candesartan (63) in heart failure patients did not show a dramatic advantage of ARBs over ACE inhibition. The Val-HeFT study [Valsartan in Heart Failure Trial] (64) showed that "valsartan significantly reduces the combined end point of mortality and morbidity and improves clinical signs and symptoms in patients with heart failure, when added to prescribed therapy".

The experimental findings that after in vivo IR, acute AT_1 receptor blockade induces cardioprotection and increases AT_2 receptor protein, $PKC\varepsilon$ and cGMP which contribute to the cardioprotective effect (24,25,27,28), are new and provocative. They support the concept that during AT_1 receptor blockade after myocardial injury, AngII stimulates AT_2 receptors which become activated and participate in cardioprotection through the BK, NO and eicosanoid pathways (31–33). Other recent in vivo studies suggest that AT_2 receptor stimulation can produce benefits via BK and NO (104,105). Although chronic AT_1 receptor blockade for 3 weeks after myocardial infarction was shown to decrease LV tissue AngII (106), long-term chronic AT_1 receptor blockade also results in increased plasma AngII (107) and presumably myocardial AngII. These increases in AngII after long-term AT_1 receptor blockade could therefore stimulate AT_2 receptors, at least in the in vivo setting. Recently PKC/NO signaling has also been implicated in ischemia-induced preconditioning (108).

CONCLUSIONS

Early coronary artery reperfusion after acute MI is becoming an established therapeutic strategy (109–111). Inhibition of the injurious effects of elevated tissue AngII levels during and after acutely reperfused MI is an attractive adjunctive therapeutic strategy (1). Cumulative evidence suggests that AT_1 receptor blockade might be more beneficial than ACE-inhibition (1). However, both chronic ACE-inhibition and chronic AT_1 receptor blockade are complicated by increased AngII (102, 107). Since AT_2 receptors are upregulated after IR and MI (23–30), and are activated after AT_1 receptor blockade (24,25,27,28), the finding that they may contribute to cardioprotection via $PKC\varepsilon$ and NO signaling is especially important. Since AT_2 receptors are pro-apoptotic (21), it is also important that during AT_1 receptor blockade, they do not seem to increase CM apoptosis (29) and might in fact inhibit apoptosis (29,87). Further experimental and clinical studies are needed to elucidate the underlying mechanisms of the beneficial effects of ARBs after IR and reperfused MI.

REFERENCES

1. Jugdutt BI. 2001. New advances in the use of AT_1 receptor blockers (ARBs). In *Proceedings, 2nd International Congress on heart Disease: New Trends in Research, Diagnosis and Treatment*. Ed. A. Kimchi Medimond, 531–538. New Jersey: Medical Publishers.

2. Brunner HR. 2001. Experimental and clinical evidence that angiotensin II is an independent risk factor for cardiovascular disease. Am J Cardiol 87:3C–9C.
3. Yusuf S, Sleight P, Pogue J, Bosch J, Davies R, Dagenais G. 2000. Effects of an angiotensin-converting-enzyme inhibitor, ramipril, on cardiovascular events in high-risk patients. The Heart Outcomes Prevention Evaluation Study Investigators. N Engl J Med 342:145–153.
4. Dahlöf B, Devereux RB, Kjeldsen SE, for the LIFE study group. 2002. Cardiovascular morbidity and mortality in the Losartan Intervention For Endpoint reduction in hypertension study (LIFE): a randomized trial against atenolol. Lancet 359:995–1003.
5. Ryan TJ, Antman EM, Brooks NH, et al. 1999. Update: ACC/AHA guidelines for the management of patients with acute myocardial infarction. A report of the American College of Cardiology/American Heart Association Task Force on Practice Guidelines (Committee on Management of Acute Myocardial Infarction). J Am Coll Cardiol 34:890–911.
6. Kleiman NS, White HD, Ohman EM, Ross AM, Woodlief LH, Califf RM, Holmes DR Jr, Bates E, Pfisterer M, Vahanian A, Topol EJ, for the GUSTO Investigators. 1994. Mortality within 24 hours of thrombolysis for myocardial infarction. The importance of early reperfusion. The GUSTO Investigators, Global Utilization of Streptokinase and Tissue Plasminogen Activator for Occluded Coronary Arteries. Circulation 90:2658–2665.
7. Braunwald E, Kloner RA. 1982. The stunned myocardium: prolonged, post-ischemic ventricular dysfunction. Circulation 66:1146–1149.
8. Kloner RA, Jennings RB. 2001. Consequences of brief ischemia: stunning, preconditioning, and their clinical implications. Part 1. Circulation 104:2981–2989.
9. Kloner RA, Jennings RB. 2001. Consequences of brief ischemia: stunning, preconditioning, and their clinical implications. Part 2. Circulation 104:3158–3167.
10. Przyklenk K, Kloner RA. 1986. Superoxide dismutase plus catalase improve contractile function in the canine model of the "stunned myocardium." Circ Res 58:148–156.
11. Bolli R, Jeroudi MO, Patel BS, et al. 1989. Marked reduction of free radical generation and contractile dysfuncrtion by antioxidant therapy begun at the time of reperfusion: evidence that myocardial "stunning" is a manifestation of reperfusion injury. Circ Res 65:607–622.
12. Bolli R. 1990. Mechanisms of myocardial "stunning." Circulation 82:723–738.
13. Fleetwood G, Boutinet S, Meier M, Wood JM. 1991. Involvement of the renin-angiotensin system in ischemic damage and reperfusion arrhythmias in the isolated perfused rat heart. J Cardiovasc Pharmacol 17:351–356.
14. Zughaib ME, Sun JZ, Bolli R. 1993. Effect of angiotensin-converting enzyme inhibitors on myocardial ischemia/reperfusion injury: an overview. Basic Res Cardiol 88:155–167.
15. Youhua Z, Shouchun X. 1995. Increased vulnerability of hypertrophied myocardium to ischemia and reperfusion injury. Relation to cardiac renin-angiotensin system. Chin Med J 108:28–32.
16. Sun Y, Weber KT. 1994. Angiotensin II receptor binding following myocardial infarction in the rat. Cardiovasc Res 28:1623–1628.
17. Francis GS, McDonald KM, Cohn JN. 1993 Neurohumoral activation in preclinical heart failure. Remodeling and the potential for intervention. Circulation 87(5 Suppl):IV90–96.
18. Dostal DE, Baker KN. 1999. The cardiac-renin-angiotensin system. Conceptual or a regulator of cardiac function? Circ Res 85:643–650.
19. Haywood GA, Gullestad L, Katsuya T, Hutchinson HG, Pratt RE, Horiuchi M, Fowler MB. 1997. AT$_1$ and AT$_2$ angiotensin receptor gene expression in human heart failure. Circulation 95:1201–1206.
20. Matsubara H. 1998. Pathophysiological role of angiotensin II type 2 receptor in cardiovascular and renal diseases. Circ Res 83:1182–1191.
21. Horiuchi M, Akishita M, Dzau VJ. 1999. Recent progress in angiotensin type 2 receptor research in the cardiovascular system. Hypertension 33:613–621.
22. Shanmugam S, Corvol P, Gasc J-M. 1996. Angiotensin II type 2 receptor mRNA expression in the developing cardiopulmonary system of the rat. Hypertension 28:91–97.
23. Xu Y, Clanachan AS, Jugdutt BI. 2000. Enhanced expression of AT$_2$R, IP$_3$R and PKC$_\varepsilon$ during cardioprotection induced by AT$_2$R blockade. Hypertension 36:506–510.
24. Xu Y, Menon V, Jugdutt BI. 2000. Cardioprotection after angiotensin II type 1 blockade involves angiotensin II type 2 receptor expression and activation of protein kinase C-ε in acutely reperfused myocardial infarction. Effect of UP269-6 and losartan on AT$_1$ and AT$_2$ receptor expression, and IP$_3$ receptor and PKC$_\varepsilon$ proteins. J Renin-Angiotensin Aldosterone System 1:184–195.
25. Jugdutt BI, Xu Y, Balghith M, Moudgil R, Menon V. 2000. Cardioprotection induced by AT$_1$R

blockade after reperfused myocardial infarction: Association with regional increase in AT_2R, IP_3R and PKC_ε proteins and cGMP. J Cardiovasc Pharmacol & Therapeut 5:301–311.

26. Moudgil R, Xu Y, Menon V, Jugdutt BI. 2001. Effect of chronic pretreatment with AT_1 receptor antagonism on postischemic functional recovery and AT_1/AT_2 receptor proteins in isolated working rat hearts. J Cardiovasc Pharmacol & Therapeut 6:183–188.

27. Jugdutt BI, Xu Y, Balghith M, Menon V. 2001. Cardioprotective effects of angiotensin II type 1 receptor blockade with candesartan after reperfused myocardial infarction: Role of angiotensin II type 2 receptor. J Renin-Angiotensin Aldosterone System 2:S162–S166.

28. Jugdutt BI, Balghith M. 2001. Enhanced regional AT_2 receptor and $PKC\varepsilon$ expression during cardioprotection induced by AT_1 receptor blockade after reperfused myocardial infarction. J Renin-Angiotensin Aldosterone System 2:134–140.

29. Moudgil R, Menon V, Xu Y, Musat-Marcu S, Jugdutt BI. 2001. Postischemic apoptosis and functional recovery after angiotensin II type 1 receptor blockade in isolated working rat hearts. J of Hypertension 19:1121–1129.

30. Nio Y, Matsubara H, Murasawa S, Kanasaki M, Inada M. 1995. Regulation and gene transcription of angiotensin II receptor subtypes in myocardial infarction. J Clin Invest 95:46–54.

31. Wiemer G, Schölkens BA, Wagner A, Heitsch H, Linz W. 1993. The possible role of angiotensin II subtype AT_2 receptors in endothelial cells and isolated ischemic rat hearts. J Hypertens 11:S234–S235.

32. Liu YH, Yang XP, Sharov VG, Nass O, Sabbah HN, Peterson E, Carretero OA. 1997. Effects of angiotensin-converting enzyme inhibitors and angiotensin II type 1 receptor antagonists in rats with heart failure: role of kinins and angiotensin type 2 receptors. J Clin Invest 99:1926–1935.

33. Jalowy A, Schulz R, Dorge H, Behrends M, Heush G. 1998. Infarct size reduction by AT_1-receptor blockade through a signal cascade of AT_2 receptor activation, bradykinin and prostaglandins in pigs. J Am Coll Cardiol 32:1787–1796.

34. Bartunek J, Weinberg EO, Tajima M, Rohrbach S, Lorell BH. 1999. Angiotensin II type 2 receptor blockade amplifies the early signals of cardiac growth response to angiotensin II in hypertrophied hearts. Circulation 99:22–25.

35. Yoshiyama M, Kim S, Yamagishi H, Omura T, Tani T, Takagi M, Toda I, Teragaki M, Akioka K, Takeuchi K, Takeda T. 1994. The deleterious effects of exogenous angiotensin I and angiotensin II on myocardial ischemia-reperfusion injury. Jpn Circ 58:362–368.

36. Yoshiyama M, Kim S, Yamagishi H, Omura T, Tani T, Yanagi S, Toda I, Teragaki M, Akioka K, Takeuchi K, Takeda T. 1994. Cardioprotective effect of the angiotensin II type 1 receptor antagonist TCV-116 on ischemia-reperfusion injury. Am Heart J 128:1–6.

37. Werrmann JG, Cohen SM. 1994. Comparison of the effects of angiotensin converting enzyme inhibition with those of angiotensin II receptor antagonism on functional and metabolic recovery in the post-ischemic working rat heart as studied by ^{31}P nuclear magnetic resonance. J Cardiovasc Pharmacol 24:573–586.

38. Werrmann JG, Cohen SM. 1996. Use of losartan to examine the role of the cardiac renin-angiotensin system in myocardial dysfunction during ischemia and reperfusion. J Cardiovasc Pharmacol 27:177–182.

39. Yang BC, Phillips MI, Ambeuhl PEJ, Shen LP, Mehta P, Mehta JL. 1997. Increase in angiotensin II type 1 receptor expression immediately after ischemia-reperfusion in isolated rat hearts. Circulation 96:922–926.

40. Ford WR, Khan MI, Jugdutt BI. 1998. Effect of the novel angiotensin II type 1 receptor antagonist L-158,809 on acute infarct expansion and acute anterior myocardial infarction in the dog. Can J Cardiol 14:73–80.

41. Becker LC, Jeremy RW, Schaper J, Schaper W. 1999. Ultrastructural assessment of myocardial necrosis occurring during ischemia and 3-h reperfusion in the dog. Am J Physiol 277:H243–H252.

42. Dörge H, Behrends M, Schulz R, Jalowy A, Heusch G. 1999. Attenuation of myocardial stunning by the AT_1 receptor antagonist candesartan. Basic Res Cardiol 94:208–214.

43. Ford WR, Clanachan AS, Jugdutt BI. 1996. Opposite effects of angiotensin receptor antagonists on recovery of mechanical function after ischemia-reperfusion in isolated working rat hearts. Circulation 94:3087–3089.

44. Ford WR, Clanachan AS, Lopaschuk GD, Schulz R, Jugdutt BI. 1998. Intrinsic AngII type 1 receptor stimulation contributes to recovery of postischemic mechanical function. Am J Physiol 274:H1524–H1531.

45. O'Brien D, Xu Y, Jugdutt BI. 2000. Efficacy of angiotensin type 1 receptor blockade in the dog model of ventricular remodeling and heart failure. J Cardiovasc Pharmacol Therapeut 5:129–137.

46. Xu Y, Dyck J, Ford WR, Clanachan AS, Lopaschuk GD, Jugdutt BI. 2002. Angiotensin II type 1 and type 2 receptor protein after acute ischemia-reperfusion in isolated working rat hearts. Am J Physiol Heart Circ Physiol 282:H1206–H1215.

47. Yang BC, Phillips MI, Zhang YC, Kimura B, Shen LP, Mehta P, Mehta JL. 1998. Critical role of AT₁ receptor expression after ischemia/reperfusion in isolated rat hearts: beneficial effect of antisense oligodeoxynucleotides directed at AT₁ receptor mRNA. Circ Res 83:552–559.

48. Liu Y-H, Yang X-P, Sharov VG, Sigmon DH, Sabbah HN, Carretero OA. 1996. Paracrine systems in the cardioprotective effect of angiotensin-converting enzyme inhibitors on myocardial ischemia/reperfusion injury in rats. Hypertension 27:7–13.

49. Sladek T, Sladkova J, Kolar F, Papousek F, Cicutti N, Korecky B, Rakusan K. 1996. The effect of AT₁ receptor antagonist on chronic cardiac response to coronary artery ligation in rats. Cardiovasc Res 31:568–576.

50. Stauss HM, Zhu Y-C, Redlich T, Adamiak D, Mott A, Kregel KC, Unger T. 1994. Angiotensin-converting enzyme inhibition in infarct-induced heart failure in rats: bradykinin versus angiotensin II. J Cardiovasc Risk 1:255–262.

51. Milavetz JJ, Raya TE, Johnson CS, Morkin E, Goldman S. 1996. Survival after myocardial infarction in rats: captopril versus losartan. J Am Coll Cardiol 27:714–719.

52. Richer C, Fornes P, Cazaubon C, Domergue V, Nisata D, Giudicelli JF. 1999. Effects of long-term angiotensin II AT1 receptor blockade on survival, hemodynamics and cardiac remodeling in chronic heart failure in rats. Cardiovasc Res 41:100–108.

53. Bastien NR, Juneau A-V, Ouellette J, Lambert C. 1999. Chronic AT₁ receptor blockade and angiotensin-converting enzyme (ACE) inhibition in (CHF 146) cardiomyopathic hamsters: effects on cardiac hypertrophy and survival. Cardiovasc Res 43:77–85.

54. Hartman JC, Hullinger TG, Wall TM, Shebuski RJ. 1993. Reduction of myocardial infarct size by ramiprilat is independent of angiotensin II synthesis inhibition. Eur J Pharmacol 234:229–236.

55. Liu Y, Tsuchida A, Cohen MV, Downey JM. 1995. Pretreatment with angiotensin II activates protein kinase C and limits myocardial infarction in isolated rabbit hearts. J Mol Cell Cardiol 27:883–892.

56. Diaz RJ, Wilson GJ. 1997. Selective blockade of AT₁ angiotensin II receptors abolishes ischemic preconditioning in isolated rabbit hearts. J Moll Cell Cardiol 29:129–139.

57. Richard V, Ghaleh B, Berdeaux A, Giudicelli J-F. 1993. Comparison of the effects of EXP3174, an angiotensin II antagonist, and enalaprilat on myocardial infarct size in anesthetized dogs. Br J Pharmacol 110:969–974.

58. McDonald KM, Garr M, Carlyle PF, Francis GS, Hauer K, Hunter DW, Parish T, Stillman A, Cohn JN. 1994. Relative effects of α₁-adrenoreceptor blockade, converting enzyme inhibitor therapy, and angiotensin II subtype 1 receptor blockade on ventricular remodeling in the dog. Circulation 90:3034–3046.

59. Schwarz ER, Montino H, Fleischhauer J, Klues HG, vom Dahl J, Hanrath P. 1997. Angiotensin II receptor antagonist EXP3174 reduces infarct size comparable with enalaprilat and augments preconditioning in the pig heart. Cardiovasc Drugs Ther 11:687–695.

60. Spinale FG, Mukherjee R, Iannini JP, Whitebread S, Hebbar L, Clair MJ, Melton DM, Cox MH, Thomas PB, de Gasparo M. 1997. Modulation of the renin-angiotensin pathway through enzyme inhibition and specific receptor blockade in pacing-induced heart failure: II. Effects on myocyte contractile processes. Circulation 96:2397–2406.

61. Pitt B, Segal R, Martinez FA, et al., on behalf of the ELITE Study Investigators: 1997. Randomized trial of losartan versus captopril in patients over 65 with heart failure (Evaluation of Losartan in Elderly Study, ELITE). Lancet 349:747–752.

62. Pitt B, Poole-Wilson PA, Segal R, Martinez FA, Dickstein K, Camm AJ, Konstam MA, Riegger G, Klinger GH, Neaton J, Sharma D, Thiyagarajan B, on behalf of the ELITE II investigators. 2000. Effect of losartan compared with captopril on mortality in patients with symptomatic heart failure: randomized trial—the Losartan Heart Failure Survival Study ELITE II. Lance 355:1582–1587.

63. McKelvie RS, Yusuf S, Pericak D, Avezum A, Burns RJ, Probstfield J, Tsuyuki RT, White M, Rouleau J, Latini R, Maggioni A, Young J, Pogue J. 1999. Comparison of candesartan, enalapril, and their combination in congestive heart failure: randomized evaluation of strategies for left ventricular dysfunction (RESOLVD) pilot study. The RESOLVD Pilot Study Investigators. Circulation 100:1056–1064.

64. Cohn JN, Tognoni G; Valsartan Heart Failure Trial Investigators. 2001. A randomized trial of the angiotensin-receptor blocker valsartan in chronic heart failure. N Engl J Med 345:1667–1675.

65. Kohya T, Yokoshiki H, Tohse N, et al. 1995. Regression of left ventricular hypertrophy prevents ischemia-induced lethal arrhythmias: Beneficial effect of angiotensin II blockade. Circ Res 76:892–899.

66. Thomas GP, Ferrier GR, Howlett SE. 1996. Losartan exerts antiarrhythmic activity independent of angiotensin II receptor blockade in simulated ventricular ischemia and reperfusion. J Pharmacol Exp Ther 278:1090–1097.

67. Vanderheyden PML, Fierens FLP, De Backer JP, Fraeyman N, Vauquelin G. 1999. Distinction between surmountable and insurmountable selective AT_1 receptor antagonists by use of CHO-K1 cells expressing human angiotensin II AT_1 receptors. Br J Pharmacol 126:1057–1065.

68. Jugdutt BI. 2001. Cardioprotection and angiotensin II type 2 receptor upregulation during angiotensin type 1 receptor blockade in dog and rat in vivo models of reperfused myocardial infarction. (Abst). J Renin-Angiotensin-Aldosterone System 2:80.

69. Haunstetter A, Izumo S. 1998. Apoptosis: Basic mechanisms and implications for cardiovascular disease. Circ Res 82:1111–1129.

70. Kang PM, Izumo S. 2000. Apoptosis and heart failure. A critical review of the literature. Circ Res 86:1107–1113.

71. Fliss H, Gattinger D. 1996. Apoptosis in ischemic and reperfused rat myocardium. Circ Res 76:949–956.

72. Gottlieb RA, Gruol DL, Zhu JY, Engler RL. 1996. Preconditioning in rabbit cardiomyocytes: Role of pH, vacuolar proton ATPase, and apoptosis. J Clin Invest 97:2391–2398.

73. Gottlieb RA, Engler RL. 1999. Apoptosis in myocardial ischemia-reperfusion. In, Heart in Stress, Ed. Das DK. Ann N Y Acad Science, New York, 874:412–426.

74. Gottlieb RA, Burleson KO, Kloner RA, Babior BM, Engler RL. 1994. Reperfusion injury induces apoptosis in rabbit cardiomyocytes. J Clin Invest 94:1621–1628.

75. Saraste A, Pulkki K, Kallajoki M, Henriksen K, Parvinen M, Voipio-Pulkki LM. 1997. Apoptosis in acute myocardial infarction. Circulation 95:320–323.

76. Bardales RH, Hailey LS, Xie SS, Schafer RF, Hsu SM. 1996. In situ apoptosis assay for the detection of early acute myocardial infarction. Am J Pathol 149:821–829.

77. Misao J, Hayakawa Y, Ohno M, Kato S, Fujiwara T, Fujiwara H. 1996. Expression of Bcl-2 protein, an inhibitor of apoptosis, and Bax, an accelerator of apoptosis, in ventricular myocytes of human hearts with myocardial infarction. Circulation 94:1505–1512.

78. Itoh G, et al. 1995. DNA fragmentation of human infarcted myocardial cells demonstrated by the nick end labeling method and DNA agarose gel electrophoresis. Am J Pathol 146:1325–1331.

79. Kanoh M, Takemura G, Misao J, et al. 1999. Significance of myocytes with positive DNA in situ nick end-labeling (TUNEL) in hearts with dilated cardiomyopathy: not apoptosis but DNA repair. Circulation 99:2757–2764.

80. Ohno M, Takemura G, Ohno A, Misao J, Hayakawa Y, Minatoguchi S, Fujiwara T, Fujiwara H. 1998. "Apoptotic" myocytes in infarct area in rabbit hearts may be oncotic myocytes with DNA fragmentation. Analysis by immunogold electron microscopy combined with in situ nick end-labeling. Circulation 98:1422–1430.

81. Katsjura J, Cheng W, Reiss K, Clark WA, Sonnenblick EH, Lrajewski S, et al. 1996. Apoptotic and necrotic myocyte cell deaths are independent variables of infarct size in rats. Lab Invest 74:86–107.

82. Yaoita H, Ogawa K, Maehara K, Maruyama Y. 1998. Attenuation of ischemia/reperfusion injury in rats by a caspase inhibitor. Circulation 97:276–281.

83. Musat-Marcu S, Gunter HE, Jugdutt BI, Docherty JC. 1999. Inhibition of apoptosis after ischemia-reperfusion in rat myocardium by cycloheximide. J Moll Cell Cardiol 31:1073–1082.

84. Leenen FHH, Skarda V, Yuan B, White R. 1999. Changes in cardiac AngII postmyocardial infarction in rats: effects of nephrotomy and ACE inhibitors. Am J Physiol 276:H317–H325.

85. Kajstura J, Cigola E, Malhotra A, Li P, Cheng W, Meggs LG, Anversa P. 1997. Angiotensin II induces apoptosis of adult ventricular myocytes in vitro. J Moll Cell Cardiol 29:859–870.

86. Cigola E, Katstura J, Li B, Meggs LG, Anversa P. 1997. Angiotensin II activates programmed myocyte cell death in vitro. Exp Cell Res 231:363–371.

87. Leri A, Claudio PP, Li Q, Wang X, Reiss K, Wang S, Malhotra A, Kajstura J, Anversa P. 1998. Stretch-mediated release of angiotensin-II induces myocyte apoptosis by activating p53 that enhances the local renin-angiotensin system and decreases the Bcl-2-Bax ratio in the cell. J Clin Invest 101:1326–1342.

88. Pollman MJ, Yamada T, Horiuchi M, Gibbons GH. 1996. Vasoactive substances regulate vascular

smooth muscle cell apoptosis. Countervailing influences of nitric oxide and angiotensin-II. Circ Res 79:748–756.

89. deBlois D, Tea BS, Dam T-V Tremblay J, Hamet P. 1997. Smooth muscle apoptosis during vascular regression in spontaneously hypertensive rats. Hypertension 29:340–349.

90. Goussev A, Sharov VG, Shimoyama H, Tanimura M, Lesch M, Goldstein S, Sabbah HN. 1998. Effects of ACE inhibition on cardiomyocyte apoptosis in dogs with heart failure. Am J Physiol 275:H626–H631.

91. Li Z, Bing OH, Long X, Robinson KG, Lakatta EG. 1997. Increased cardiomyocyte apoptosis during the transition to heart failure in the spontaneously hypertensive rat. Am J Physiol 272: H2313–H2319.

92. Masaki H, Kurihara T, Yamaki A, Inomata N, Nozawa Y, Mori Y, Murasawa S, Kizima K, Maruyama K, Horiuchi M, Dzau VJ, Takahashi H, Iwasaka T, Inada M, Matsubara H. 1998. Cardiac-specific overexpression of angiotensin II AT$_2$ receptor causes attenuated response to AT$_1$ receptor-mediated pressor and chronotropic effects. J Clin Invest 101:527–535.

93. Zhu YC, Zhu YZ, Gohlke P, Stauss HM, Unger T. 1997. Effects of angiotensin-converting enzyme inhibition and angiotensin II AT1 receptor antagonism on cardiac parameters in left ventricular hypertrophy. Am J Cardiol 80:110A–117A.

94. Opie LH, Sack MN. 2001. Enhanced angiotensin II activity in heart failure. Reevaluation of the counter-regulatory hypothesis of receptor subtypes. Circ Res 88:654–658.

95. Schmieder RE, Erdmann J, Delles C, Jacobi J, Fleck E, Hilgers K, Regitz-Zagrosek V. 2001. Effect of the angiotensin II type 2-receptor gene (+1675 G/A) on left ventricular structure in humans. J Am Coll Cardiol 37:175–182.

96. Sugino H, Ozono R, Kurisu S, Matsuura H, Ishida M, Oshima T, Kambe M, Teranishi Y, Masaki H, Matsubara H. 2001. Apoptosis is not increased in myocardium overexpressing type 2 angiotensin II receptor in transgenic mice. Hypertension 37:1394–1398.

97. Regitz-Zagrosek V, Friedel N, Heymann A, Bauer P, Neuss M, Rolfs A, Steffen C, Hildebrandt A, Hetzer R, Fleck E. 1995. Regulation, chamber localization, and subtype distribution of angiotensin II receptors in human hearts. Circulation 91:1461–1471.

98. Biollaz J, Brunner HR, Gavras I, Waeber B, Gavras H. 1982. Antihypertensive therapy with MK 421: angiotensin-renin relationships to evaluate efficacy of converting enzyme blockade. J Cardiovasc Pharmacol 4:966–972.

99. Mento PF, Wilkes BM. 1987. Plasma angiotensins and blood pressure during converting enzyme inhibition. Hypertension 9 (Suppl III): III42–III48.

100. Rousseau MF, Konstam MA, Benedict CR, Donckier J, Galanti L, Melin J, Kinan D, Ahn S, Ketelslegers J-M, Pouleur H. 1994. Progression of left ventricular dysfunction secondary to coronary artery disease, sustained neurohormonal activation and effects of ibopamine therapy during long-term therapy wth angiotensin-converting enzyme inhibitor. Am J Cardiol 73:488–493.

101. Baruch L, Anand I, Cohen IS, Zeische S, Judd D, Cohn JN, for the Vasodilator Heart Failure Trial (V-HeFT) Study Group. 1999. Augmented short- and long-term hemodynamic and hormonal effects of an angiotensin receptor blocker added to angiotensin converting enzyme inhibitor therapy in patienst with heart failure. Circulation 99:2658–2664.

102. Goldberg MR, Bradstreet TE, McWilliams EJ, et al. 1995. Biochemical effects of losartan, a non-peptide angiotensin II receptor antagonist, on the renin-angiotensin-aldosterone system in hypertensive patients. Hypertension 25:37–46.

103. Urata HB, Healy B, Stewart RW, Bumpus FM, Husain A. 1990. Angiotensin II-forming pathways in normal and failing hearts. Circ Res 66:883–890.

104. Seyedi N, Xu XB, Nasjletti A, Hintze TH. 1995. Coronary kinin generation mediates nitric oxide release after angiotensin receptor stimulation. Hypertension 26:164–170.

105. Tsutsumi Y, Matsubara H, Masaki H, Kurihara H, Murasawa S, Takai S, Miyazaki M, Nozawa Y, Ozono R, Nakagawa K, Miwa T, Kawada N, Mori Y, Shibasaki Y, Tanaka Y, Fujiyama S, Koyama Y, Fujiyama A, Takahashi H, Iwasaka T. 1999. Angiotensin II type 2 receptor overexpression activates the vascular kinin system and causes vasodilation. J Clin Invest 104:925–935.

106. Yamagishi H, Kim S, Nishikimi T, Takeuchi K, Takeda T. 1993. Contribution of cardiac renin-angiotensin system to ventricular remodelling in myocardial-infarcted rats. J Mol Cell Cardiol 25: 1369–1380.

107. Hübner R, Högemann AM, Sunzel M, Riddell JG. 1997. Pharmacokinetics of candesartan after single and repeated doses of candesartan cilexetil in young and elderly human volunteers. J Hum Hypertens 11:S19–S25.

108. Ping P, Takano H, Zhang J, Tang X-L, Qiu Y, Li RCX, Banerjee S, Dawn B, Balafonova Z, Bolli

R. 1999. Isoform-selective activation of protein kinase C by nitric oxide in the heart of conscious rabbits. A signaling mechanism for both nitric oxide-induced and ischemia-induced preconditioning. Circ Res 84:587–604.

109. Cannon CP, Gibson CM, Lambrew CT, Shoultz DA, Levy D, French WJ, Gore JM, Weaver WD, Rogers WJ, Tiefenbrunn AJ. 2000. Relationship of symptom-onset-to-balloon time and door-to-balloon time with mortality in patients undergoing angioplasty for acute myocardial infarction. JAMA 283:2941–2947.

110. Topol EJ. 1996. Early myocardial reperfusion: an assessment of current strategies in acute myocardial infarction. Eur Heart J 17 (Suppl E):42–48.

111. Ross AM, Coyne KS, Reiner JS, Greenhouse SW, Fink C, Frey A, Moreyra E, Traboulsi M, Racine N, Riba AL, Thompson MA, Rohrbeck S, Lundergan CF. 1999. A randomized trial comparing primary angioplasty with a strategy of short-acting thrombolysis and immediate planned rescue angioplasty in acute myocardial infarction: the PACT trial. PACT investigators. Plasminogen-activator Angioplasty Compatibility Trial. J Am Coll Cardiol 34:1954–1962.

Signal Transduction and Cardiac Hypertrophy,
edited by N.S. Dhalla, L.V. Hryshko,
E. Kardami & P.K. Singal
Kluwer Academic Publishers, Boston, 2003

Relation between Intracellular Ca^{2+} Concentration and Contraction in Tetanized Myocytes of Rat and Mouse

Kenichi Hongo,[1] Yoichiro Kusakari,[2] Makoto Kawai,[1] Masato Konishi,[3] Seibu Mochizuki,[1] and Satoshi Kurihara[2]

Division of Cardiology
Department of Internal Medicine[1]
and Department of Physiology (II)[2]
The Jikei University School of Medicine
3-25-8 Nishishinbashi, Minato-ku
Tokyo 105-8461, Japan
Department of Physiology[3]
Tokyo Medical University
6-1-1 Shinjuku, Shinjuku-ku
Tokyo 160-8402, Japan

Summary. To investigate the characteristics of Ca^{2+} responsiveness of myofibrils in isolated myocytes of rats and mice, we used the relation between intracellular Ca^{2+} concentration ($[Ca^{2+}]_i$) and cell shortening during tetanus. Single ventricular myocytes were isolated from rat and mouse using enzymatic dispersion technique. Isolated myocytes were loaded with fura-2 AM, and the resultant fluorescence ratio signals excited at 340 nm and 380 nm wave length [F(340)/F(380)] were measured simultaneously with cell length. To produce tetanus, myocytes were treated with thapsigargin (0.2 μM) and the repetitive electrical stimulation of 10 Hz was applied to the myocytes. An instantaneous plot of the fluorescence ratio signal versus cell length (R-L trajectory) during tetanus was constructed. The R-L trajectory was extended without a substantial shift by an increase in the extracellular Ca^{2+} concentration in rat and mouse ventricular myocytes. Myofibrillar responsiveness to Ca^{2+} of mouse ventricular myocytes seems to be less than that of rat ventricular myocytes. In both rat and mouse ventricular myocytes, the trajectory was shifted rightward by the non-selective phosphodiesterase inhibitor, 3-isobutyl-1-methylxantine (IBMX) (desensitization of the myofibrils to

Address for Correspondence: Dr. Kenichi Hongo, Division of Cardiology, Department of Internal Medicine, The Jikei University School of Medicine, 3-25-8 Nishishinbashi, Minato-ku, Tokyo 105-8461, Japan. Tel: 81-3-3433-1111 ex)3261, Fax: 81-3-3459-6043 E-mail: hongo@jikei.ac.jp.

Ca^{2+}) and was shifted leftward by the Ca^{2+} sensitizing thiadiazinone derivative, EMD57033 (sensitization of the myofibrils to Ca^{2+}). In mouse ventricular myocytes, β-adrenergic stimulant, isoproterenol shifted the R-L trajectory to the right (desensitization of the myofibrils to Ca^{2+}). These results suggest that the R-L trajectory is a useful method to estimate the myofibrillar responsiveness to Ca^{2+} in mammalian ventricular myocytes, and that mouse myocytes might have different characteristics of Ca^{2+} responsiveness compared to that of rat myocytes.

Key words: 1) ventricular myocyte, 2) myofibrillar responsiveness to Ca^{2+}, 3) tetanus.

INTRODUCTION

Cardiac contractility can be modulated by various mechanisms in physiological condition (1). Myofilament responsiveness to Ca^{2+} (Ca^{2+} sensitivity) is one of the important mechanisms in the regulation of contractility (2). There are a number of studies to estimate myofibrillar responsiveness to Ca^{2+} using cardiac skinned preparations in which intracellular ion concentrations can be altered to the desired values easily (3). However, it is also important to estimate this mechanism in intact preparations because skinned preparations lost membrane receptors or ion transporters, which could modulate myofibrillar responsiveness to Ca^{2+} (4). We and other investigators reported the use of tetanus to estimate the Ca^{2+} sensitivity of the myofilament in multicellular preparations [5,6], however, no report has been published in the use of tetanus in isolated myocytes except for our previous study (7).

In the present study, we used the relation between intracellular Ca^{2+} concentration ($[Ca^{2+}]_i$) and cell length during tetanus (R-L trajectory) of isolated ventricular myocytes to estimate myofibrillar responsiveness to Ca^{2+}. In both rat and mouse ventricular myocytes, we observed the expected shift of the R-L trajectory with inotropic interventions. In addition, myofibrillar responsiveness to Ca^{2+} of mouse ventricular myocytes might be less than that of rat ventricular myocytes. We conclude that the R-L trajectory is a useful method to estimate myofibrillar responsiveness to Ca^{2+} in intact cardiac myocytes and can be applied to various animal models.

MATERIALS AND METHODS

Cell isolation

Single ventricular myocytes were isolated from rats (Wistar, 250–350 g) or mice (ICR 25–30 g) using an enzymatic dispersion technique that has been published previously (7,8). Animal was killed by cervical dislocation after stunning and the heart was excised and mounted on a Langendorff apparatus. After perfusion with Ca^{2+} free HEPES (N-2-hydroxyethyl-piperazine-N'-2-ethanesulfonic acid) Tyrode's solution, the heart was perfused with the solution containing collagenase (Nitta Zerachin, Tokyo, Japan for rats; type X, Wako, Tokyo, Japan for mice) and protease (Sigma type XIV, St. Louis, MO, USA). Myocytes were dissociated from ventricular tissue and were kept in 1 mM Ca^{2+} Tyrode's solution until used.

Fluorescence measurement and cell length detection

Fluorescence measurement and cell length detection was essentially the same as the previous report (7,8). Briefly, myocytes were loaded with fura-2 AM and the fluorescence signals, excited with 340 nm and 380 nm wavelength light at 400 Hz using an epifluorescence system (CAM-230, JASCO, Tokyo, Japan), were passed through a 500 ± 20 nm bandpass filter before being detected with a photomultiplier tube (Hamamatsu Photonics, Hamamatsu, Japan). The fluorescence ratio signals [F(340)/F(380)] were calculated after subtraction of the background fluorescence as an indicator of $[Ca^{2+}]_i$. To monitor cell length, myocytes were illuminated with long wavelength light (>600 nm) and cell image was projected onto a linear 612-element photodiode array. The cell length was automatically detected from the cell image using an edge detection device (MOS-SPL46A001, Hamamatsu Photonics). All experiments were performed at room temperature (22 ± 2°C).

Solutions and chemicals

The composition of the HEPES Tyrode's solution was (mM): NaCl, 136.9; KCl, 5.4; $MgCl_2$, 0.5; NaH_2PO_4, 0.33; HEPES, 5; glucose, 5; and pH was adjusted to 7.40 ± 0.05 with NaOH at 22°C. Ca^{2+} concentration of the solution was adjusted by adding a $CaCl_2$ stock solution (1M). All chemicals were reagent grade; fura-2 AM (Molecular Probe Inc., Eugene, OR, USA); thapsigargin (Calbiochem Novabiochem Corp., La Jolla, CA, USA); EMD57033 (a kind gift from Pharmaceutical Research, E. Merck, Darmstadt, Germany); 3-isobutyl-1-methylxantine (IBMX) (Sigma Chemicals Co.); L-isoproterenol D-bitartrate (Nacalai Tesque, Inc., Tokyo).

Statistical analysis

The averaged values were expressed as the mean ± standard error of the mean (SEM). Statistical comparisons were carried out using paired or unpaired t-test with the significance level set at $p < 0.05$.

RESULTS

1. Fluorescence ratio signals versus cell shortening plot during tetanus in rat and mouse ventricular myocytes

We applied a repetitive electrical stimulation of 10 Hz to the myocytes under treatment with thapsigargin (0.2 μM) (an inhibitor of Ca^{2+} pump of sarcoplasmic reticulum) (9) to produce tetanus in intact preparations. In rat ventricular myocytes, fluorescence ratio signals gradually increased (Figure 1A) and cell length gradually shortened (Figure 1B) during tetanus. We then plotted fluorescence signals against cell length during entire tetanus, which made a narrow loop (R–L trajectory, Figure 1C). When extracellular Ca^{2+} concentration ($[Ca^{2+}]_o$) was increased the R–L trajectory extended along the same slope without a significant shift. Tetanus was also produced in mouse ventricular myocytes (Figure 2A and 2B), and the R–L trajectory was constructed (Figure 2C). The R–L trajectory did not shift when extracellular Ca^{2+} concentration was increased in mouse ventricular myocytes.

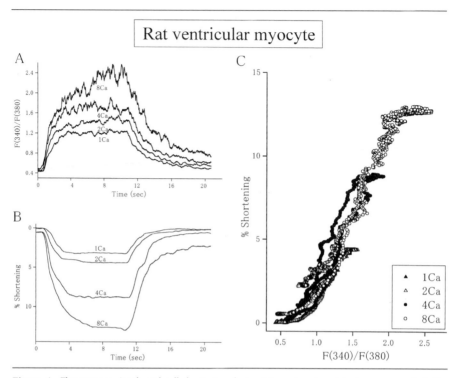

Figure 1. Fluorescence signals and cell shortening during tetanus in rat ventricular myocyte. A & B. Fura-2 fluorescence ratio signals [F(340)/F(380)] (A) and cell shortening (downward deflection) (B) during tetanus in solutions of varied $[Ca^{2+}]_o$ (labelled in mM). C. An instantaneous plot of fluorescence signals and cell length (R-L trajectory) in rat ventricular myocyte. Abscissa: Fluorescence ratio signals [F(340)/F(380)] corresponding to changes in F(340)/F(380) in A. Ordinate: Cell shortening, corresponding to changes in cell length in B (upward deflection). ▲ : 1 mM $[Ca^{2+}]_o$, △ : 2 mM $[Ca^{2+}]_o$, ● : 4 mM $[Ca^{2+}]_o$, ○ : 8 mM $[Ca^{2+}]_o$. Reproduced from Hongo et al. (1998) [7] with the permission of Pflügers Archiv—European Journal of Physiology.

For statistical comparison, we calculated the value of fluorescence ratio to produce 5% shortening from the resting cell length during falling phase of the R-L trajectory (R5%). In the same experimental condition (2 mM $[Ca^{2+}]_o$), R5% of mouse ventricular myocytes (1.664 ± 0.154, n = 9) was significantly larger than R5% of rat ventricular myocytes (1.173 ± 0.032, n = 10).

2. Effect of IBMX and EMD57033 on the R-L trajectory in rat ventricular myocytes

To test whether the R-L trajectory would shift upon changes in myofibrillar responsiveness to Ca^{2+}, we used two compounds known to change myofibrillar responsiveness to Ca^{2+}. Non-selective phosphodiesterase inhibitor, IBMX is known

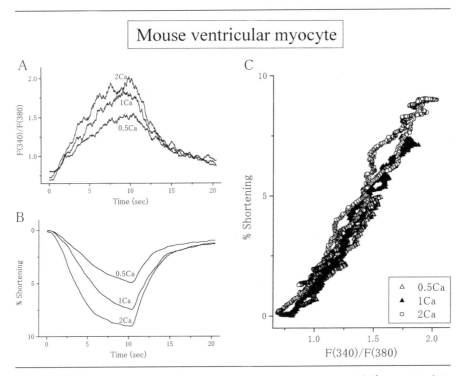

Figure 2. Fluorescence signals and cell shortening during tetanus in mouse ventricular myocyte. A & B. Fura-2 fluorescence ratio [F(340)/F(380)] (A) and cell shortening from resting length (B) during tetanus in solutions of varied [Ca²⁺]$_o$ (labeled in mM). C. The R-L trajectory obtained from A and B. Abscissa: Fluorescence ratio signals [F(340)/F(380)]. Ordinate: Cell shortening. $\triangle$: 0.5 mM [Ca²⁺]$_o$, $\blacktriangle$: 1 mM [Ca²⁺]$_o$, $\bigcirc$: 2 mM [Ca²⁺]$_o$. Reproduced from Hongo et al. (2002) [8] with the permission of the Japanese Physiological Society.

to decrease myofibrillar responsiveness to Ca²⁺ through an increase in cyclic AMP concentration and protein kinase A dependent phosphorylation of troponin I (10). In rat ventricular myocytes, IBMX (200 μM) shifted the R-L trajectory to the right, which corresponded to a decrease in myofibrillar responsiveness to Ca²⁺ (Figure 3A). R5% was significantly increased from 1.228 ± 0.037 to 1.494 ± 0.093 with 200 μM IBMX (n = 5). Ca²⁺ sensitizing agent, EMD57033 is known to increase myofibrillar responsiveness to Ca²⁺ by direct interaction with myofilament (11). EMD57033 (1 μM) shifted the trajectory to the left in rat myocytes and this leftward shift reflected an increase in myofibrillar responsiveness to Ca²⁺ (Figure 3B). R5% was significantly decreased from 0.926 ± 0.072 to 0.682 ± 0.050 by 1 μM EMD57033 (n = 5). These results suggest that the R-L trajectory can be shifted to the expected direction by maneuvers to change the myofibrillar responsiveness to Ca²⁺.

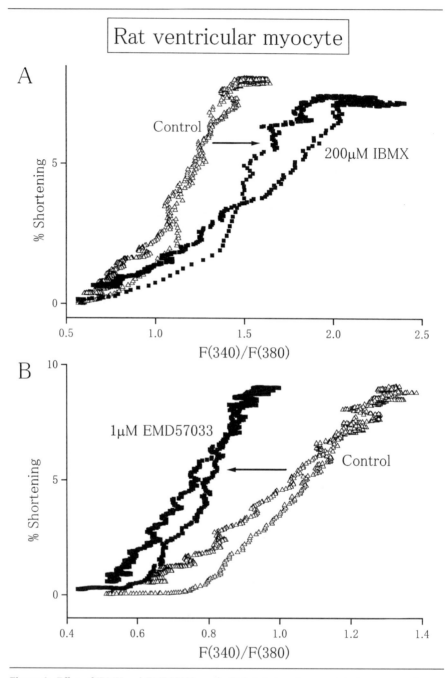

Figure 3. Effect of IBMX and EMD57033 on the R–L trajectory in rat ventricular myocyte. A. IBMX (200 μM) shifted the R–L trajectory to the right (→) in tetanized rat ventricular myocyte. △ : Control. ■ : 200 μM IBMX. B. EMD 57033 (1 μM) shifted the R–L trajectory to the left (←) in rat ventricular myocyte. △ : Control. ■ : 1 μM EMD 57033. Reproduced from Hongo et al. (1998) [7] with the permission of Pflügers Archiv—European Journal of Physiology.

3. Effect of IBMX and EMD57033 on the R-L trajectory in mouse ventricular myocytes

We then tested the effect of IBMX and EMD57033 on the R-L trajectory in mouse ventricular myocytes. The R-L trajectory was shifted to the right by 200 μM IBMX in mouse ventricular myocytes (Figure 4A) and R5% was significantly increased from 1.477 ± 0.081 to 1.731 ± 0.149 with IBMX (n = 5). EMD57033 (0.5 μM) shifted the R-L trajectory to the left in mouse myocytes (Figure 4B) and R5% was significantly decreased from 1.264 ± 0.070 to 0.988 ± 0.038 with EMD57033 (n = 5). This indicates that the R-L trajectory can be used to investigate myofibrillar responsiveness to Ca^{2+} in isolated mouse ventricular myocytes.

4. Effect of isoproterenol on the R-L trajectory in mouse ventricular myocytes

To test whether membrane receptor and second messenger system can be preserved in our method, we used β-adrenergic stimulant, isoproterenol. Beta-adrenergic stimulation is known to activate adenylate cyclase and protein kinase A through an increase in cyclic AMP concentration, which desensitizes the myofibrils to Ca^{2+} (10). Isoproterenol (5 nM) shifted the R-L trajectory to the right in mouse ventricular myocytes (Figure 5) and R5% was significantly increased from 2.104 ± 0.204 to 2.359 ± 0.232 (n = 5).

DISCUSSION

1. Advantages and disadvantages of the present method

In the present study, we examined a method to estimate myofibrillar responsiveness to Ca^{2+} in isolated myocytes. This method has advantages over the previously reported methods. Using skinned preparations is easy to change environment surrounding myofibrillar proteins, however, various important factors which affect contractility, such as membrane receptor or second messenger system, have been eliminated in skinned preparations (4). In the present study, we confirmed the effect of β-adrenergic stimulation on the myofibrillar responsiveness to Ca^{2+} in mouse ventricular myocytes using the R-L trajectory method. Although some investigators used skinned preparations pretreated with receptor agonist to estimate the effect of the agonist on the myofilament (12), it is questionable whether alteration of the myofibrillar proteins by the agonist could be preserved after skinning procedure. We and other investigators reported the use of tetanus to investigate the Ca^{2+} sensitivity of the myofilament in multicellular preparations (5,6). In these studies, however, it is necessary to change extracellular Ca^{2+} concentration at least 4–5 steps to require pCa-tension relationship. In contrast, we can estimate a rather wide range of [Ca^{2+}]$_i$–contraction relation with one concentration of extracellular Ca^{2+} using the R-L trajectory.

There are some disadvantages in the use of the R-L trajectory. Because we did not measure maximal contraction, it is hard to know the alteration of the maximal contraction with inotropic interventions. We measured cell shortening instead of

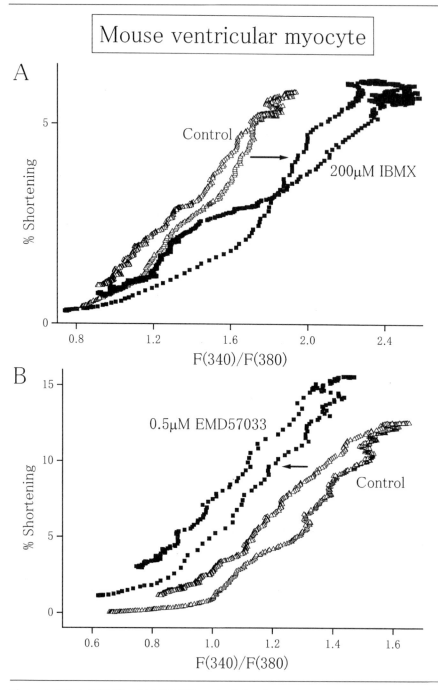

Figure 4. Effect of IBMX and EMD57033 on the R-L trajectory in mouse ventricular myocyte. A. IBMX (200 μM) shifted the R-L trajectory to the right (→) in tetanized mouse ventricular myocyte. △ : Control. ■ : 200 μM IBMX. B. EMD 57033 (0.5 μM) shifted the R-L trajectory to the left (←) in mouse ventricular myocyte. △ : Control. ■ : 0.5 μM EMD 57033. Reproduced from Hongo et al. (2002) [8] with the permission of the Japanese Physiological Society.

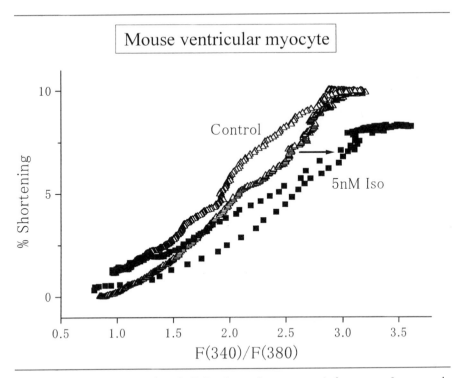

Figure 5. Effect of isoproterenol on the R-L trajectory in mouse ventricular myocyte. Isoproterenol (5 nM) shifted the R-L trajectory to the right (→) in tetanized mouse ventricular myocyte. △ : Control. ■ : 5 nM isoproterenol (Iso). Reproduced from Hongo et al. (2002) [8] with the permission of the Japanese Physiological Society.

isometric tension because measurement of isometric tension of a single intact myocyte is extremely difficult. Since the myofibrillar responsiveness to Ca²⁺ is dependent on sarcomere length (13), changes in cell length during shortening would alter the myofibrillar responsiveness to Ca²⁺ (possibly desensitization of the myofilament). Therefore, it should be cautious that the R-L trajectory would reflect myofibrillar responsiveness to Ca²⁺, which differs from that measured by the pCa-tension relation of the isometric contraction. In spite of these disadvantages, however, the R-L trajectory is still a useful method to estimate myofibrillar responsiveness to Ca²⁺, because there has been no established method to estimate Ca²⁺ responsiveness of myofilament in intact myocytes.

2. Myofibrillar responsiveness to Ca²⁺ of rat and mouse

Although we did not calibrate the fluorescence signals into [Ca²⁺]ᵢ in the present study, if the in vivo calibration of fura-2 fluorescence is the same between rat and mouse ventricular myocytes, it is possible to compare myofibrillar responsiveness to

Ca^{2+} of rat and mouse. In the same experimental conditions, we found the R5% in mouse ventricular myocytes was significantly larger than that in rat ventricular myocytes. This might indicate that myofibrillar responsiveness to Ca^{2+} of mouse myocytes is less than that of rat myocytes. Recently, we observed similar results using aequorin injected papillary muscles of rat and mouse, in which Ca^{2+} sensitivity of the myofilament is less in mouse muscle than that in rat muscle (Kusakari, Ishikawa, Hirano, Hongo, Kurihara; unpublished data). If the myofibrillar responsiveness to Ca^{2+} is less in mouse, this is reasonable to maintain fast heart beats of mouse because the time course of contraction, in particular relaxation, would be accelerated by a decrease in myofibrillar responsiveness to Ca^{2+} (6). Thus, the present result also suggests that extrapolation of the results obtained from mouse heart to other mammalian species should be cautious.

We found similar changes in the R-L trajectory with the inotropic interventions in rat and mouse ventricular myocytes. Relative changes in R5% by inotropic interventions in rat and mouse are qualitatively the same (21.4 % increase in rat and 16.7 % increase in mouse for IBMX; 26.1 % decrease in rat and 21.3 % decrease in mouse for EMD57033). These results indicate that the qualitative estimation of the myofibrillar responsiveness to Ca^{2+} using the R-L trajectory can be preserved in rat and mouse. Although there have been various models of heart diseases in rat, recent advances in genetic technology have enabled the use of various models of heart diseases in genetically engineered mice (14). Estimation of Ca^{2+} responsiveness of myofibril in various animal models is required to characterize the regulatory mechanisms of contraction. The present study indicates that this method can be applied to various models of heart diseases including genetically altered mice, and is useful for the estimation of Ca^{2+} responsiveness of the contractile elements as well as pCa-tension relation in tetanic contraction.

ACKNOWLEDGEMENTS

The authors thank Miss N. Tomizawa for her technical support. This work was supported by a Grant-in-Aid for Scientific Research from the Ministry of Education, Culture, Sports, Science and Technology, Japan and by a Uehara Memorial Foundation Research Grant.

REFERENCES

1. Bers DM. 2001. Excitation-Contraction Coupling and Cardiac Contractile Force. 2nd ed. Dordrecht, Netherlands, Kluwer Academic Publishers.
2. Blinks JR, Endoh M. 1986. Modification of myofibrillar responsiveness to Ca^{++} as an inotropic mechanism. Circulation 73 [Suppl III]: 85–89.
3. Strauss JD, Rüegg JC, Lues I. 1993. In search of calcium sensitizer compounds; from subcellular models of muscle to in vivo positive inotropic action. In: Modulation of Cardiac Calcium Sensitivity. Ed. JA Lee and DG Allen, 37–66. Oxford: Oxford University Press.
4. Blinks JR. 1993. Analysis of the effects of drugs on myofibrillar Ca^{2+} sensitivity in intact cardiac muscle. In: Modulation of Cardiac Calcium Sensitivity. Ed. JA Lee and DG Allen, 242–282. Oxford: Oxford University Press.
5. Yue DT, Marban E, Wier WG. 1986. Relationship between force and intracellular $[Ca^{2+}]$ in tetanized mammalian heart muscle. J Gen Physiol 87:223–242.

6. Hongo K, Tanaka E, Kurihara S. 1993. Alterations in contractile properties and Ca^{2+} transients by β- and muscarinic receptor stimulation in ferret myocardium. J Physiol (Lond) 461:167–184.

7. Hongo K, Kusakari Y, Konishi M, Kurihara S, Mochizuki S. 1998. Estimation of myofibrillar responsiveness to Ca^{2+} in isolated rat ventricular myocytes. Pflügers Arch 436:639–645.

8. Hongo K, Kusakari Y, Kawai M, Konishi M, Kurihara S, Mochizuki S. 2002. Use of tetanus to investigate myofibrillar responsiveness to Ca^{2+} in isolated mouse ventricular myocytes. Jpn J Physiol, 52:121–127.

9. Janczewski AM, Lakatta EG. 1993. Thapsigargin inhibits Ca^{2+} uptake, and Ca^{2+} depletes sarcoplasmic reticulum in intact cardiac myocytes. Am J Physiol 265:H517-H522.

10. Kurihara S, Konishi M. 1987. Effects of beta-adrenoceptor stimulation on intracellular Ca transients and tension in rat ventricular muscle. Pflügers Arch 409:427–437.

11. Lues I, Beier N, Jonas R, Klockow M, Haeusler G. 1993. The two mechanisms of action of racemic cardiotonic EMD 53998, calcium sensitization and phosphodiesterase inhibition, reside in different enantiomers. J Cardiovasc Pharmacol 21:883–892.

12. Puceat M, Clement O, Lechene P, Pelosin JM, Ventura-Clapier R, Vassort G. 1990. Neurohormonal control of calcium sensitivity of myofilaments in rat single heart cells. Circ Res 67:517–524.

13. Kentish JC, ter Keurs HEDJ, Ricciardi L, Bucx JJJ, Noble MIM. 1986. Comparison between the sarcomere length-force relations of intact and skinned trabeculae from rat right ventricle. Circ Res 58:755–768.

14. Kadambi VJ, Kranias EG. 1998. Genetically engineered mice: model for left ventricular failure. J Card Fail 4:349–361.

Signal Transduction and Cardiac Hypertrophy,
edited by N.S. Dhalla, L.V. Hryshko,
E. Kardami & P.K. Singal
Kluwer Academic Publishers, Boston, 2003

The Role of Hydrogen Peroxide as a Signaling Molecule

Michael P. Czubryt and Grant N. Pierce

Cell Biology Laboratory
Division of Stroke and Vascular Disease
St. Boniface General Hospital Research Centre and the Dept. of Physiology
University of Manitoba, Winnipeg, Canada

Summary. Hydrogen peroxide is conventionally regarded as a molecule that is generated in disease conditions and is responsible for inducing significant functional and structural derangement. However, it is becoming increasingly evident that H_2O_2 is also expressed in normal healthy tissue and functions as an important signaling molecule. It is involved in complex transcriptional processes that ultimately play a role in inducing cell proliferation or apoptosis. Indeed, it is this unusual dual capacity to serve as a signaling molecule in both promoting and inhibiting cell growth that makes it a particularly interesting focal point for regulatory processes. Ultimately, this results in hydrogen peroxide having an important clinical significance to affect the direction of signaling pathways that will be beneficial or deleterious to the tissue. This paper reviews the present state of our knowledge regarding hydrogen peroxide as a signaling molecule in this context.

Key words: signal transduction, vascular smooth muscle, free radicals, review.

INTRODUCTION

Hydrogen peroxide (H_2O_2) is a reactive oxygen species generated under both physiological and pathological conditions in a wide variety of cells. For many years, the conventional wisdom was that H_2O_2 was simply another toxic byproduct of cellular metabolism. Antioxidant enzymes such as catalase and glutathione

Address for Correspondence: Dr. Grant N. Pierce, Division of Stroke and Vascular Disease, St. Boniface General Hospital Research Centre, 351 Tache Avenue, Winnipeg, Manitoba, Canada R2H 2A6. Tel: (204) 235-3003, Fax: (204) 231-1151, E-mail: *gpierce@sbrc.ca*

peroxidase had evolved to ensure that cells did not become victims of their own biological wastes. The reasons for the deliberate generation of H_2O_2 or other reactive oxygen species were simply for fatty acid metabolism or to facilitate immune responses.

Over the past ten years, however, convincing evidence has accumulated revealing that H_2O_2 serves an important role as a signaling molecule in a wide variety of cell types. Studies to support this contention have often involved identifying existing signaling pathways that are activated or inactivated in response to exogenously added H_2O_2. Alternatively, the formation of H_2O_2 could be quenched by the addition of free radical scavengers or the overexpression of cellular antioxidants such as catalase, and the impact of these actions on well-understood signaling cascades examined. The development of reactive dyes for *in vitro* fluorescent studies of H_2O_2 formation and breakdown has led to new insights and ideas about the role played by H_2O_2 and other free radicals in cell metabolism.

As our understanding of the metabolism of H_2O_2 developed, it was found that H_2O_2 could also dramatically affect cell fate. The decision by cells to divide, migrate or die was found to be at least partially dependent on H_2O_2. The importance of these processes in the development of various diseases, coupled with reports that H_2O_2 is generated in a number of pathologies, has led to the idea that control of H_2O_2 production and metabolism may provide important new therapeutic targets in these diseases.

This review describes the generation and breakdown of H_2O_2 in the cell, and presents recent data demonstrating the important role of H_2O_2 in intracellular signaling pathways, particularly those involved in mitogenesis and apoptosis. Special attention is paid to data focusing on the role of H_2O_2 in smooth muscle, a tissue in which a large body of research in this area has been carried out and in which H_2O_2 appears to be a highly important regulator of cell function. Although evidence has been reported that cellular redox status and other reactive oxygen species play roles in intracellular signaling (1), the focus of the present review is on H_2O_2. The reasons for this focus are two-fold: first, the majority of the data on reactive oxygen species and intracellular signaling comes from studies of H_2O_2; and second, after H_2O_2 the most widely-studied reactive oxygen species is superoxide. Although superoxide appears to mediate some signaling pathways in its own right, the greater stability of H_2O_2, its ability to readily cross cell membranes and the fact that superoxide is usually rapidly dismutated into H_2O_2 makes H_2O_2 likely to be a more important mediator of cell function and dysfunction (see below).

PHYSIOLOGICAL AND PATHOLOGICAL SOURCES OF HYDROGEN PEROXIDE

Although it is often described as a free radical, H_2O_2 lacks unpaired electrons and is therefore more properly called a reactive oxygen species (2,3). Because it lacks unpaired electrons, H_2O_2 is much less reactive than true free radicals such as the hydroxyl radical, which makes H_2O_2 generally much less toxic to cells and results in a relatively long half-life, on the order of minutes or longer (2,4,5). H_2O_2 is also readily membrane permeable, which allows H_2O_2 to easily move within and between

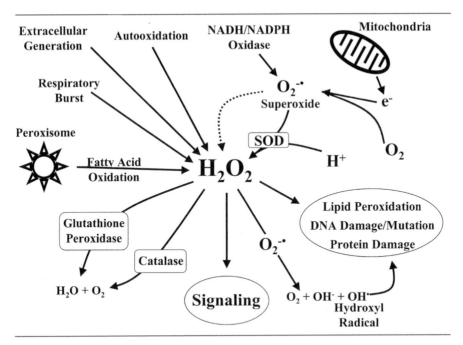

Figure 1. Sources and fates of H₂O₂ in the cell.

cells (3,6). Together, the membrane permeability and long half-life make for a molecule that is able to exert effects distal to the site of production.

Hydrogen peroxide can be generated *in vivo* in a variety of ways (Figure 1). Two major sources of intracellular H_2O_2 are leakage of electrons out of the electron transport chain (7) and autoxidation of various intracellular compounds (2). Unchecked, H_2O_2 can produce reactive free radicals, initiating chain reactions that generate lipid peroxides and other peroxide byproducts, and leading to destruction or alteration of proteins, lipid membranes and nucleic acids (2,6,8). Endogenous scavengers of H_2O_2, such as glutathione peroxidase and catalase, ensure that the redox status of the cell is maintained at an appropriate level and prevent H_2O_2 from damaging cell components (2,6,8).

H_2O_2 can also be produced by superoxide dismutase (SOD). SOD breaks down the free radical superoxide, which is generated by a membrane-bound NADH/NADPH oxidase, by combining it with free protons (or hydronium ions) to produce H_2O_2 and O_2 (9,10). This oxidase/SOD pathway appears to be a major synthesis pathway for H_2O_2 in vascular smooth muscle cells (11). Generation of H_2O_2 by SOD prevents superoxide from combining with H_2O_2 to produce the highly toxic hydroxyl radical (2,6). H_2O_2 can also arise from the spontaneous dismutation of superoxide (3). Oxidation of fatty acids in peroxisomes produces H_2O_2 as a byproduct, and can be a major source of peroxide in fat metabolizing tissues like the liver (2,7). Cells such as monocytes and macrophages purposefully produce large amounts of free radicals and H_2O_2 for microbial killing during the respiratory burst (12).

H_2O_2 is also produced in a variety of pathological conditions, particularly those in which redox balance is compromised. For example, H_2O_2 is generated during ischemia/reperfusion of the heart (13–17) and brain (18–20), and may contribute significantly to ischemia/reperfusion damage. Indeed, prevention of H_2O_2 generation by exogenous addition or overexpression of catalase is a potential therapy in the management of ischemic damage (21–24).

Generation of H_2O_2 and other reactive oxygen species by endothelial and vascular smooth muscle cells, as well as monocytes and macrophages infiltrating the vascular intima, contribute to the formation of atherosclerotic plaques. These species act by oxidizing low density lipoproteins and stimulating proliferation of smooth muscle (see below) (25,26). Other pathologies in which H_2O_2 generation plays an important causative role include cataract formation (27), inflammation (28,29) and Alzheimer's disease (30).

EFFECTS OF HYDROGEN PEROXIDE ON INTRACELLULAR SIGNALING

Until recently, the mode of action of H_2O_2 was believed to be simple oxidation of various cellular components, eventually leading to cell necrosis. H_2O_2 is now known to be a mitogen for many cell types, including smooth muscle cells (31–33), in which it also causes apoptosis (34–36). H_2O_2 interacts with a number of intracellular signaling pathways to exert its effects, and parallels have been drawn between H_2O_2 and nitric oxide (NO). Both molecules are small, relatively stable reactive oxygen species (but not free radicals) that are readily membrane permeable (9). Both molecules also seem to be produced in either high concentrations by phagocytic cells to mediate immune responses, or in low concentrations by non-phagocytic cells to mediate signal transduction (9,37). There may even be cross-talk between the H_2O_2 and NO signaling pathways, since catalase (after reacting with H_2O_2) is able to activate guanylate cyclase, which is directly activated by NO (38), and since expression of endothelial nitric oxide synthase is regulated by H_2O_2 (100). Furthermore, NO may feed back and inhibit catalase (39).

The last several years have shown H_2O_2 to be involved in many intracellular signaling pathways. Smooth muscle cells, in particular, appear to employ H_2O_2 as a signaling molecule. For example, a variety of responses by smooth muscle following angiotensin II stimulation involve the generation of H_2O_2. Activation of protein kinase B (Akt) by angiotensin II appears to depend upon the generation of intracellular H_2O_2, since this activation could be mimicked by the addition of exogenous H_2O_2 and blocked by overexpression of catalase (40). Similarly, transcription of insulin-like growth factor 1 receptor mRNA is activated by angiotensin II, and is blocked by catalase but activated by H_2O_2 (41). Angiotensin II–induced hypertrophy of smooth muscle cells also requires the generation of H_2O_2 (11). H_2O_2 may also be involved in negative feedback regulation of angiotensin II signaling, since AT1 receptor mRNA is apparently destabilized in response to peroxide (42).

Like angiotensin II signal transduction, the mediation of responses of vascular smooth muscle cells to platelet-derived growth factor (PDGF) is also dependent upon the generation of H$_2$O$_2$. The effects of PDGF on tyrosine phosphorylation, MAPK stimulation, DNA synthesis and chemotaxis could be mimicked by the addition of exogenous H$_2$O$_2$, and were inhibited when the production of H$_2$O$_2$ was blocked (43). Similarly, H$_2$O$_2$ production is required for TGF-β1 induced signal transduction leading to IL-6 gene expression in human lung fibroblasts (44). Signaling through the EGF receptor may also be mediated by H$_2$O$_2$ (45).

The number of intracellular signaling cascades in which H$_2$O$_2$ is involved is steadily growing. Activation of extracellular-regulated kinase (ERK) in vascular smooth muscle in response to angiotensin II may involve H$_2$O$_2$ generation (46). The ERK1/2 mitogen-activated protein kinase (MAPK) pathway is strongly and rapidly activated by H$_2$O$_2$ in vascular smooth muscle (47,48), as well as in other cell types including cardiomyocytes (49–51) and airway smooth muscle (52). The p90 ribosomal S6 kinase, a downstream effector of the ERK1/2 pathway and activator of several transcription factors, is also activated by H$_2$O$_2$ in several cell types, but this activation is apparently independent of ERK1/2 activation (53), suggesting that other pathways are involved. The c-Jun NH$_2$-terminal kinase pathway is directly activated by H$_2$O$_2$ in bovine chondrocytes (54). The p38 MAPK pathway is activated by H$_2$O$_2$ (55), and is also a critical component of angiotensin II signaling in vascular smooth muscle (56). Finally, H$_2$O$_2$ has been shown to open BK$_{Ca}$ potassium channels using a pathway that involves signaling through phospholipase A2 and arachidonic acid (57).

Exactly how H$_2$O$_2$ interacts with these pathways is unclear, but one possibility is that H$_2$O$_2$ inhibits the activity of tyrosine phosphatases involved in regulation of these pathways. These phosphatases normally maintain components of these pathways in inactive hypophosphorylated states, but are inactivated by oxidation of critical cysteine residues by H$_2$O$_2$ (58). Endogenous kinases are then free to phosphorylate the signaling pathway components, resulting in activation of the pathway. The oxidation of cysteine residues by H$_2$O$_2$ has been demonstrated to be specific for tyrosine phosphatases and not serine/threonine phosphatases (59). It has been proposed that reduction of the phosphatase cysteine residues by reducing enzymes or glutathione would restore phosphatase activity, turning off the activation of the signaling pathways (37,59). This brings up a potential important difference between H$_2$O$_2$ and NO signaling: NO acts specifically via guanylate cyclase whereas H$_2$O$_2$, by using a cysteine oxidation mechanism of action, is able to affect a wide variety of targets, including phosphatases, caspases and transcription factors.

H$_2$O$_2$ mediates the activity of several transcription factors. One of these, NF-κB, is normally anchored in the cytoplasm by its inhibitor, IkB. NF-κB is activated by a variety of stimuli, particularly immune or inflammatory responses (60). Upon appropriate stimulation, IκB is proteolyzed, permitting entry of NF-κB into the nucleus and binding to DNA promoters (61). Exogenous or endogenous H$_2$O$_2$ is able to activate NF-κB (60,62), therefore NF-κB appears to act as a redox-sensing transcription factor. This activation is mediated by the small GTPases Rac1 and Rho

(63,64). H_2O_2 also mediates the interaction of NF-κB with DNA in a tissue and gene-specific manner (65–67).

The expression of a variety of other transcription factors is affected by H_2O_2 c-fos, and in smooth muscle, c-myc, c-jun, egr-1 and fra-1 expression is strongly upregulated by H_2O_2 exposure (33,48,68,69). In the cases of c-jun, egr-1 and fra-1, this increase in expression is mediated by tyrosine kinase activity (68), possibly via a cysteine oxidation mechanism as described above. It is noteworthy that expression of both c-jun and c-fos is upregulated by ERK2 activation, which is also induced by H_2O_2 (see above) (70). H_2O_2 also appears able to influence the binding of transcription factors to DNA. Binding of the AP-1 fos/jun dimer to DNA is mediated by H_2O_2 in a tissue-dependent fashion (66,71), and H_2O_2 has also been shown to affect DNA binding of Sp-1, egr-1 and the glucocorticoid receptor (69).

The way in which H_2O_2 modulates the specific interaction between transcription factors and DNA is unknown, but may be similar in mechanism to how H_2O_2 mediates protein phosphatase activity. Key cysteine residues in the DNA-binding domain of transcription factors may be oxidized by reactive oxygen species such as H_2O_2, inhibiting interaction with DNA (72). An intriguing regulatory mechanism for the redox state of these cysteine residues involving the nuclear protein Ref-1 and the antioxidant protein thioredoxin has been proposed. Oxidant stress of the cell causes the nuclear localization of thioredoxin, where it interacts with and activates Ref-1. Ref-1 is then able to reduce cysteine residues to permit interaction with transcription factors (37). This mechanism provides a potential feedback mechanism for the regulation of transcription factor binding to DNA by H_2O_2.

A novel way in which H_2O_2 may affect intracellular signaling is by modulating trafficking of molecules between the cytosol and the nucleus via the nuclear pore. Our laboratory has recently reported that H_2O_2 inhibits nuclear import of a fluorescent reporter protein bearing a classical nuclear localization signal in aortic vascular smooth muscle cells (73). This inhibition was specifically mediated by activation of ERK2 and could be attenuated either by catalase or by PD98059, which blocks the activation of MEK1/2, the upstream activator of ERK2 (Figure 2). H_2O_2 exerted its effect on a cytosolic factor and not the nuclear pore or membrane, in contrast to superoxide and hydroxyl radicals, which were only able to inhibit import by interaction with non-soluble cellular structures. It is likely that these highly toxic reactive oxygen species inhibited import simply by oxidizing structures required for import to occur or by compromising nuclear integrity. Therefore, it appears that H_2O_2 is able to specifically modulate nuclear protein import, which may affect translocation of molecules such as transcription factors into the nucleus and provide the cell with a level of generalized transcriptional control.

ROLE OF HYDROGEN PEROXIDE IN PROLIFERATION AND APOPTOSIS

Considering the ability of H_2O_2 to activate a wide variety of intracellular signaling pathways, many of which are involved in mediating mitogenic responses, it is not surprising that H_2O_2 has been reported to act as a mitogen for vascular smooth muscle cells (31–33). Increased proliferation of smooth muscle cells in response to

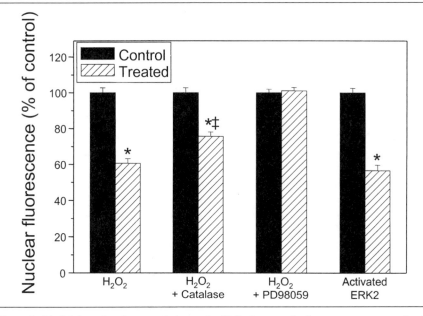

Figure 2. Modulation of nuclear protein import by H_2O_2. Import of a fluorescent reporter molecule in vascular smooth muscle cells was significantly inhibited by treatment of cell cytosol with 1 mM H_2O_2. This effect could be reversed partially by catalase (1.4 mg/ml), and completely by the MEK1/2 inhibitor PD98059 (20 μM). Inhibition of import by H_2O_2 could be reproduced by treating cell cytosol with 40 ng/ml activated ERK2. Data are adapted from Czubryt et al. (73). ⋆$P < 0.05$ vs. control. ‡$P < 0.05$ vs. H_2O_2-treated.

H_2O_2 exposure is associated with activation of the ERK1/2 MAP kinases, and DNA replication (33,74). Several vascular smooth muscle cell mitogens also generate H_2O_2 as a mediator of action, including angiotensin II (11), PDGF (43), basic fibroblast growth factor (FGF-2) (32), thrombin (75), oleic acid (76) and phenylephrine and arachidonic acid (77).

Some groups have reported, however, that H_2O_2 exposure also mediates programmed cell death, or apoptosis, of vascular smooth muscle cells (34–36). The confusion surrounding the apparent dual role of H_2O_2 in mediating vascular smooth muscle cell fate is compounded by the fact that, as in proliferation, the ERK1/2 MAP kinases and DNA replication are also stimulated in H_2O_2-mediated apoptosis (34,35). The degree of exposure of the cell to H_2O_2 does not seem to be the main determinant of cell fate, at least in *in vitro* experiments. Concentrations of H_2O_2 demonstrated to cause smooth muscle proliferation range from 100–200 μM (32,33), while concentrations shown to cause DNA replication and ERK1/2 activation range from 5–200 μM (33,47,51,74). The times of exposure to H_2O_2 to produce these effects range from 5 minutes to 12 hours (33,47,51,74). At the same time, concentrations of H_2O_2 demonstrated to cause apoptosis have been reported to be 10–

150 μM, with exposure times of 1–5 hours (34,36). Thus there is considerable overlap between the concentrations and times of exposure of cells to H_2O_2 demonstrated to cause both apoptosis and proliferation.

It is unclear why H_2O_2 exhibits this dual role and exactly what mechanism is responsible for the individual responses. The mechanism, however, may involve protein kinase C (PKC). The activation of apoptosis by H_2O_2 in vascular smooth muscle cells is mediated by PKC (78), but activation of MAPK in response to H_2O_2 appears to be independent of PKC in vascular smooth muscle (79) and dependent on PKC in airway smooth muscle (80). These findings suggest that multiple signaling pathways, some dependent on PKC and some independent, are likely to be involved in the apoptotic response, and may be precisely tissue-specific. Another pathway which may be involved in mediating apoptosis in response to H_2O_2 is NF-κB, which is activated in microglial cells in response to H_2O_2 exposure in conjunction with increased expression of the death ligand Fas (CD95L) (81). Furuke et al., however, have shown that in activated NK cells, exposure to H_2O_2 inhibited Fas ligand expression, suggesting that the modulation of Fas by H_2O_2 may be cell type-specific (82).

The apoptosis inhibitor Bcl-2 may protect cells by increasing cellular glutathione levels to counteract exposure to H_2O_2, again implicating H_2O_2 as a causative factor in apoptosis (83). This hypothesis is in agreement with earlier data showing that overexpression of Bcl-2 may cause cells to shift to a more reduced redox state (84) and may attenuate increased H_2O_2 levels (85). Release of cytochrome c from mitochondria, an early step in apoptosis induction, may be caused by H_2O_2 (86) and is blocked by Bcl-2 (87).

Caspases involved in apoptosis are cysteine containing proteins and, like tyrosine phosphatases, may be subject to regulation by cellular redox status. Evidence for redox regulation of caspases includes the finding that caspase-3 is activated by increased intracellular peroxide levels (86). However, in the leukemia cell line HL-60, the opposite finding was reported, that caspase-3 activation was accompanied by decreased levels of intracellular H_2O_2 (88). Prolonged exposure of cells to hydrogen peroxide may actually inactivate caspases and therefore block apoptosis (89). This novel finding is in agreement with recent data showing that overexpression of catalase in vascular smooth muscle cells reduces intracellular H_2O_2 concentration and results in inhibition of cell proliferation and increased apoptosis (31).

Agents that cause apoptosis themselves may use H_2O_2 as a mediator of action. The antioxidant BHT causes apoptosis of U937 cells in a time- and dose-dependent manner, and appears to act through H_2O_2 (90). The DNA alkylating agent duocarmycin A induces H_2O_2 generation, which eventually leads to apoptosis (91).

From these results, it is obvious that the role of H_2O_2 in mediating either proliferation or apoptosis of smooth muscle involves complicated intracellular signaling pathways that likely interact with one another in ways that are not yet completely defined. The ultimate decision made by the cell to reproduce or perish probably involves precise temporal regulation and a balance between many factors determining the overall stress or health of the cell, or the cellular redox state. This may be further complicated by the possibility that some cells may be under constant exposure to H_2O_2 derived from intracellular metabolic pathways. This basal $[H_2O_2]$ may induce a response in the cell that differs from that observed when the $[H_2O_2]$ is modulated acutely by an external stimulus.

CLINICAL RELEVANCE OF HYDROGEN PEROXIDE

Proliferation and apoptosis of vascular smooth muscle play critical roles in vascular remodeling in both physiological situations like angiogenesis and pathological situations like restenosis or tumorigenesis (92). It is therefore critical that a rigorous understanding of factors that influence rates of cell growth and death be well understood before novel therapies are tested.

Restenosis is one of the most common complications following cardiac bypass surgery and angioplasty, which are among the most widely used cardiac therapies in North America (92). Up to 50% of patients undergoing angioplasty will present with significant restenosis within one year of surgery when smooth muscle cells from the vascular intima proliferate and grow into the vessel lumen (93). Possible treatments to improve the success rate of angioplasty may include the use of inhibitors of smooth muscle cell growth (94), which would have minimal effects on normal blood vessels since smooth muscle in vessel walls turns over very slowly (92). These inhibitors may also be useful in blocking angiogenesis evoked by developing tumors (92,101). Therapeutic angiogenesis is currently being explored as a possible treatment to restore or improve cardiac function following myocardial infarct (95). By shifting smooth muscle towards proliferation or apoptosis using clinical interventions that modulate cellular redox state, it may be possible to optimize these therapeutic strategies.

Besides its role in mediating smooth muscle cell fate, H_2O_2 has also been found to have other distinct effects on cardiovascular function. Migration of smooth muscle cells and infiltration of macrophages and monocytes into the vascular intima are well-established early steps in atherogenic plaque formation. Recently, chemotaxis of vascular smooth muscle cells in response to lysyl oxidase activity, which initiates cross-linking of elastin and collagen, has been reported to be mediated by H_2O_2 (46). Infiltration of macrophages into the vascular intima may also be facilitated directly by an enhancement of macrophage spreading in response to H_2O_2 (55). Overproduction of H_2O_2 in the vasculature may therefore result in mitogenesis and migration of smooth muscle, contributing to atherogenesis and possibly restenosis. At the same time, the recent identification of H_2O_2 as an endothelium-derived hyperpolarizing factor suggests that H_2O_2 may play a role in the development of hypertension independently of its role in mediating smooth muscle cell proliferation (97). Any effect on blood pressure may have negative consequences for patients with atherosclerosis or restenosis.

A recent study by Penn et al. implicated H_2O_2 and low density lipoprotein (LDL) in a two-step pathway resulting in activation of tissue factor, a possible contributory agent in atherosclerotic plaque and thrombus formation (98). In this schema, LDL caused inactive tissue factor to accumulate on smooth muscle cell surfaces.

Table 1. Signaling pathways modulated by H_2O_2

Extracellular Ligands	References
Angiotensin II	(11,40,41,46)
PDGF	(43)
TGF-β1	(44)
EGF	(45)
FGF-2	(32)
Thrombin	(75)
Oleic Acid	(76)
Phenylephrine	(77)
Arachidonic Acid	(57,77)
Intracellular Signal Cascades	
ERK1/2	(46–52)
NF-κB	(60,62,65,66,67,81)
p38 MAPK	(48,55)
c-Jun-NH$_2$ Kinase	(48,54)
Phospholipase A$_2$	(57)
Protein Kinase B/Akt	(40)
Protein Kinase C	(48,78)
p90 Ribosomal S6 Kinase	(53)
Rac1	(63,64)
Rho	(81,82)
Fas	(83,85)
Bcl-2	(86,88,89)
Caspase-3	
Transcription Factors	
c-fos	(33)
c-jun	(48,68)
AP-1	(66,71)
c-myc	(33)
egr-1	(68,48)
fra-1	(48)
Sp-1	(69)
Glucocorticoid Receptor	(69)

H_2O_2 then activated the latent tissue factor. At the same time, it has been reported that H_2O_2 is able to induce expression of scavenger receptors via a mechanism involving activation of JNK and increased AP-1 transcription factor binding (99). Together, these data suggest a critical role for H_2O_2 in the process of atherogenesis, making H_2O_2 a possible therapeutic target for treatment of atherosclerosis and restenosis.

CONCLUSIONS

In order to improve the success of current therapies, a better understanding of the factors that regulate smooth muscle cell growth and death is required. The recent emergence of H_2O_2 as an apparently widely used signaling molecule in smooth muscle physiology, including proliferation and apoptosis, necessitates the investigation of the modes of action of H_2O_2. Further research is required to delineate the exact pathways in which H_2O_2 is involved, how these pathways interact with one another, and whether antioxidants may be a useful intervention in regulating smooth muscle proliferation in diseases of the vasculature.

ACKNOWLEDGEMENTS

This work was supported by the Canadian Institutes for Health Research. G.N.P. is a Senior Scientist of the Canadian Institutes for Health Research. M.P.C. was supported by a Research Traineeship from the Heart and Stroke Foundation of Canada.

REFERENCES

1. Griendling KK, Sorescu D, Lassègue B, Ushio-Fukai M. 2000. Modulation of protein kinase activity and gene expression by reactive oxygen species and their role in vascular physiology and pathophysiology. Arterioscler Thromb Vasc Biol 20:2175–2183.
2. Cheeseman KH, Slater TF. 1993. An introduction to free radical biochemistry. Br Med Bull 49:481–493.
3. Rubanyi GM. 1988. Vascular effects of oxygen-derived free radicals. Free Radic Biol Med 4:107–120.
4. Barnard ML, Matalon S. 1992. Mechanisms of extracellular reactive oxygen species injury to the pulmonary microvasculature. J Appl Physiol 72:1724–1729.
5. Sies H. 1991. Oxidative stress: from basic research to clinical application. Am J Med 91:31S–38S.
6. Halliwell B, Gutteridge JMC. 1990. Role of free radicals and catalytic metal ions in human disease: an overview. Meth Enzymol 186:1–85.
7. Boveris A. 1977. Mitochondrial production of superoxide radical and hydrogen peroxide. Adv Exp Med Biol 78:67–82.
8. Kehrer JP. 1993. Free radicals as mediators of tissue injury and disease. Crit Rev Toxicol 23:21–48.
9. Griendling KK, Harrison DG. 1999. Dual role of reactive oxygen species in vascular growth. Circ Res 85:562–563.
10. McCord JM, Fridovich I. 1968. The reduction of cytochrome c by milk xanthine oxidase. J Biol Chem 243:5753–5760.
11. Zafari AM, Ushio-Fukai M, Akers M, Yin Q, Shah A, Harrison DG, Taylor WR, Griendling KK. 1998. Role of NADH/NADPH oxidase-derived H_2O_2 in angiotensin II-induced vascular hypertrophy. Hypertension 32:488–495.
12. Babior BM. 1978. Oxygen-dependent microbial killing by phagocytes. N Engl J Med 298:659–668.
13. Bast A, Haenen GRMM, Doelman CJA. 1991. Oxidants and antioxidants: State of the art. Am J Med 91:2S–13S.
14. Burton KP, McCord JM, Ghai G. 1984. Myocardial alterations due to free-radical generation. Am J Physiol 246:H776–H783.
15. Kaul N, Siveski-Iliskovic N, Hill M, Slezak J, Singal PK. 1993. Free radicals and the heart. J Pharmacol Toxicol Meth 30:55–67.
16. Kloner RA, Przyklenk K, Whittaker P. 1989. Deleterious effects of oxygen radicals in ischemia/reperfusion: Resolved and unresolved issues. Circulation 80:1115–1127.
17. Vanden Hoek TL, Li C, Shao Z, Schumacker PT, Becker LB. 1997. Significant levels of oxidants are generated by isolated cardiomyocytes during ischemia prior to reperfusion. J Mol Cell Cardiol 29:2571–2583.
18. Fullerton HJ, Ditelberg JS, Chen SF, Sarco DP, Chan PH, Epstein CJ, Ferriero DM. 1998. Copper/zinc superoxide dismutase transgenic brain accumulates hydrogen peroxide after perinatal hypoxia ischemia. Ann Neurol 44:357–364.
19. Hyslop PA, Zhang Z, Pearson DV, Phebus LA. 1995. Measurement of striatal H_2O_2 by microdialysis following forebrain ischemia and reperfusion in the rat: correlation with the cytotoxic potential of H_2O_2 in vitro. Brain Res 671:181–186.
20. Watanabe S. 1998. In vivo fluorometric measurement of cerebral oxidative stress using 2′-7′-dichlorofluorescein (DCF). Keio J Med 47:92–98.

21. Baker K, Marcus CB, Huffman K, Kruk H, Malfroy B, Doctrow SR. 1998. Synthetic combined superoxide dismutase/catalase mimetics are protective as a delayed treatment in a rat stroke model: a key role for reactive oxygen species in ischemic brain injury. J Pharmacol Exp Ther 284:215–221.

22. Woo YJ, Zhang JC, Vijayasarathy C, Zwacka RM, Englehardt JF, Gardner TJ, Sweeney HL. 1998. Recombinant adenovirus-mediated cardiac gene transfer of superoxide dismutase and catalase attenuates postischemic contractile dysfunction. Circulation 98:II255–II260.

23. Yabe Y, Koyama Y, Nishikawa M, Takakura Y, Hashida M. 1999. Hepatocyte-specific distribution of catalase and its inhibitory effect on hepatic ischemia/reperfusion injury in mice. Free Radic Res 30:265–274.

24. Yabe Y, Nishikawa M, Tamada A, Takakura Y, Hashida M. 1999. Targeted delivery and improved therapeutic potential of catalase by chemical modification: combination with superoxide dismutase derivatives. J Pharmacol Exp Ther 289:1176–1184.

25. Morel DW, DiCorleto PE, Chisolm GM. 1984. Endothelial and smooth muscle cells alter low density lipoprotein in vitro by free radical oxidation. Arteriosclerosis 4:357–364.

26. Parthasarathy S, Printz DJ, Boyd D, Joy L, Steinberg D. 1986. Macrophage oxidation of low density lipoprotein generates a modified form recognized by the scavenger receptor. Arteriosclerosis 6:505–510.

27. Sanderson J, McLauchlan WR, Williamson G. 1999. Quercetin inhibits hydrogen peroxide-induced oxidation of the rat lens. Free Radic Biol Med 26:639–645.

28. Bragt PC, Bonta IL. 1980. Oxidant stress during inflammation: anti-inflammatory effects of anti-oxidants. Agents Actions 10:536–539.

29. Shimada T, Watanabe N, Hirashi H, Terano A. 1999. Redox regulation of interleukin-8 expression in MKN28 cells. Dig Dis Sci 44:266–273.

30. Huang X, Cuajungco MP, Atwood CS, Hartshorn MA, Tyndall JD, Hanson GR, Stokes KC, Leopold M, Multhaup G, Goldstein LE, Scarpa RC, Saunders AJ, Lim J, Moir RD, Glabe C, Bowden EF, Masters CL, Fairlie DP, Tanzi RE, Bush AI. 1999. Cu(II) potentiation of alzheimer abeta neurotoxicity. Correlation with cell-free hydrogen peroxide production and metal reduction. J Biol Chem 274:37111–37116.

31. Brown MR, Miller FJJ, Li W-G, Ellingson AN, Mozena JD, Chatterjee P, Engelhardt JF, Zwacka RM, Oberley LW, Fang X, Spector AA, Weintraub NL. 1999. Overexpression of human catalase inhibits proliferation and promotes apoptosis in vascular smooth muscle cells. Circ Res 85:524–533.

32. Herbert JM, Bono F, Savi P. 1996. The mitogenic effect of H_2O_2 for vascular smooth muscle cells is mediated by an increase of the affinity of basic fibroblast growth factor for its receptor. FEBS Lett 395:43–47.

33. Rao GN, Berk BC. 1992. Active oxygen species stimulate vascular smooth muscle cell growth and proto-oncogene expression. Circ Res 70:593–599.

34. Cantoni O, Boscoboinik D, Fiorani M, Staüble B, Azzi A. 1996. The phosphorylation state of MAP-kinases modulates the cytotoxic response of smooth muscle cells to hydrogen peroxide. FEBS Lett 389:285–288.

35. Fiorani M, Cantoni O, Tasinato A, Boscoboinik D, Azzi A. 1995. Hydrogen peroxide- and fetal bovine serum-induced DNA synthesis in vascular smooth muscle cells: positive and negative regulation by protein kinase C isoforms. Biochim Biophys Acta 1269:98–104.

36. Li P-F, Dietz R, von Harsdorf R. 1997. Differential effect of hydrogen peroxide and superoxide anion on apoptosis and proliferation of vascular smooth muscle cells. Circulation 96:3602–3609.

37. Finkel T. 1998. Oxygen radicals and signaling. Curr Opin Cell Biol 10:248–253.

38. Mohazzab HK-M, Agarwal R, Wolin MS. 1999. Influence of glutathione peroxidase on coronary artery responses to alterations in PO_2 and H_2O_2. Am J Physiol 276:H235–H241.

39. Wolin MS, Davidson CA, Kaminski PM, Fayngersh RP, Mohazzab HK-M. 1998. Oxidant-nitric oxide signaling mechanisms in vascular tissue. Biochemistry-Mosc 63:810–816.

40. Ushio-Fukai M, Alexander RW, Akers M, Yin Q, Fujio Y, Walsh K, Griendling KK. 1999. Reactive oxygen species mediate the activation of Akt/protein kinase B by angiotensin II in vascular smooth muscle cells. J Biol Chem 274:22699–22704.

41. Du J, Peng T, Scheidegger KJ, Delafontaine P. 1999. Angiotensin II activation of insulin-like growth factor 1 receptor transcription is mediated by a tyrosine kinase-dependent redox-sensitive mechanism. Arterioscler Thromb Vasc Biol 19:2119–2126.

42. Nickenig G, Strehlow K, Baumer AT, Baudler S, Wabetamann S, Sauer H, Bohm M. 2000. Negative feedback regulation of reactive oxygen species on AT1 receptor gene expression. Br J Pharmacol 131:795–803.

43. Sundaresan M, Yu Z-X, Ferrans VJ, Irani K, Finkel T. 1995. Requirement for generation of H$_2$O$_2$ for platelet-derived growth factor signal transduction. Science 270:296–299.

44. Junn E, Lee KN, Ju HR, Han SH, Im JY, Kang HS, Lee TH, Bae YS, Ha KS, Lee ZW, Rhee SG, Choi I. 2000. Requirement of hydrogen peroxide generation in TGF-beta 1 signal transduction in human lung fibroblast cells: involvement of hydrogen peroxide and Ca^{2+} in TGF-beta 1-induced IL-6 expression. J Immunol 165:2190–2197.

45. Kamata H, Shibukawa Y, Oka SI, Hirata H. 2000. Epidermal growth factor receptor is modulated by redox through multiple mechanisms. Effects of reductants and H$_2$O$_2$. Eur J Biochem 267:1933–1944.

46. Frank GD, Eguchi S, Yamakawa T, Tanaka S, Inagami T, Motley ED. 2000. Involvement of reactive oxygen species in the activation of tyrosine kinase and extracellular signal-regulated kinase by angiotensin II. Endocrinology 141:3120–3126.

47. Guyton KZ, Liu Y, Gorospe M, Xu Q, Holbrook NJ. 1996. Activation of mitogen-activated protein kinase by H$_2$O$_2$. J Biol Chem 271:4138–4142.

48. Zhang J, Jin N, Liu Y, Rhoades RA. 1998. Hydrogen peroxide stimulates extracellular signal-regulated protein kinases in pulmonary arterial smooth muscle cells. Am J Respir Cell Mol Biol 19:324–332.

49. Bogoyevitch MA, Ng DC, Court NW, Draper KA, Dhillon A, Abas L. 2000. Intact mitochondrial electron transport function is essential for signaling by hydrogen peroxide in cardiac myocytes. J Mol Cell Cardiol 32:1469–1480.

50. Clerk A, Michael A, Sugden PH. 1998. Stimulation of multiple mitogen-activated protein kinase sub-families by oxidative stress and phosphorylation of the small heat shock protein, HSP25/27, in neonatal ventricular myocytes. Biochem J 333:581–589.

51. Sabri A, Byron KL, Samarel AM, Bell J, Lucchesi PA. 1998. Hydrogen peroxide activates mitogen-activated protein kinases and Na$^+$-H$^+$ exchange in neonatal rat cardiac myocytes. Circ Res 82:1053–1062.

52. Abe MK, Chao T-SO, Solway J, Rosner MR, Hershenson MB. 1994. Hydrogen peroxide stimulates mitogen-activated protein kinase in bovine tracheal myocytes: implications for human airway disease. Am J Respir Cell Mol Biol 11:577–585.

53. Abe J, Okuda M, Huang Q, Yoshizumi M, Berk BC. 2000. Reactive oxygen species activate p90 ribosomal S6 kinase via Fyn and Ras. J Biol Chem 275:1739–1748.

54. Lo YYC, Wong JMS, Cruz TF. 1996. Reactive oxygen species mediate cytokine activation of c-Jun NH$_2$-terminal kinases. J Biol Chem 271:15703–15707.

55. Ogura M, Kitamura M. 1998. Oxidant stress incites spreading of macrophages via extracellular signal-regulated kinases and p38 mitogen-activated protein kinase. J Immunol 161:3569–3574.

56. Ushio-Fukai M, Alexander RW, Akers M, Griendling KK. 1998. p38 Mitogen-activated protein kinase is a critical component of the redox-sensitive signaling pathways activated by angiotensin II. Role in vascular smooth muscle cell hypertrophy. J Biol Chem 273:15022–15029.

57. Barlow RS, El-Mowafy AM, White RE. 2000. H$_2$O$_2$ opens BK$_{Ca}$ channels via the PLA$_2$-arachidonic acid signaling cascade in coronary artery smooth muscle. Am J Physiol 279:H475–H483.

58. Hecht D, Zick Y. 1992. Selective inhibition of protein tyrosine phosphatase activities by H$_2$O$_2$ and vanadate *in vitro*. Biochem Biophys Res Commun 188:773–779.

59. Denu JM, Tanner KG. 1998. Specific and reversible inactivation of protein tyrosine phosphatases by hydrogen peroxide: evidence for a sulfenic acid intermediate and implications for redox regulation. Biochemistry 37:5633–5642.

60. Schreck R, Rieber P, Baeuerle PA. 1991. Reactive oxygen intermediates as apparently widely used messengers in the activation of the NF-κB transcription factor and HIV-1. EMBO J 10:2247–2258.

61. Foo SY, Nolan GP. 1999. NF-κB to the rescue: RELs, apoptosis and cellular transformation. Trends Genet 15:229–235.

62. Schmidt KN, Amstad P, Cerutti P, Baeuerle PA. 1996. Identification of hydrogen peroxide as the relevant messenger in the activation pathway of transcription factor NF-kappaB. Adv Exp Med Biol 387:63–68.

63. Perona R, Montaner S, Saniger L, Sanchez PI, Bravo R, Lacal JC. 1997. Activation of the nuclear factor-κB by Rho, CDC42, and Rac-1 proteins. Genes Dev 11:463–475.

64. Sulciner DJ, Irani K, Yu ZX, Ferrans VJ, Goldschmidt-Clermont PJ, Finkel T. 1996. rac1 regulates a cytokine-stimulated, redox-dependent pathway necessary for NF-κB activation. Mol Cell Biol 16:7115–7121.

65. Carballo M, Marquez G, Conde M, Martin-Nieto J, Monteseirin J, Conde J, Pintado E, Sobrino F. 1999. Characterization of calcineurin in human neutrophils. Inhibitory effect of hydrogen peroxide on its enzymatic activity and on NF-kappaB DNA binding. J Biol Chem 274:93–100.

66. Lakshminarayanan V, Drab-Weiss EA, Roebuck KA. 1998. H_2O_2 and tumor necrosis factor-alpha induce differential binding of the redox-responsive transcription factors AP-1 and NF-kappaB to the interleukin-8 promoter in endothelial and epithelial cells. J Biol Chem 273:32670–32678.

67. Salminen A, Liu PK, Hsu CY. 1995. Alteration of transcription factor binding activities in the ischemic rat brain. Biochem Biophys Res Commun 212:939–944.

68. Jin N, Hatton ND, Harrington MA, Xia X, Larsen SH, Rhoades RA. 2000. H_2O_2-induced egr-1, fra-1, and c-jun gene expression is mediated by tyrosine kinase in aortic smooth muscle cells. Free Radic Biol Med 29:736–746.

69. Sun Y, Oberley LW. 1996. Redox regulation of transcriptional activators. Free Radic Biol Med 21:335–348.

70. Shimizu N, Yoshiyama M, Omura T, Hanatani A, Kim S, Takeuchi K, Iwao H, Yoshikawa J. 1998. Activation of mitogen-activated protein kinases and activator protein-1 in myocardial infarction in rats. Cardiovasc Res 38:116–124.

71. Staüble B, Boscoboinik D, Tasinato A, Azzi A. 1994. Modulation of activator protein-1 (AP-1) transcription factor and protein kinase C by hydrogen peroxide and D-α-tocopherol in vascular smooth muscle cells. Eur J Biochem 226:393–402.

72. Cimino F, Esposito F, Ammendola R, Russo T. 1997. Gene regulation by reactive oxygen species. Curr Top Cell Regul 35:123–148.

73. Czubryt MP, Austria JA, Pierce GN. 2000. Hydrogen peroxide inhibition of nuclear protein import is mediated by the mitogen-activated protein kinase, ERK2. J Cell Biol 148:7–15.

74. Rao GN. 1996. Hydrogen peroxide induces complex formation of SHC-Grb2-SOS with receptor tyrosine kinase and activates Ras and extracellular signal-regulated protein kinases group of mitogen-activated protein kinases. Oncogene 13:713–719.

75. Patterson C, Ruef J, Madamanchi NR, Barry-Lane P, Hu Z, Horaist C, Ballinger CA, Brasier AR, Bode C, Runge MS. 1999. Stimulation of a vascular smooth muscle cell NAD(P)H oxidase by thrombin. Evidence that p47(phox) may participate in forming this oxidase in vitro and in vivo. J Biol Chem 274:19814–19822.

76. Lu G, Greene EL, Nagai T, Egan BM. 1998. Reactive oxygen species are critical in the oleic acid-mediated mitogenic signaling pathway in vascular smooth muscle cells. Hypertension 32:1003–1010.

77. Nishio E, Watanabe Y. 1997. The involvement of reactive oxygen species and arachidonic acid in alpha 1-adrenoceptor-induced smooth muscle cell proliferation and migration. Br J Pharmacol 121:665–670.

78. Li PF, Maasch C, Haller H, Dietz R, von Harsdorf R. 1999. Requirement for protein kinase C in reactive oxygen species-induced apoptosis of vascular smooth muscle cells. Circulation 100:967–973.

79. Taher MM, Mahgoub MA, Abd-Elfattah AS. 1998. Redox regulation of signal transduction in smooth muscle cells: distinct effects of PKC down regulation and PKC inhibitors on oxidant induced MAP kinase. J Recept Signal Transduct Res 18:167–185.

80. Abe MK, Kartha S, Karpova AY, Li J, Liu PT, Kuo WL, Hershenson MB. 1998. Hydrogen peroxide activates extracellular signal-regulated kinase via protein kinase C, Raf-1, and MEK1. Am J Respir Cell Mol Biol 18:562–569.

81. Vogt M, Bauer MK, Ferrari D, Schulze-Osthoff K. 1998. Oxidative stress and hypoxia/reoxygenation trigger CD95 (APO-1/Fas) ligand expression in microglial cells. FEBS Lett 429:67–72.

82. Furuke K, Shiraishi M, Mostowski HS, Bloom ET. 1999. Fas ligand induction in human NK cells is regulated by redox through a calcineurin-nuclear factors of activated T cell-dependent pathway. J Immunol 162:1988–1993.

83. Rimpler MM, Rauen U, Schmidt T, Moroy T, de Groot H. 1999. Protection against hydrogen peroxide cytotoxicity in rat-1 fibroblasts provided by the oncoprotein Bcl-2: maintenance of calcium homeostasis is secondary to the effect of Bcl-2 on cellular glutathione. Biochem J 340:291–297.

84. Ellerby LM, Ellerby HM, Park SM, Holleran AL, Murphy AN, Fiskum G, Kane DJ, Testa MP, Kayalar C, Bredesen DE. 1996. Shift of the cellular oxidation-reduction potential in neural cells expressing Bcl-2. J Neurochem 67:1259–1267.

85. Chau Y-P, Shiah S-G, Don M-J, Kuo M-L. 1998. Involvement of hydrogen peroxide in topoisomerase inhibitor B-lapachone-induced apoptosis and differentiation in human leukemia cells. Free Radic Biol Med 24:660–670.

86. Chen Y-C, Lin-Shiau S-Y, Lin J-K. 1998. Involvement of reactive oxygen species and caspase 3 activation in arsenite-induced apoptosis. J Cell Physiol 177:324–333.

87. Cai J, Jones DP. 1998. Superoxide in apoptosis. J Biol Chem 273:11401–11404.

88. DiPietrantonio AM, Hsieh TC, Wu JM. 2000. Specific processing of poly(ADP-ribose) polymerase, accompanied by activation of caspase-3 and elevation/reduction of ceramide/hydrogen peroxide levels, during induction of apoptosis in host HL-60 cells infected by the human granulocytic ehrlichiosis (HGE) agent. IUBMB Life 49:49–55.

89. Hampton MB, Fadeel B, Orrenius S. 1998. Redox regulation of the caspases during apoptosis. Ann NY Acad Sci 854:328–335.

90. Palomba L, Sestili P, Cantoni O. 1999. The antioxidant butylated hydroxytoluene induces apoptosis in human U937 cells: the role of hydrogen peroxide and altered redox state. Free Radic Res 31:93–101.

91. Tada-Oikawa S, Oikawa S, Kawanishi M, Yamada M, Kawanishi S. 1999. Generation of hydrogen peroxide precedes loss of mitochondrial membrane potential during DNA alkylation-induced apoptosis. FEBS Lett 442:65–69.

92. Moses MA, Klagsbrun M, Shing Y. 1995. The role of growth factors in vascular cell development and differentiation. Int Rev Cytol 161:1–48.

93. Kurbaan AS, Bowker TJ, Rickards AF. 1998. Differential restenosis rate of individual coronary artery sites after multivessel angioplasty: implications for revascularization strategy. CABRI Investigators. Coronary Angioplasty versus Bypass Revascularisation Investigation. Am Heart J 135:703–708.

94. Laitinen M, Yla-Herttuala S. 1998. Vascular gene transfer for the treatment of restenosis and atherosclerosis. Curr Opin Lipidol 9:465–469.

95. Losordo DW, Vale PR, Isner JM. 1999. Gene therapy for myocardial angiogenesis. Am Heart J 138:S132–S141.

96. Li W, Liu G, Chou IN, Kagan HM. 2000. Hydrogen peroxide-mediated, lysyl oxidase-dependent chemotaxis of vascular smooth muscle cells. J Cell Biochem 78:550–557.

97. Matoba T, Shimokawa H, Nakashima M, Hirakawa Y, Mukai Y, Hirano K, Kanaide H, Takeshita A. 2000. Hydrogen peroxide is an endothelium-derived hyperpolarizing factor in mice. J Clin Invest 106:1521–1530.

98. Penn MS, Patel CV, Cui MZ, DiCorleto PE, Chisolm GM. 1999. LDL increases inactive tissue factor on vascular smooth muscle cell surfaces: hydrogen peroxide activates latent cell surface tissue factor. Circulation 99:1753–1759.

99. Mietus-Snyder M, Glass CK, Pitas RE. 1998. Transcriptional activation of scavenger receptor expression in human smooth muscle cells requires AP-1/c-jun and C/EBPbeta: both AP-1 binding and JNK activation are induced by phorbol esters and oxidative stress. Arterioscler Thromb Vasc Biol 18:1440–1449.

100. Drummond GR, Cai H, Davis ME, Ramasamy S, Harrison DG. 2000. Transcriptional and post-transcriptional regulation of endothelial nitric oxide synthase expression by hydrogen peroxide. Circ Res 86:347–354.

101. Hamby JM, Showalter HD. 1999. Small molecule inhibitors of tumor-promoted angiogenesis, including protein tyrosine kinase inhibitors. Pharmacol Ther 82:169–193.

Signal Transduction and Cardiac Hypertrophy,
edited by N.S. Dhalla, L.V. Hryshko,
E. Kardami & P.K. Singal
Kluwer Academic Publishers, Boston, 2003

Localized Control of Oxidative Phosphorylation within Intracellular Energetic Units in Heart Cells: A Possible Solution of Some Old Problems

Valdur Saks,[1,2] Florence Appaix,[1] Yves Usson,[3]
Karen Guerrero,[1] Jose Olivares,[1] Enn Seppet,[4] Mayis Aliev,[5]
Raimund Margreiter,[6] and Andrey Kuznetsov[6]

[1] Laboratory of Bioenergetics
Joseph Fourier University
Grenoble, France
[2] Laboratory of Bioenergetics
National Institute of Chemical Physics and Biophysics
Tallinn, Estonia
[3] Equipe RFMQ, Laboratory TIMC UMR5525 CNRS
Institute Albert Bonniot, Grenoble
[4] Department of Pathophysiology
Tartu University, Tartu, Estonia
[5] Cardiology Research Center
Moscow, Russia
[6] Department of Transplant Surgery
University Hospital Innsbruck
Innsbruck, Austria

Summary. Experimental and *in silico* studies of regulation of mitochondrial respiration in permeabilized muscle fibers have revealed functional complexes of mitochondria with myofibrils and sarcoplasmic reticulum—intracellular energetic units—as basic pattern of organization of cell energy metabolism in oxidative muscle cells (*Saks et al. Biochem. J. 356, 643–657, 2001*). In this paper we review new data showing that in the cells *in vivo* there are at least two major factors of the control of mitochondrial function which are lost in experiments *in vitro*: mitochondrial position in the cell with respect to other cellular structures, and the tightly controlled mitochondrial outer membrane. Because of this, the local concentration of ADP available in

Address for Correspondence: V.A.Saks, Laboratory of Bioenergetics, Joseph Fourier University, 2280, Rue de la Piscine, BP53X—38041, Grenoble Cedex 9, France. E-mail: *Valdur.Saks@ujf-grenoble.fr*

the vicinity of ATP/ADP translocase is strictly controlled by the organized metabolic networks of energy transfer including the creatine kinase and adenylate kinase systems within the intracellular energetic units. Mathematical modelling of energy fluxes within these units satisfactorily explains the linear relationship between heart work and oxygen uptake under conditions of metabolic stability, and allows to quantitatively analyse the mechanism of the regulation of mitochondrial function in the cells *in vivo*. The knowledge of metabolic changes within the functional complexes of mitochondria with MgATPases in normal and pathological conditions may help to explain the mechanism of acute ischemic cardiac failure.

Key words: heart, respiration, contraction, mitochondria, regulation, ischemia.

INTRODUCTION: THE UNSOLVED PROBLEMS

The main mechanisms of the regulation of mitochondrial activity became clear soon after successful isolation of mitochondria in 1949 by Pallade, Lehninger and Kennedy due to development of the method of differential centrifugation and application of isoosmotic solutions. Lardy and Wellmann (1) and then Chance (2) discovered soon the phenomenon of the respiratory control: the respiration rate of isolated mitochondria was shown to depend strongly on the availability of ADP. This phenomenon is used for the classification of the functional states of mitochondria, the ratio of rate of respiration in the State 3 (presence of ADP) to that in the State 4 (all ADP is converted to ATP), the respiratory control index, RCI, being used as a quantitative indicator of the efficiency of coupling between mitochondrial reactions of oxidation and phosphorylation. This ratio is also a very useful practical index of the quality of the experimental work with isolated mitochondria, especially when mitochondria are isolated and studied in the presence of Mg^{2+} (necessary cofactor of all kinases, as well as ATPases): if mitochondria are damaged during isolation, the MgATPase activity is increased due to its exposure to the bulk medium, this decreases the respiratory control index, RCI. With the discoveries of the chemiosmotic nature of the oxidative phosphorylation by Peter Mitchell (3) and of the rotary "binding change" mechanism of the ATP synthesis by Boyer and Walker (4,5), the regulatory role of ADP over respiration became clear in molecular terms: this is due to the decrease of the transmembrane electrochemical potential of protons used for rephosphorylation of ADP by the F_0F_1 complex. Thus, there is no doubt that mitochondrial respiration rate is regulated by ADP available for adenine nucleotide translocator and thus for F_0F_1 complex within the mitochondrial matrix.

For the regulation of mitochondrial activity in the cells *in vivo* the question is: where this ADP comes from? The conventional theory of homogenous distribution of ADP, due to its rapid diffusion within the cells, where the ADP levels are controlled by the equilibrium creatine kinase reaction (6) was overthrown first by Balaban et al. (7) and then by others (reviewed in ref. 8) by showing that the rate of oxygen consumption by working heart can be increased by order of magnitude without any changes of ATP and phosphocreatine levels (the phenomenon of metabolic stability), and consequently, without any changes in the average ADP concentration in the cells. To date the question of the mechanism of regulation of mitochondrial respiration in the cells *in vivo* remains still open. The problems with the alternative theory of parallel regulation of respiration by calcium ions are discussed below.

The second, even more profound mystery of cardiac cell energetics and physiology, in particular of its pathophysiology, is an observation by Gudbjarnason et al. (9), Neely et al. (10), Koretsune and Marban (11) and many others that when the mitochondrial respiration is inhibited in the cells *in vivo* due to the lack of perfusion (ischemia) or oxygen in the perfusate (anoxia), the contraction stops in the presence of high levels of ATP (about 5 mM, or 70–80% of its normal level, much higher than the affinities for this substrate of the ATP-sensitive systems, as actomyosin ATPase, ATP-sensitive K^+ channel etc.), leading to the conclusion that these systems should still be saturated by ATP. The intuitive logical explanation was the compartmentation theory that led to the quantitative description of the phosphocreatine-creatine kinase and adenylate kinase pathways of energy transfer described in details in many recent reviews and publications (12–16). What remained to elucidate in the framework of these theories is the cellular basis of compartmentation of ATP and ADP in the heart cells, and thus the basis for the phosphocreatine pathway of energy transfer. How this pathway helps to explain the phenomenon of metabolic stability was recently well analysed by Keith Garlid (17).

The aim of this article is to summarize the recent experimental data showing that the possible answer, the possible solution of these important problems are to be found in the structural organization of the oxidative muscle cells and its consequences for the energy metabolism.

MATHERIALS AND METHODS

Animals

Wistar rats (200–250 g) were used in all experiments. The investigation conforms with the Guide for the Care and Use of Laboratory Animals published by the National Institutes of Health (NIH Publication No. 85-23, revised 1985).

Isolation of mitochondria from cardiac muscle

Mitochondria were isolated from rat hearts by a proteolytic procedure described earlier (18).

Preparation of skinned muscle fibers

Skinned fibers were prepared from rat hearts by the careful mechanical dissection and saponin treatment according to the method described previously (19).

Determination of the rate of mitochondrial respiration in skinned fibers and cardiomyocytes

The rates of oxygen uptake were recorded by using the two-channel high resolution respirometer (OROBOROS *Oxygraph*, Paar KG, Graz, Austria) or a Yellow

Spring Clark oxygen electrode in solution B (for respiration kinetics, composition see below).

Confocal microscopy

a) Imaging of mitochondrial flavoproteins: Isolated saponin-permeabilized fiber bundles or cardiomyocytes were fixed in a Heraeus flexiperm chamber (Hanau, Germany) with microscopic glass slide. Then 200 µl of respiration medium were immediately added into the chamber. Fully oxidized state of mitochondrial flavoproteins was achieved by substrate deprivation and equilibration of the medium with air (20). The digital video images of mitochondrial flavoproteins in the fiber bundle were acquired using a confocal microscope (LSM510NLO, Zeiss) with a 40× water immersion lens (NA 1.2). The use of such a water immersion prevented from geometrical aberations when observing in vitro living cells. The autofluorescence of flavoproteins was excited with the 488 nm line of an Argon laser, the laser output power was set to an average power of 8 mW. The fluorescence was collected through a 510 nm dichroic beam-splitter and a 505–550 nm band pass filter. The pinhole aperture was set to one Airy disk unit.

b) Simultaneous imaging of flavoproteins and NADH: Autofluorescence of flavoproteins was imaged using a confocal microscope (LSM510NLO, Zeiss) with a 40× water immersion lens (NA 1.2) as described above. The autofluorescence of NADH was excited by two-photon absorption using a femto-second pulsed infra-red laser (Tsunami + MilleniaVIII, SpectraPhysics). The pulse frequency was set at 100 MHz with a pulse width of 100 femto-second. The infra-red line was tuned to 720 nm giving a maximum two-photon absorption at 360 nm. The laser output power was set to an average power of 400 mW. The fluorescence signals were collected through a multiline beam splitter with maximum refexions at 488 nm ± 10 nm (for rejection of the 488 nm line) and above 700 nm (for rejection of infra-red excitation). A second 490 nm beam splitter was used to discriminate the NADH signal from the flavoprotein signal. Then the flavoprotein signal passed through a 500–550 nm band-pass filter with an additional infra-red rejection filter before being collected through a pinhole (one Airy disk unit). The NADH signal was redirected to a 390–465 nm band-pass filter with an additional infra-red rejection filter.

Determination of the pyruvate kinase activity

The activity of pyruvate kinase in the stock solutions was assessed by a coupled lactate dehydrogenase system. The decrease in the NADH level was determined spectrophotometrically in Uvikon 941 plus spectrophotometer (Kontron Instruments, UK) in solution B supplimented with 0.3 mM NADH, 2 m MADP, 1 mM phosphoenolpyruvate and 4–5 IU/ml of lactate dehydrogenase in response to addition of different amounts of PK. Recordings were performed at a wavelength of 340 nm.

Protein concentration determination

Protein concentration in mitochondrial preparations was determined by the ELISA method using the EL_x800 Universal Microplate Reader from Bio-Tek instruments and a BCA kit (Protein Assay Reagent) from Pierce (USA).

Solutions. Composition of the solutions used for preparation of skinned fibers and for oxygraphy was based on the information of the ionic contents in the muscle cell cytoplasm ().

Solution A contained, in mM: CaK_2EGTA 1.9, K_2EGTA 8.1, $MgCl_2$ 9.5, dithiothreitol (DTT) 0.5, potassium 2-(N-morpholino)ethanesulfonate (K-Mes) 53.3, imidazole 20, taurine 20, Na_2ATP 2.5, phosphocreatine 19, pH 7.1 adjusted at 25°C.

Solution B contained, in mM: CaK_2EGTA 1.9, K_2EGTA 8.1, $MgCl_2$ 4.0, DTT 0.5, K-Mes 100, imidazole 20, taurine 20, K_2HPO_4 3 and pyruvate 5 (or glutamate 5) + malate 2, pH 7.1 adjusted at 25°C.

Solution KCl contained, in mM: KCl 125, Hepes 20, glutamate 4, malate 2, Mg-acetate 3, KH_2PO_4 5, EGTA 0.4 and DTT 0.3, pH 7.1 adjusted at 25°C and 2mg/ml of BSA was added.

Reagents. All reagents were purchased from Sigma (USA) except ATP and ADP, which were obtained from Boehringer (Germany).

Analysis of the experimental results

The values in tables and figures are expressed as means ± S.D. The apparent Km for ADP was estimated from a linear regression of double-reciprocal plots. Statistical comparisons were made using the Anova test (variance analysis and Fisher test), and $P < 0.05$ was taken as the level of significance.

RESULTS AND DISCUSSION

1. Regulation of mitochondrial activity in vitro versus in vivo

One of the experimental techniques that allows to study the function of mitochondria without their isolation from the cell, *in situ*, is the permeabilized cell technique (19). The experiments with this technique have shown that mitochondrial properties *in vitro* and *in situ* are very different (21–28). This is illustrated in Figure 1, which shows the oxygraph recordings of the different responses of isolated rat heart mitochondria and mitochondria *in situ* in the skinned cardiac fibers to the addition of exogenous ADP. The recording were made in both cases in solution B with high K^+ concentration to maintain normal matrix volume of mitochondria (29,30). While the isolated mitochondria were saturated rapidly by the addition of exogenous ADP in micromolar concentrations (Figure 1A), the mitochondria *in situ* in the permeabilzed cells (skinned fibers) responded only to the addition of ADP in concentrations in the millimolar range (Figure 2B). Correspondingly, the apparent affinities of mitochondria to ADP were very different: apparent Km for exogenous ADP was 12μM in the case of isolated mitochondria and 300μM in the case of mitochondria *in situ* in this particular experiment (Figure 1C). (For statistics, see Table 1). These differences cannot be explained by the differences in the matrix volume of mitochondria, as proposed recently by Dos Santos et al. (29), since all experiments were performed in the solution B with high concentration of K^+ in the presence of respiratory substrates, and therefore the matrix volume was equally expanded in both cases due to the entry of K^+ into mitochondrial matrix via ATP-dependent channel (30). In addition, Table 1 shows that when

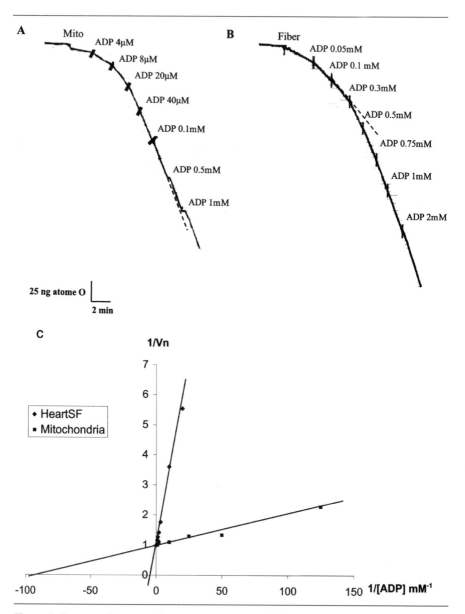

Figure 1. Representative traces of oxygen consumption at different ADP concentrations in the solution B. A—isolated rat heart mitochondria (60 μg/ml protein); B—permeabilized myocardial fibers (1 mg of dry weight) in the presence of glutamate and malate as substrates. C—presentation of the data in the Lineweaver—Burk plots. Respiration traces illustrate a remarkably different responses to the addition of increasing concentration of ADP and as a result, clearly different affinities for ADP in isolated and *in situ* mitochondria. Respiration was measured at 25°C as described in "Methods".

Table 1. Changes of apparent kinetic parameters of mitochondrial respiration in skinned cardiac fibers by hypo-osmotic shock and proteolysis

Conditions	Apparent Km for exogenous ADP, µM	Reference
Control		
a) in solution B	320 ± 26	(21,22,25,27,28)
b) in sucrose, 240 mM	306 ± 16	
Hypoosmotic solution, 40 mOsM	32 ± 5	(22,26)
Treatment by 5 µM trypsin, 15 min	98 ± 8	(24,28)
Isolated heart mitochondria in solution B	14 − 28	(21,22−29,31)

skinned fibers were placed into sucrose solution without K^+ and according to the hypothesis by Dos Santos et al. (29), the mitochondrial matrix should have contracted as a result of loss of K^+, nevertheless the apparent Km for exogenous ADP in skinned fibers stayed very high. Thus, there is no direct connection between high apparent Km for ADP in skinned cardiac fibers and intramitochondrial volume changes. These conclusions are in concord with data of Liobikas et al. (31), who also did not observe the changes on apparent Km for exogenous ADP with the changes in oncotic pressure of solution. At the same time, multiple investigations have shown that there are two different experimental methods to decrease the apparent Km for exogenous ADP in the permeabilized cardiac fibers, which may help us to understand the mechanism of regulation of mitochondrial activity in the cells *in vivo*. These data are summarized in Table 1. The apparent Km for exogenous ADP of mitochondria *in situ* may be decreased by: 1) disruption of the mitochondrial outer membrane by hypo-osmotic treatment (22,26); 2) by rather short selective proteolysis of some fiber proteins (24–28). Remarkably, in these two cases the structural changes in the cells revealed by the confocal microscopy, are very different, as it is shown below.

2. Confocal microscopic imaging of the intracellular energetic units in the oxidative muscle cells: two major procedures which change the mitochondrial properties in vivo

Figure 2 shows the confocal imaging of mitochondrial localization in isolated cardiomyocytes by recording the autofluorescence of mitochondrial flavoproteins (Figure 2A) and by autofluorescence of NADH (Figure 2B). In both cases the remarkably regularity of position of mitochondria in the cells with characteristic striations (25) is seen. Similar observation was made for the skinned cardiac fibers (Figure 3). In the oxidized state of mitochondrial respiratory chain (achieved by substrate deprivation in the aerated open chamber) one observes intensive fluorescence of flavoproteins, but not NADH (Figure 3A and 3B). Addition of respiratory substrates (glutamate + malate) reduces the flavoproteins and diminishes their autofluorescence, but increases that of NADH. Thus, both methods of autofluorescence

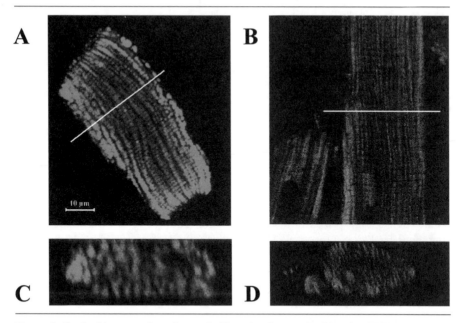

Figure 2. Confocal laser-scanning micrographs illustrating flavoprotein (A) and NAD(P)H (B) auto-fluorescence in isolated cardiomyocytes. Corresponding cross-sections (XZ scanning) are shown in (C, D). Note the very regular position of mitochondria between myofibrils, with characteristic striations between them at the level of Z-lines. In cross-section (C and D) mitochondrial distribution follows random pattern.

registration give rather precise information of the position of mitochondria inside the cells. Moreover, confocal laser-scanning micrographs illustrate clear co-localization of the flavoprotein autofluorescence and the fluorescence of the mitochondrial NADH across myocardial fibers.

Figure 4 shows that two different procedures which change the apparent affinity (apparent Km) for exogenous ADP in the oxidative muscle fibers—hypoosmotic treatment of permeabilized cells or skinned fibers and their short-time treatment with proteases, see Table 1—have very different effects on the mitochondrial position in the cells. The regular mitochondrial position is not changed after treatment of skinned cardiac fibers under hypo-osmotic conditions (Figure 4B and C), which induce only the swelling of the matrix space and results in rupture of the outer mitochondrial membrane with the release of cytochrome c (22,26). On the contrary, Figures 4D–G show that the regular arrangement of mitochondria in the cells is completely changed by short proteolytic treatment using optimal trypsin concentration, but the outer mitochondrial membrane in this case stays intact (24,28).

Thus, there are at least two important intracellular factors which influence the

Mito flavoproteins   Mito NAD(P)H

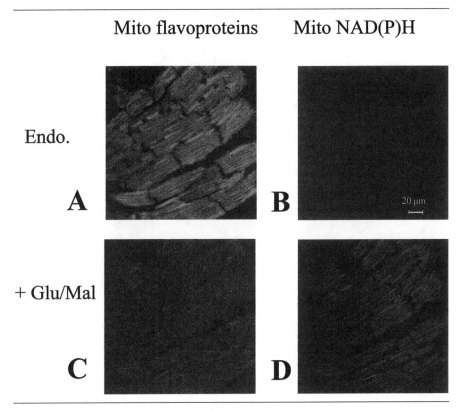

Endo.

A   **B**

+ Glu/Mal

C   **D**

Figure 3. Simultaneous confocal imaging of the autofluorescence of mitochondrial flavoproteins (A, C) and NAD(P)H (B, D) within saponin permeabilized myocardial fibers. A and B: Confocal laser-scanning micrographs in the oxidized state. C and D: Corresponding flavoprotein and NAD(P)H autofluorescence images after addition of 5 mM glutamate and 2 mM malate. Bar, 20 μm. The autofluorescence of flavoproteins diminishes with reduction of the respiratory chain, and that of NAD(P)H increases.

affinity of mitochondria for exogenous ADP in the cells *in situ*: 1) the obviously altered (decreased) permeability of the mitochondrial outer membrane (the VDAC channels) for this substrate, which may be increased by rupture of this membrane under hypo-osmotic conditions; 2) the position of mitochondria in the cells and their interactions with other cellular structures presumably due to the presence of some distribution proteins connected to the cytoskeleton, which may be altered by trypsin (28).

3. Metabolic channelling of ADP in the cells in situ: the competitive enzyme metod

The precise structural organisation of the cell by the cytoskeleton may create conditions for effective interactions between mitochondria and energy-consuming

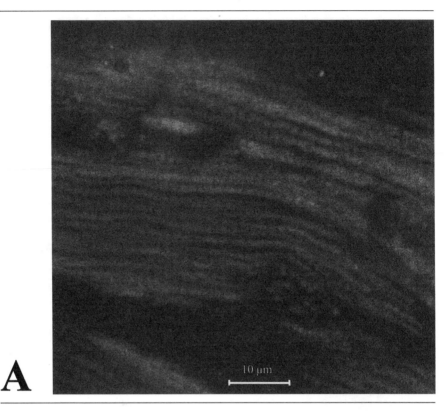

Figure 4. Confocal imaging of the autofluorescence of mitochondrial flavoproteins within saponin permeabilized myocardial fibers in the oxidized state. A: Control fibers. B: after hypo-osmotic treatment (30 mOsm/L) and cytochrome c depletion. C: after selective treatment with 5 μM trypsin for 5 min. A corresponding 3.5-fold magnification of the areas from B and C are shown in D and E. Bar, 20 μm.

systems which may form effective functional complexes of mitochondria with sarcoplasmic reticulum and sarcomeres in muscle cells (27,28). The channeling of ADP within these complexes may be studied by using a competitive coupled enzyme method (32,33). When ATP in the concentration of 1 or 2 mM is added to the permeabilized fibers, intracellular MgATPase reactions produce endogenous ADP. This ADP can be released into the medium or supplied to mitochondria to support the oxidative phosphorylation. Addition of pyruvate kinase (PK) to the system in sufficiently high activity together with its substrate phosphoenol pyruvate (PEP) will allow to measure spectrophotometrically the rate of ADP production, if it is coupled to lactate dehydrogenase reaction in the presence of NADH. This protocol is shown in Figure 5A. When mitochondrial substrates are absent, all ADP could be released into the medium. Addition of the substrates (glutamate-malate in the presence of phosphate) significantly decreases the rate of coupled reactions leading to NADH

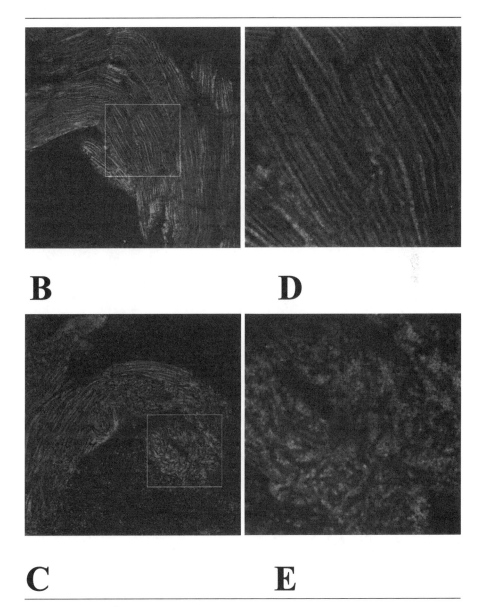

Figure 4. Continued.

oxidation (Figure 5A), demonstrating that the endogenous ADP is directly chan-nelled to mitochondria before its release into the bulk medium. Inhibition of the adenine nucleotide translocase by its specific inhibitor atractyloside results in inhi-bition of utilization of endogenous ADP by mitochondria and restores the rate of ADP flux into the medium. This conclusion is supported the data in Figure 5B

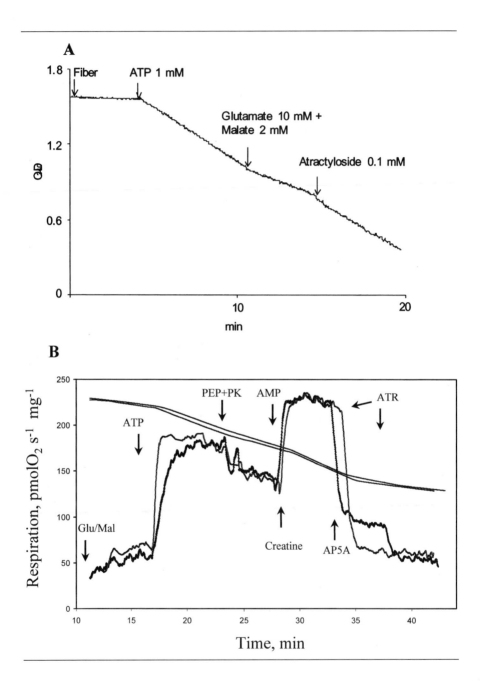

◀

Figure 5. A. Competition between mitochondria and the external PK-PEP system for ADP generated in ATPase reactions by measurements of the PK reaction in skinned cardiac fibers of normal rat. The experiments were performed at 25°C in solution B complemented with 5 mg/ml BSA, 5 mM PEP, 20 IU/ml PK, 20 IU/ml LDH, and 250 μM NADH. The experiment was started by addition of 1.9 mg skinned fibers into the spectrophotometric quvette. Then 1 mM MgATP was added to initiate ATPase reactions monitored as a decrease in NADH concentration in the medium due to flux of ADP through the PK. Further addition of glutamate and malate resulted in inhibition of PK reaction because of the mitochondrial control over ADP produced by ATPases. This is confirmed by observation that inhibition of oxidative phosphorylation by atractyloside reactivated the flux through the PK. B. Representative traces of oxygen concentration and flux in permeabilized myocardial fibers illustrating a Pyruvate kinase/PEP protocol with particular emphasis on creatine (normal line) and AMP (bold line) stimulations. Additions: Glu/Mal, 5 mM glutamate and 2 mM malate; 2 mM ATP; 2 mM PEP and 20 IU/ml pyruvate kinase; 1 mM AMP; 30 mM creatine; AP5A, 50 μM diadenosinepentaphosphate; ATR, 100 μM atractyloside. Respiration was measured at 25°C as described in "Methods".

showing that PK-PEP system is not able to suppress more than 40% of the mitochondrial respiration activated by endogenous ADP, pointing to the existence of locally non-accessible ADP due to its fast recycling and channelling. The addition of creatine into the system in presence of high activity of the PK allows to maximally activate the respiration (Figure 5B) due to the local ADP production by the mitochondrial creatine kinase in the vicinity of the adenine nucleotide translocator (18), behind the outer mitochondrial membrane. This ADP is not accessible at all to the PK, clearly illustrating the importance of the mitochondrial creatine kinase in the regulation of the rate of respiration and oxidative phosphorylation. It follows from these experiments that an important mechanism of the ADP and ATP compartmentation in the cells may be the control of the mitochondrial outer membrane VDAC channels by some still non-identified proteins, probably connected to cytoskeleton and also responsible for mitochondrial distribution and formation of mitochondrial functional complexes in the cardiac cells (27,28). All these data support the view that the organized networks of ADP channelling within functional complexes of mitochondria with Ca, MgATPases of myofibrils and sarcoplasmic reticulum is an important mechanism of feedback regulation of mitochondrial activity in the cardiac cells in vivo, as illustrated by the general scheme in Figure 6.

These localized metabolic events in these structural and functional units have been analyzed and described quantitatively by the original reaction—diffusion mathematical models of compartmentalized energy transfer (34,35). The results of the modelling showed that in mitochondria the creatine kinase reaction is continuously out of equilibrium, and in the cytoplasm it approaches the equilibrium state only in the diastolic phase. Mathematical modelling of energy fluxes within these units satisfactorily explains the experimentally observed linear dependence of the rate of oxygen consumption by heart muscle upon the workload under conditions of metabolic stability, and allows to quantitatively analyze in silico the mechanism of regulation of mitochondrial function in the cells in vivo (34,35). The contradictory explanation of heart muscle metabolic stability is considered in section 5.

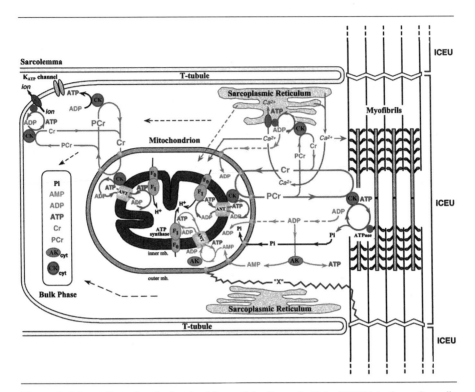

Figure 6. Scheme illustrating the functional Intracellular Energetic Units (ICEUs) in the cardiac cell. By interaction with cytoskeletal elements, the mitochondria and sarcoplasmic reticulum (SR) are precisely fixed with respect to the structure of sarcomere of myofibrils between two Z-lines and correspondingly between two T-tubules. Calcium is released from SR into the space in ICEU in the vicinity of mitochondria and sarcomeres to activate contraction and mitochondrial dehydrogenases. Adenine nucleotides within ICEU do not equilibrate rapidly with adenine nucleotides in the bulk water phase. The mitochondria, SR and MgATPase of myofibrils and ATP sensitive systems in sarcolemma are interconnected by metabolic channeling of reaction intermediates and energy transfer within ICEU by the creatine kinase—phosphocreatine and myokinase systems. The protein factors (still unknown and marked as "X"), most probably connected to cytoskeleton, fix the position of mitochondria and probably also controls the permeabilty of the VDAC channels for ADP and ATP. Adenine nucleotides within ICEU and bulk water phase may be connected by some more rapidly diffusing metabolites as Cr–PCr. Synchronization of functioning of ICEUs within the cell may occur by the same metabolites (for example, Pi or PCr) or/and synchronized release of calcium during excitation—contraction coupling process.

4. The consequences of the structural organization of heart cells for regulation of mitochondrial function and contraction: possible solution of the old problems?

The data described above are summarized in the scheme in the Figure 6. This scheme shows the possible rather complex interactions between mitochondria, sarcoplasmic reticulum and the contractile apparatus in sarcomeres, involving channelling and facilitated diffusion of ADP via the creatine kinase and adenylate kinase networks (8,12–18,36–42). It shows the structure and function of one intracellular energetic unit which may probably be a basic pattern of organization of cardiac cell energy metabolism (28,35). According to this hypothesis, structural organization of the cell is one of important factors which may determine the mechanism of regulation of both energy production and utilization. It may be assumed that: 1) the local concentrations of adenine nucleotides, from the point of view of enzyme kinetics, and 2) local values of phosphorylation potential, from the point of view of chemical thermodynamics, which are controlled by the creatine kinase and adenylate kinase networks, are the most important factors of regulation of energetic processes. The macromolecular crowding and structural organization of the cells is obviously the reason for compartmentation of adenine nucleotides as described above, and the phosphocreatine-creatine system might play a role in synchronizing the activities of these units in the cell. If this is true, it becomes clear that inhibition of mitochondrial oxidative phosphorylation by lack of oxygen results first in inhibition of phosphocreatine production in the coupled mitochondrial creatine kinase reaction (8,15,16,18), leading to the rapid fall of local phosphorylation potentials in the intracellular energetic units and thus inhibition of contraction and to rapid alterations in transmembrane ion currents responsible for excitation-contraction coupling (38,42). If there is some local restriction for free exchange of ATP between its bulk phase in cytoplasm and local functionally important pools, due to the phenomena of structural or/and kinetic microcompartmentation, the inhibition of contraction in the presence of high cellular ATP level could be easily understood. This mechanism corresponds to the original proposal by Gudbjarnason et al. (9).

While verification of this hypothesis still requires further intensive work, there is already abundant and still growing evidence that important consequences of cardiac ischemia are: 1) the loss of the integrity of the precise structural organization of cardiac cell and its energy transport network (36,39–41); 2) destruction or rupture of the barrier function of the outer mitochondrial membrane (43,44); 3) impairment of functional coupling between mitochondrial creatine kinase and oxidative phosphorylation leading to damage of intracellular metabolic channelling (16,19,43). Understanding and further investigation of these processes will be important as an effective basis for new diagnostic approaches in the ischemia-reperfusion injury and for evaluation of efficiency of cardioprotection by the analysis of *in situ* mitochondria using permeabilized cell and skinned fiber technique.

5. An analysis of the parallel activation theory

The alternative explanation of the regulation of mitochondrial respiration in dependence upon the workload is the parallel activation theory of both contraction and respiration by calcium ions (45–47). This hypothesis, proposed to explain the metabolic stability of cardiac muscle was examined quantitatively by Korzeniewski also by methods of mathematical modelling (45), and critically checked in experiments by Brandes and Bers (48). Taking into account the importance of problem, we will consider the hypothesis of parallel activation in more details. In 1998 Korzeniewski tried to explain the known experimental fact: in white skeletal muscle an increase in oxygen consumption rate on rest-activity transition is 18-fold while the increase in ATP/ADP ratio is only 3-fold (45). To analyze these data, he used original dynamic model of skeletal muscle bioenergetics based on formal description of chemical reactions by adjustable parameters. This simplified approach allows to consider a wide range of particular mitochondrial reactions, including substrate dehydrogenation, complex I, complex II, complex IY (cytochrome oxidase), proton leak, ATP synthase, ATP/ADP and phosphate carriers. Three main sets of simulations were performed.

In the first set of simulations, increasing ATP utilization and ATP/ADP ratio by 3.3-fold and 2.9-fold, respectively, he revealed only 2.3-fold increase in muscle respiration rate. Moreover, an increase in ATP utilization up to 100-fold followed by dramatic decrease in ATP/ADP ratio to 0.1 allowed only 4.5-fold increase in muscle respiration rate. These results lead directly to conclusion that the negative feedback mechanism by Chance "cannot account for the 18-fold increase in the respiration rate and explains the only 3-fold changes in ATP/ADP ratio".

In the second set of simulations, mitochondrial substrate dehydrogenation reactions were allowed to increase up to 50-fold. At this background, an increase in ATP utilization up to 20-fold was followed by the severe decrease in ATP/ADP ratio to 0.4 and only 5.2-fold increase in respiration rate. These results lead directly to conclusion "that the parallel activation of only NADH supply and ATP usage cannot account for the observed changes in the respiration rate and the ATP/ADP ratio".

In the third set of simulations, the background was the 8.5-fold parallel activation of mitochondrial substrate dehydrogenation reactions, activities of mitochondrial complexes I, II and IY, ATP synthase, ATP/ADP and phosphate carriers. At this background, the 29-fold increase in ATP utilization rate allowed to obtain the necessary 17.8-fold simulation of muscle respiration rate. An increase in ATP/ADP ratio was only 2.9-fold, like in vivo. These results lead to final conclusion, that the metabolic stability of muscle supposes the parallel activation of all steps of mitochondrial oxidative phosphorylation and ". . . not only of the ATP-consuming block and ATP-producing block as a whole". The nature of the universal external parallel activator (like, for example, calcium ions or protein phoshorylation) is unknown; it should be searched and discovered (45).

In the framework of parallel activation hypothesis the mechanism of Chance, named as negative feedback via ADP concentration, acts at very low work intensities, "while at medium and high work intensities the parallel activation mechanism is recruited and begins to predominate". If really the case, then direct mitochondrial activation by ADP and Pi will constitute only a fraction of maximal oxidative phosphorylation capacity of the heart and skeletal muscles.

This issue was explored by Robert Balaban and his coworkers (49). Authors isolated well coupled mitochondria (respiratory control ratios between 8 and 15 at 37°C; ADP-to-O ratio for respiration in 5 mM glutamate-malate of 2.9 ± 0.2 from homogenates of dog and pig hearts. A special care was taken to eliminate calcium ions during isolation procedure. Respiration rates at state 3, measured at 37°C in medium with 0.5 mM ADP, 6 mM K_2HPO_4, 6 mM glutamate-malate and without added calcium, were 676 ± 31 and 665 ± 65 nmol O2*min^{-1}*nmol cytochrome a^{-1} for dog and pig heart mitochondria, respectively. With measured contents of cytochrome a in myocardium, 43.6 ± 2.4 and 36.6 ± 3.1 nmol/g wet mass of tissue, myocardial respiratory capacities were estimated as 29.5(30.6) and 24.3(25.1) μmol O_2*min^{-1}*g wet $mass^{-1}$ for dog and pig hearts, respectively. Values in brackets indicate the uncoupled respiration rates.

These values may be even higher when taking into account that samples of myocardial tissue in the work of Balaban were hydrated, with wet mass-to-dry mass ratio of 4.62 ± 0.45 g/g. Assuming, that wet mass-to-dry mass ratio in intact dog and pig hearts is similar to that in intact rat hearts, 3.25 g/g (50), the measured respiratory capacity for dog and pig hearts will be 41.9 and 33.4 μmol O_2*min^{-1}*g wet mass of intact $heart^{-1}$, respectively (4.62/3.25*29.5 and 4.62/3.25*24.3). The obtained estimates are in line with maximal respiratory capacity for rat heart, 31.25 μmol O_2*min^{-1}*g wet $mass^{-1}$, taken in mathematical model of Aliev and Saks on the basis of multiple biochemical and physiological data (34).

The biochemical estimates for respiratory capacity of heart tissue, 31–42 μmol O_2*min^{-1}*g wet mass of intact $heart^{-1}$, are even higher when compared with reported respiration rates for in vivo dog hearts at high workload levels, 25.4 μmol O_2*min^{-1}*g wet $mass^{-1}$ (51). Huang and Feigl had some dogs that approached 43 μmol O_2*min^{-1}*g wet $mass^{-1}$ (52).

Taken together, all these data clearly indicate that direct mitochondrial activation by ADP and Pi ensures maximal oxidative phosphorylation capacity of the heart muscle, but not only a fraction of it, as proposed by parallel activation hypothesis of Korzeniewski (45). Therefore, the parallel activation hypothesis has no basis at least for heart muscle.

Concerning the model of Korzeniewski, it should be pointed that its module for cytoplasm is extremely simple; it neglects the time dynamics of ATP hydrolysis by myofibrils and ignores cellular CK (45). Obviously, this model is incomplete even for description of white skeletal muscle bioenergetics: in this tissue, ATP consumption by myofibrils and its oxidative regeneration are separated in time and CK buffers the ATP pool (34). The data from this modeling cannot be directly related to analysis of heart muscle bioenergetics, as in heart the ATP hydrolysis by myofibrils and its regeneration must be accomplished in each steady state contraction cycle, the compartmented CK system plays an important role in the control of respiration (15,34,41). It is important that Vendelin et al. (36), supplementing the mathematical model of Korzeniewski by the modules for dynamics of myofibrillar ATP hydrolysis, compartmented cellular CK and two-dimensional diffusion of metabolites between cell compartments, essentially confirmed all our data. It is also important that in the work of Vendelin et al. (36) all calculations have been made for the constant maximal activity of mitochondrial oxidative phosphorylation. The calcium is important to achieve this maximal activity (46,47), but the real value of respiration rate is determined by the metabolic feedback signal from cytoplasm (48).

ACKNOWLEDGEMENTS

This work was supported by grants from Association Francaise contre les Myopathies (AFM), Estonian Science Foundation grant N. 4928, and by the Russian Foundation for Basic Research grant 00-04-48480. Skillful participation of Laurence Kay, Tatiana Andrienko and Marina Panchishkina, University of Joseph Fourier, Grenoble, France, and Peeter Sikk, Tuuli Kaambre, Toomas Tiivel and Maire Peitel, Tallinn, in the experiments and preparation of this manuscript is gratefully acknowledged.

REFERENCES

1. Lardy HA, Wellmann H. 1952. Oxidative phosphorylation: role of the inorganic phosphate and acceptor systems in control of metabolic reactions. J Biol Chem 1955:215–224.
2. Chance B, Williams GR. 1955. Respiratory enzymes in oxidative phosphorylation. I Kinetics of oxygen utilization. J Biol Chem 217:383–393.
3. Mitchell P. 1996. Coupling of phosphorylation to electron and hydrogen transfer by a chemiosmotic type of mechanism. Nature 191:144–148.
4. Boyer P. 1997. The ATP—synthase—a splendid molecular machine. Ann Rev Biochem 66:717–749.
5. Abrahams JP, Leslie AGW, Lutter R, Walker, J. 1994. Structure at 2.8 A resolution of F_1—ATPase from bovine heart mitochondria. Nature 370:621–628.
6. Kushmerick MJ. 1987. Energetic studies of muscles of different types. Basic Res Cardiol 82 Suppl 2:17–30.
7. Balaban RS, Kantor HL, Katz LA, Briggs RW. 1986. Relation between work and phosphate metabolite in the *in vivo* paced mammalian heart. Science 232:1121–1123.
8. Saks VA, Khuchua ZA, Vasilyeva EV, Belikova YO, Kuznetsov AV. 1994. Metabolic compartmentation and substrate channeling in muscle cells. Role of coupled creatine kinases in in vivo regulation of cellular respiration. A synthesis. Mol Cell Biochem 133/134:155–192.
9. Gudbjarnason S, Mathes P, Raven KG. 1970. Functional compartmentation of ATP and creatine phosphate in heart muscle. J Mol Cell Cardiol 1:325–339.
10. Neely JR, Rovetto MJ, Whitmer JT, Morgan H. 1973. Effects of ischemia on function and mtabolism of the isolated working rat heart. Am J Physiol 225:651–658.
11. Koretsune Y, Marban E. 1990. Mechanism of ischemic contracture in ferret hearts: relative roles of $[Ca^{2+}]_i$ elevation and ATP depletion. Am J Physiol 258:H9–H16.
12. Ross Ellington W. 2001. Evolution and physiological roles of phosphagen systems. Annu Rev Physiol 63:289–325.
13. Wyss M, Kaddurah-Daouk R. 2000. Creatine and creatinine metabolisme. Physiological Reviews 80:1107–1213.
14. Bessman SP, Geiger PJ. 1981. Transport of energy in muscle: the phosphorylcreatine shuttle. Science 211:448–452.
15. Walliman TM, Wyss D, Brdiczka K, Nicolay H, Eppenberger. 1992. Transport of energy in muscle:the phosphorylcreatine shuttle. Biochem J 281:21–40.
16. Dzeja PP, Zelenznikar RJ, Goldberg ND. 1998. Adenylate kinase: kinetic behaviour in intact cells indicates it is integral to multiple cellular processes. Mol Cell Biochim 184:169–182.
17. Garlid K. 2001. Physiology of mitochondria. In: Nicolas Sperelakis (Ed.) Cell Physiology Sourcebook. A Molecular Approach. Academic Press, New York-Boston, p. 139–151.
18. Saks VA, Chernousova GB, Gukovsky DE, Smirnov VN, Chazov EI. 1975. Studies of Energy Transport in heart cells. Mitochondrial isoenzyme of creatine phosphokinase: kinetic properties and regulatort action of Mg $^{2+}$ ions. Eu J Biochem 57:273–290.
19. Saks VA, Veksler VI, Kuznetsov AV, Kay L, Sikk P, Tiivel T, Tranqui L, Olivares J, Winkler K, Wiedemann F, Kunz WS. 1998. Permeabilized cell and skinned fiber techniques in studies of mitochondrial function in vivo. Mol Cell Biochem 184:81–100.
20. Kuznetsov AV, Mayboroda O, Kunz D, Winkler K, Schubert W, Kunz WS. 1998. Functional imaging of mitochondria in saponin-permeabilized mice muscle fibers. J Cell Biol 140:1091–1099.
21. Saks VA, Belikova Yu O, Kuznetsov AV. 1991. *In vivo* regulation of mitochondrial respiration in cardiomyocytes: Specific restrictions for intracellular diffusion of ADP. Biochimica and Biophysica Acta 1074:302–311.
22. Saks VA, Vassilyeva EV, Belikova Yu O, Kuznetsov AV, Lyapina SA, Petrova L, Perov NA. 1993.

Retarded diffusion of ADP in cardiomyocytes: Possible role of outer mitochondrial membrane and creatine kinase in cellular regulation of oxidative phosphorylation. Biochim Biophys Acta 1144:134–148.

23. Saks VA, Kuznetsov AV, Khuchua ZA, Vasilyeva EV, Belikova Yu O, Kesvatera T, Tiivel T. 1995. Control of cellular respiration *in vivo* by mitochondrial outer membrane and by creatine kinase. A new speculative hypothesis: possible involvement of mitochondrial-cytoskeleton interactions. J Mol Cell Cardiol 27:625–645.

24. Kuznetsov AV, Tiivel T, Sikk P, Käämbre T, Kay L, Daneshrad Z, Rossi A, Kadaja L, Peet N, Seppet E, Saks V. 1996. Striking difference between slow and fast twitch muscles in the kinetics of regulation of respiration by ADP in the cells in vivo. Eur J Biochem 241:909–915.

25. Kay L, Li Z, Fontaine E, Leverve X, Olivares J, Tranqui L, Tiivel T, Sikk P, Kaambre T, Samuel JL, Rappaport L, Paulin D, Saks VA. 1997. Study of functional significance of mitochondrial—cytoskeletal interactions. In vivo regulation of respiration in cardiac and skeletal muscle cells of desmin—deficient transgenic mice. Biochim Biophys Acta 132241–132259.

26. Saks VA, Tiivel T, Kay L, Novel-Chate V, Daneshrad Z, Rossi A, Fontaine E, Keriel C, Leverve X, Ventura-Clapier R, Anflous K, Samuel J-L, Rappaport L. 1996. Mol. Cell Biochem 160/161:195–208.

27. Seppet E, Kaambre T, Sikk P, Tiivel T, Vija H, Kay L, Appaix F, Tonkonogi M, Sahlin K, Saks VA. 2001. Functional complexes of mitochondria with MgATPases of myofibrils and sarcoplasmic reticulum in muscle cells. Biochim Biophys Acta 1504:379–395.

28. Saks VA, Kaambre T, Sikk P, Eimre M, Orlova E, Paju K, Piirsoo A, Appaix F, Kay L, Regiz-Zagrosek V, Fleck E, Seppet E. 2001. Intracellular energetic units in red muscle cells. Biochem J 356:643–657.

29. Dos Santos P, Kowaltowski AJ, Laclau M, Subramanian S, Paucek P, Boudina S, Thambo JB, Tariosse L, Garlid K. 2002. Am J Physiol In Press Feb14 DOI 10.1152/ajpheart.

30. Garlid KD. 1994. Mitochondrial cation transport: a progress report. J Bioenerg Biomembr 26:537–542.

31. Liobikas J, Kopustinskiene DM, Toleikis A. 2001. What controls the outer mitochondrial membrane permeability for ADP: facts for and against the oncotic pressure. Biochim Biophys Acta 1505:220–225.

32. Gellerich F, Saks VA. 1982. Control of heart mitochondrial oxygen consumption by creatine kinase: the importance of enzyme localization. Biochem Biophys Res Comm 105:1473–1481.

33. Saks VA, Ventura–Clapier R, Khuchua ZA, Preobrazensky AN, Emelin IV. 1984. Creatine kinase in regulation of heart function and metabolism. I Further evidence for compartmentation of adenine nucleotides in cardiac myofibrillar and sarcolemmal coupled ATPase-creatine kinase systems. Biochim Biophys Acta 803:254–264.

34. Aliev MK, Saks VA. 1997. Compartmentalised energy transfer in cardiomyocytes. Use of mathematical modeling for analysis of *in vivo* regulation of respiration. Biophys J 73:428–445.

35. Vendelin M, Kongas O, Saks VA. 2000. Regulation of mitochondrial respiration in heart cells analyzed by reaction—diffusion model of energy transfer. Am J Physiol 278:C747–C764

36. Saks VA, Dos Santos P, Gellerich FN, Diolez P. 1998. Quantitative studies of enzyme—substrate compartmentation, functional coupling and metabolic channeling in muscle cells. Mol Cell Biochem. 184:291–307.

37. Janssen E, Dzeja PP, Oerlemans F, Simonetti AW, Heerschap A, de Haan A, Rush PS, Terjung RR, Wieringa B, Terzic A. 2000. Adenylate kinase 1 gene deletion disrupts muscle energetic economy despite metabolic rearrgement. EMBO Journal 19:6371–6381.

38. Carrasco AJ, Dzeja PP, Alekseev AE, Pucar D, Zingman LV, Abracham MR, Hodgson D, Bienengraeber M, Puceat M, Janssen E, Wieringa B, Terzik A. 2001. Adenylate kinase phosphotransfer communicates cellular energetics signals to ATP sensitive—potassium channels. Proc Natl Acad Sci US 98:7623–7628.

39. Dzeja PP, Vitkevicius KT, Redfield MM, Burnett JC, Terzik A. 1999. Adenylate-kinase catalyzed phosphotransfer in the myocardium: increased contribution in heart failure. Circ Res 84:1137–1143.

40. Pucar D, Dzeja PP, Bast P, Juranic N, Macura S, Terzik A. 2001. Cellular energetics in the preconditioned state. Protective role for phosphotransfer reactions captured by ^{18}O- assisted ^{31}PNMR. J Biol Chem 276:44812–44819.

41. Kay L, Nicolay K, Wieringa B, Saks V, Wallimann T. 2000. Direct evidence of the control of mitochondrial respiration by mitochondrial creatine kinase in muscle cells *in situ*. J Biol Chem 275:6967–6944.

42. Sasaki N, Sato T, Marban E, O'Rourke B. 2001. ATP consumption by uncoupled mitochondria activates sarcolemmal KATP channels in cardiac myocytes. Am J Physiol 280:H1882–H1888.

43. Rossi A, Kay L, Saks VA. 1998. Early ischemia-induced alterations of the outer mitochondrial membrane and the intermembrane space: a potential cause for altered energy transfer in cardiac muscle? Mol Cell Biochem 184:209–229.

44. Boudina S, Laclau MN, Tariosse L, Daret D, Gouverneur G, Boron-Adele S, Saks VA, Dos Santos P. 2002. Alteration of mitochondrial function in a model of chronic ischemia in vivo in rat heart. Am J Physiol 282(2):H821–H831.

45. Korzeniewski B. 1998. Regulation of ATP supply during muscle contraction: theoretical studies. Biochem J 330:1189–1195.

46. McGormack JG, Halestrap AP, Denton RM. 1990. Role of calcium ions in regulation of mammalian intramitochondrial metabolism. Physiol Rev 70:391–425.

47. Hansford RG, Zorov D. 1998. Role of mitochondrial calcium transport in the control of substrate oxidation. Mol Cell Biochem 184:359–369.

48. Brandes R, Bers DM. 1999. Analysis of the mechanisms of mitochondrial NADH regulation in cardiac trabeculae. Biophys Journal 77:1666–1682.

49. Mootha VK, Arai AE, Balaban RS. 1997. Maximum oxidative phosphorylation capacity of the mammalian heart. Am J Physiol 272:H769–H775.

50. Aliev MK, Dos Santos P, Hoerter JA, Soboll S, Tikhonov AN, Saks VA. 2002. The water content and its intracellular distribution in intact and saline perfused rat hearts revisited. Cardiovasc Res 53:48–58.

51. von Restorff W, Holtz J, Bassenge E. 1977. Exercise induced augmentation of myocardial oxygen extraction in spite of normal dilatory capacity in dogs. Pfluegers Arch 372:181–185.

52. Huang AH, Feigl EO. 1988. Adrenergic coronary vasoconstriction helps maintain uniform transmural blood flow distribution during exercise. Circ Res 62:286–298.

Signal Transduction and Cardiac Hypertrophy,
edited by N.S. Dhalla, L.V. Hryshko,
E. Kardami & P.K. Singal
Kluwer Academic Publishers, Boston, 2003

Role of High Molecular Weight Calmodulin Binding Protein in Cardiac Muscle

Lakshmikuttyamma Ashakumary, Rakesh Kakkar,
Ponniah Selvakumar, Mohammed Khysar Pasha, and
Rajendra K. Sharma

*Department of Pathology
College of Medicine
University of Saskatchewan
and Cancer Research Unit
Health Research Division
Saskatchewan Cancer Agency
20 Campus Drive, Saskatoon
Canada S7N 4H4*

Summary. High molecular weight calmodulin binding protein (HMWCaMBP) was originally discovered and purified in our laboratory and identified as a homologue of the calpains inhibitor, calpastatin. Calpains are Ca^{2+}-dependent cysteine proteases that regulate various enzymes, transcription factors and structural proteins through limited proteolysis. Decreased expression of HMWCaMBP in ischemia suggests that it may be susceptible to proteolysis by calpains during ischemia and reperfusion. HMWCaMBP may protect its substrates from calpains in the normal myocardium, however during an early phase of ischemia and reperfusion with increased Ca^{2+} influx calpain activity exceeds HMWCaMBP activity leading to its proteolysis and of other substrates resulting in cellular injury. This study will lead to a better understanding of the pathology of disease states and the development of novel therapeutics. The exact role of HMWCaMBP in ischemia and reperfusion is not clear because most of the studies have been carried out *in vitro*. Therefore, it is essential that further research should be directed to *in vivo* studies. The nucleic acid and amino acid sequence information of HMWCaMBP will help us to do further characterization of this protein.

Key words: calcium, calmodulin, high molecular weight calmodulin-binding protein, calpastatin, calpains, ischemia.

Address for Correspondence: Dr. Rajendra K. Sharma, Department of Pathology, College of Medicine, University of Saskatchewan, Research Unit, Saskatchewan Cancer Agency, 20, Campus Drive, Saskatoon, Canada S7N 4H4. Tel: (306) 966-7733, Fax: (306) 655-2635, E-mail: rsharma@scf.sk.ca.

INTRODUCTION

Calcium ions regulate many cellular processes that are usually achieved through their interaction by binding to receptor proteins such as calmodulin (CaM), troponin C, S-100 proteins, calcyclin and calregulin to transmit the Ca^{2+} signal (1–3). However, CaM is a primary receptor for Ca^{2+} (4–7). CaM is a heat stable acidic protein, which was originally discovered as an activator of cyclic nucleotide phosphodiesterase by Cheung (8,9). One of the characteristics of CaM is it's ability to associate with many different proteins in a Ca^{2+}-dependent and reversible manner (3–9). A number of enzymes and several proteins were found to be regulated by CaM (4–7). Figure 1 summarizes the many processes in which CaM plays a crucial role. Identifying and characterizing these CaM-binding target proteins are essential to define the pathways by which Ca^{2+}-regulated signals are transduced. The distribution of CaM-regulated proteins appears to vary among tissues and their biological functions are largely unknown. A number of CaM-dependent enzymes and proteins have been purified as CaM-binding proteins before their intrinsic biological activity was established. For example, originally calcineurin was discovered and purified as an inhibitor of CaM-dependent cyclic nucleotide phosphodiesterase (10–11). Homogeneous calcineurin was obtained from bovine brain extract by use of CaM-affinity chromatography (12,13). Calcineurin had been extensively characterized (14,15) before it was found to be a CaM-stimulated phosphatase (16). Similarly caldesmon, a CaM-binding protein abundant in smooth muscle and involved in smooth muscle contraction (17–19) was initially discovered as a CaM-binding protein (20).

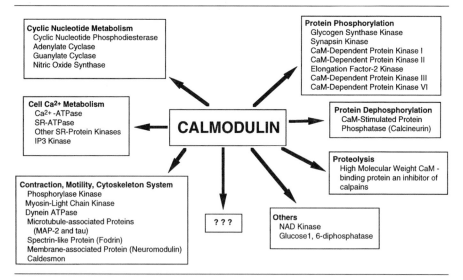

Figure 1. Calmodulin-regulated cellular processes.

It has become clear that many other proteins, in addition to known CaM-dependent enzymes and the CaM-binding proteins, are capable of specific associa-

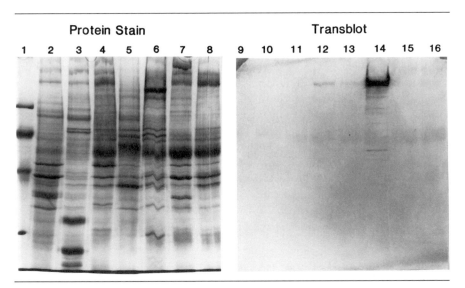

Figure 2. The distribution of total CaM-binding proteins in different bovine tissues. Protein stain; lane 1, protein molecular weight markers: phosphorylase *b*, 97,000; bovine serum albumin, 67,000; ovalbumin, 43,000; soybean trypsin inhibitor, 20,100. Total CaM-binding proteins: lanes 2, spleen; 3, skeletal muscle; 4, lung; 5, brain; 6, heart; 7, uterus and 8, kidney: 9–16, respective transblot of lanes 1–8. For details see Sharma (27).

tion with CaM. Using CaM–Sepharose 4B-affinity column, Sharma has isolated total CaM-binding proteins from various bovine tissues and these proteins are capable of Ca^{2+}-dependent association with the affinity gel (21). These fractions contain several proteins besides the known CaM-dependent enzymes and CaM-binding proteins. In this article, the discovery of a high molecular weight CaM-binding protein (HMWCaMBP) from cardiac muscle and its biological function in the area of ischemia and reperfusion are described. The illustrations used are from the author's work.

DISCOVERY OF HMWCaMBP

During purification of bovine heart CaM–dependent cyclic nucleotide phosphodiesterase from CaM–Sepharose 4B affinity column chromatography, we discovered that EGTA samples contained several CaM-binding proteins including HMW-CaMBP, which displayed a molecular weight of 140,000 Da under denaturing conditions (Figure 2, lane 6). CaM deficient samples were prepared from several bovine tissues including heart, spleen, lung, skeletal muscle, uterus and brain by the use of DEAE–Sepharose CL-6B column chromatography and CaM-binding protein fractions were isolated by CaM–Sepharose 4B affinity column chromatography (21). Such preparations are expected to contain most, if not all, proteins, which are capable of reversible interaction with CaM. A major HMWCaMBP was observed in cardiac muscle, whereas a CaM-binding protein of similar apparent molecular weight was not observed in any of the other tissues examined suggesting that HMWCaMBP was a heart–specific CaM-binding protein (Figure 2, lane 6). It has been shown that CaM-dependent proteins exist in multiple isoforms (22–26). Furthermore, the distribution of HMWCaMBP in bovine tissues was compared on the basis of immunoreactivity using a polyclonal antibody to this protein by Western blotting analysis in the total CaM-binding protein fractions. A major protein with an apparent molecular weight of 140,000 Da in the heart was observed (Figure 2, lane 14). In addition to heart, this protein was present in lung and brain (Figure 2, lane 12, 13) at much lower concentrations but was not present in skeletal muscle, spleen, kidney or uterus (27). The total CaM-binding protein fractions were prepared in an identical manner from each tissue assuming that the HMWCaMBP antibody cross-reacted equally with HMWCaMBP from each tissue. These results suggested that, in addition to heart, the lung and brain also contained this protein but at much lower levels.

PURIFICATION, CHARACTERIZATION AND IDENTIFICATION OF HMWCaMBP

Endogenous CaM was removed from crude extracts of bovine heart by using DEAE-Sepharose CL-6B column chromatography as described by Sharma (21). Further purification of HMWCaMBP was accomplished by altering the elution conditions during CaM-Sepharose 4B affinity column chromatography to resolve the HMWCaMBP from many other CaM-binding proteins (Figure 3A). The purified HMWCaMBP was shown to be a highly asymmetric protein with a sedimentation coefficient of approximately 5.0 S and Stokes radius of 83.0 Å (Figure 3B). The molecular weight of the HMWCaMBP was determined to be 175,000 Da from the sedimentation constant and Stokes radius of the protein, whereas on SDS-PAGE this protein showed a single polypeptide band with an apparent molecular weight of 140,000 Da. This suggests that this protein is monomeric (21). However, HMW-CaMBP was highly susceptible to proteolysis. HMWCaMBP could be purified by phenyl Sepharose 4B column chromatography after gel filtration chromatography, if the purified sample contains any contaminants (28).

The electrophoretic properties of HMWCaMBP resembled caldesmon (Figure 4A), which has molecular weight varying from 135,000 to 150,000 Da, a major CaM-binding protein originally discovered in chicken gizzard (20) and is also present in the heart (29,30). To test the possibility that the HMWCaMBP is bovine heart caldesmon, immunoblotting of this protein using polyclonal antibodies against chicken gizzard caldesmon was carried out. HMWCaMBP from bovine heart did not react with the polyclonal antibodies raised against chicken gizzard caldesmon suggesting that the protein from bovine heart was not caldesmon (Figure 4B, lane 4). However, the possibility that the lack of cross-reactivity was due to a tissue and/or species specificity of the chicken gizzard antibody could not be ruled out. To test for this possibility, an immunoblotting experiment was carried out using the partially purified caldesmon from bovine heart (30). HMWCaMBP exhibited no cross-reactivity (Figure 4C, lane 6) whereas bovine cardiac caldesmon was

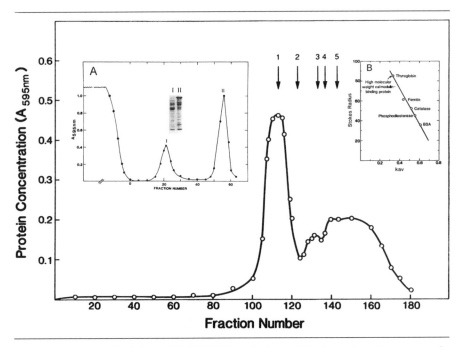

Figure 3. Protein profile elution of HMWCaMBP on Sepharose 6B column. *Insert* A, separation of CaM-binding proteins from CaM-Sepharose 4B column. Peak I, protein eluted with 1 mM EGTA alone and peak II, protein eluted with 1 mM EGTA containing 0.2 M NaCl and SDS-PAGE of peak I and II. Arrows indicate protein molecular weight markers. Arrows: 1, thyroglobin; 2, ferritin; 3, catalase; 4, CaM-dependent phosphodiesterase and 5, bovine serum albumin. *Insert* B, Stokes radius of HMWCaMBP is indicated by an arrow. For details see Sharma (21).

visualized in the immunoblot (Figure 4C, lane 7). These experiments suggested that the HMWCaMBP is an apparently different protein from those reported previously.

BIOLOGICAL FUNCTION OF HMWCaMBP

In order to establish the biological function of HMWCaMBP, the protein was digested with lysyl endopeptidase and three peptides (H1, H2, H3) were purified for partial peptide sequencing. Two peptides H1 and H2 shared 88–100% and 50–65% homology to calpastatin, respectively but H3 did not have any similarity to the known protein sequence (Table 1). These results revealed that HMWCaMBP could be a distinct protein, which shares homology with calpastatin (28). Furthermore, polyclonal antibodies against HMWCaMBP cross-reacted with calpastatin from bovine cardiac muscle, suggesting that the HMWCaMBP and calpastatin may have common antigenic epitopes (Figure 5). Calpastatin is an inhibitor protein of Ca^{2+}-dependent cysteine proteases, calpains which act as mediators for Ca^{2+} signals in many biological systems (28,31–35). Calpains exist in two distinct forms; μ-calpain (calpain I) and *m*-calpain (calpain II), which are stimulated by micromolar

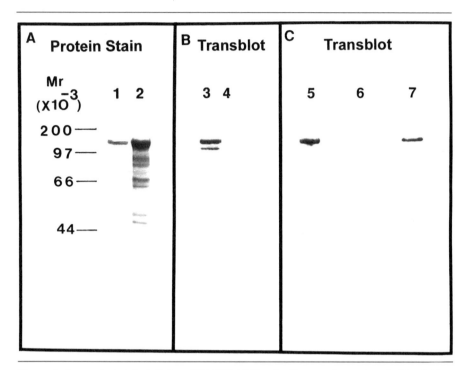

Figure 4. Immunological dissimilarity of HMWCaMBP and caldesmon. A, protein stain; B and C, Western blot using anti-chicken gizzard caldesmon. Lanes 1, 3 and 5, purified chicken gizzard caldesmon; 2, 4 and 6, bovine heart CaM-binding protein; 7, purified bovine heart caldesmon. For details see Sharma (21).

Table 1. Homology of partial peptide sequence of HMWCaMBP to calpastatin

Species	Peptide H1	Peptide H2
HMWCaMBP	ELDDALDQLSDSLGQRQP	DNTTYXGPEVSXGMFXXTIE
Bos taurus	25 ELDDALDQLSDSLGQRQP 42 [100%]	153 DNTTYTGPEVSDPMSSTYIE 172 [65%]
	554 ELDDALDQLSDTLGQRQP 571 [94%]	
Porcine	566 KLDDALDQLSDSLGQRQP 583 [94%]	174 DNTTYTGPEVLDPMSSTYIE 193 [60%]
Oryctolagus cuniculus	570 ELDDALDKLSDSLGQRQP 587 [94%]	173 DSTAYTGP E ISDPMSSTYIE 192 [50%]
Homo sapiens	531 DLDDALDKLSDSLGQRQP 548 [88%]	151 ENTTYTGPEVSDPMSSTYIE 170 [60%]

The amino acids marked with asterisks are different from those of HMWCaMBP. The third HMWCaMBP peptide (H3) DAMTAGALEALSESL-----SEGIEHPG showed no homology. The data presented in parenthesis indicates percent homology to HMWCaMBP. [for details see Kakkar et al (28)].

kDa
Mr 10⁻³

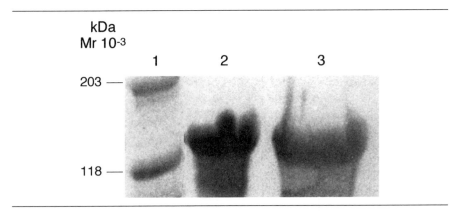

Figure 5. Western blot analysis of HMWCaMBP and calpastatin from bovine cardiac muscle. Lanes 1, protein molecular weight markers (myosin, 203,000 and β-galactosidase 118,000); 2, bovine cardiac HMWCaMBP; 3, bovine cardiac calpastatin. For details see Kakkar et al. (28)

and millimolar concentrations of Ca^{2+}, respectively (33). To test further the possibility that HMWCaMBP contains calpastatin activity, an inhibition study of μ-calpain and *m*-calpain was carried out. HMWCaMBP inhibited both forms of calpains in a concentration dependent manner. In the case of calpain II, the maximal inhibition was observed at the concentration of 1.5 μg/ml and half maximal inhibition was at 0.3 μg/ml (Figure 6A). In addition, HMWCaMBP was also found to inhibit purified human erythrocyte calpain I (Figure 6B). It is noteworthy that HMWCaMBP produced an essentially linear inhibition *vs* concentration relationship until at least 70% inhibition of calpain. This is typical of calpastatins, which are rapid, tightly binding inhibitors of calpains. In addition, these results suggest that HMWCaMBP appeared to possess four inhibitory domains per 80 kDa mass unit as predicted for calpastatin. Furthermore, this rules out the co-purification of small amounts of contaminating calpastatin in the preparation suggesting that HMW-CaMBP has the same number of calpain inhibitory domains as characterized for calpastatin (36–38). Several other structural proteins such as neurofilament, spectrin, microtubule associated protein, Tau and calspectin act as substrates for calpains, which suggests that calpains play a role in maintaining cellular structural integrity (39–42). These results suggesting HMWCaMBP is homologous to calpastatin and may be a CaM-dependent isoform of calpastatin.

Immunohistochemical localization of HMWCaMBP from autopsy specimens of human heart revealed a strong staining of myocardium muscle fiber with polyclonal antibodies against HMWCaMBP, and immunostaining was observed throughout the cytoplasm of myocardial cells (Figure 7) (43). Similar distribution of bovine myocardial calpastatin was obtained by Mellgren *et al.* (44). Further ultra structural studies indicated that in human cardiomyocyte, HMWCaMBP is distributed in the cytoplasm and myofilaments (43). Our observations suggest that HMWCaMBP exists predominantly in cardiac muscle and binds to CaM and has a potential role in the regulation of calpain activity in cardiac muscle (28).

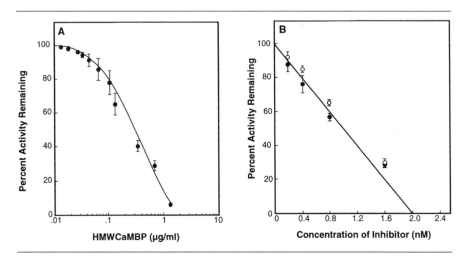

Figure 6. Inhibition of calpain I and calpain II by HMWCaMBP and calpastatin. A, inhibition of calpain II by bovine cardiac HMWCaMBP. B, inhibition of calpain I by either bovine cardiac HMW-CaMBP or bovine cardiac calpastatin (●–●) (O–O), respectively. For details see Kakkar et al. (28).

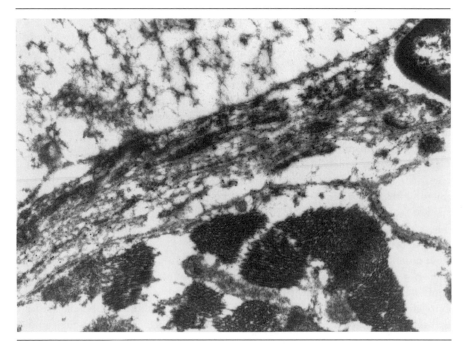

Figure 7. Ultra structural localization of HMWCaMBP in human cardiac myocyte. For details see Kakkar et al. (43).

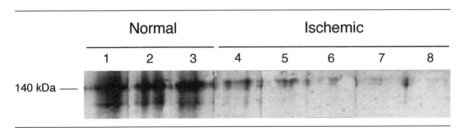

Figure 8. Western blot analysis of HMWCaMBP from human normal and ischemic cardiac tissue. Lanes 1–3, normal; 4–8, ischemic cardiac tissue samples. For details see Kakkar et al. (43).

The involvement of calpains has been implicated in myocardial ischemia and reperfusion injury (45,46), myocardial stunning (47) and cardiac hypertrophy (48). Intracellular Ca^{2+} overloading is the cause of myocardial injury during ischemia and reperfusion and is considered to be a pivotal event in cell death (47). An increase in Ca^{2+} influx can activate dormant Ca^{2+}-dependent enzymes, including calpains causing damage to structural proteins [myocardial troponin, calspectin (fodrin), microtubules] leading to membrane breakdown and eventually cell death (36,40). Cell death is believed to occur via two pathways, necrosis or apoptosis. Apoptosis is considered to be a significant contributor to myocardial cell death as a result of ischemia and reperfusion injury (48). It has been reported that cardiomyocytes undergo apoptosis in patients with ischemic cardiomyopathy (48) but the role of HMWCaMBP and calpains in ischemia and reperfusion is not known.

ROLE OF HMWCaMBP IN ISCHEMIA AND REPERFUSION

Western blot analysis of human normal and ischemic cardiac tissue from autopsy specimens indicated that HMWCaMBP expression was higher in normal cardiac tissue than in ischemic cardiac tissue which had very little or no expression of HMWCaMBP (Figure 8). Furthermore, the immunohistochemical localization of HMWCaMBP from normal autopsy specimen showed strong staining in myocardial muscle fibres (Figure 7). Immunoreactivity was observed throughout the cytoplasm of the myocardial cell whereas in ischemic tissue staining with HMWCaMBP showed poor to negative immunoreactivity (Figure 9) (43). From this study, it was not clear what effect post-mortem autolysis of tissues may have had on the most severely affected area and what was its possible contribution to the myocardial damage as a result of hypoxia. Therefore, the role of HMWCaMBP along with calpains during ischemia and reperfusion was investigated in a rat model.

Regional ischemia was induced in the male Sprague Dawley rats and immunohistochemical studies were performed (49). Normal rat heart muscle showed strong expression of HMWCaMBP in myocardial cells (Figure 10, group 1) and this expression decreased as the duration of ischemia and reperfusion increased (Figure 10, group 2, 3, 4, 5, 6 and 7). However, almost a lack of expression of HMW-CaMBP after 30 min ischemia and 30 min reperfusion was observed (Figure 10,

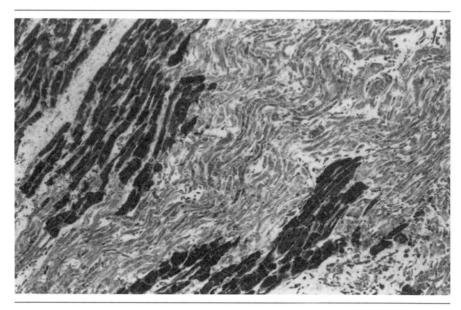

Figure 9. Expression of HMWCaMBP in human ischemic cardiac tissue. For details see Kakkar et al. (43).

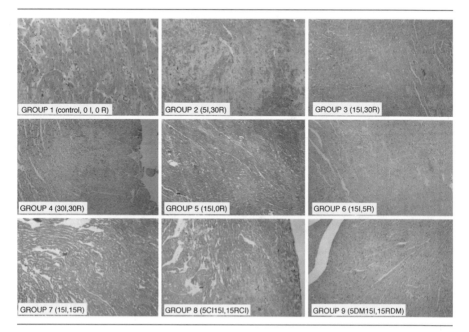

Figure 10. Expression of HMWCaMBP in rat cardiac tissues after ischemia and reperfusion. For details see Kakkar et al. (49).

group 4). It has been reported that synthetic calpain inhibitors prevent proteolysis and contractile dysfunction during reperfusion, suggesting the involvement of calpains in proteolysis that characterizes reperfusion injury (46). Therefore, we examined the protective effect of cell-permeable inhibitor (N-Ac-Leu-Leu-methioninal, ALLM) on the pre-ischemic and post-ischemic perfused heart. The findings suggest that the expression of HMWCaMBP is increased with the calpain inhibitor, ALLM treatment (Figure 10, group 8). In contrast to HMWCaMBP the μ-calpain and m-calpain expression increased during ischemia and reperfusion compared to control, (Figure 11, group 2 to 7 compared with control, group 1) whereas pre-ischemic perfusion and post-ischemic reperfusion with ALLM caused inhibition in the increase in μ-calpain and m-calpain expression (Figure 11, group 8). It is interesting to note that during ischemia alone calpain expression did not increase significantly (Figure 11, group 5), however with reperfusion a significant increase in calpain expression was observed (Figure 11, group 6 and 7) suggesting that the majority of calpain activity occurs during reperfusion. In addition, μ-Calpain expression was increased after a shorter period of ischemia than was the case for m-calpain. μ-calpain requires a much lower Ca^{2+} concentration for activity in intact cells as compared to skinned cells (33). The K_m of μ-calpain for Ca^{2+} has been reported to be 1–20 μM and 1–3 μM *in vitro* and *in vivo*, respectively (33). μ-Calpain is activated when the short-lived elevation of Ca^{2+} concentration increased to 1–3 μM during myocardial ischemia. Therefore, μ-calpain is activated and it can cleave m-calpain thereby lowering its Ca^{2+} requirement to micro molar levels. In ischemic heart HMWCaMBP expression was low, which may be due to the rise in calpain activity.

The HMWCaMBP can be proteolysed *in vitro* by both of the calpains in the presence of Ca^{2+} (Figure 12). Therefore, the low expression of HMWCaMBP may be due to the proteolysis by calpains during cardiac ischemia and reperfusion. In the calpain inhibitory activity study, 8 nM μ-calpain is inhibited by 2 nM HMW-CaMBP in a ratio of 4:1. Similarly the normal cardiac muscle HMWCaMBP expression was abolished when the calpain to HMWCaMBP ratio was greater than 4:1. Therefore, this suggests that HMWCaMBP may protect their substrates from calpains in the normal myocardium. Once calpain activity prevails over HMWCaMBP activity, it causes proteolysis of HMWCaMBP and other substrates resulting in cellular injury.

In some cases of cardiac ischemia, HMWCaMBP was highlighted in the contraction band necrosis, but in surviving muscle, intact staining was observed. Contraction band necrosis develops almost immediately on reperfusion of irreversibly injured myocytes (50,51). Degradation of HMWCaMBP may partly account for the contraction band necrosis and contractile failure of the myocardium after post ischemic reperfusion injury. Calpains are concentrated in the Z-disk, the site were myofibril disassembly begins (52). It has been reported that Ca^{2+} activates calpains and treatment of purified myofibrils with Ca^{2+} causes rapid and complete loss of the Z-disk and partial degradation of M-lines (53). One of the physiological functions of Z-disks and M-lines is to maintain the architecture of myofibrils; their

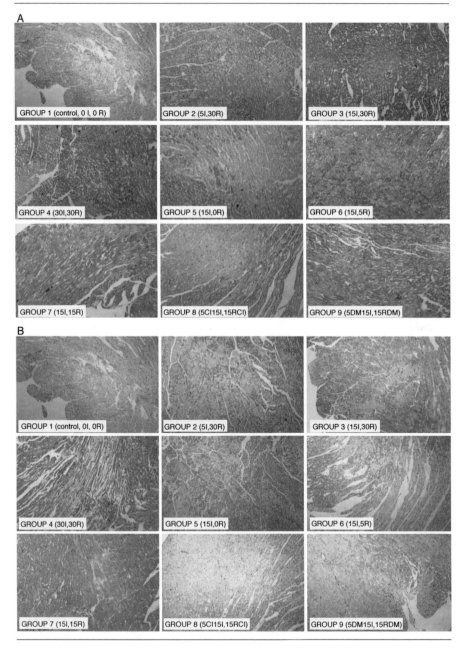

Figure 11. Expression of calpains in rat cardiac tissues after ischemia and reperfusion. A, μ-calpain and B, *m*-calpain. For details see Kakkar et al. (49).

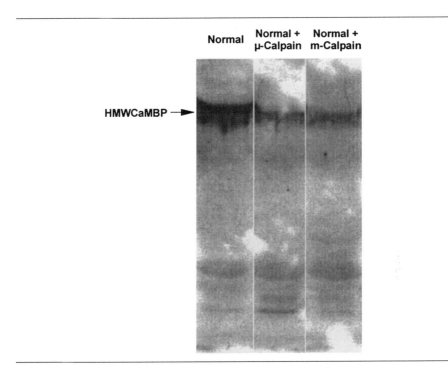

Figure 12. Proteolysis of HMWCaMBP by calpains. Lanes 1, normal cardiac supernatant fraction; 2, normal cardiac supernatant fraction and μ-calpain; 3, normal cardiac supernatant fraction and m-calpain. For details see Kakkar et al. (49).

disintegration can lead to masses of disorganized filaments (53,54). Calpains degrade tropomyosin and C-protein, which contribute to the stability of thin and thick filaments and some other cardiac contractile proteins (desmin, troponin T, C and I, filamen, nebulin, gelosin, titin, alpha-actin and myosin) (55–60). Calpains therefore, have a unique specificity for degradation of those structural proteins that serve to keep actin myosin assembled in the form of myofibrils. The decrease in HMW-CaMBP expression could be responsible for an increased activity of cytoplasmic calpains, causing a subsequent increase in myofibrillar turnover that comprises about 60% of the total protein in myocardium. Disruption of myofibrils can cause functional deficiencies, structural deformations, and mechanical stress to the cell, resulting in membrane breakdown, which serves as an early marker of cell death. The balance between calpains and HMWCaMBP may determine whether the myofibril proteins are targeted for degradation

REGULATION OF HMWCaMBP

The possible regulation of HMWCaMBP by phosphorylation was investigated because protein phosphorylation is one of the most prevalent and best-understood

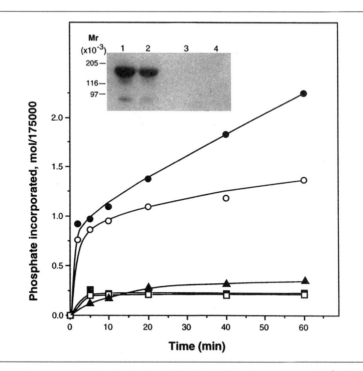

Figure 13. Time course of phosphorylation of HMWCaMBP in the presence of Ca²⁺ (O–O), EGTA (●–●), without cAMP-dependent protein kinase in the presence of EGTA (■–■) or Ca²⁺/CaM (□–□), cAMP-dependent protein kinase alone (▲–▲). *Insert*, autoradiography of phosphorylated samples. Lanes 1 and 2 are HMWCaMBP phosphorylated by cAMP-dependent protein kinase in the presence of 0.1 mM EGTA and 0.1 mM Ca²⁺, respectively. Lanes 3 and 4 are in the absence of cAMP-dependent protein kinase. For details see Kakkar et al. (61).

mechanisms employed in cellular regulation. Incubation of HMWCaMBP with cAMP-dependent protein kinase and [³²P] ATP, followed by SDS-PAGE and autoradiography revealed that the HMWCaMBP was phosphorylated. The time course and stoichiometry of phosphorylation of HMWCaMBP showed that 2.0 mol of phosphate were incorporated per mol of HMWCaMBP in the presence of EGTA. However, in the presence of Ca²⁺ and CaM the incorporation of phosphate to HMWCaMBP was reduced to 1.0 mol of phosphate per mole of HMWCaMBP (Figure 13) suggesting that CaM exerts its effects on the phosphorylation through binding to HMWCaMBP rather than acting on the kinase (61). The phosphorylation of the HMWCaMBP by cAMP-dependent protein kinase is accompanied by a decrease in the affinity of HMWCaMBP for CaM. The phosphorylated HMW-CaMBP can be dephosphorylated by a CaM-dependent protein phosphatase (calcineurin). Whether dephosphorylation of HMWCaMBP is accompanied by an increase in the affinity for CaM is difficult to demonstrate, since calcineurin is present in the dephosphorylation reaction of HMWCaMBP and this calcineurin in turn can directly affect CaM affinity. In the case of calpastatin, cAMP–dependent protein kinase is involved in the regulation, gene transcription and also its phosphorylation (62). A phosphorylated form of calpastatin isolated from rat skeletal muscle has been reported to have lower K_i for inhibition of m-calpain than for inhibition of μ-calpain, whereas a non-phosphorylated form preferentially inhibited μ-calpain (63). Since it has been established in our laboratory that HMWCaMBP is homologous to calpastatin, the effect of phosphorylation on calpain inhibition will be examined. This definitely merits a further in-depth study. The partial sequence information suggested similarity at the amino acid level with calpastatin and present studies on the sequence analysis of HMWCaMBP are underway in our laboratory. This study will greatly enhance the further characterization of HMWCaMBP.

ACKNOWLEDGEMENT

This work was supported by the Heart and Stroke Foundation of Saskatchewan, Canada. The authors are thankful to Dr. John Tuchek, Department of Pharmacology, College of Medicine, University of Saskatchewan for his helpful suggestion and critical evaluation of the manuscript. The authors are thankful to Mr. Todd Reichert for photographic work.

REFERENCES

1. Clapham DE. 1995. Calcium signalling. Cell 80:259–268.
2. Rogers MS, Strechler EE. 1996. Calmodulin. In: Guide Book to the Calcium-Binding Proteins. Ed. MR Celoi, T Pauls and B Schwaller, 34–40. Sambrook 2 Tooze, Oxford, United Kingdom: Oxford University Press.
3. Berridge MJ, Bootman MD, Lipp P. 1998. Calcium-a life and death signal. Nature 395:645–648.
4. Wang JH, Waisman DM. 1979. Calmodulin and it's role in the second-messenger system. Curr Top Cell Regul 15:47–107.
5. Cheung WY. 1980. Calmodulin plays a pivotal role in cellular regulation. Science 207:19–27.
6. Klee CB, Vanaman TC. 1982. Calmodulin. Adv Protein Chem 35:213–321.
7. Klee CB. 1988. Interaction of calmodulin with Ca^{2+} and target proteins. In: Mol Aspects Cell Regul P. Cohen and CB Klee, 5:35–56. New York: Elsevier Science Publishing Co.
8. Cheung WY. 1970. Cyclic 3',5'-nucleotide phosphodiesterase. Demonstration of an activator. Biochem Biophys Res Commun 38:533–538.
9. Cheung WY. 1971. Cyclic 3',5'-nucleotide phosphodiesterase. Evidence for and properties of a protein activator. J Biol Chem 246:2859–2869.
10. Wang JH, Desai R. 1976. A brain protein and its effect on the Ca^{2+} and protein modulator–activated cyclic nucleotide phosphodiesterase. Biochem Biophys Res Commun 72:926–932.
11. Sharma RK, Desai R, Waisman DM, Wang JH. 1979. Purification and subunit structure of bovine brain modulator binding protein. J Biol Chem 254:4276–4282.
12. Watterson DM, Vanaman TC. 1976. Affinity chromatography purification of a cyclic nucleotide phosphodiesterase using immobilized modulator protein, a troponin C-like protein from brain. Biochem Biophys Res Commun 73:40–46.
13. Klee CB, Krinks MH. 1978. Purification of cyclic 3',5'-nucleotide phosphodiesterase inhibitory protein by affinity chromatography on activator protein coupled to Sepharose. Biochemistry 17:120–126.
14. Pallen CJ, Sharma RK, Wang JH. 1988. Regulation of Calcineurin: a multifunctional calmodulin stimulated phosphatase. In: Calcium Binding Protein. Ed. MP Thompson, 51–83. Boca Raton, FL: CRC Press, Inc.

15. Klee CB. 1991. Concerted regulation of protein phosphorylation and dephosphorylation by calmodulin. Neurochem Res 16:1059–1065.
16. Stewart AA, Ingebritsen TS, Manalan A, Klee CB, Cohen P. 1982. Discovery of a Ca^{2+} and calmodulin–dependent protein phosphatase: Probable identity with calcineurin (CaM-BP80). FEBS Lett 137:80–84.
17. Adelstein RS, Eisenberg E. 1980. Regulation and kinetics of the actin-myosin—ATP interaction. Annu Rev Biochem 49:921–956.
18. Walsh MP, Hartshorne DJ. 1982. Actomyosin in smooth muscle calcium and cell. In: Calcium and Cell Function. Ed. WY. Cheung, vol.3, 223–269. Orlando FL: Academic Press.
19. Walsh MP. 1985. Calcium regulation of smooth muscle contraction. In: Calcium and Cell Physiology Ed. D. Marme, 170–203. Springer-Verlag, Berlin.
20. Sobue K, Muramoto Y, Fujita M, Kakiuchi S. 1981. Purification of a calmodulin—binding protein from chicken gizzard that interacts with F-actin. Proc Natl Acad Sci USA 78:5652–5655.
21. Sharma RK. 1990. Purification and characterization of novel calmodulin-binding protein from cardiac muscle. J Biol Chem 265:1152–1157.
22. Kakkar R, Raju RVS, Sharma RK. 1999. Calmodulin-dependent cyclic nucleotide phosphodiesterase (PDE1). Cell Mol Life Sci 55:1164–1186.
23. Stull JT. 1988. Myosin light chain kinases and caldesmon: biochemical properties and roles in skeletal muscle contractions. In: Molecular Aspects of Cellular Regulation. Ed. P Cohen and CB Klee, 99–122. New York, NY: Elesevier Science publishing.
24. Cohen P. 1988. The calmodulin-dependent multikinases. In: Molecular Aspects of Cellular Regulation. Ed. P Cohen and CB Klee, 145–193. New York, NY: Elesevier Science publishing.
25. Nishizuka Y. 1988. The molecular heterogeneity of protein kinase C and its implications for cellular regulation. Nature 334:661–665.
26. Rusnak F, Mertz P. 2000. Calcineurin: form and function. Physiol Rev 80:1483–1521.
27. Sharma R.K. 1991. Tissue distribution of high molecular weight calmodulin-binding protein. Biochem Biophys Res Commun 181:493–497.
28. Kakkar R, Raju RVS, Mellgren RL, Radhi J, Sharma RK. 1997. Cardiac high molecular weight calmodulin binding protein contains calpastatin activity. Biochemistry 36:11550–11555.
29. Clark T, Ngai PK, Sutherland C, Groschel-Stewart U, Walsh MP. 1986. Vascular smooth muscle caldesmon. J Biol Chem 261:8028–8035.
30. Ngai PK, Walsh MP. 1985. Properties of caldesmon isolated from chicken gizzard. Biochem J 230:695–707.
31. Saido TC, Sorimachi H, Suzuki K. 1994. Calpain: new perspectives in molecular diversity and physiological and pathological involvement. FASEB J 8:814–822.
32. Hata S, Sorimachi H, Nakagawa K, Maeda T, Abe K, Suzuki K. 2001. Domain II of m-calpain is a Ca^{2+} dependent cysteine protease. FEBS Lett 501:111–114.
33. Croall DE, DeMartino GN. 1991. Calcium-activated neutral protease (calpain) system: structure, function and regulation. Physiol Rev 71:813–847.
34. Blomgren K, Hallin U, Anderson AL, Puka-Sundvall M, Bahr BA, McRae A, Saido TC, Kawashima S, Hagberg H. 1999. Calpastatin is up-regulated in response to hypoxia and is a suicide substrate to calpain after neonatal cerebral hypoxia-ischemia. J Biol Chem 274:14046–14052.
35. Villa PG, Henzel WJ, Sensenbrenner M, Henderson CE, Pettmann B. 1998. Calpain inhibitors, but not caspase inhibitors, prevent actin proteolysis and DNA fragmentation during apoptosis. J Cell Sci 111:713–722.
36. Maki M, Hatanaka M, Takano E, Murachi T. 1990. Structure-function relationship of calpastain. In: Intracellular Calcium-Dependent proteolysis. Ed. RL Mellgren and T Murachi, 37–54. Boca Raton, FL: CRC press
37. Takano E, Maki M, Mori H, Hatanaka M, Marti T, Titani K, Kannagi R, Ooi T, Murachi T. 1988. Pig heart calpastatin: identification of repetitive domain structures and anomalous behavior in polyacrylamide gel electrophoresis. Biochemistry 27:1964–1972.
38. Mellgren RL, Carr TC. 1983. The protein inhibitor of calcium-dependent proteases: purification from bovine heart and possible mechanisms of regulation. Arch Biochem Biophys 225:779–786.
39. Saito K, Elce JS, Hamos JE, Nixon RA. 1993. Widespread activation of calcium-activate neutral proteinase (calpain) in the brain in Alzheimer disease: a potential molecular basis for neuronal degeneration. Proc Natl Acad Sci USA 90:2628–2632.

40. Yoshida K, Inui M, Harada K, Saido TC, Sorimachi Y, Ishihara T, Kawashima S, Sobue K. 1995. Reperfusion of rat heart after brief ischemia induces proteolysis of calspectin (nonerythroid spectrin or fodrin) by calpain. Circ Res 77:603–610.
41. Nath R, Raser KJ, Stafford D, Hajimohammadreza I, Posner A, Allen H, Talanian RV, Yuen P, Gilbertsen RB, Wang KK. 1996. Non-erythroid alpha-spectrin breakdown by calpain and interleukin 1 beta-converting-enzyme-like protease(s) in apoptotic cells: contributory roles of both protease families in neuronal apoptosis. Biochem J 319:683–690.
42. Deshpande RV, Goust JM, Hogan EL, Banik NL 1995. Calpain secreted by activated human lymphoid cells degrades myelin. J Neurosci Res 42:259–265.
43. Kakkar R, Radhi JM, Rajala RV, Sharma RK. 2000. Altered expression of high molecular weight calmodulin binding protein in human ischemic myocardium. J Pathol 191:208–216.
44. Mellgren RL, Renno W, Lane RD. 1989. The non-lysosomal, calcium-dependent proteolytic system of mammalian cells. Revis Biol Celular 20:139–159.
45. Iizuka K, Kawaguchi H, Kitabatake A. 1993. Effects of thiol protease inhibitors on fodrin degradation during hypoxia in cultured myocytes. J Mol Cell Cardiol 25:1101–1109.
46. Yoshida K, Sorimachi Y, Fujiwara M, Hironaka K. 1995. Calpain is implicated in rat myocardial injury after ischemia or reperfusion. Jpn Circ J 59:40–48.
47. Gao WD, Liu Y, Mellgren R, Marban E. 1996. Intrinsic myofilament alterations underlying the decreased contractility of stunned myocardium: A consequence of Ca^{2+} dependent proteolysis. Circ Res 78:455–465.
48. Arthur GD, Belcastro AN. 1997. A calcium stimulated cysteine protease involved in isoproterenol induced cardiac hypertrophy. Mol Cell Biochem 176:241–248.
49. Kakkar R, Wang X, Radhi JM, Rajala RVS, Wang R, Sharma RK. 2001. Decreased expression of high-molecular-weight calmodulin-binding protein and its correlation with apoptosis in ischemia-reperfused rat heart. Cell Calcium 29:59–71.
50. Beltrami CA, Finato N, Rocco M, Feruglio GA, Puricelli C, Cigola E, Sonnenblick EH, Olivetti G, Anversa P. 1995. The cellular basis of dilated cardiomyopathy in humans. J Mol Cell Cardiol 27:291–305.
51. Steenbergen C, Murphy E, Watts JA, London RE. 1990. Correlation between cytosolic free calcium, contracture, ATP and irreversible ischemic injury in perfused rat heart. Cir Res 66:135–146.
52. Bird JW, Carter JH, Triemer RE, Brooks RM, Spanier AM. 1980. Proteinases in cardiac and skeletal muscle. Fed Proc 39:20–25.
53. Goll DE, Kleese WC, Okitani A, Kumamoto T, Cong J, Kapprell HP. 1990. Historical background and current status of the Ca^{2+} dependent protease system. In: Intracellular Calcium Dependent Proteolysis Ed. RL Mellgren and T Murachi, 3–24. Boca Raton, FL: CRC Press.
54. Dayton WR, Reville WJ, Goll DE, Stromer MH. 1976. A Ca^{2+} activated protease possibly involved in myofibrillar protein turnover. Partial characterization of purified enzyme. Biochemistry 15:2159–2167.
55. Koohmaraie M. 1992. Ovine skeletal muscle multicatalytic proteinase complex (proteosome): Purification, characterization and comparison of it's effect on myofibrils with mu-calpains. J Anim Sci 70:3697–3708.
56. Sorimachi H, Kimura S, Kinbara K, Kazama J, Takahashi M, Yajima H, Ishiura S, Sasagawa N, Nonaka I, Sugita H, Maruyama K, Suzuki K. 1996. Structure and physiological functions of ubiquitous and tissue-specific calpain species. Muscle-specific calpain, p94, interacts with connectin/titin. Adv Biophys 131–122.
57. Tan FC, Goll DE, Otsuka Y. 1988. Some properties of the millimolar Ca^{2+} dependent proteinase from bovine cardiac muscle. J Mol Cell Cardiol 20:983–987.
58. Huang J, Forsberg NE. 1998. Role of calpain in skeletal-muscle protein degradation. Proc Natl Acad Sci USA 95:12100–12105.
59. Papp Z, van der Velden J, Stienen GJ. 2000. Calpain-I induced alterations in the cytoskeletal structure and impaired mechanical properties of single myocytes of rat heart. Cardiovasc Res 45:981–993.
60. Feng J, Schaus BJ, Fallavollita JA, Lee TC, Canty JM Jr. 2001. Preload induces Troponin I degradation independently of myocardial ischemia. Circulation 103:2035–2037.
61. Kakkar R, Taketa S, Raju RVS, Proudlove S, Colquhoun P, Grymaloski K Sharma RK. 1997. In vitro phosphorylation of bovine cardiac muscle high molecular weight calmodulin binding protein by cyclic AMP-dependent protein kinase and dephosphorylation by calmodulin-dependent phosphatase. Mol Cell Biochem 177:215–219.

62. Cong M, Thompson VF, Goll DE, Antin PB. 1998. The bovine calpastatin gene promoter and a new N- terminal region of the protein are targets for cAMP-dependent protein kinase activity. J Biol Chem 273:660–666.
63. Salamino F, De Tullio R, Michetti M, Mengotti P, Melloni E, Pontremoli S. 1994. Modulation of calpastatin specificity in rat tissues by reversible phosphorylation and dephosphorylation. Biochem Biophys Res Commun 199:1326–1332.

Signal Transduction and Cardiac Hypertrophy,
edited by N.S. Dhalla, L.V. Hryshko,
E. Kardami & P.K. Singal
Kluwer Academic Publishers, Boston, 2003

β-Adrenergic Signaling in Chronic Heart Failure—Friend or Foe?

Christoph Maack★ and Michael Böhm

Medizinische Universitätsklinik u. Poliklinik
Innere Medizin III
66421 Homburg/Saar
Germany

Summary. In chronic heart failure, a number of compensatory mechanisms are activated in order to maintain circulation and thus supply of the body with blood and oxygen. One important mechanism is the activation of the sympathetic nervous system, resulting in increased β-adrenergic signaling. This leads to both adaptive and pathological processes within the cell, including a desensitization of the β-adrenergic signal transduction cascade, the induction of hypertrophy, apoptosis and necrosis. It is currently a matter of debate whether a desensitization of the β-adrenergic signal transduction cascade is adaptive or maladaptive. In other words, it is not entirely clear whether in heart failure, decreased β-adrenergic signaling due to desensitization of the signaling cascade per se is a cause for cardiac dysfunction. In order to elucidate this issue, this review will focus on the consequences of increased β-adrenergic signaling, investigated by selective overexpression of distinct cascade components in mouse models. Furthermore, the impact of partial and inverse agonism of β-blockers on β-adrenergic signaling in human myocardium *in vitro* as well as *in vivo* in the clinical situation in patients with heart failure is highlighted. It is discussed whether the fact that not all β-blockers improve survival in heart failure patients may be due to their respective degree of inverse agonism.

Key words: β-adrenergic receptors, heart failure, β-blockers, inverse agonism.

★ Address for Correspondence: Christoph Maack, M.D., Medizinische Universitätsklinik u. Poliklinik, Innere Medizin III, 66421 Homburg/Saar, Germany. Tel. (00)49-6841-16 23433, Fax. (00)49-6841-16 23434, E-mail: maack@med-in.uni-sb.de

INTRODUCTION

Congestive heart failure is a major public health problem in most Western countries. In the United States, approximately three million people suffer from heart failure, 10% of whom are admitted to hospital each year (1). Heart failure is defined as the inability of the heart to supply the body with sufficient amounts of blood and oxygen. In response, a number of compensatory mechanisms are activated in order to maintain blood flow to vital organs. Besides activation of the renin-angiotensin-aldosterone system, increased activity of the sympathetic nervous system is a hallmark of heart failure. Chronic sympathetic activation leads to both adaptive and pathological processes within the cell, including alterations of the β-adrenergic signal transduction cascade, the induction of hypertrophy and cell death. It is currently a matter of debate whether alterations of the β-adrenergic signal transduction cascade are adaptive or maladaptive. To further elucidate this issue, in its first part, this review will focus on the consequences of increased β-adrenergic signaling, investigated by creation of transgenic mouse models, in order to delineate mechanisms leading to rescue or deterioration of cardiac function.

The inhibition of β-adrenergic signaling by pharmacological intervention with β-blockers has proven to exert beneficial effects on cardiac function and survival of patients with chronic heart failure. However, these benefits are not a class-effect of β-blockers, since some agents did not prolong survival in heart failure patients. Thus, the impact of partial and inverse agonism of β-blockers on β-adrenergic signaling in human myocardium *in vitro* as well as *in vivo* in the clinical situation in patients with heart failure is highlighted in the second part of the review.

FIRST PART

Chronic sympathetic activation in heart failure

In patients with chronic heart failure, plasma norepinephrine levels are substantially elevated, and the amount of elevation correlates with the poor prognosis of this syndrome (2). As a consequence of chronic activation of the β-adrenergic system, β-adrenergic receptors (β-ARs) are desensitized and down-regulated (3). While β_1-ARs are down-regulated, β_2-AR density is unchanged but desensitized by uncoupling from the stimulatory G-protein (G_s). Thus, the normal relation of β_1/β_2-ARs ($\approx 80/20$) is changed towards higher relative amounts of β_2-ARs in heart failure (65/35) (4). β-AR desensitization and down-regulation is due to phosphorylation of receptors by the β-AR kinase (β-ARK), the activity and expression of which is increased in heart failure (5). While expression of G_s is unchanged, the α-subunit of the inhibitory G-protein ($G_{i\alpha}$) is up-regulated in chronic heart failure (6). The functional consequence of these processes in concert is a decreased responsiveness of human failing myocardium to β-adrenergic stimulation *in vitro* (6) and *in vivo* (7).

The question that arises from these results is whether desensitization of the β-adrenergic system is the predominant mechanism leading to cardiac dysfunction in heart failure. This hypothesis is supported by the observation that in patients with

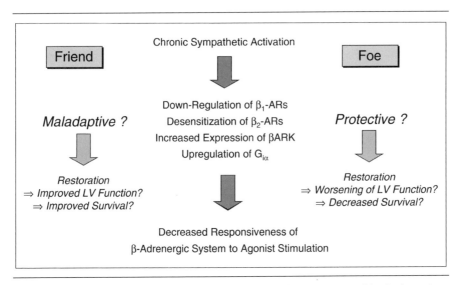

Figure 1. Pathophysiological changes in chronic heart failure. If desensitization of the β-adrenergic system was maladaptive, then restoration would improve cardiac function, and enhanced β-adrenergic signaling would be the *friend*. If desensitization was protective, then restoration would be detrimental and pronounced signaling would be the *foe* in chronic heart failure.

heart failure, a restoration of β-AR density and post-receptor events by treatment with the β-blocker metoprolol is associated with an improvement of left ventrcular (LV) function (8,9) and prognosis (10). On the other hand, treatment with the β-blocker carvedilol does not lead to an up-regulation of ventricular β-AR density but does improve LV function (8) and prognosis in heart failure patients (11,12). In this context, decreased β-adrenergic signaling may protect the heart from harmful effects of catecholamines (13). In order to systematically investigate the impact of β-adrenergic signaling on cardiac morphology and cellular function, a number of transgenic animal models have been created to selectively enhance or inhibit signaling via different components of the β-adrenergic signaling cascade. These transgenic models include overexpression of β_1- and β_2-ARs and $G_{s\alpha}$ as well as inhibition of βARK-activity. The short- and long-term results of these transgenic interventions could resolve the question whether β-adrenergic signaling is a friend or a foe in chronic heart failure (Figure 1).

β_1-AR overexpression

Using the α-myosin heavy chain promotor, Engelhardt et al. (14) transfected mice with human β_1-ARs at a level of 5- to 15-fold overexpression of receptor density in wild-type animals. At an early stage (8–12 weeks), β_1-AR overexpression resulted in increased *in vivo* contractility (dP/dt_{max}) as well as increased sensitivity and

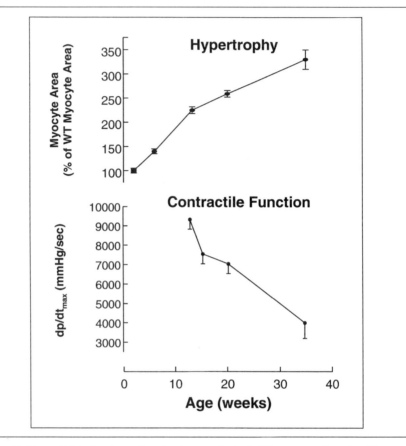

Figure 2. Myocardial dysfunction and cardiac hypertrophy in β_1-AR overexpressing mice. Hypertrophy preceeds the onset of myocardial dysfunction (from 14).

efficacy of isoproterenol in enhancing spontaneous right atrial beating frequency *in vitro*. On the other hand, this improvement of cardiac function and β-adrenergic coupling was associated with a rise in cross-sectional myocyte area, indicating compensated cardiac hypertrophy at this early stage. Long-term follow-up of these animals revealed that after 16 weeks, LV function continuously decreased, resulting in overt heart failure with LV ejection fraction decreasing from 65% to 20% after 35 weeks. It is noteworthy that hypertrophy preceeded the onset of cardiac dysfunction in these animals (Figure 2). Despite progressive myocyte hypertrophy over the 35 weeks of follow-up, overall weight of transgenic hearts increased only by 10%, compatible with myocyte cell death and replacement by fibrous tissue. Taken together, the results of this important study reveal that signaling via β_1-ARs leads to functional improvement in the short term, but to deterioration of myocardial morphology and function in the long term.

$G_{s\alpha}$ overexpression

The β_1-AR is coupled to adenylate cyclase via the α-subunit of the stimulatory G-protein ($G_{s\alpha}$). 5-fold overexpression of this component of the β-adrenergic signal transduction cascade has similar effects as β_1-AR overexpression. At 10 months of age, echocardiography of these animals displays increased sensitivity of cardiac function to isoproterenol stimulation (15). On the other hand, after 16 months, an increase of myocyte cross-sectional area and myocardial collagen content compared to control animals reveals pronounced cardiac hypertrophy and fibrosis in these animals. Furthermore, an increase of cardiomyocyte apoptosis is observed in transgenic animals at this late age (16). Treatment of transgenic animals with the β-blocker propranolol from month 9 (when heart failure begins to develop) to month 16 inhibits hypertrophy, ameliorates fibrosis and suppresses apoptosis to levels of wild-type animals (16). Accordingly, propranolol treatment clearly improved LV function and survival of transgenic animals during the 8 months of follow-up after treatment initiation. These data clearly demonstrate that pronounced signaling via the β_1-AR and $G_{s\alpha}$ results in short-term benefit with detrimental effects on cardiac function and survival in the long-term. Pharmacologic intervention with β-blockers may improve cardiac function and survival by reducing β-adrenergic signaling.

β_2-AR overexpression

While relatively low levels of β_1-AR overexpression (5- to 15-fold) result in cardiac dysfunction after 4 months (14), early studies on mice overexpressing β_2-ARs up to 200-fold revealed enhanced cardiac function without apparent detrimental long-term effects (17). Thus, β_2-AR overexpression was used to "rescue" mice from cardiac dysfunction and death induced by different pathological events. The results of these studies were ambiguous. Low-level β_2-AR overexpression (30-fold) normalized the characteristic resting systolic dysfunction in the $G\alpha q$ transgenic mouse model of hypertrophy (18), whereas higher-level β_2-AR overexpression failed to improve a murine transgenic model of dilated cardiomyopathy (19). Furthermore, while 200-fold overexpression of β_2-ARs improved ventricular contractility in mice up to 9 weeks after myocardial infarction without adverse consequences on survival (20), the same mouse line (TG4) experienced excessive mortality after aortic banding (21). In these animals, the functional deterioration after aortic banding was associated with more extensive fibrosis and hypertrophy compared to banded wild-type animals (21). These data indicate that β_2-AR overexpression may be beneficial even in the longer-term, depending on the model of initial cardiac dysfunction. In this context, the duration and degree of receptor overexpression are of critical importance. This is suggested by a study of Liggett et al. (22), who followed animals with different degrees of β_2-AR overexpression (60- to 350-fold) up to an age of 50 weeks. They observed that the mice of the highest-expressing line (350-fold) developed a rapidly progressive fibrotic dilated cardiomyopathy and died of heart failure at 25 ± 1 weeks of age. The lowest-expressing line (60-fold) exhibited enhanced basal cardiac function without increased mortality when followed for 1

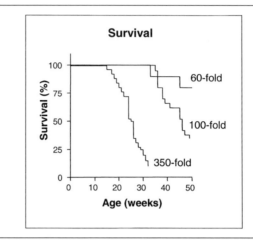

Figure 3. Impaired survival of high-level β₂-AR overexpressors. Kaplan-Meier survival curves of β₂-AR-overexpressing mouse lines followed for 50 weeks (from 22).

year, whereas 100-fold overexpression developed fibrotic cardiomyopathy and heart failure, with death occuring at 41 ± 1 weeks of age. Cardiac function was enhanced in the 3 lower-expressing β₂-AR lines (60-, 100- and 150-fold), while 350-fold overexpressing mice exhibited impaired LV function and ventricular enlargement. Only in the highest-expressing line, gene expression of markers of cardiac hypertrophy (β-myosin heavy chain (β-MHC) and atrial natriuretic factor (ANF)) were increased. Mortality rates of the different lines of β₂-AR overexpression were substantially different. The higher β₂-ARs were overexpressed, the higher was the mortality rate (Figure 3). Thus, adverse effects of β₂-AR overexpression on cardiac morphology and function are dependent on time and the level of overexpression, with low levels of β₂-AR overexpression leading to enhancement of cardiac function without adverse effects on longer-term outcome.

Different coupling of β₁- and β₂-adrenergic receptors

Taken together, the results from β₁- and β₂-AR-overexpressing mice suggest that β₁-AR overexpression is more harmful than β₂-AR overexpression. This implicates that different signaling pathways may be activated by β₁- and β₂-AR stimulation. First functional evidence of differential β₁- and β₂-AR signaling pathways came from a study of Xiao et al. (23), where β₂-AR-induced augmentations in intracellular Ca^{2+}-transient and contractility were dissociated from cellular cyclic adenosine monophosphate (cAMP) accumulation and protein kinase A (PKA)-mediated protein phosphorylation in rat ventricular myocytes, whereas the classical linear G_s/adenylate cyclase/cAMP/PKA signaling cascade was corroborated for β₁-AR stimulation. Further studies revealed that while the β₁-AR is primarily coupled to the stimulatory G-protein (Gs), the β₂-AR is coupled to both G_s and G_i. Disrupting G_i

signaling by pertussis toxin (PTX)-mediated ribosylation enhances $β_2$-AR-induced contractile response in rat ventricular myocytes (24) and unmasks the $β_2$-AR positive inotropic effect in mouse cardiac myocytes, in which G_i signaling fully negates $β_2$-AR/G_s-mediated contractile response (25). Similar results were obtained in human myocardium, where $β_2$-AR stimulation activates both G_s and G_i, whereas $β_1$-AR activates only G_s (26).

Different G-protein coupling of $β_1$- and $β_2$-ARs is of importance not only for regulation of contractility, but also apoptotic pathways are differently activated by β-adrenergic stimulation. Norepinephrine-induced decrease of cardiomyocyte viability is mediated by β-adrenergic rather than α-adrenergic pathways (27). This decreased viability is mediated by a PKA-dependent increase of cellular Ca^{2+}-influx and is due to, at least in part, the induction of apoptosis (28). Inhibition of $β_2$-adrenergic signaling potentiates, inhibition of $β_1$-adrenergic signaling ameliorates norepinephrine-induced apoptosis (29), indicating that activation of $β_1$-ARs induces apoptosis while activation of $β_2$-ARs inhibits apoptosis. $β_2$-AR-mediated anti-apoptotic effects are inhibited by PTX-induced inactivation of G_i (29). Further studies indicate that the anti-apoptotic effects of $β_2$-AR-G_i coupling are mediated by dissociation of $G_{βγ}$-subunits, activating phosphatidylinositol 3'-kinase (PI-3K) which in turn activates Akt, a key regulator of cell survival (30,31). This anti-apoptotic pathway is suggested to counteract G_s-mediated apoptosis. In situations of pronounced β-adrenergic activation, the balanced dual G-protein coupling of the $β_2$-AR is shifted towards G_i by PKA-dependent $β_2$-AR phosphorylation (32) and may therefore be regarded as a potentially protective adaptation of the cell in response to sympathetic activation.

β-adrenergic signaling—friend or foe?

In chronic heart failure, decreased cardiac $β_1$-AR density and thus increased relative amounts of $β_2$-ARs as well as enhanced expression of G_i may facilitate this anti-apoptotic pathway (Figure 4). Nevertheless, the fact that in chronic heart failure, continual β-adrenergic activation leads to a progression of the disease (2) and increased rate of apoptosis (33,34) without the ability of the heart to rescue itself by anti-apoptotic mechanisms suggests that the pro-apoptotic signaling pathways outweigh the protective ones. In this context, sympathetic activation and thus β-adrenergic signaling in chronic heart failure has to be regarded as the *foe*, leading to a desensitization of the β-adrenergic system on the one hand and to pronounced hypertrophy, fibrosis and apoptosis and thus cardiac remodeling on the other hand (Figure 5). While a desensitization of the β-adrenergic system may affect cardiac contractility especially during exercise, progressive ventricular remodeling may be the critical mechanism leading to an impairment of ventricular function already at rest. Worsening of cardiac contractile function by both processes leads to a decrease of peripheral perfusion. As a response, the activation of the sympathetic nervous system initiates a vicious cycle with progressive deterioration of cardiac function and heart failure as the final result. Thus, therapeutic intervention of this vicious cycle by inhibiting the effects of sympathetic activation by the application of a β-AR antagonist may be the *friend* in chronic heart failure.

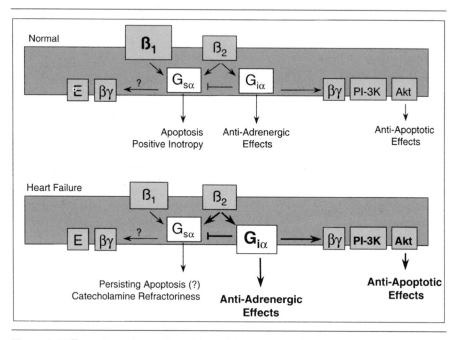

Figure 4. Different G-protein coupling of β_1- and β_2-ARs with different pro- and anti-apoptotic effects. In chronic heart failure, G_i-mediated signaling may be pronounced by a decrease of β_1-AR density and an increase of G_i expression. By this route, anti-apoptotic effects may be enhanced. PI-3K, phosphatidylinositol 3'-kinase.

SECOND PART

β-AR antagonist treatment of patients with chronic heart failure

Treatment of patients with chronic heart failure with most β-blockers leads to an improvement of symptoms and left ventricular (LV) function. However, while treatment with carvedilol (11,12), metoprolol (10), and bisoprolol (35) improved prognosis, bucindolol led only to a non-significant 10% reduction of overall mortality in patients of New York Heart Association (NYHA) class III-IV in the BEST-trial (36). The BEST-trial was the first to involve a considerable amount of black patients. In these patients, bucindolol had even adverse effects on mortality, while in non-black patients, a significant reduction of mortality was observed. However, even in non-black patients risk reduction by bucindolol was only 18%, which is clearly below the 35% reduction of mortality provided by carvedilol in an even sicker population (36). Thus, the different results in outcome suggest that among β-blockers, different pharmacological properties, i.e. different intrinsic activity, may have an important impact on prognosis of heart failure patients.

Agonist and inverse agonist activity of β-AR antagonists

According to the ternary complex model of receptor activation established by De Lean et al. in 1980 (37), the binding of an agonist to the β-AR leads to an

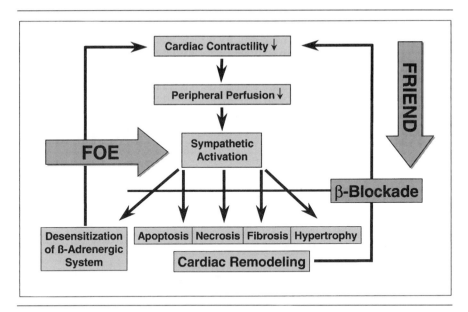

Figure 5. Vicious cycle of sympathetic activation in chronic heart failure. Pharmacological intervention by β-blockade is the friend in chronic heart failure.

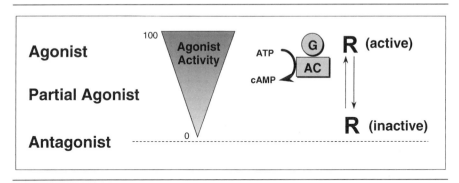

Figure 6. Ternary complex model of receptor activation, established by De Lean et al. in 1980 (37).

activation of the receptor and allows the coupling to G_s and adenylate cyclase. In this context, the binding of a partial agonist leads to partial activation, whereas the binding of an antagonist merely inhibits agonist-induced activation of the receptor (Figure 6). The development of transgenic mouse models with overexpression of the $β_2$-AR provided further insight to the mechanisms of receptor action in response to antagonists. In mice with 200-fold overexpression of the $β_2$-AR, baseline cardiac function was found to be maximally activated already under baseline conditions (17). In contrast to wild-type animals, no further increase of left atrial isometric tension could be induced by isoprenaline. The authors concluded that unoccupied β-ARs

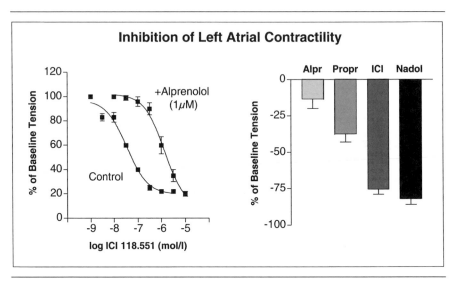

Figure 7. Inhibition of contractility in β_2-AR overexpressing mice by inverse agonists (from 17). Alpr, alprenolol; Propr, propranolol; ICI, ICI 118.551; Nadol, nadolol.

consist of a certain amount of receptors in an activated state (R*) that maintain a baseline degree of adenylate cyclase activation. When overexpressing β_2-ARs, the fraction of receptors in the activated state is sufficient to account for complete activation of adenylate cyclase, since further distal components of the signal transduction cascade (G_s, adenylate cyclase) were not overexpressed. In this mouse model (TG4), application of the selective β_2-AR antagonist ICI 118.551 led to an 80% reduction of baseline contractility (38, Figure 7). Different β-AR antagonists lead to different degrees of inhibition of contractility (Figure 7). These data indicate that unoccupied β-ARs already exert a basal amount of intrinsic activity. The ability of β-AR antagonists to reduce this basal β-AR activity is termed "inverse agonist activity". The action of a strong inverse agonist (i.e. ICI 118.551) on β_2-AR activity can be antagonized by a weak inverse agonist (i.e. alprenolol, Figure 7). According to these new findings, the ternary complex model had to be modified by establishing the allosteric ternary complex model of receptor activation (Figure 8), in which the β-AR exists in an equilibrium between the inactivated (R) and the activated state of the receptor (R*). The binding of an agonist leads to a conformational change of the receptor, allowing it to interact with G_s and adenylate cyclase. In contrast, the binding of an inverse agonist stabilizes the receptor in its inactive conformation, thereby maximally inhibiting interaction of the receptor with G_s. The binding of a neutral antagonist leaves the equilibrium more or less unchanged.

Impact of β-AR signaling on receptor regulation

The activation state of the β-AR is of importance not only for contractility, but also for receptor regulation. Only receptors in the activated state (R*) are a

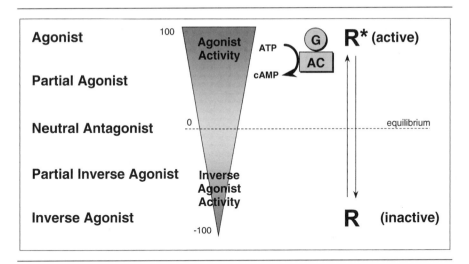

Figure 8. Allosteric ternary complex model of receptor activation. In contrast to the model of De Lean et al. (37), a second dimension of inverse agonist activity has to be considered.

substrate for phosphorylation by the β-AR kinase and thus desensitization and down-regulation. The intrinsic activity of several partial and full agonists was shown to correlate with the degree of receptor phosphorylation and in turn desensitization and down-regulation (39). Accordingly, also inverse agonism has an impact on receptor regulation. When transfecting mice with a constitutively active mutant of the β_2-AR (CAM β_2), no overexpression of this receptor could be achieved in these animals (40). Only when treating these animals with the inverse agonist ICI 118.551, robust levels of CAM β_2-AR density could be achieved. These results indicate that inverse agonist-induced inactivation of receptors leads to inhibition of phosphorylation of receptors by βARK and thus to sensitization and up-regulation of receptor density, while agonist-induced activation facilitates phosphorylation and thus desensitization and down-regulation of receptors (Figure 8).

Inverse agonism of β-AR antagonists in human myocardium

Inverse agonism is a phenomenon that is observed not only in experimental animal models with artificial β-AR overexpression, but also in human myocardium. In vitro application of the β-AR antagonist metoprolol to human ventricular myocardium leads to inhibition of contractility by about 85%, an effect that could be antagonized by co-incubation with bucindolol (41; Figure 9). In contrast, application of bucindolol alone led to no significant change of cardiac contractility. This was due to the fact that bucindolol had a positive inotropic effect in one part and a weak negative inotropic effect in the other part of experiments (Figure 10). When comparing the effects of various β-AR antagonists on cardiac contractility in human

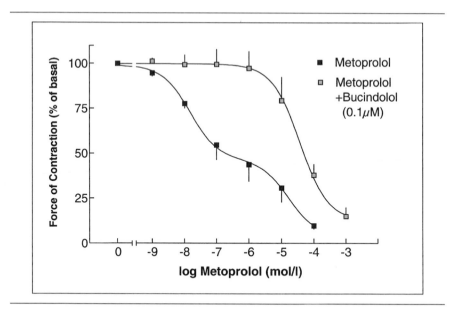

Figure 9. Inverse agonist activity of metoprolol in human ventricular myocardium. The negative inotropic effect of metoprolol can be antagonized in the presence of bucindolol (from 41).

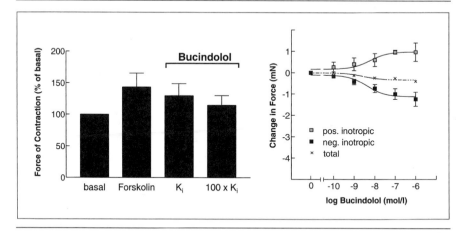

Figure 10. Bucindolol does not reduce force of contraction in human ventricular myocardium. This is due to the fact that it had a slight negative inotropic effect in one part of experiments and a positive inotropic effect in the other part (from 41). Coupling of $G_{s\alpha}$ to adenylate cyclase was facilitated by the addition of forskolin. K_i, $100 \times K_i$: Concentration at which 50% (K_i) and 100% β-AR ($100 \times K_i$) occupation by β-AR antagonist occurs.

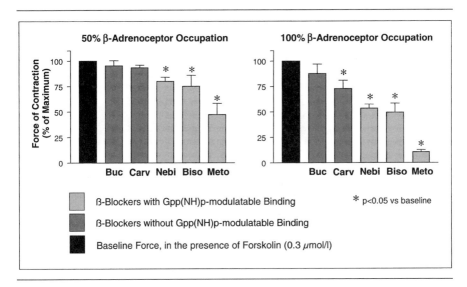

Figure 11. Different inverse agonist activity of different β-AR antagonists in human ventricular myocardium. Metoprolol (Meto) is a strong-, carvedilol (Carv) a weak inverse agonist. In human myocardium, bucindolol (Buc) is a "neutral" antagonist. β-AR antagonists that displayed Gpp(NH)p-modulatable binding, which indicates β-adrenoceptor-G-protein interaction, have less inverse agonist activity compared to agents that do not have this feature. Biso, bisoprolol; Nebi, nebivolol.

myocardium, effects range from strong inverse agonist activity of metoprolol over weak inverse agonists (bisoprolol, carvedilol) to the merely neutral antagonist bucindolol (Figure 11).

Clinical implications of inverse agonist activity of β-AR antagonists

In chronic heart failure, plasma catecholamine levels are elevated (2). The question is whether in this situation, different inverse agonist activity of β-AR antagonists may lose importance since at agonist-occupied receptors, any β-blocker primarily antagonizes agonist-induced activation of receptors. Nevertheless, even at agonist-occupied receptors, the degree of inactivation by β-blockers is variable. While bucindolol lowers contractility to baseline values, metoprolol reduces contractility beyond baseline (Figure 12). Thus, any β-AR ligand may "fix" the receptor at a certain conformation and thus activity, which is independent of the initial state of the receptor. This implicates that in the clinical situation, net β-adrenergic signaling may be dependent on the intrinsic activity of the β-blocker that is applied.

What clinical parameter is an indicator of β-adrenergic signaling? Going back to transgenic animal studies, a characteristic hallmark of increased β-adrenergic signaling is an elevation of heart rate at rest. Overexpression of β_1- and β_2-ARs as well as $G_{s\alpha}$ leads to elevated baseline heart rate in these animals (14,42,15). Also in patients with heart failure, heart rate is increased due to sympathetic activation. Thus, the

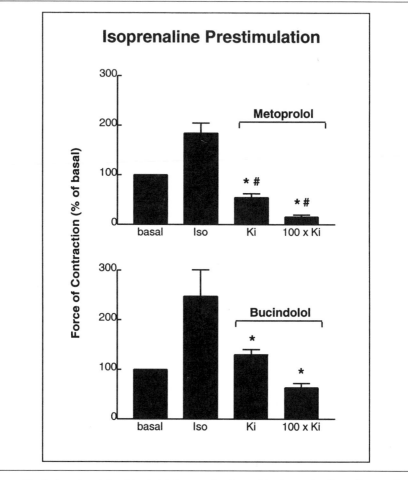

Figure 12. Both metoprolol and bucindolol antagonize the positive inotropic effect of isoprenaline (Iso) in human ventricular myocardium. Metoprolol, but not bucindolol decreases force below baseline values. K_i, $100 \times K_i$: Concentration at which 50% (K_i) and 100% β-AR ($100 \times K_i$) occupation by β-AR antagonist occurs.

effect of a β-blocker on heart rate could be considered as its effect on β-adrenergic signaling. Especially in situations of decreased adrenergic stimulation, i.e. during the night, heart rate mirrors intrinsic activity of the respective β-blocker. In patients with heart failure, heart rate at night is increased by the partial agonist xamoterol (43), decreased by the inverse agonist metoprolol (44) and unchanged by bucindolol (45). Interestingly, mortality is affected in a similar way by these three agents. While xamoterol treatment of heart failure patients increased mortality (43), metoprolol reduced it (10) and bucindolol neither increased nor decreased it significantly (36). Of course, in vitro data cannot readily be transferred to results of clinical studies,

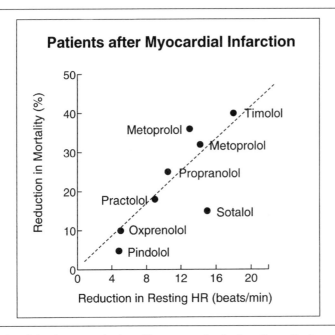

Figure 13. Correlation between reduction of heart rate and reduction of mortality in patients after myocardial infarction (from 48).

however increased heart rate is associated with excess mortality in patients with arterial hypertension (46), coronary artery disease (47) and chronic heart failure. A metaanalysis of trials in patients after myocardial infarction indicates that there is a close correlation between the degree of heart rate reduction and mortality reduction (48, Figure 13). It is of note that agents displaying intrinsic sympathomimetic activity (i.e., pindolol or oxprenolol) have lesser effects on mortality compared to inverse agonists (i.e., metoprolol). These authors even postulate that a reduction of heart rate by 1 beat/min reduces mortality by 2% (48). Similar results were obtained in patients with chronic heart failure. Figure 14 illustrates the correlation between heart rate reduction and mortality reduction in large pharmacological intervention trials in heart failure patients (49).

These data suggest that

1. reduction of heart rate in patients with cardiovascular disorders is associated with reduced mortality and
2. inverse agonists, neutral antagonists and partial agonists affect heart rate and thus β-adrenergic signalling in different ways.

Furthermore, intrinsic activity of β-AR antagonists is of importance for receptor regulation. Activated β-ARs (R*) are phosphorylated, uncoupled from G_s and

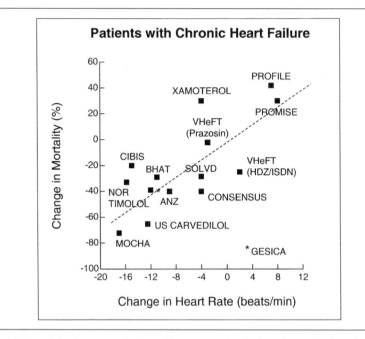

Figure 14. Correlation between reduction of heart rate and reduction of mortality in patients with chronic heart failure (from 49).

down-regulated. In contrast, inactivated receptors are dephosphorylated, resensitized and upregulated. Accordingly, in patients with chronic heart failure, β-AR density was upregulated by the strong inverse agonist metoprolol but not by the weak inverse agonist carvedilol (8). In patients with heart failure, ventricular β-AR density is positively correlated with the maximum increase of heart rate as well as maximum oxygen consumption at exertion (50). This may explain why in clinical trials with β-blockers, maximum exercise tolerance was improved in most studies with metoprolol but not carvedilol (51).

CONCLUSION

Taken together, increased β-adrenergic signaling is a hallmark of chronic heart failure and substantially contributes to the development of cardiac dysfunction by the induction of hypertrophy, fibrosis and finally apoptotic or necrotic cell death. Desensitization of the β-adrenergic signaling cascade may be regarded as an adaptive mechanism. Whether this is beneficial or maladaptive remains a matter of debate. In this context, different coupling of β$_1$- and β$_2$-ARs to heterotrimerous G-proteins and other downstream signal transduction components has to be considered, since in chronic heart failure, a shift from G$_s$- to G$_i$-mediated signaling may occur. Apparently, deleterious G$_s$-mediated effects still outweigh potentially protective G$_i$-related ones. Thus, pharmacological intervention with β-AR antagonists is beneficial due to a reduction of overall β-adrenergic signaling. The degree of β-AR inactivation is dependent on the degree of inverse agonist activity of the respective β-AR antagonist, which may have an impact on β-AR regulation, exercise tolerance, heart rate and finally survival in patients with chronic heart failure. The conclusion is that β-adrenergic signaling may be regarded as the *foe*, while pharmacological intervention of the vicious cycle of sympathetic activation with β-blockers is the friend in the treatment of chronic heart failure.

REFERENCES

1. Smith WM. 1985. Epidemiology of congestive heart failure. Am J Cardiol 55:3–8A.
2. Cohn JN, Levine TB, Olivari MT, Gerberg V, Lura D, Francis GS, Simon AB, Rector T. 1984. Plasma norepinephrine as a guide to prognosis in patients with chronic congestive heart failure. N Engl J Med 311:819–823.
3. Bristow MR, Ginsburg R, Minobe W, Cubiciotti RS, Sageman WS, Lurie K, Billingham ME, Harrison DE, Stinson EB. 1982. Decreased catecholamine sensitivity and β-adrenergic receptor density in failing human hearts. N Engl J Med 307:205–211.
4. Bristow MR, Anderson FL, Port JD, Skerl L, Hershberger RE, Larrabee P, O'Connell JB, Renlund DG, Volkman K, Murray J, et al. 1991. Differences in beta-adrenergic neuroeffector mechanisms in ischemic versus idiopathic dilated cardiomyopathy. Circulation 84:1024–1039.
5. Ungerer M, Böhm M, Elce JS, Erdmann E, Lohse MJ. 1993. Altered expression of β-adrenergic receptor kinase and β₁-adrenergic receptors in the failing human heart. Circulation 87:454–463.
6. Böhm M, Gierschik P, Jakobs KH, Pieske B, Schnabel P, Ungerer M, Erdmann E. 1990. Increase of $G_{i\alpha}$ in human hearts with dilated but not ischemic cardiomyopathy. Circulation 82:1249–1265.
7. Gage J, Rutman H, Lucido D, Le Jemtel TH. 1986. Additive effects of Dobutamine and amrinone on myocardial contractility and ventricular performance in patients with severe heart failure. Circulation 74:367–373.
8. Gilbert EM, Olsen SL, Renlund DG, Bristow MR. 1993. Beta-adrenergic receptor regulation and left ventricular function in idiopathic dilated cardiomyopathy. Am J Cardiol 71:23C–29C.
9. Böhm M, Deutsch HJ, Hartmann D, La Rosée K, Stäblein A. 1997. Improvement of postreceptor events by metoprolol treatment in patients with chronic heart failure. J Am Coll Cardiol 30:992–996.
10. MERIT-HF Investigators. 1999. Effect of metoprolol CR/XL in chronic heart failure: Metoprolol CR/XL Randomised Intervention Trial in Congestive Heart Failure (MERIT-HF). Lancet 353:2001–2007.
11. Packer M, Bristow MR, Cohn JN, Colucci W, Fowler MB, Gilbert EM, Shusterman NH, for the US Carvedilol Heart Failure Study Group. 1996. The effect of carvedilol on morbidity and mortality in patients with chronic heart failure. N Engl J Med 334:1349–1355.
12. Packer M, Coats AJ, Fowler MB, Katus HA, Krum H, Mohacsi P, Rouleau JL, Tendera M, Castaigne A, Roecker EB, Schultz MK, DeMets DL. 2001. Effect of carvedilol on survival in severe chronic heart failure. N Engl J Med 344:1651–1658.
13. Bristow MR. 2000. β-Adrenergic receptor blockade in chronic heart failure. Circulation 101:558–569.
14. Engelhardt S, Hein L, Wiesmann F, Lohse MJ. 1999. Progressive hypertrophy and heart failure in β₁-adrenergic receptor transgenic mice. Proc Natl Acad Sci USA 96:7059–7064.
15. Iwase M, Bishop SP, Uechi M, Vatner DE, Shannon RP, Kudej RK, Wight DC, Wagner TE, Ishikawa Y, Homcy CJ, Vatner SF. 1996. Adverse effects of chronic endogenous sympathetic drive induced by cardiac $G_{s\alpha}$ overexpression. Circ Res 78:517–524.
16. Asai K, Yang GP, Geng YJ, Takagi G, Bishop S, Ishikawa Y, Shannon RP, Wagner TE, Vatner DE, Homcy CJ, Vatner SF. 1999. β-Adrenergic receptor blockade arrests myocyte damage and preserves cardiac function in the transgenic $G_{s\alpha}$ mouse. J Clin Invest 104:551–558.
17. Milano CA, Allen LF, Rockman HA, Dolber PC, McMinn TR, Chien KR, Johnson TD, Bond RA, Lefkowitz RJ. 1994. Enhanced myocardial function in transgenic mice overexpressing the β₂-adrenergic receptor. Science 264:582–586.
18. Dorn GW 2nd, Tepe NM, Lorenz JN, Koch WJ, Liggett SB. 1999. Low- and high-level transgenic expression of β₂-adrenergic receptors differentially affect cardiac hypertrophy and function in $G_{\alpha q}$-overexpressing mice. Proc Natl Acad Sci USA 96:6400–6405.

19. Rockman HA, Chien KR, Choi DJ, Iaccarino G, Hunter JJ, Ross J Jr, Lefkowitz RJ, Koch WJ. 1998. Expression of a β-adrenergic receptor kinase 1 inhibitor prevents the development of myocardial failure in gene-targeted mice. Proc Natl Acad Sci USA 95:7000–7005.

20. Du XJ, Gao XM, Jennings GL, Dart AM, Woodcock EA. 2000. Preserved ventricular contractility in infarcted mouse heart overexpressing β₂-adrenergic receptors. Am J Physiol 279:H2456–H2463.

21. Du XJ, Autelitano DJ, Dilley RJ, Wang B, Dart AM, Woodcock EA. 2000. β₂-adrenergic receptor overexpression exacerbates development of heart failure after aortic stenosis. Circulation 101:71–77.

22. Liggett SB, Tepe NM, Lorenz JN, Canning AM, Jantz TD, Mitarai S, Yatani A, Dorn GW 2nd. 2000. Early and delayed consequences of β₂-adrenergic receptor overexpression in mouse hearts: critical role for expression level. Circulation 101:1707–1714.

23. Xiao RP, Hohl C, Altschuld R, Jones L, Livingston B, Ziman B, Tantini B, Lakatta EG. 1994. β₂-Adrenergic receptor-stimulated increase in cAMP in rat heart cells is not coupled to changes in Ca²⁺ dynamics, contractility, or phospholamban phosphorylation. J Biol Chem 269:19151–19156.

24. Xiao RP, Ji X, Lakatta EG. 1995. Functional coupling of the β₂-adrenoceptor to a pertussis toxin-sensitive G protein in cardiac myocytes. Mol Pharmacol 47:322–329.

25. Xiao RP, Avdonin P, Zhou YY, Cheng H, Akhter SA, Eschenhagen T, Lefkowitz RJ, Koch WJ, Lakatta EG. 1999. Coupling of β₂-adrenoceptor to Gᵢ proteins and its physiological relevance in murine cardiac myocytes. Circ Res 84:43–52.

26. Kilts JD, Gerhardt MA, Richardson MD, Sreeram G, Mackensen GB, Grocott HP, White WD, Davis RD, Newman MF, Reves JG, Schwinn DA, Kwatra MM. 2000. β₂-adrenergic and several other G protein-coupled receptors in human atrial membranes activate both Gₛ and G₂i. Circ Res 87:705–709.

27. Mann DL, Kent RL, Parsons B, Cooper G 4th. 1992. Adrenergic effects on the biology of the adult mammalian cardiocyte. Circulation 85:790–804.

28. Communal C, Singh K, Pimentel DR, Colucci WS. 1998. Norepinephrine stimulates apoptosis in adult rat ventricular myocytes by activation of the β-adrenergic pathway. Circulation 98:1329–1334.

29. Communal C, Singh K, Sawyer DB, Colucci WS. 1999. Opposing effects of β₁- and β₂-adrenergic receptors on cardiac myocyte apoptosis: role of a pertussis toxin-sensitive G-protein. Circulation 100:2210–2212.

30. Chesley A, Lundberg MS, Asai T, Xiao RP, Ohtani S, Lakatta EG, Crow MT. 2000. The β₂-adrenergic receptor delivers an antiapoptotic signal to cardiac myocytes through Gᵢ-dependent coupling to phosphatidylinositol 3'-kinase. Circ Res 87:1172–1179.

31. Zhu WZ, Zheng M, Koch WJ, Lefkowitz RJ, Kobilka BK, Xiao RP. 2001. Dual modulation of cell survival and cell death by β₂-adrenergic signaling in adult mouse cardiac myocytes. Proc Natl Acad Sci USA 98:1607–1612.

32. Daaka Y, Luttrell LM, Lefkowitz RJ. 1997. Switching of the coupling of the β₂-adrenergic receptor to different G proteins by protein kinase A. Nature 390:88–91.

33. Narula J, Haider N, Virmani R, Di ST, Kolodgie FD, Hajjar RJ, Schmidt U, Semigran MJ, Dec GW, Khaw BA. 1996. Apoptosis in myocytes in end-stage heart failure. N Engl J Med 335:1182–1189.

34. Olivetti G, Abbi R, Quaini F, Kajstura J, Cheng W, Nitahara JA, Quaini E, Di LC, Beltrami CA, Krajewski S, Reed JC, Anversa P. 1997. Apoptosis in the failing human heart. N Engl J Med 336:1131–1141.

35. CIBIS II Investigators. 1999. The Cardiac Insufficiency Bisoprolol Study II (CIBIS-II): a randomised trial. Lancet 353:9–13.

36. The Beta-Blocker Evaluation of Survival Trial Investigators. 2001. A trial of the beta-blocker bucindolol in patients with advanced chronic heart failure. N Engl J Med 344:1659–1667.

37. De Lean A, Stadel JM, Lefkowitz RJ. 1980. A ternary complex model explains the agonist-specific binding properties of the adenylate cyclase-coupled β-adrenergic receptor. J Biol Chem. 255:7108–7117.

38. Bond RA, Leff P, Johnson TD, Milano CA, Rockman HA, McMinn TR, Apparsundaram S, Hyek MF, Kenakin TP, Allen LF. 1995. Physiological effects of inverse agonists in transgenic mice with myocardial overexpression of the β₂-adrenoceptor. Nature 374:272–276.

39. Benovic JL, Staniszewski C, Mayor FJ, Caron MG, Lefkowitz RJ. 1988. β-Adrenergic receptor kinase. Activity of partial agonists for stimulation of adenylate cyclase correlates with ability to promote receptor phosphorylation. J Biol Chem 263:3893–3897.

40. Samana P, Bond RA, Rockman HA, Milano CA, Lefkowitz RJ. 1997. Ligand-induced overexpression of a constitutively active β₂-adrenergic receptor: pharmacological creation of a phenotype in transgenic mice. Proc Natl Acad Sci USA 94:137–141.

41. Maack C, Flesch M, Südkamp M, Böhm M. 2000. Different intrinsic activities of bucindolol, carvedilol and metoprolol in human ventricular myocardium. Br J Pharmacol 130:1131–1139.

42. Bond RA, Leff P, Johnson TD, Milano CA, Rockman HA, McMinn TR, Apparsundaram S, Hyek MF, Kenakin TP, Allen LF. 1995. Physiological effects of inverse agonists in transgenic mice with myocardial overexpression of the β₂-adrenoceptor. Nature 374:272–276.

43. Nicholas G, Oakley C, Pouleur H, Rousseau MF, Rydén LE, Wellens H for The Xamoterol In Heart Failure Study Group. 1990. Xamoterol in severe heart failure. Lancet 336:1–6.

44. Tuininga YS, Crijns HJ, Brouwer J, van den Berg MP, Man in't Veld AJ, Mulder G, Lie KI. 1995. Evaluation of importance of central effects of atenolol and metoprolol measured by heart rate variability during mental performance tasks, physical exercise, and daily life in stable postinfarct patients. Circulation 92:3412–3415.

45. Bristow MR, Roden RL, Lowes BD, Gilbert EM, Eichhorn EJ. 1998. The role of third-generation β-blocking agents in chronic heart failure. Clin Cardiol 21:I3–I13.

46. Gillman MW, Kannel WB, Belanger A, D'Agostino RB. 1993. Influence of heart rate on mortality among persons with hypertension: the Framingham Study. Am Heart J 125:1145–1148.

47. Wilhelmsen L, Berglund G, Elmfeldt D, Tibblin G, Wedel H, Pennert K, Vedin A, Wilhelmsson C, Werko L. 1986. The multifactor primary prevention trial in Goteborg, Sweden. Eur Heart J 7:278–279.

48. Kjekshus JK. 1986. Importance of heart rate in determining β-blocker efficacy in acute and long-term acute myocardial infarction intervention trials. Am J Cardiol 57:43F–49F.

49. Kjekshus J, Gullestad L. 1999. Heart rate as a therapeutic target in heart failure. Eur Heart J 1(Suppl. H), H64–H69.

50. White HD, Norris RM, Brown MA, Brandt PW, Whitlock RM, Wild CJ. 1987. Left ventricular end-systolic volume as the major determinant of survival after recovery from myocardial infarction. Circulation 76:44–51.

51. Hash TW, Prisant LM. 1997. β-Blocker use in systolic heart failure and dilated cardiomyopathy. J Clin Pharmacol 37:7–19.

Signal Transduction and Cardiac Hypertrophy,
edited by N.S. Dhalla, L.V. Hryshko,
E. Kardami & P.K. Singal
Kluwer Academic Publishers, Boston, 2003

Compartmentation to Lipid Rafts as a Mechanism to Regulate β-adrenergic Receptor Signaling in Cardiomyocytes

Departments of Pharmacology and Medicine
College of Physicians and Surgeons
Columbia University
New York, NY, USA

Summary. The traditional notion that cardiomyocyte β_1- and β_2-adrenergic receptors signal in an identical fashion to adenylyl cyclase and the accumulation of cAMP has been challenged by recent studies demonstrating that: (1) β_1- and β_2-adrenergic receptors promote a marked increase in cAMP accumulation and exert positive inotropic/lusitropic responses in neonatal rat cardiomyocytes; β_1-adrenergic receptors increase cAMP in adult rat cardiomyocytes, but β_2-adrenergic receptors increase twitch amplitude, without inducing a detectable elevation of intracellular cAMP or accelerating the kinetics of relaxation, in adult rat cardiomyocytes. (2) In neonatal rat cardiomyocytes (where both β_1- and β_2-adrenergic receptors increase cAMP accumulation), the β_1-adrenergic receptor pathway is highly sensitive to inhibitory modulation by muscarinic cholinergic agonists, whereas the β_2-adrenergic receptor-dependent increase in cAMP accumulation is not. (3) Overexpression of type VI adenylyl cyclase in neonatal rat cardiomyocytes leads to a selective increase in β-adrenergic receptor-dependent signaling to cAMP formation, without changing cAMP accumulation by agonists of prostenoid, adenosine, glucagon, or histamine receptors. This type of specificity for β-adrenergic receptor subtype signaling cannot be explained by traditional concepts that focus on high-affinity protein-protein interactions between receptors, G proteins, and effectors (freely mobile in the plasma membrane) as the prime determinants of signaling specificity. This chapter summarizes recent studies that identify spatial localization to membrane subdomains (caveolae/lipid rafts) as a mechanism to calibrate β-adrenergic receptor signaling

Address for Correspondence: Susan F. Steinberg, M.D., Associate Professor of Pharmacology and Medicine, Department of Pharmacology, College of Physicians and Surgeons, Columbia University, 630 West 168 Street, New York, New York 10032. Tel: 212-305-4297, Fax: 212-305-8780, E-mail: sfs1@columbia.edu

in cardiomyocytes. This mechanism might be pertinent to the pathogenesis of heart failure, where β-adrenergic receptor signaling is augmented.

Key words: β-adrenergic receptors, caveolae, cardiomyocytes.

INTRODUCTION

It is almost two decades since the first reports linking high circulating levels of norepinephrine with an unfavorable long-term prognosis in heart failure (1). The role of prolonged sympathetic nervous system activation in the progression of heart failure remains an important topic of heart failure research. Original studies focused on desensitization of the β-adrenergic receptor (β-AR) signaling pathway (downregulation of β-ARs themselves as well as changes in other elements of the β-AR signaling pathway such as G proteins, adenylyl cyclase [AC], and GRKs) as a mechanism whereby chronic sympathetic nervous system activation limits the efficacy of inotropic therapies directed at enhancing the performance of the failing heart. However, multiple clinical trials provided consistent and disappointing evidence that the short-term benefits of positive inotropic agents ultimately are replaced by long-term adverse effects, which accelerate the natural history of heart failure. The evidence that these agents aversely affect the heart by directly or indirectly activating cardiotoxic neurohormonal pathways forced a reversal in the prevailing concept regarding the role of the sympathetic nervous system in the biology of heart failure (2). Current thinking is that long-term β-AR activation leads to abnormalities in cardiomyocyte growth, energy utilization, and calcium regulation, leading to a progressively dysfunctional and mechanically inefficient heart. In contrast, β-AR blocking drugs prevent many of the structural/functional changes that develop during the progression of heart failure (2). Consequently, β-AR antagonists have come to be included in current regimens for the therapy of heart failure.

The traditional concept that β_1- and β_2-AR signal in an identical fashion to the Gs-cAMP pathway has been challenged by recent evidence that β_1- and β_2-ARs display distinct biological actions in cardiomyocytes (both to acutely modulate contractile function and to chronically regulate cardiac muscle cell biology). The most dramatic evidence that individual β-AR subtypes exert distinct cardiac actions comes from studies in transgenic mice. Here, cardiac β_2-AR overexpression enhances contractile function without deleterious effects, unless β_2-AR overexpression is driven to very high levels or sustained for protracted intervals (3). Nevertheless, the "therapeutic window" for β_2-AR overexpression is relatively wide. In contrast, the salutary effects of even low-levels of transgenic β_1-AR overexpression are very transient, with even relatively low levels of β_1-AR overexpression leading to an aggressive cardiomyopathy that is not tolerated (4,5). Collectively, these studies support the notion that signals emanating from β_1-ARs are highly cardiotoxic, whereas β_2-AR stimulation is much better tolerated. The severe deleterious biological consequences of β_1-AR overexpression (relative to β_2-ARs, which even may be protective in some settings (6)) provides a rationale to consider β-AR subtype blockers in heart failure therapy. Accordingly, this paper focuses on recent progress towards understanding mechanisms that impart specificity to transmembrane signaling by β_1- and β_2-ARs.

DIFFERENCES IN β_1- AND β_2-AR ACTIVATION OF cAMP ACCUMULATION IN CARDIOMYOCYTES

The traditional teaching held that acute catecholamine-dependent changes in cardiomyocyte contractile function are mediated in large part by the predominant β_1-AR subtype which couples to the stimulatory GTP regulatory protein (G_s), activation of AC, accumulation of cAMP, stimulation of cAMP-dependent protein kinase A (PKA), and phosphorylation of key target proteins (including L-type calcium channels, phospholamban, and troponin I). β_1-AR actions are attributable to a cAMP pathway in all cardiomyocyte preparations (regardless of age or species studied). Cardiomyocytes also express pharmacologically distinct β_2-ARs, which assume increased functional importance in heart failure (where β_1-ARs become down-regulated). Until quite recently, most studies were wedded to the concept that β_2-AR signaling also is confined to the traditional Gs/cAMP pathway (and functionally equivalent to that elicited by β_1-ARs). However, in the course of studies to explore potential developmental changes in β-AR subtype action in the rat ventricle, we identified striking differences in β-AR subtype signaling to cAMP and regulation of contractile function (Figure 1). Specifically, the β_2-AR agonist zinterol promotes a marked increase in cAMP accumulation (and exerts positive inotropic and lusitropic responses) in neonatal rat cardiomyocytes; similar results have been obtained in studies on tissues from failing human ventricles or normal human atrium (7–10). In contrast, β_2-AR agonists increase the amplitude of the twitch, without accelerating the kinetics of relaxation or inducing a detectable elevation of intracellular cAMP (under conditions where control experiments identify a pronounced elevation of cAMP by β_1-ARs) in adult rat cardiomyocytes (10–13, as well as ventricular cells isolated from embryonic mouse or adult dog hearts (14,15)); zinterol provides inotropic support to adult cardiomyocytes only at very high agonist concentrations (in the presence of a β_1-AR antagonist). The failure to detect a β_2-AR-dependent rise in cAMP is not due to β_2-AR linkage to inhibitory G_i proteins (offsetting the effects of the stimulatory G_s pathway); β_2-ARs do not induce a global elevation of cAMP levels following pretreatment with PTX (Ref #16 and unpublished observations). Although these studies do not rule out the possibility that β_2-ARs induce a small, functionally important increase in cAMP that is confined to the sarcolemmal (as espoused by Xiao/Lakatta (17)), we have identified an alternative cAMP-independent pathway for β_2-AR-dependent inotropic support involving β_2-AR-dependent intracellular alkalinization leading to enhanced myofibrillar calcium sensitivity (18). A mechanism that would restrict β_2-AR-dependent activation of cAMP in adult rat cardiomyocytes (that maintain a robust increase in cAMP in response to β_1-AR agonists) is not obvious. Certainly, differences in β-AR subtype signaling to cAMP are not readily explained by the traditional "random collision model" that considers receptors, G-proteins, and effectors freely mobile in

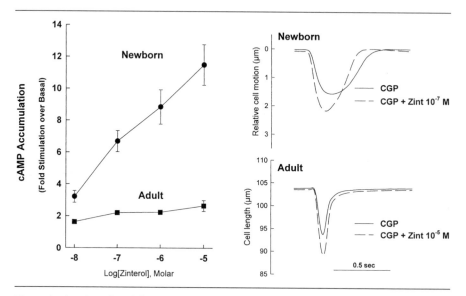

Figure 1. Age-dependent differences in β_2-adrenergic receptor function in rat ventricle. *Left:* Effects of the β_2-AR agonist zinterol on cAMP accumulation in neonatal and adult rat ventricular myocytes. A significant increase in cAMP accumulation in newborn contrasts with the minimal increase in cAMP accumulation in the adult. *Right:* Representative tracings comparing the effect of zinterol on the amplitude and kinetics of the twitch in neonatal and adult cardiomyocytes. In neonate, a low concentration of zinterol increases the amplitude and accelerates the kinetics of the twitch. In adult, β_2-AR responses are identified only with 100-fold higher zinterol in the presence of CGP20712A 10^{-7} M to prevent any β_1-AR activation. Here, zinterol increases with amplitude, without hastening the kinetics of relaxation. Cell shortening is recorded as microns of motion, depicted as downward deflections. Adapted from Ref #11.

the plasma membrane. This constituted the first set of experimental results that forced a re-evaluation of prevailing models of β-AR subtype signaling.

Almost simultaneous with the studies depicted in Figure 1, we obtained a separate set of experimental observations that argued for differences in the molecular organization of β_1- and β_2-AR pathways leading to cAMP accumulation in cardiomyocytes (19). These studies focused on the interaction of β-adrenergic and muscarinic cholinergic receptor (mAChR) signaling pathways, the phenomenon termed accentuated antagonism. Figure 2 shows that the β_1-AR pathway for cAMP accumulation is highly sensitive to inhibition by mAChR agonists in neonatal rat cardiomyocyte cultures. However, the effect of β_2-ARs to promote cAMP accumulation (in neonatal rat cardiomyocytes, where both β_1- and β_2-ARs are linked to an increase in cAMP accumulation) is not susceptible to inhibitory regulation by mAChR agonists. These unpredicted results provided additional evidence that heretofore-unrecognized mechanisms must contribute to the regulation of β-AR subtype signaling in cardiomyocytes.

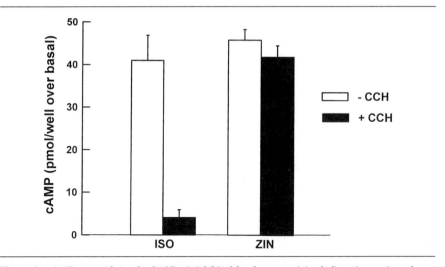

Figure 2. cAMP accumulation by β_1-ARs is inhibited by the muscarinic cholinergic agonist carbachol (10^{-5} M, starting 5 min prior to β-agonist exposure), but cAMP accumulation by β_2-ARs is not. Adapted from Ref #19.

Finally, the Insel laboratory reported that overexpression of type VI AC in neonatal rat cardiomyocytes selectively enhances β-AR-dependent signaling to cAMP formation, without changing the cAMP response to agonists at prostenoid, adenosine, glucagon, or histamine receptors (20). Again, the results suggest distinct modes of G protein-coupled receptor signaling to AC in cardiomyocytes.

MECHANISMS THAT COULD CONFER DISTINCT COUPLING PHENOTYPES FOR β_1- VS β_2-AR (AND FOR β_2-AR IN NEONATAL AND ADULT CARDIOMYOCYTES).

One potential molecular mechanism that could impart specificity to β-AR subtype signaling is compartmentalization to membrane subdomains such as lipid rafts or caveolae (21). Lipid rafts are ubiquitous features of mammalian cells; rafts may be small and dispersed over the cell surface or may coalesce into caveolae, flask-shaped uncoated invaginations on the surface of highly differentiated cells. The distinct lipid and protein composition of lipid rafts or caveolae results in biophysical features that favor local sequestration of certain cytoplasmically-oriented signal transduction molecules (22). In particular, there is evidence that certain GPCRs, their associated G protein α and β subunits, certain AC isoforms, one member of the G protein-coupled receptor kinase family (GRK2, which phosphorylates agonist-activated β-ARs), and the catalytic subunit of protein kinase A (PKA) accumulate in caveolae at steady state and/or following ligand-induced activation (Ref #21 and references cited therein). Localization of these diverse signaling molecules to caveolae provides a mechanism to preassemble membrane-bound oligomeric complexes and thereby facilitate efficient and rapid transmission of signals from agonist-occupied receptors to effectors. Such a mechanism would be particularly pertinent for sympathetic regulation of cardiomyocyte contractility, where delays in β-AR signaling to AC—due to low, potentially limiting, levels of AC expression—would be poorly tolerated. Caveolae also may sequester and/or dampen signaling as a result of the properties of its principle structural protein, caveolin. The mammalian caveolin gene family consists of caveolin-1, caveolin-2 and the muscle-specific caveolin-3 (22). Domain-mapping studies identify a cytosolic membrane-proximal region (designated the "caveolin-scaffolding domain") in caveolin-1 (as well as the structurally homologous caveolin-3) that interacts with putative caveolin-binding motifs in a wide range of signaling molecules (including G protein α subunits and the catalytic domains of certain adenylyl cyclase isoforms, GRK2, and the catalytic subunit of PKA (22,23)). Interactions of signaling proteins with the scaffolding domains of caveolin-1 or -3 may subserve two seemingly contradictory functions. On the one hand, interactions with caveolins serve to sequester signaling molecules and enhance the efficiency (and kinetics) of signal transmission. However, interactions with caveolins also return Gα subunits to the inactive GDP-liganded conformation following cycles of activation and (with notable exceptions) inhibit the kinase activity of many signaling enzymes. The importance of caveolae as a mechanism to dampen signaling through growth regulatory pathways is underscored by observations that [1] caveolin-1 is downregulated in tumor cell lines, [2] forced caveolin-1 reexpression abrogates anchorage-independent growth of transformed cells, and [3] caveolin-1 maps to a tumor suppressor gene locus on chromosome 7q3.1 that is frequently deleted in breast and other epithelial cell cancers.

In view of the aforementioned evidence that GPCRs reside in caveolae either at steady state or following ligand-induced activation, we and others have focused on targeting to caveolin-enriched vesicles as a mechanism to impart specificity for β-AR subtype signaling in cardiomyocytes (20,24,25). Results of recent studies that identify distinct β_1- and β_2-AR targeting to membrane subdomains in neonatal rat cardiomyocyte cultures (a preparation where both β_1- and β_1-ARs promote cAMP accumulation, but only β_1-ARs are susceptible to inhibitory regulation by mAChRs) are schematized in Figure 3. β_1-ARs partition between caveolae, non-caveolar cell surface membranes, and internal membranes, with the vast majority of the β_1-AR excluded from caveolae at rest; β_1-AR partitioning is not detectably altered by agonist activation. In contrast, β_2-AR reside exclusively in caveolae isolated from quiescent cardiomyocytes and egress upon activation. These results fully accommodate the prevailing paradigm for clathrin-dependent endocytosis of β_2-AR following activation by agonist. These results also emphasize the distinct modes for β_1-AR (the predominant β-AR subtype in cardiomyocytes) and β_2-AR regulation in cardiomyocytes. Drastic domain-specific differences in the stoichiometry of β_1- vs. β_2-AR in caveolae (which contain all of the β_2-AR and only a fraction of the β_1-AR) and the remainder of the plasma membrane (which contains only β_1-ARs) are predicted to contribute to the apparent difference in compartmentation of β_1- and β_2-AR responses. Differences in the local stoichiometry of β-AR subtypes and their

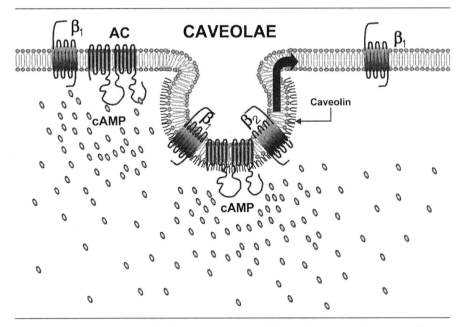

Figure 3. Compartmentation of β-adrenergic receptor signaling pathways in cardiomyocytes. Caveolae are depicted as cave-like indentations of the sarcolemma coated with caveolin. The cartoon depicts β$_1$-ARs and AC in caveolae as well as non-caveolae surface membranes; β$_2$-ARs are confined to caveolae in resting cardiomyocytes. Upon activation, β$_2$-ARs exit from caveolae, whereas β$_1$-AR partitioning is not detectably altered. The cartoon depicts spatial compartmentation of the cAMP signal (the small droplets emanating from the membrane represent cAMP molecules).

signaling partners (including AC) in caveolae also could contribute to the inherently "more efficient" coupling of β$_2$-ARs to AC (relative to β$_1$-ARs, a difference previously ascribed to structural differences between the third intracellular loop structure of β-AR subtypes (26)).

Other studies indicated that spatial constraints, imposed by localization to caveolae, regulate β-AR activation of AC (16). Specifically, β$_2$-AR-dependent activation of exogenous type VI AC (which localizes to caveolae when overexpressed in neonatal rat cardiomyocytes) is facilitated by strategies that promote a local increase in β$_2$-AR density in caveolae. These include β$_2$-AR overexpression or expression of the C-terminal peptide of βARK to sequester G protein βγ dimers and prevent β$_2$-AR desensitization. The observation that exogenous type VI AC in caveolae is not activated by prostenoids is consistent with the existence of spatial constraints that restrict the interactions between prostenoid EP$_2$ receptors (which are excluded from caveolae) and type VI AC. Similarly, spatial co-localization of m$_2$-mAChRs (which are largely are excluded from caveolae) and β$_1$-ARs would be permissive for interactions at the level of cAMP formation. In contrast, the observation that β$_2$-AR-dependent cAMP formation is refractory to inhibitory modulation by mAChRs could be explained by the segregation of β_2-ARs and m_2-mAChRs to separate membrane subdomains. Collectively, these studies support the notion that local changes in the stoichiometry of components of the cAMP-generating pathway critically calibrate β-AR responsiveness.

In keeping with the concept that caveolae function as a platform to nucleate signaling pathways, downstream components of the β-AR signaling machinery required to generate, propagate, or down-regulate the cAMP signal display pronounced differences in subcellular targeting. For example, $G\alpha_i$ is confined to caveolae, whereas $G\alpha_s$ is detected in caveolae and other membrane fractions. This could provide a mechanism to generate a gradient in cAMP levels in cells exposed to catecholamines and is of interest, given the early evidence that local pools of cAMP may differentially activate PKA-dependent functions (27). Similarly, the functional consequences of the cAMP signal may be modulated by local differences in the PKA enzyme, since the RII subunit of PKA is abundant in caveolae but RI is excluded from this site. High concentrations of RII in caveolae would effectively increase local concentrations of the PKA II holoenzyme and promote phosphorylation of proteins in the vicinity of this structure. In contrast, RI at other sites would phosphorylate a distinct spectrum of target proteins (and subserve functions that are distinct from PKAII) in the heart.

As noted above, caveolae also sequester cardiac type V/VI AC. Studies in cardiomyocytes suggest that localization of type V/VI AC to caveolae provides a mechanism to tonically inhibit AC enzyme activity. These studies used cyclodextrin (a membrane-impermeable cholesterol-binding drug) to disrupt the functional integrity of the very cholesterol-enriched caveolae membrane. Cyclodextrin releases AC from caveolae membrane and augments AC activity (25,28). Two possible inhibitory mechanisms have been proposed. AC is reported to be tonically repressed in caveolae through a direct molecular interaction with caveolin (AC co-immunoprecipitates with caveolin and peptides based upon the scaffolding-domain of caveolin inhibit the catalytic activity of cardiac AC isoforms (29,30)). However, there is also evidence for another mechanism involving calcium-dependent local inhibition of the calcium-sensitive cardiac AC isoforms, as a results of co-localization of AC and capacitative calcium entry channels in caveolae (28); both mechanisms may be contributory. Membrane partitioning of channels that serve as effectors for β-ARs has not been considered in any detail. However, evidence that Shaker-like potassium channels reside in caveolae and are regulated by the local lipid microenvironment suggests that channel localization might be an as yet another generalized mechanism to regulate β-AR signaling in excitable tissues (31).

CHALLENGES FOR FUTURE STUDIES

Identify the mechanisms that target β-ARs, G proteins and AC to caveolae/lipid rafts

The mechanism(s) regulating β-AR partitioning between caveolae and the remainder of the PM is not known, but inferences can be deduced from studies of other signaling proteins. There is recent evidence that the biophysical features of lipid rafts and caveolae (an evironment highly enriched in cholesterol and saturated gly-cosphingolipids) favors local sequestration of certain lipid-modified signaling molecules. Saturated acyl chains covalently attached to Gα subunits (myristate and/or palmitate) pack well into this highly-ordered lipid milieu; in contrast, the prenyl groups that modify γ subunits (which are bulky, branched structures) do not pack well and appear to be excluded from rafts (consistent with studies of the βγ dimer crystal structure, which place the γ subunit isoprenyl group between propellers of the β subunit rather than in an orientation that could intercalate in the PM as initially assumed (32)). Hence, lipid modifications of signaling molecules (including β-ARs) may contribute to subcellular targeting. Direct interactions between the cytosolic membrane-proximal region (designated the "caveolin-scaffolding domain") of caveolin-1 and caveolin-3 and putative caveolin-binding motifs in a wide range of signaling molecules (including Gα subunits and the catalytic domains of certain AC isoforms, GRK2, and PKA) provide an alternative mechanism that is predicted to favor the targeting, sequestration, and regulation of signaling molecules in lipid rafts/caveolae (21). Both should be considered in future studies.

Resolve the functional significance of β-AR, G protein and AC targeting to caveolae/lipid rafts in the heart

Currently, the strongest evidence that caveolae/lipid rafts play a functionally important role in muscle biology comes from studies of patients with skeletal muscle dystrophies. The evidence that caveolin-3 associates with components of the dystrophin complex, and is required for the structural integrity of skeletal muscle, has fueled studies of the role of caveolin-3 in muscle dystrophy. Recent studies identify mutations within the coding region of caveolin-3 in several independent kindreds with autosomal dominant limb-girdle muscular dystrophy (LGMD, type 1C (33)). The first two LGMD-1C mutants (a missense mutation in the transmembrane domain and an inframe deletion in the caveolin scaffolding domain) block wild-type caveolin-3 trafficking to the plasma membrane in a dominant-negative fashion; since wild-type caveolin-3 is retained intracellularly and is degraded via the proteosome system, this defect can be ameliorated by inhibitors of proteosomal degradation (34). Three other pathogenic heterozygous missense mutations have been identified in unrelated patients with muscle disease (LGMD-1C, idiopathic hyperCKemia, and rippling muscle disease), further emphasizing the importance of caveolin-3 in muscle cell biology (35). However, it is noteworthy that studies to date have largely explored caveolin-3 function in skeletal muscle; its role in the heart has not been considered in any detail. In this regard, it is noteworthy that caveolin-3 null mice have been generated to explore the role of caveolin-3 in mammalian physiology. Caveolin-3 mice are viable, but display a loss of caveolae and myopathic changes (with abnormalities in the organization of the T-tubule system) in skeletal muscle (36,37). In initial studies, no noticeable pathologic changes were detected in the heart of these animals. It is anticipated that more detailed studies of the role of caveolae/caveolin-3 in transmembrane signaling and cardiomyocyte biology will be revealing.

Finally, a potential role for caveolae (and caveolin-3 expression) in heart failure should be considered, given the recent evidence for reciprocal regulation of caveolin-3 expression and β-AR function in heart failure syndromes (38,39). Insofar as caveolae provide a mechanism to calibrate β-AR signaling to AC, changes in caveolin-3 expression (and the associated alterations in the structural integrity of cardiomyocyte caveolae) would be predicted to alter autonomic regulation of heart. These studies suggest a novel strategy to exploit in further efforts to design therapies to modify the pathogenesis of heart failure.

ACKNOWLEDGMENTS

This work was supported by U.S.P.H.S.-N.H.L.B.I. grant HL-28958.

REFERENCES

1. Cohn JN, Levine TB, Olivari MT, Garberg V, Lura D, Francis GS, Simon AB, Rector T. 1984. Plasma norepinephrine as a guide to prognosis in patients with chronic congestive heart failure. N Engl J Med 311:819–823.
2. Packer M. 1998. Beta-blockade in heart failure. Basic concepts and clinical results. Am J Hypertens 11:23S–37S.
3. Liggett SB, Tepe NM, Lorenz JN, Canning AM, Jantz TD, Mitarai S, Yatani A, Dorn GW. 2000. Early and delayed consequences of β_2-adrenergic receptor overexpression in mouse hearts: critical role for expression level. Circulation 101:1707–1714.
4. Engelhardt S, Hein L, Wiesmann F, Lohse MJ. 1999. Progressive hypertrophy and heart failure in β_1-adrenergic receptor transgenic mice. Proc Natl Acad Sci U S A 96:7059–7064.
5. Bisognano JD, Weinberger HD, Bohlmeyer TJ, Pende A, Raynolds MV, Sastravaha A, Roden R, Asano K, Blaxall BC, Wu SC, Communal C, Singh K, Colucci W, Bristow MR, Port DJ. 2000. Myocardial-directed overexpression of the human β_1-adrenergic receptor in transgenic mice. J Mol Cell Cardiol 32:817–830.
6. Chesley A, Lundberg MS, Asai T, Xiao RP, Ohtani S, Lakatta EG, Crow MT. 2000. The β_2-adrenergic receptor delivers an anti-apoptotic signal to cardiac myocyte through G_i-dependent coupling to phosphatidylinositol 3'-kinase. Circ Res 87:1172–1179.
7. Kaumann AJ, Sanders L, Lynham J, Bartel S, Kuschel M, Karczewski P, Krause EG. 1996. β_2-adrenoceptor activation by zinterol causes protein phosphorylation, contractile effects and relaxant effects through a cAMP pathway in human atrium. Mol Cell Biochem 163/164:113–123.
8. Kaumann A, Bartel S, Molenaar P, Sanders L, Burrell K, Vetter D, Hempel P, Karczewski P, Krause EG. 1999. Activation of β_2-adrenergic receptors hastens relaxation and mediates phosphorylation of phospholamban, troponin I. and C-protein in ventricular myocardium from patients with terminal heart failure. Circulation 99:65–72.
9. Stamatelopoulou SI, Mittmann C, Eschenhagen T. 1999. β-Adrenergic stimulation of azidoanilido [^{32}P]-GTP binding to Gs and Gi/Go proteins in human myocardial membranes. Circulation 100:I-487.
10. Steinberg SF. 2000. The cellular actions of β-adrenergic receptor agonists: Looking beyond cAMP. Circ Res 87:1079–1082.
11. Kuznetsov V, Pak E, Robinson RB, Steinberg SF. 1995. β_2-Adrenergic receptor actions in neonatal and adult rat ventricular myocytes. Circ Res 76:40–52.
12. Steinberg SF. 1999. The molecular basis for distinct β-adrenergic receptor subtype actions in cardiomyocytes. Circ Res 85:1101–1111.
13. Laflamme MA, Becker PL. 1998. Do β_2-adrenergic receptors modulate Ca^{2+} in adult rat ventricular myocytes? Am J Physiol 274:H1308–H1314.
14. Sabri A, Pak E, Alcott SA, Wilson BA, Steinberg SF. 2000. Coupling function of endogenous α_1- and β-adrenergic receptors in mouse cardiomyocytes. Circ Res 86:1047–1053.
15. Altschuld RA, Starling RC, Hamlin RL, Billman GE, Hensley J, Castillo L, Fertel RH, Hohl CM, Robitaille PML, Jones LR, Xiao RP, Lakatta EG. 1995. Response of failing canine and human heart cells to β_2-adrenergic stimulation. Circulation 92:1612–1618.

16. Ostrom RS, Gregorian C, Drenan RM, Xiang Y, Regan JW, Insel PA. 2001. Receptor number and caveolar co-localization determine receptor coupling efficiency to adenylyl cyclase. J Biol Chem 276:42063–42069.
17. Xiao RP, Cheng H, Zhou YY, Kuschel M, Lakatta EG. 1999. Recent advances in cardiac β$_2$-adrenergic signal transduction. Circ Res 85:1092–1100.
18. Jiang T, Steinberg SF. 1997. β$_2$-adrenergic receptors enhance contractility by stimulating HCO$_3^-$-dependent intracellular alkalinization. Am J Physiol 273:H1044–H1047.
19. Aprigliano O, Rybin VO, Pak E, Robinson RB, Steinberg SF. 1997. β$_1$- and β$_2$-adrenergic receptors exhibit differing susceptibility to muscarinic accentuated antagonism. Am J Physiol 272:H2726–H2735.
20. Ostrom RS, Violin JD, Coleman S, Insel PA. 2000. Selective enhancement of beta-adrenergic receptor signaling by overexpression of adenylyl cyclase type 6: colocalization of receptor and adenylyl cyclase in caveolae of cardiac myocytes. Mol Pharmacol 57:1075–1079.
21. Steinberg SF, Brunton LL. 2001. Compartmentalization of G-protein-mediated signal transduction components in the heart. Ann Rev Pharm Tox 41:751–773.
22. Okamoto T, Schlegel A, Scherer PE, Lisanti MP. 1998. Caveolins, a family of scaffolding proteins for organizing "preassembled signaling complexes" at the plasma membrane. J Biol Chem 273:5419–5422.
23. Razani B, Schlegel A, Lisanti MP. 2000. Caveolin proteins in signaling, oncogenic transformation and muscular dystrophy. J Cell Sci 113:2103–2109.
24. Schwencke C, Okumura S, Yamamoto M, Geng YJ, Ishikawa Y. 1999. Colocalization of beta-adrenergic receptors and caveolin within the plasma membrane. J Cell Biochem 75:64–72.
25. Rybin VO, Xu X, Lisanti MP, Steinberg SF. 2000. Differential targeting of beta-adrenergic receptor subtypes and adenylyl cyclase to cardiomyocyte caveolae: A mechanism to functionally regulate the cAMP signaling pathway. J Biol Chem 275:41447–41457.
26. Green SA, Liggett SB. 1994. A proline-rich region of the third intracellular loop imparts phenotypic β$_1$-versus β$_2$-adrenergic receptor coupling and sequestration. J Biol Chem 269:26215–26219.
27. Hohl CM, Li Q. 1991. Compartmentation of cAMP in adult canine ventricular myocytes: Relation to single-cell free Ca^{2+} transients. Circ Res 69:1369–1379.
28. Fagan KA, Smith KE, Cooper DMF. 2000. Regulation of the Ca^{2+}-inhibitable adenylyl cyclase type VI by capacitative Ca^{2+} entry requires localization in cholesterol-rich domains. J Biol Chem 275:26530–26537.
29. Schwencke C, Yamamoto M, Okumura S, Toya Y, Kim SJ, Ishikawa Y. 1999. Compartmentation of cyclic adenosine 3′,5′-monophosphate signaling in caveolae. Mol Endocrinol 13:1061–1070.
30. Toya Y, Schwencke C, Couet J, Lisanti MP, Ishikawa Y. 1998. Inhibition of adenylyl cyclase by caveolin peptides. Endocrinology 139:2025–2031.
31. Martens JR, Navarro-Polanco R, Coppock EA, Nishiyama A, Parshley L, Grobaski TD, Tamkun MM. 2000. Differential targeting of Shaker-like potassium channels to lipid rafts. J Biol Chem 275:7443–7446.
32. Melkonian KA, Ostermeyer AG, Chen JZ, Roth MG, Brown DA. 1999. Role of lipid modifications in targeting proteins to detergent-resistant membrane rafts. Many raft proteins are acylated, while few are prenylated. J Biol Chem 274:3910–3917.
33. Minetti C, Sotgia F, Bruno C, Scartezzini P, Broda P, Bado M, Masetti E, Mazzocco M, Egeo A, Donati MA, Volonté D, Galbiati F, Cordone G, Bricarelli FD, Lisanti MP, Zara F. 1998. Mutations in the caveolin-3 gene cause autosomal dominant limb-girdle muscular dystrophy. Nature Genetics 18:365–368.
34. Galbiati F, Volonte D, Minetti C, Chu JB, Lisanti MP. 1999. Phenotypic behavior of caveolin-3 mutations that cause autosomal dominant limb girdle muscular dystrophy (LGMD-1C). Retention of LGMD-1C caveolin-3 mutants within the golgi complex. J Biol Chem 274:25632–25641.
35. Schlegel A, Lisanti MP. 2001. The caveolin triad: caveolae biogenesis, cholesterol trafficking, and signal transduction. Cytokine Growth Factor Rev 12:41–51.
36. Galbiati F, Engelman JA, Volonte D, Zhang XL, Minetti C, Li M, Hou H, Jr., Kneitz B, Edelmann W, Lisanti MP. 2001. Caveolin-3 null mice show a loss of caveolae, changes in the microdomain distribution of the dystrophin-glycoprotein complex, and T-tubule abnormalities. J Biol Chem 276:21425–21433.
37. Hagiwara Y, Sasaoka T, Araishi K, Imamura M, Yorifuji H, Nonaka I, Ozawa E, Kikuchi T. 2000. Caveolin-3 deficiency causes muscle degeneration in mice. Hum Mol Genet 9:3047–3054.

38. Yamamoto M, Okumura S, Oka N, Schwencke C, Ishikawa Y. 1999. Downregulation of caveolin expression by cAMP signal. Life Sci 64:1349–1357.
39. Hare JM, Lofthouse RA, Juang GJ, Colman L, Ricker KM, Kim B, Senzaki H, Cao S, Tunin RS, Kass DA. 2000. Contribution of caveolin protein abundance to augmented nitric oxide signaling in conscious dogs with pacing-induced heart failure. Circ Res 86:1085–1092.

Signal Transduction and Cardiac Hypertrophy,
edited by N.S. Dhalla, L.V. Hryshko,
E. Kardami & P.K. Singal
Kluwer Academic Publishers, Boston, 2003

Role of Renin-Angiotensin System in Phospholipase C-Mediated Signaling in Congestive Heart Failure

Paramjit S. Tappia, Nina Aroutiounova, and Naranjan S. Dhalla

Institute of Cardiovascular Sciences
St. Boniface General Hospital Research Centre
Departments of Human Nutritional Sciences and
Physiology, Faculties of Human Ecology and Medicine
University of Manitoba
Winnipeg, Canada

Summary. The molecular events underlying the cardiac contractile dysfunction in congestive heart failure are not fully understood. Although different drugs such as angiotensin converting enzyme inhibitors and angiotensin receptor antagonist have been shown to improve cardiac function, the mechanisms of these agents in the failing heart remain largely unexplored. Since phospholipase C (PLC) is known to generate signaling molecules which are critical in increasing contractile force development, it is likely that changes in PLC may be responsible in altering cardiac contractile force in congestive heart failure. This article reviews the role of the renin angiotensin system in PLC signal transduction mechanisms as well as discussion of the potential of such signaling events as additional targets for the action of angiotensin converting enzyme inhibitors and angiotensin receptor antagonists.

Key words: Congestive Heart Failure; Sarcolemma; Renin-Angiotensin System; Angiotensin Converting Enzyme Inhibitors; Angiotensin Receptor Antagonist.

INTRODUCTION

Congestive heart failure (CHF) is a complex syndrome where the heart is unable to pump sufficient blood to meet the needs of the body as a consequence of its inability to contract and relax normally (1–3). The heart failure is invariably preceded by cardiac hypertrophy as an adaptive mechanism due to a wide variety of

Address for Correspondence: Dr. Paramjit S. Tappia, Institute of Cardiovascular Sciences, St. Boniface General Hospital Research Centre (R3020), 351 Tache Avenue, Winnipeg, Manitoba, Canada R2H 2A6. Tel: 204-235-3681, Fax: 204-233-6723, E-mail: ptappia@sbrc.ca

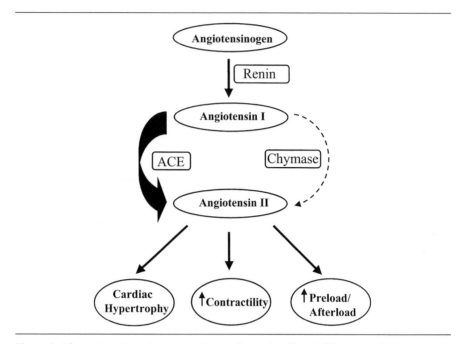

Figure 1. The renin-angiotensin system and its cardiovascular effects. ACE; angiotensin converting enzyme.

neurohumoral changes including the activation of renin-angiotensin system (RAS) (4–6); however, the mechanisms for the transition of cardiac hypertrophy to heart failure are poorly understood. Although substantial information exists regarding the abnormalities in cardiac subcellular organelles in different types of cardiac hypertrophy and heart failure, the role of sarcolemmal (SL) changes is poorly understood. In this regard, a wide variety of SL defects in Ca^{2+}-related transport processes have been identified in different models of heart failure (7–11). Since the domain of the cation-transporting systems is in the hydrophobic region of the membrane (12), abnormalities in the phiosphoipid component of the membrane bilayer and specifically, in signaling phospholipid, may be involved in the SL defects in the heart failure. For example, the decreased number of SL phosphatidylinositol 4,5-bisphosphate (PIP_2) molecules observed by us in CHF (13,14) was suggested to compromise the contractile performance of the heart by causing a depression of the inward rectifier K^+ channel (15–17), as well as of the SL Ca^{2+}-pump (18) and Na^+-Ca^{2+} exchanger activities (19,20). Thus, SL cation-transporting systems are characterized by complex phospholipid requirements and/or phospholipid modulatory mechanisms which remain to be clarified but would appear to involve phospholipid signaling molecules. One of these modulatory mechanisms is the cardiac renin-angiotensin system (RAS) which is known to produce different but marked cardiovascular effects via angiotensin II (Figure 1). Since the RAS is activated in

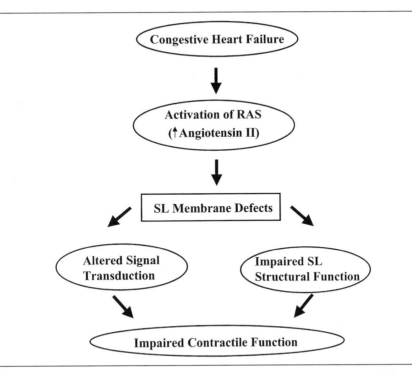

Figure 2. Role of the renin-angiotensin system in the pathogenesis of impaired contractile function during congestive heart failure.

heart failure (4–6) and since prolonged exposure of the heart to angiotensin II has shown to cause changes in cardiac gene expression (21), it is likely that alterations in phospholipid-mediated signaling as well as membrane phospholipid composition in the heart may be due to excessive amounts of circulating angiotensin II and or/ activated cardiac RAS (Figure 2).

RAT MODEL OF CONGESTIVE HEART FAILURE
DUE TO MYOCARDIAL INFRACTION

A great deal of attention has been directed to limiting the infarct size due to coronary occlusion, relatively little is known about the pathophysiology of congestive heart failure which occurs in subjects with 30% or more infarcted left ventricle (22,23). Several animals such as rabbits, cats and dogs exhibit varying degrees of myocardial infarction upon occlusion of the coronary artery (24–32); however, due to high mortality and relatively small infarct size, these animals do not form good experimental models of congestive heart failure. On the other hand, the rat is considered to be an excellent model for studying changes in the viable uninfarcted myocardium following occlusion of the left coronary artery. A wide spectrum of scar formation (15–60% of the left ventricle) has been reported to occur upon occluding the coronary artery in rats; the scar is healed within 3 weeks of the coronary occlusion (33–37). Hypertrophy of the left ventricle (38), as well as of the right ventricle (39,40) which accompanies large infarction in the rat, is considered to be a compensation for preserving the cardiac function as a consequence of the loss of the tissue from the left ventricle. The degree of depression in the left ventricle function was found to depend upon the myocardial infarct size as well as the duration of the disease (41,42). It should be noted that studies concerning the time-course changes in heart function have revealed that mild, moderate and severe stages of congestive heart failure occur at 4, 8 and 16 weeks after inducing myocardial infarction in rats, respectively (43).

Extensive efforts have been made to improve heart function in the infracted animals upon treatments with various pharmacological interventions. In view of the activation of the renin-angiotensin system due to myocardial infraction, treatment of rats with various angiotensin converting enzyme (ACE) inhibitors and angiotensin receptor antagonists have been shown to prevent ventricular remodeling, improve heart function, change hormone profile and reduce mortality in the infracted animals (44–46). It should be noted that interventions such as ACE inhibitors and angiotensin receptor antagonists are used for treatment of patients with different types of heart failure including ischemic cardiomyopathy. In fact there is good experimental evidence showing improved cardiac function and ventricular remodeling in different types of animal models of cardiac hypertrophy and heart failure upon treatment with ACE inhibitors and angiotensin receptor antagonists (47–52). The cellular and molecular mechanisms by which these drugs improve cardiac function in heart failure have not yet been clearly defined.

ALTERATIONS IN PHOSPHOINOSITIDE-SPECIFIC PHOSPHOLIPASE C IN HEART FAILURE

Phosphoinositide-specific phospholipase C (PLC) is a modular monofunctional enzyme, which is involved in numerous transmembranal signals (53). Its most common physiological substrate, PIP_2, is synthesized in the SL membrane by the coordinated and successive action of phosphotidylinositol 4 kinase (PI 4 kinase) and phosphatidylinositol 4-phosphate 5 kinase, (PI4-P 5 kinase) (13,14), PIP_2 is converted into two messenger molecules, inositol 1,4,5-trisphosphate (IP_3) and sn-1, 2 diacylglycerol (DAG), which participate in many different physiological processes (53). The membrane level of PIP_2 is also an important signaling factor as this phosphoinositide is a membrane-attachment site and/or and essential requirement for the function of several proteins (15–17,54–56). The four known classes of mammalian PLC (β, γ, δ and ε) compromise at least eleven isoforms (53) and display differences in structure, function and activation mechanisms in response to stimulation of specific cell-surface receptors (53,57–62). Angiotensin II, $α_1$-adrenergic agonists and endothelin-1 are relevant stimulators of PLC β isoenzymes via the α subunits of the heterotrimeric Gq subfamily (53,61); PLC β has also been shown to be activated by Gβγ dimer (63). Binding of polypeptide growth factors, which are related to angiotensin II (64), to their receptors with intrinsic or associated tyrosine kinase

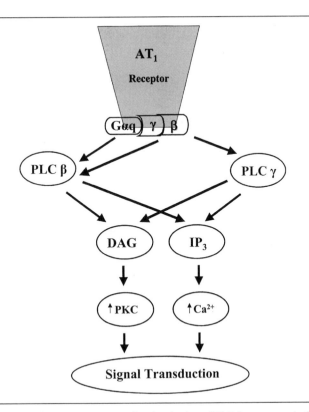

Figure 3. Angiotensin II type 1 receptor mediated activation of PLC isoenzymes via G protein α and βγ subunits.
The α subunit of heterotrimeric Gq stimulates phospholipase (PLC) β isoenzymes, whereas Gβγ subunit activates both PLC β and γ isoenzymes. PLC hydrolytic activity produces 1,2-diacyglycerol (DAG), which in turn activates some isoenzymes of protein kinase C (PKC), and inositol 1,4,5-trisphosphate (IP₃) that can mobilize Ca²⁺ from intracellular stores.

activity activates PLC γ and PLC β isoenzymes (53,65). Figure 3 shows angiotensin II type 1 receptor activation of PLC isoenzymes via Gqα and βγ subunits. A non-tyrosine kinase mediated activation as well as G protein coupled receptor via non-receptor tyrosine kinase activation of PLC γ isoenzymes has also been reported (66). The receptor (α₁-adrenergic, oxytocin, thromboxane)-initiated events for the activation of PLC δ isoenzymes are mediated via transglutaminase II, G_h, a new class of GTP binding protein (67,68). The recently identified PLC ε isoenzymes are activated by Gα₁₂ (69).

It should be noted that PLC γ₁, is activated by intramembranal signaling lipid molecules such as phospholipase D (PLD)-derived phosphatidic acid (PA) which also stimulates PLC δ₁ (70,71). Phospholipase A₂ (PLA₂)—released arachidonic acid (in combination with the microtubule-associated τ protein), as well as phosphatidylinositol 3,4,5-trisphosphate (PIP₃) which is known to specifically interact with the Src homology (SH) 2 domains that are unique to PLC γ_1 (62). PA was found to stimulate SL PLC γ_1 by PA (70,71). Also, it has been shown that: (a) PIP_3 can activate PLC γ_1 but not PLC β_1 and δ_1 isoenzymes (53,62,72); (b) Gqα-coupled PLC β_1 has the distinct feature of being a GTPase activating protein for Gqα (53,60) and it regulates the rate of termination of its signal (60); and c) the mechanisms of recruitment to the plasma membrane differ among the three PLC classes (58). Indeed, the N-terminal part of the pleckstrin homology domain of PLC δ_1 possesses a critical region rich in basic amino acid residues which bind with high affinity to the polar head of PIP_2 (59,73). This property confers on the δ_1 isoenzyme a unique capacity of association with the plasma membrane, which is lost with single basic amino acid replacement by a neutral or acidic amino acid (59). Furthermore, defects in the SH 2 and 3 domains of PLC γ_1 may impair the enzyme association with, and phosphorylation by activated growth factor receptors and its subsequent localization to the cytoskeleton (58). Thus specific responses may occur depending on the type, quantity and activity of the isoenzymes present in the membrane. This is exemplified by the irreplaceable role of PLC γ_1 in mammalian growth and development.

Although little is known about the number and characteristics of PLC isoforms in normal cardiac cells, β_1, β_2, β_3, δ_1, δ_3, γ_1 and two forms of ϵ are expressed in adult vertricular cardiomyocytes (13,74–77). It is pointed out that PLC δ_1 is the predominant SL PLC isoenzyme (13,75). The distinct functions of each PLC isoenzyme in the cardiomyocytes, and the extent of their overlap have yet to be established. However, recently by using adenovirus infection, the α_1-adrenoceptor mediated IP_3 generation in rat neonatal cardiomyocytes has been shown to be mediated by PLC β_1 (78). In spite of the fact that the role of PLC in the development of some types of cardiac hypertrophy and cardiomyopathies is documented, very little is known regarding the status of PLC isoenzymes in CHF. While the hypertrophic stage is associated with an increase in PLC activity (79), the failing stage is associated with downregulation of PLC activity (80). In this regard, the development of cardiac hypertrophy has been suggested to involve and increase in the PLC signaling pathway in stroke-prone spontaneously hypertensive rats (81,82). Studies with the cardiomyopathic hamster (BIO 14.6) have shown that cardiac hypertrophy is due to increase in PLC activity as a consequence of an enhanced responsiveness to angiotensin II (83). With respect to this, it is interesting to note that angiotensin II receptor type 1 overexpression has been reported to induce cardiac hypertrophy (84). The development of hypertrophy in cultured rat neonatal cardiomyocytes induced by endothelin-1 has been reported to be due to activation of PLC β isoenzymes (85). In addition, recent studies in neonatal rat cardiomyocytes stimulated with different hypertrophic stimuli, have shown an increased mRNA expression of PLC β isoenzymes (86). However, the precise mechanisms involved in the transition from hypertrophy to failure have not yet been elucidated, although the targeted overexpression of α subunits of Gq in transgenic mice has been observed to evoke hypertrophy and failure (87–90). We have found differential changes in SL PLC isoenzyme activities and their SL abundance in the failing heart of the

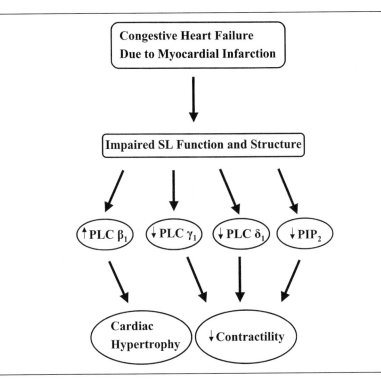

Figure 4. Possible role of phospholipase C isoenzymes in the pathogenesis of congestive heart failure. PLC; phospholipase C.

cardiomyopathic hamster (UM X7.1) (14). Although a depressed total SL PLC activity has been reported in moderate and chronic stage of CHF due to MI, there is an over-abundance and hyperactivity of the SL PLC β_1 isoenzyme; this finding is in direct contrast to a drastic reduction of PLC γ_1 and δ_1 activity and protein mass (5–17% of control values) (13). It is pointed out that while the right ventricle is hypertrophied at moderate as well as in chronic CHF (80), a depressed total SL has been observed only at chronic CHF stage (80). However, differential changes in PLC isoenzymes cannot be excluded and remain to be determined.

CONSEQUENCES OF PLC ISOENZYME CHANGES IN THE FAILING HEART

PLC isoenzyme changes, which would translate into an amplification of the PLC β_1-dependent function with almost complete loss of the PLC γ_1- and δ_1-related signaling, are shown in Figure 4. Specifically, the increase in myocardial catecholamines (91), high density of α_1-adrenoceptors (67,92), normal $G_q\alpha$ level (93), and high mass/activity of PLC β_1, have been observed in the surviving LV tissue of failing hearts, subsequent to MI (13,93). These alterations are consistent with an activation of the $\alpha_1/G_q\alpha/$PLC β_1 pathway and may explain the augmented responsiveness of the failing hearts to $\alpha 1$-agonists in this model of CHF (67). High plasma and myocardial catecholamines selectively downregulate β_1-adrenoceptors in the failing heart, leading to subsensitivity of the β_1 agonist-mediated biochemical and mechanical responses (8). In this context, the $\alpha_1/G_q\alpha/PLC$ β_1 pathway may serve as an efficient source of cardiac positive inotropy in the failing heart. Others have reported unchanged PLC β_1 abundance in a membranous fraction comprising all the membranes of diverse cells present in the failing LV tissue during pressure overload CHF in guinea pigs; however, it was suggested that PLC β_1 activity was increased (94). Also, it is pointed out that signaling via $G_q\alpha/PLC$ β is not only implicated in stimulating cardiac hypertrophy, but also a sustained or excessive activation of the signaling pathway results in apoptotic loss of cardiomyocytes; this change is associated with decreased ventricular function in the failing heart (95). However, a detailed examination of all the components of the pathway will ascertain the relevance of this possibility in human CHF due to MI. An upgrade of the biological functions of angiotensin II and of the other agonists that operate mainly (if not exclusively) via $G_q\alpha/PLC$ β_1 may also be expected.

Many functions may be severely impaired in CHF as a direct consequence of the reduction of PLC γ_1 and δ_1, which are prominent isoforms in normal heart SL. In fact, (a) A significant attenuation of the myocardial responsiveness to polypeptide growth factors, which activate downstream PLC γ_1 as a specific effector enzyme (62), may be expected. The possible action of angiotensin II via this isoenzyme in the heart may also be downgraded, such that angiotensin II would act through the hyperactive $AT_1/G_q\alpha/PLC$ β_1 axis. (b) The stimulation of PLC γ_1 by intramembranal signaling lipid molecules [e.g., PA (formed by PLD), arachidonic acid (released by PLA_2), and PIP_3 (53,67,68)] would be limited. (c) The striking decrease of SL PLC γ_1, which is also stimulated by PA (70,71), may preclude the possibility of valid interactions between SL PLC and PLC in CHF (71,96). (d) Because G_h (transglutaminase II) seems to transfer the signal from α_1-adrenoceptors to PLC δ_1 (53,67,68), this signal be markedly depressed in failing hearts. Accordingly, it should be noted that downregulation of G_h activity is associated with human cardiac failure (97). Also, recently it has been demonstrated that the targeted overexpression of $\alpha 1_A$-adrenoceptor induces a positive inotropic effect (98). Taken together, these observations suggest that a depressed PLC δ_1 activity could compromise cardiac contractile performance. We also observed that PLC isoenzyme protein mass and activity were partially reversed by an *in vivo* delayed monotherapy with an angiotensin converting enzyme (ACE) inhibitor, imidapril (13). This may be seen to confer pathophysiological significance to PLC isoenzymes and may be related to the mechanism of action of this ACE inhibitor. We have also detected a diminished amount of PIP_2 in the SL membranes in CHF due to myocardial infarction, which seems to be due, at least partially, to its decreased synthesis by PI 4 kinase and PI 4-phosphate 5 kinase (13). This may limit the *in vivo* activity of PLC isoenzymes and affect the formations of another membrane-messenger, PIP_3, by PI3 kinase. It should be noted that angiotensin II has been shown to induce activation of PI3 kinase in cardiomyocytes (99). It is conceivable that this effect may occur in the failing heart and therefore could also contribute to the reduced amount of PIP_2.

CONCLUDING REMARKS

Activation of the RAS is considered a hallmark of CHF. The presented evidence indicates that alterations in PLC-mediated signaling mechanisms in the heart may be due to excessive amounts of circulating angiotensin II and or/ activated cardiac RAS and may contribute to cardiac dysfunction. Although the cellular and molecular mechanisms by which ACE inhibitors and angiotensin II receptor antagonists improve the function of the failing heart have not yet been clearly defined, it is likely that PLC may constitute an additional therapeutic target whereby these agents exert their beneficial effects.

ACKNOWLEDGEMENTS

The work reported in this article was supported by a grant from the Canadian Institutes of Health Research (CIHR Group in Experimental Cardiology). NSD holds a CIHR/Pharmaceutical Research and Development Chair in Cardiovascular Research supported by Merck Frosst Canada.

REFERENCES

1. Dhalla NS, Afzal N, Beamish RE, Naimark B, Takeda N, Nagano M. 1993. Pathophysiology of cardiac dysfunction in congestive heart failure. Can J Cardiol 9:873–887.
2. Baig MK, Mahon N, McKenna WJ, Caforio AL, Bonow RO, Francis GS, Gheorghiade M. 1998. The pathophysiology of advanced heart failure. Am Heart J 135:S216–S230.
3. Piano MR, Bondmass M, Schwartz DW. 1998. The molecular and cellular pathophysiology of heart failure. Heart Lung 27:3–19.
4. Weber KT, Sun Y, Guarda E. 1994. Structural remodeling in hypertensive heart disease and the role of hormones. Hypertension 23:869–867.
5. Serneri GG, Boddi M, Cecioni I, Vanni S, Coppo M, Papa ML, Bandinelli B, Bertoolozzi I, Polidori G, Toscano T, Maccherini M, Modesesti PA. 2001. Cardiac angiotensin II formation in the clinical course of heart failure and its relationship with left ventricular function. Circ Res 88:861–863.
6. Barlucchi L, Leri A, Dostal DE, Fiordaliso F, Tada H, Hintze TH, Kajstura J, Nadal-Ginard B, Anversa P. 2001. Canine ventricular myocytes possess a renin-angiotensin system that is upregulated with heart failure. Circ Res 88:298–304.
7. Dhalla NS, Shao Q, Panagia V. 1998. Remodeling of cardiac membranes during the development of congestive heart failure. Heart Failure Reviews 2:261–272.
8. Bristow MR. 1997. Mechanism of action of beta-blocking agents in heart failure. Am J Cardiol 80:26L–40L.
9. Hasenfuss G. 1998. Alterations of calcium-regulatory proteins in heart failure. Cardiovasc Res 37:279–89.
10. deTombe PP. 1998. Altered contractile function in heart failure. Cardiovasc Res 37:367–380.
11. Gomez AM, Valdivia HH, Cheng H, Lederer MR, Santana LF, Cannell MB, McCune SA, Altschuld RA, Lederer WJ. 1997. Defective excitation-contraction coupling in experimental cardiac hypertrophy and heart failure. Science 276:800–806.
12. Hanahan DJ, Nelson DR. 1984. Phospholipids as dynamic participants in biological processes. J Lipid Res 25:1528–1535.
13. Tappia PS, Liu SY, Shatadal S, Takeda N, Dhalla NS, Panagia V. 1999. Changes in sarcolemmal PLC isoenzymes in postinfarct congestive heart failure: partial correction by imidapril. Am J Physiol 277:H40–H49.
14. Ziegelhoffer A, Tappia PS, Mesaeli N, Sahi N, Dhalla NS, Panagia V. 2001. Low level of sarcolemmal phosphatidylinositol 4,5-bisphosphate in cardiomyopathic hamster (UM-X7.1) heart. Cardiovasc Res 49:118–126.
15. Huang CL, Feng S, Hilgemann DS. 1998. Direct activation of inward rectifier potassium channels by PIP_2 and its stabilization by $G\beta\gamma$. Nature 391:803–806.
16. Kobrinsky E, Mirshahi T, Zhang H, Jin T, Logothetis DE. 2000. Receptor-mediated hydrolysis

of plasma membrane messenger PIP_2 leads to K^+-current desensitization. Nat Cell Biol 2:507–514.

17. Hilgemann DW, Ball R. 1996. Regulation of cardiac Na^+, Ca^{2+} exchange and K_{ATP} potassium channels by PIP_2. Science 273:956–959.

18. Caroni P, Zurlini M, Clark A. 1982. The calcium-pumping ATPase of heart sarcolemma. Ann NY Acad Sci 402:402–421.

19. He Z, Feng S, Tong Q, Hilgemann DW, Philipson KD. 2000. Interaction of PIP(2) with the XIP region of the cardiac Na/Ca exchanger. Am J Physiol 278:C661–C666.

20. Asteggiano C, Berberian C, Beauge L. 2001. Phosphatidyl inositol-4,5-bisphosphate bound to bovine cardiac Na+/Ca2+ exchanger displays a MgATP regulation similar to that of the exchange fluxes. Eur J Biochem 268:437–442.

21. Ju H, Scammel-LaFleur T, Dixon IMC. 1996. Altered mRNA abundance of calcium transport genes in cardiac myocytes induced by angiotensin II. J Mol Cell Cardiol 28:1119–1128.

22. Dhalla NS, Dixon IM, Rupp H, Barwinsky J. 1991. Experimental congestive heart failure due to myocardial infarction: sarcolemmal receptors and cation transporters. Basic Res Cardiol 86 (Suppl. 3):13–23.

23. Cheng TO. 1990. Cardiac failure in coronary heart disease. Am Heart J 120:396–412.

24. Lerman RH, Asptein CA, Kagan HM, Osmers EL, Chichester CO, Vogel WM, Connelly CM, Steffee WP. 1983. Myocardial healing and repair after experimental infarction in the rabbit. Circ Res 53:378–388.

25. Cox MM, Berman I, Myerburg RJ, Smets MJ, Kozlovskis PL. 1991. Morphometric mapping of regional myocyte diameters after healing of myocardial infarction in cats. J Mol Cell Cardiol 23:127–135.

26. Vanoli E, De Ferrari GM, Stramba-Badiale M, Hull SS Jr, Foreman RD, Schwartz PJ. 1991. Vagal stimulation and prevention of sudden death in conscious dogs with a healed myocardial infarction. Circ Res 68:1471–1481.

27. Sabbah HN, Kono T, Stein PD, Mancini GB, Goldstein S. 1992. Left ventricular shape changes during the course of evolving heart failure. Am J Physiol 263:H266–H270.

28. McDonald KM, Francis GS, Carlyle PF, Hauer K, Matthews J, Hunter DW, Cohn JN. 1992. Hemodynamic, left ventricular structural and hormonal changes after discrete myocardial damage in the dog. J Am Coll Cardiol 19:460–467.

29. Jugdutt BI, Schwarz-Michorowski BL, Khan MI. 1992. Effect of long-term captopril therapy on left ventricular remodeling and function during healing of canine myocardial infarction. J Am Coll Cardiol 19:713–721.

30. Connelly CM, Ngoy S, Schoen FJ, Apstein CS. 1992. Biomechanical properties of reperfused transmural myocardial infarcts in rabbits during the first week after infarction. Implications for left ventricular rupture. Circ Res 71:401–413.

31. Knowlton AA, Connelly CM, Romo GM, Mamuya W, Apstein CS, Brecher P. 1992. Rapid expression of fibronectin in the rabbit heart after myocardial infarction with and without reperfusion. J Clin Invest 89:1060–1068.

32. Kozlovaskis PL, Gerdes AM, Smets M, Moore JA, Bassett AL, Myerburg RJ. 1991. Regional increase in isolated myocyte volume in chronic myocardial infarction in cats. J Mol Cell Cardiol 23:1459–1466.

33. Johns TNP, Olson BJ. 1954. Experimental myocardium infarction: method of coronary occlusion in small animals. Ann Surg 140:675–682.

34. Selye H, Bajusz E, Grasso S, Mendell P. 1960. Simple techniques for the surgical occlusion of coronary vessels in the rat. Angiology 11:398–407.

35. Pfeffer MA, Pfeffer JM, Fletcher PJ, Braunwald E. 1991. Progressive ventricular remodeling in rat with myocardial infarction. Am J Physiol 260:H1406–H1414.

36. Gopalkrishnan M, Triggle DJ, Rutledge A, Kwon YW, Bauer JA, Fung HL. 1991. Regulation of K^+ and Ca^{2+} channels in experimental cardiac failure. Am J Physiol 261:H1979–H1987.

37. Chasteney EA, Liang CS, Hood WB Jr. 1992. β-adrenoceptor and adenylate cyclase function in the infarct model of rat heart failure. Proc Soc Exp Biol Med 200:90–94.

38. Anversa P, Beghi C, Kikkawa Y, Olivetti G. 1986. Myocardial infarction in rats. Infarct size, myocyte hypertrophy, and capillary growth. Circ Res 58:26–37.

39. Anversa P, Beghi C, McDonald SL, Levicky V, Kikkawa Y, Olivetti G et al. 1984. Morphometry of right ventricular hypertrophy induced by myocardial infarction in the rat. Am J Pathol 116:504–513.

40. Zimmer HG, Gerdes AM, Lorlet S, Mall G. 1990. Changes in heart function and cardiac cell size in rats with chronic myocardial infarction. J Mol Cell Cardiol 22:1231–1243.
41. Fletcher PJ, Pfeffer JM, Pfeffer MA, Braunwald E. 1981. Left ventricular diastolic pressure-volume relations in rats with healed myocardial infarction. Effects on systolic function. Circ Res 49:618–626.
42. Pfeffer JM, Pfeffer MA, Fletcher PJ, Braunwald E. 1984. Ventricular performance in rats with myocardial infarction and failure. Am J Med 76:99–103.
43. Dixon IMC, Lee S-L, Dhalla NS. 1990. Nitrendipine binding in congestive heart failure due to myocardial infarction. Circ Res 66:782–788.
44. Ren B, Lukas A, Shao Q, Guo M, Takeda N, Aitken RM, Dhalla NS. 1998. Electrocardiographic changes and mortality due to myocardial infarction in rats with or without imidapril treatment. J Cardiovasc Pharmacol Therapeut 3:11–22.
45. Kuizinga MC, Smits JF, Arends JW, Daemen MJAP. 1998. AT$_2$ receptor blockade reduces cardiac interstitial cell DNA synthesis and cardiac function after rat myocardial infarction. J Mol Cell Cardiol 30:425–434.
46. Liu Y-H, Yang X-P, Sharov VG, Nass O, Sabbah HN, Peterson E, Carretero OA. 1997. Effects of angiotensin-converting enzyme inhibitors and angiotensin II type 1 receptor antagonists in rats with heart failure. Role of kinins and angiotensin II type 2 receptors. J Clin Invest 99:1926–1935.
47. Ruzicka M, Skarda V, Leenen FHH. 1995. Relevance of blockade of cardiac and circulatory angiotensin-converting enzyme for the prevention of volume overload-induced cardiac hypertrophy. Circulation 92:3568–3573.
48. Gervais M, Fornes P, Richer C, Nisato D, Giudicelli JF. 2000. Effects of angiotensin II AT1-receptor blockade on coronary dynamics, function, and structure in postischemic heart failure in rats. J Cardiovasc Pharmacol 36:329–337.
49. Fischer TA, Singh K, O'Hara DS, Kaye DM, Kelly RA. 1998. Role of AT1 and AT2 receptors in regulation of MAPKs and MKP-1 by ANG II in adult cardiac myocytes. Am J Physiol 275:H906–H916.
50. Yang X, Zhu Q, Fong J, Gu X, Hicks GL Jr, Bishop SP, Wang T. 1996. Enalaprilat, an angiotensin-converting enzyme inhibitor, enhances functional preservation during long-term cardiac preservation. Possible involvement of bradykinin and PKC. J Mol Cell Cardiol 28:1445–1452.
51. Flesch M, Schiffer F, Zolko O, Pinto Y, Stasch JP, Knorr A, Ettelbruck S, Bohm M. 1997. Angiotensin receptor antagonism and angiotensin converting enzyme inhibition improve diastolic dysfunction and Ca^{2+}-ATPase expression in the sarcoplasmic reticulum in hypertensive cardiomyopathy. J Hypertension 15:1001–1009.
52. Shao Q, Ren B, Zarain-Herzberg A, Ganguly PK, Dhalla NS. 1999. Captopril treatment improves the sarcoplasmic reticular Ca^{2+} transport in heart failure due to myocardial infarction. J Mol Cell Cardiol 31:1663–1672.
53. Rhee SG. 2001. Regulation of phosphoinositide-specific phospholipase C. Annu Rev Biochem 70:281–312.
54. Toker A. 1998. The synthesis and cellular roles of phosphatidylinositol 4,5-bisphosphate. Curr Opin Cell Biol 10:254–261.
55. Buckland AG, Wilton DC. 2000. Anionic phospholipids, interfacial binding and the regulation of cell functions. Biochim Biophys Acta 1483:199–216.
56. Downes CP, Currie RA. 1998. Lipid signaling. Curr Biol 8:R865–R867.
57. Ji QS, Winnier GE, Niswender KD, Hortsman D, Wisdom R, Magnuson MA, Carpenter G. 1997. Essential role of the tyrosine kinase substrate phospholipase C-γ1 in mammalian growth and development. Proc Natl Acad Sci USA 94:2999–3003.
58. Singer WD, Brown HA, Sternweis PC. 1997. Regulation of eukaryotic phosphatidylinositol-specific phospholipase C and phospholipase D. Annu Rev Biochem 66:475–509.
59. Yagisawa H, Sakuma K, Paterson HE, Cheung R, Allen V, Hirata H, Watanabe Y, Hirata M, Williams RL, Katan M. 1998. Repalcements of single basic amino acids in the pleckstrin homology domain of phospholipase C-δ$_1$ alter the ligand binding, phospholipase activity and interaction with the plasma membrane. J Biol Chem 273:417–424.
60. James SR, Downes CP. 1997. Structural and mechanistic features of phospholipase C: effectors of inositol phospholipid-mediated signal transduction. Cell Signal 9:329–336.
61. Katan M. 1998. Families of phosphoinositide-specific phospholipase C: structure and function. Biochim Biophys Acta 1436:5–17.
62. Rhee SG, Bae YS. 1997. Regulation of phosphoinositide-specific phospholipase C isoenzymes. J Biol Chem 272:15045–15048.

63. Lee CW, Lee KH, Lee SB, Park D, Rhee SG. 1994. Regulation of phospholipase C-β_4 by ribonucleotides and the α subunit of Gq. J Biol Chem 269:25335–25338.

64. van Bilsen, 1997. M. Signal transduction revisited: recent developments in angiotensin II signaling in the cardiovascular system. Cardiovasc Res 36:310–322.

65. Tappia PS, Padua RR, Panagia V, Kardami E. 1999. Fibroblast growth factor-2 stimulates phospholipase Cβ in adult cardiomyocytes. Biochem Cell Biol 77:569–575.

66. Sekiya F, Bae Y-S, Rhee SG. 1999. Regulation of phospholipase C isoenzymes: activation of phospholipase C-γ in the absence of tyrosine-phosphorylation. Chem Phys Lipids 98:3–11.

67. Im H-J, Russell MA, Feng J-F. 1997. Transglutaminase II: a new class of GTP-binding protein with new biological functions. Cell Signal 9:477–482.

68. Park H, Park ES, Lee HS, Yun HY, Kwon NS, Baek KJ. 2001. Distinct characteristic of Gαh (transglutaminase II) by compartment: GTPase and transglutaminase activities. Biochem Biophys Res Commun 284:496–500.

69. Lopez I, Mak EJ, Ding J, Hamm HE, Lomasney JW. 2001. A novel bifunctional phopsholipase C that is regulated by Gα12 and stimulates the Ras/mitogen-activated protein kinase pathway. J Biol Chem 276:2758–2765.

70. Henry RA, Boyce SY, Kurz T, Wolf RA. 1995. Stimulation and binding of myocardial phospholipase C by phosphatidic acid. Am J Physiol 269:C349–C358.

71. Tappia PS, Yu C-H, Di Nardo P, Pasricha AK, Dhalla NS, Panagia V. 2001. Depressed responsiveness of phospholipase C isoenzymes to phosphatidic acid in congestive heart failure. J Mol Cell Cardiol 33:431–440.

72. Bony C, Roche S, Shuichi U, Sasaki T, Crackower MA, Penninger J, Mano H, Puceat M. 2001. A specific role of phosphatidylinositol 3-kinase γ. A regulation of autonomic Ca^{2+} oscillations in cardiac cells. J Cell Biol 152:717–728.

73. Tall E, Dormán G, Garcia P, Runnels L, Shah S, Chen J, Profit A, Gu Q-M, Chaudhary A, Prestwich GD, Rebecchi MJ. 1997. Phosphoinositide binding specificity among phospholipase C isoenzymes as determined by photo-cross-linking to novel substrate and product analogs. Biochemistry 36:7239–7248.

74. Wolf RA. 1993. Specific expression of phospholipase C-δ_1 and γ_1 by adult cardiac ventricular myocytes (Abstract) Circulation 88 (Suppl. 1):I–241.

75. Wolf RA. 1992. Association of phospholipase C-δ with a highly enriched preparation of canine sarcolemma. Am J Physiol 263:C1021–C1028.

76. Gonzalez-Yanes C, Santos-Alvarez J, Sanchez-Margalet V. 2001. Pancreastatin, a chromogranin A-derived peptide, activates Gα_{16} and phospholipase C-β2 by interacting with specific receptors in rat heart membranes. Cell Signal 13:43–49.

77. Song C, Hu CD, Masago M, Kariyai K, Yamawaki-Kataoka Y, Shibatohge M, Wu D, Satoh T, Kataoka T. 2001. Regulation of a novel human phospholipase C, PLCε, through membrane targeting by Ras. J Biol Chem 276:2752–2757.

78. Arthur JF, Matkovich SJ, Mitchell CJ, Biden TJ, Woodcock EA. 2001. Evidence for selective coupling of α_1- adrenergic receptors to phospholipase C-β_1 in rat neonatal cardiomyocytes. J Biol Chem 276:37341–37346.

79. Dhalla NS, Xu Y-J, Sheu S-S, Tappia PS, Panagia V. 1997. Phosphatidic acid: a potential signal transducer for cardiac hypertrophy. J Mol Cell Cardiol 29:2865–2871.

80. Meij JTA, Panagia V, Mesaeli N, Peachell JL, Afzal N, Dhalla NS. 1997. Identification of changes in cardiac phospholipase C activity in congestive heart failure. J Mol Cell Cardiol 29:237–246.

81. Shoki M, Kawaguchi H, Okamoto H, Sano H, Sawa H, Kudo T, Hirao N, Sakata Y, Yasuda H. 1992. Phosphatidylinositol and inositolphosphatidate metabolism in hypertrophied rat heart. Jpn Circ J 56:142–147.

82. Kawaguchi H, Sano H, Iizuka K, Okada H, Kudo T, Kageyama K, Muramoto S, Murakami T, Okamoto H, Mochizuki N, Kitabatke A. 1993. Circ Res 72:966–972.

83. Sakata Y. 1993. Tissue factors for contributing to cardiac hypertrophy in cardiomyopathic hamsters (Bio14.6): involvement of transforming growth factor-β1 and tissue rennin-angiotensin system in the progression of cardiac hypertrophy. Hokkaido Igaku Zasshi 68:18–23.

84. Paradis P, Dali-Youcef N, Paradis FW, Thibault G, Nemer M. 2000. Overexpression of angiotensin II type 1 receptor in cardiomyocytes induces cardiac hypertrophy and remodeling. Proc Natl Acad Sci USA 97:931–936.

85. Lamers JM, Eskildesen-Helmond YE, Resink AM, DeJonge HW, Bezstarosti K, Sharma HS, van Heugten HA. 1995. Endothelin-1-induced phospholipase C-β and D and protein kinase C

isoenzyme in sigmaling leading to hypertrophy in rat cardiomyocytes. J Cardiovasc Pharmacol 26 (Suppl. 3):S100–S103.

86. Schnabel P, Mies F, Nohr T, Geisler M, Bohm M. 2000. Differential regulation of phospholipase C-beta isozymes in cardiomyocyte hypertrophy. Biochem Biophys Res Commun 275:1–6.

87. D'Angelo DD, Sakata Y, Lorenz JN, Boivin GP, Walsh RA, Dorn G. 1997. Transgenic Gαq overexpression induces contractile failure in mice. Proc Natl Acad Sci USA 94:8121–8126.

88. Sakata Y, Hoit BD, Liggett SB, Walsh RA, Dorn GW. 1998. Decompensation of pressure-overload hypertrophy in Gαq-overexpressing mice. Circulation 97:1488–1495.

89. Mende U, Kagen A, Cohen A, Aramburu J, Schoen FJ, Neer EJ. 1998. Transient cardiac expression of constitutively active Gαq leads to hypertrophy and dilated cardiomyopathy by calcineurin-dependent and independent pathways. Proc Natl Acad Sci USA 95:13893–13898.

90. Dorn GW, Tepe NM, Wu G, Yatani A, Liggett SB. 2000. Mechanisms of impaired β-adrenergic receptor signaling in Gαq-mediated cardiac hypertrophy and ventricular dysfunction. Mol Pharmacol 57:278–287.

91. Esler M, Kaye D, Lambert G, Esler D, Jennings G. 1997. Adrenergic nervous system in heart failure. Am J Cardiol 80:7L–14L.

92. Dixon IMC, Dhalla NS. 1991. Alterations in cardiac adrenoceptors in congestive heart failure secondary to myocardial infarction. Coronary Artery Dis 2:805–814.

93. Ju H, Zaho S, Tappia PS, Panagia V, Dixon IMC. 1998. Expression of Gqα and PLC-β in scar and border tissue in heart failure due to myocardial infarction. Circulation 97:892–898.

94. Jalili T, Takeishi Y, Song G, Ball NA, Howles G, Walsh RA. 1999. PKC translocation without changes in Gαq and PLC-β protein abundance in cardiac hypertrophy and failure. Am J Physiol 277: H2298–H22304.

95. Adams JW, Brown JH. 2001. G-proteins in growth and apoptosis: lessons from the heart. Oncogene 20:1626–1634.

96. Panagia V, Tappia PS, Yu C, Takeda N, Dhalla NS. 1999. Abnormalities in sarcolemmal phospholipase D and phospholipase C isoenzymes and in their interactions in post-infarcted failing hearts. Lipids 34:S73–S74.

97. Hwang K-C, Gray C, Sweet WE, Moravec CS, Im MJ. 1996. α_1-adrenergic receptor coupling with Gh in the failing human heart. Circulation 94:718–726.

98. Lin F, Owens WA, Chen S, Stevens ME, Kesteven S, Arthur JF, Woodcock EA, Feneley MP, Graham RM. 2001. Targeted α_{1A}-adrenergic receptor overexpression induces enhanced cardiac contractility but not hypertrophy. Circ Res 89:343–350.

99. Rabkin SW, Goutsouliak V, Kong JY. 1997. Angiotensin II induces activation of phosphatidylinositol 3-kinase in cardiomyocytes. J Hypertens 15:891–899.

Signal Transduction and Cardiac Hypertrophy,
edited by N.S. Dhalla, L.V. Hryshko,
E. Kardami & P.K. Singal
Kluwer Academic Publishers, Boston, 2003

JAK/Stat Signaling in Cardiac Diseases

M.A.Q. Siddiqui* and Eduardo Mascareno

Center for Cardiovascular and Muscle Research
Department of Anatomy and Cell Biology
State University of New York
Downstate Medical Center
450 Clarkson Avenue
Brooklyn, New York 11203

Summary. The molecular mechanisms that initiate and propagate myocardial diseases are known to involve participation of distinct signaling pathways. The onset of myocardial hypertrophy and ischemia followed by reperfusion, hypoxia/reoxygenation and oxygen radicals is accompanied by an upregulated level of the heart tissue-localized renin-angiotensin system (RAS). The major signaling events attributed to the RAS are the G-protein receptor signaling and those that are associated with the redox regulated system. The cross-talk likely to occur between these pathways may reach a putative focal point needed to program the execution of the disease related transcriptional events. In this context, the JAK2/Stat proteins play a pivotal role. Our studies support the notion that signals induced by diverse stimuli are somehow linked to the activated Janus Kinase-2 (JAK2) which appears to be the determining factor in triggering the execution of the disease related genetic program in cardiomyocytes. If this signaling pathway in cardiomyocyte plays a role in initiation and progression of cardiac diseases, specific inhibitors of the components of the pathway might be important as therapeutic agents. Selective inhibition of JAK2 by AG490 caused a reduction of cardiac hypertrophy, ischemic injury and cell death and a simultaneous increase in cardiac function. These observations thus provide new conceptual paradigms in heart disease research making it possible to develop novel cardioprotective agents mechanistically based on modulation in signaling events.

Key words: Janus Kinase 2, G-protein receptor signaling, cardiac hypertrophy, renin-angiotensin system, redox regulated system.

* Corresponding Author. Phone: 718-270-1014, Fax: 718-270-3732, E-mail:msiddiqui@netmail.hscbklyn.edu.

SIGNAL TRANSDUCTION IN MYOCARDIAL HYPERTROPHY

Cardiovascular researchers have long been intrigued by the possibility of gene based therapy for treatment of cardiovascular disorders. In a large segment of adult population at risk for hypertension, hemodynamic pressure overload of the heart leads to enlargement (hypertrophy) of the heart and its functional deterioration. Initially, the enlargement results from an adaptive response on the part of the heart to alleviate pressure overload. Interestingly, many aspects of pathological cardiac hypertrophy in adult animals and in human appear to be similar to those of fetal cardiac development, leading to the notion that adult heart cells respond to pressure overload by calling upon the fetal growth program to provide compensatory growth and increase contractility. Indeed, many contractile protein genes originally expressed during myofibrillogenesis in fetal cardiomyocytes are re-expressed during adaptive hypertrophic growth in the adult heart. The similarities in gene expression profiled between fetal and adult hypertrophic myofibrillogenic programs suggest that many of the transcription factors, signal transduction proteins, and other regulatory proteins responsible for fetal growth may also be active in adult cardiac hypertrophy.

Given the different demands placed upon the cardiac muscle cells, it is likely that two different genetic programs are operating to bring about hyperplasia and hypertrophic growth. It is apparent that the adaptive response of cardiac muscle cells to pressure overload is directed towards increasing contractility through re-expression of the developmental programs of cardiac growth and myofibrillogenesis. The re-expression of a developmental growth program during hypertrophy suggests that all the regulatory molecules responsible for coordinated and controlled gene expression within the program are also re-expressed during adaptive growth.

The most widely accepted model of the genetic and sub-cellular events underlying hypertrophy of cardiac muscle cells suggests that hypertrophic stimuli, either mechanical or hormonal, activate a variety of cell surface receptors that are linked to signal transducers (1). The molecular mechanism(s) that leads to the onset and maintenance of cardiac hypertrophy is still unknown and is under intense investigation. So far, four main signal transduction pathways are implicated in relaying the extracellular signals that mediate myocardial hypertrophy, namely the mitogen activated protein kinases (MAPK) pathway (1–3), the janus kinase/signal transducers and activators of transcription (Jak/Stat) pathway (2–4), the Ca++/calmodulin (CaM)-dependent calcineurin pathway (5–6), and phosphoinositide 3-kinase (7–8). It is well documented that mechanical stretch (9) and several known hypertrophic ligands, such as, cardiotrophin-1 (10), IL-6 (11), Leukemia inhibitory factor (12), and angiotensin II (13), mediate the hypertrohic response. These transducers can directly activate and cross activate multiple signal transduction pathways that lead to the nucleus where they activate nuclear genes. In addition to the proto-oncogene and contractile protein genes, growth factors and signaling molecules such as angiotensin II are also expressed by hypertrophic cardiac muscle cells. These molecules sustain the adaptive response of hypertrophic cardiac muscle cells by acting in an autocrine fashion to maintain the hypertrophic state. Although the signal transduction pathway responsible for transmitting the hypertrophic signal from membrane to nucleus have been the subject of intense study, how these pathways lead to activation of genes involved in implementing and in maintaining hypertrophic growth is only now being addressed. Our laboratory has focused on this aspect of cardiac hypertrophy by examining the genetic mechanism controlling expression of the gene involved in this process, such as for angiotensinogen. We have taken an approach that first seeks to identify the transacting factors that interact with the target elements in the responding genes to mediate the signal-to-gene interactions.

RENIN ANGIOTENSIN SYSTEM AND THE JAK/STAT SIGNAL TRANSDUCTION PATHWAY

It is becoming increasingly clear that aberrations in the RAS are significant contributors to the etiology of hypertension and cardiac hypertrophy (14). The RAS controls blood pressure through complex biochemical and signal transduction pathways that together regulate the production of angiotensinogen and its conversion to the signaling peptide angiotensin II. It is angiotensin II that acts as a first messenger by binding to its receptor, the AT1 receptor, on the surface of target cells that increases intracellular calcium levels and activates second messenger such as protein kinase C as well as other signaling pathways (15). Although it has been known for some time that angiotensinogen produced by the liver acts to control blood pressure and may be involved in hypertension, more recent evidence suggest that regulation of angiotensinogen expression is tissue specific and the local sites of synthesis, such as the heart, may play a biological role independent of the circulating angiotensinogen from liver. When cardiac cells are treated with angiotensin II, not only is angiotensinogen gene expression is stimulated, but the cardiac cells become hypertrophic. At the molecular level, these findings suggest a number of differences between local RAS and systemic RAS. First, angiotensin II receptors reside in heart cells and unlike the kidney form the basis of an autocrine type of RAS for the heart (16). Secondly, it appears that angiotensin II stimulation of heart cells lead primarily to expression of the angiotensinogen gene whereas in noncardiac cells, such as renal cells, angiotensin II stimulates a protein kinase C signaling pathway that promotes sodium uptake. This would suggest that while heart and renal cells express the same type of cell surface angiotensin II receptors, these receptors are linked to different signal transduction pathways that mediate different effector functions.

Our laboratory has focused on angiotensin II and has provided new insights into how angiotensin II activates a normal cellular signaling pathway to bring about activation of angiotensinogen gene (4). Angiotensin II promotes myocardial hypertrophy via activation of the RAS. When angiotensin II binds to the cell surface receptor it activates G proteins that trigger a cascade of multiple second messenger system (17). This second messenger cascade leads to the nucleus where it ultimately causes the activation of the angiotensinogen gene which leads to more production of angiotensinogen II and activation of RAS. Our laboratory has shown that angiotensin II activates the angiotensinogen gene through the JAK/Stat pathway of signal transduction and gene activation. The mechanism by which the JAK/Stat pathway signals from the cell membrane to the cell nucleus has been elucidated by Ihle (18) and Darnell's laboratory (19). The specificity of the JAK/Stat signal transduction pathway resides at different levels. For instance, there are reports indicating that the Stat proteins regulate specificity through the amino terminus (20), the DNA binding domain (21) the Sh2 domain (22), the phosphorylation levels (23,24), and the cis element recognized by the activated Stats (25,26). Sequence analysis of the angiotensinogen gene promoter has revealed the presence of a conserved sequence element (ST-domain) originally found in the promoter of the Gamma Interferon gene and required for its activation by Stat proteins. By using the Stat binding domain as a probe in gel electrophoretic mobility shift assay, this promoter element was shown to bind Stat proteins in cardiomyocytes treated with angiotensin II (13).

Our studies support the idea that normal cell signal transduction pathways such as the JAK/Stat pathways are used by hypertrophic agents to transmit signals where they activate nuclear genes. Our results document that the peptide hormone angiotensin II turns on the angiotensinogen gene through activation of JAK/Stat pathway. Activation of the angiotensinogen gene by angiotensin II to produce more of the angiotensinogen prohormone for processing could lead to the formation of an autocrine loop that positively reinforces production of angiotensin II in cardiomyocytes. This feedback loop may lead to an overactive RAS which, in turn, maintains the hypertrophic state. Our hypothesis was supported independently by analysis of another cytokine, cardiotrophin-1. It was observed that cardiotrophin-1 activates Stat3 in cardiomyocytes which in turn activates the angiotensinogen promoter via the conserved St-domain and maintains the autocrine loop. This activation is blocked by losartan, an AT1 inhibitor, thus establishing the role of the Jak/Stat pathway in the RAS mediated maintenance of myocardial hypertrophy (27).

In our subsequent study, we used the transverse aortic constriction (TAC) model, well-established as an experimental model in mice, to study the effect of subjecting mice to pressure overload hypertrophy in presence of tyrphostin AG490, a specific inhibitor of the Jak2 kinase. Mice subjected to TAC showed induction of the hypertrophic phenotype with concomitant activation of the Jak2/STAT signaling pathway. However, when mice were chronically treated with tyrphostin AG490, we observed an attenuation of the hypertrophic response as characterized by morphological, histological and molecular markers. Thus, it appears that activation of Jak2 kinase during pressure overload hypertrophy represents an early step that perhaps controls the downstream signaling events involved in promoting or maintaining the hypertrophic response. Further support for a convergence point of Jak2 kinase is the fact other established hypertrophic transducer, such as, mechanical stretch, cardiotrophin-1, IL-6, Leukemia inhibitory factor, and angiotensin II, all activate Jak2 kinase, which, therefore, is likely to play a pivotal role in the etiology of hypertrophy-mediated cardiac disorders.

JAK/STAT SIGNALING IN ISCHEMIA/REPERFUSION INJURY

Several studies using isolated working heart as an in vivo model have documented the involvement of AT1 in the pathogenesis of ischemia/reperfusion injury and in the consequent myocardial dysfunction (28). Administration of losartan, the AT1 receptor antagonist, causes functional recovery of the ischemic heart suggesting that the signaling pathway mediated through the AT1 receptor is indeed involved in cardiovascular dysfunction. In a recent study (29), we reported that when rat hearts are subjected to ischemia/reperfusion there is a significant increase in the activated Stat 5A and Stat 6 binding to angiotensinogen promoter with a concommitant increase in the angiotensinogen mRNA level. Treatment of the hearts with losartan resulted in loss of Stat protein interactions with angiotensinogen promoter DNA and consequently the loss of activated angiotensinogen mRNA levels. Likewise, inhibition of Jak2 which phosphorylates Stat 5A and Stat 6 by tyrphostin AG490 caused reduction in Stat angiotensinogen promoter interaction and in the level of angiotensinogen mRNA. AG490 treatment also caused a marked reduction in the infarct size and in apoptotic cell death of cardiomyocytes which is accompanied by an improvement in the hemodynamic performance of the heart. Thus, our results provide, for the first time, the evidence that JAK/STAT signaling plays a pivotal role in stimulation of the RAS in ischemia reperfusion injury. Our evidence establishes that the activation of Stats and their binding to ST domain in the angiotensinogen promoter are linked to activation of the heart tissue RAS, a documented regulator of physiological function of the heart including in ischemic injury. Evidence was presented in support of the causal relationship between the angiotensinogen mRNA level in ischemic heart and activation of JAK2. Secondly, inhibition of AT1 receptor function by losartan resulted in loss of Stat/ST domain complex formation and caused reduction in the angiotensingen mRNA level. These effects are mimicked by AG490. In addition the inhibitor AG490, selective for JAK2 inhibition at low concentration, caused recovery in cardiac performance suggesting that JAK 2 activation is involved in ischemia induced dysfunction of the heart.

PIVOTAL ROLE OF JAK2 SIGNALING IN INDUCTION OF APOPTOSIS

Apoptosis is defined as the end result of a tightly regulated series of biochemical events, which are controlled by the cellular transcriptional machinery (30). Apoptosis represents the cellular phenotype resulting from activation of the genomic programs that lead to DNA damage and cell death (31). Apoptosis has been unequivocally identified in cardiomyocytes in ischemic and dilated cardiac myopathy associated with clinical heart failure, acute myocardial infarction, congenital arrhythmogenic dysplasias, myocarditis and arrhythmias, although the contribution of cardiomyocyte apoptosis to initiation of these diseases cannot be precisely evaluated. A significant amount of data was derived from the in vitro studies using adult cardiomyocytes. Stress conditions imposed such as in ischemia followed by reperfusion and oxygen radicals elicit cardiomyocyte apoptotic cell death (32). Indeed, it is believed that diverse stimuli are capable of producing apoptosis in cardiac myocytes, many of which co-exist in advanced heart failure. Several possible pro-apoptotic signaling pathways have been proposed for apoptotic cell death in cardiomyocyte which may undergo cross-talk among themselves. The apoptotic process is likely to be aborted by inhibitors of the pathway and other anti-apoptotic regulatory events. The identification and characterization of these molecular signals and the associated pathways may provide novel therapeutic strategies for diverse cardiac ailments.

Two prominent pathways, the stress activated protein kinase (SAPK) and mitogen activated protein kinase (MAPK) have been proposed to be involved in promoting apoptotic signaling. In a rabbit model of in vivo ischemia, robust activation of SAPK pathway occurred that was accompanied by the onset of apoptosis (33). Carvedilol significantly reduced the infarct size and the administration of propranolol provided significant protection against ischemia induced apoptosis. Likewise, the activation of SAPK was also inhibited significantly by administration of these drugs. Thus, the association of the kinase pathway suppression to apoptosis inhibition and the consequential improved function of the myocardium suggest a role of these kinases in ischemia induced apoptotic cell death and injury. Myocardial ischemia and reperfusion was also shown to activate the p38 MAPK in vivo (34). The use of potent and selective inhibitors of p38 MAPK in a rabbit heart model of ischemia and reperfusion thus suggested that p38 MAPK inhibition and the markedly diminished consequences, that include apoptosis, are causally related. Recent experiments have also shown that over-expression of tumor suppressor p53 in cardiomyocyte results in the up-regulation of mRNA specific for angiotensinogen (35). At the same time, the mRNA for the pro-apoptotic gene Bax is also up-regulated. The induction of p53 activated apoptosis can be also be abolished by losartan, demonstrating that there is a direct linkage between the activated RAS and the apoptotic signaling cascade.

We also showed that when isolated rat hearts are subjected to ischemia reperfusion, Stat proteins are activated accompanied by an increase in apoptosis (29). These observations led us to propose that JAK2 activation may play a pivotal role in mediating the signaling events intrinsic to apoptosis. We tested the hypothesis that if AG490 effectively blocks the AngII mediated signaling of the heart RAS system besides attenuating hypertrophy and ischemia (as discussed above), it may block angiotensin II induced apoptosis of cardiac myocytes. Using the adult rat primary cardiomyocytes in culture we observed that angiotensin II alone or ectopically expressed constitutively active JAK2 alone were sufficient to induce apoptosis. The apoptotic effect was abolished by either losartan or the inhibitor of JAK2, AG490. It appears that the proapoptotic role of angiotensin II is achieved via induction of Bax expression by JAK2 kinase. Thus, angiotensin II and constitutively active Jak2 mediate transcriptional induction of the promoters of the established pro-apoptotic gene, the rat angiotensinogen and the mouse Bax genes. An examination of the promoter sequence of Bax gene revealed the presence of two distinct St-domains suggesting an involvement of Stat proteins in transcriptional modulation of Bax promoter. We also found that in cardiomyocytes subjected to hypoxia and reoxygenation, which is known to produce an oxidative stress state where apoptosis predominates, both losartan and AG490 were effective in abolishing apoptotic cell death. It would appear that AngII activated JAK2 can deliver the pro-apoptotic signal that causes a change in the Bax/BCL2 ratio that, in turn, determines the susceptibility to the pro-apoptotic program. Inhibition of JAK2 phosphorylation afforded a remarkable recovery in the survival of cells subjected to hypoxia reoxygenation, a finding that may prove to be of significant clinical benefit.

REFERENCES

1. Shaub MHC, Hefti MA, Harder BA, Eppenberger HM. 1997. Various hypertrophic stimuli I induce distinct phenotypes in cardiomyocytes. J Mol Med 75:901–920.
2. Ruwhof C, Laarse A. 2000. Mechanical stress-induced cardiac hypertrophy: mechanisms and signal transduction pathways. Card Res 47:23–37.
3. Sugden PH, Signaling in myocardial hypertrophy-Life after Calcineurin? 1999. Circ Res 84:633–646.
4. Mascareno E, Siddiqui MAQ. 2000. The role of Jak/STAT signaling in heart tissue renin-angiotensin system. Mol Cell Biochem 212:171–175.
5. Chien KR. 2000. Meeting Koch's postulates for calcium signaling in cardiac hypertrophy. J Clin Invest 105:1339–1342.
6. Molkentin J, Dorn II G. 2001. Cytoplasmic signaling pathways that regulate cardiac hypertrophy. Annu Rev Physiol 63:391–426.
7. Naga Prasad SV, Esposito G, Mao L, Koch WJ, Rockman HA. 2000. Gbetagamma-dependent phosphoinositide 3-kinase activation in hearts with in vivo pressure overload hypertrophy. J Biol Chem 275(7):4693–4698.
8. Schluter KD, Goldberg Y, Taimor G, Schafter M, Piper HM. 1998. Role of phosphatidylinositol 3-kinase activation in the hypertrophic growth of adult ventricular cardiomyocytes. Cardiovasc Res 40(1):174–181.
9. Pan J, Fukuda K, Saito M, Matsuzaki J, Kodama H, Sano M, Takahashi T, Kato T, Ogawa S. 1999. Mechanical stretch activates the JAK/STAT pathway in rat cardiomyocytes. Circ Res 84:1127–1136.
10. Sheng Z, Knowlton K, Chen J, Hoshijima M, Brown JH, Chien KR. 1997. Cardiotrophin 1 (CT-1) inhibition of cardiac myocyte apoptosis via a mitogen-activated protein kinase-dependent pathway. Divergence from downstream CT-1 signals for myocardial cell hypertrophy. J Biol Chem 272: 5783–5791.
11. Hirota H, Yoshida K, Kishimoto T, Taga T. 1995. Continuous activation of gp130, a signal-transducing receptor component for interleukin 6-related cytokines, causes myocardial hypertrophy in mice. Proc Natl Acad Sci USA 92:4862–4866.
12. Murata M, Fukuda K, Ishida H, Miyoshi S, Koura T, Kodama H, Nakazawa HK, Ogawa S. 1999. Leukemia inhibitory factor, a potent cardiac hypertrophic cytokine, enhances L-type Ca2+ current and [Ca2+]i transient in cardiomyocytes. J Mol Cell Cardiol 31:237–245.
13. Mascareno E, Dhar M, Siddiqui MAQ. 1998. Signal transduction and activator of transcription (STAT) protein-dependent activation of angiotensinogen promoter: a cellular signal for hypertrophy in cardiac muscle. Proc Natl Acad Sci USA 95:5590–5594.
14. Raizada M, Phillips M, Summers C. 1993. Cellular and Molecular Biology of the Renin Angiotensin System, CRC Press, Boca Raton, FL.
15. Braunwald E. 1992. E. Braunwald, Editor, Heart Disease—A Textbook of Cardiovascular Medicine, Volume 1, 4th Edition, WB Saunders Co., Phila, PA USA.
16. Lee AA, Dillmann WH, McCulloch AD, Villareal EJ. 1995. Angiotensin II stimulates the autocrine production of transforming growth factor—beta 1 in adult rat cardiofibroblast. J Mol Cardiol 27:2347–2357.
17. Marrero MB, Schieffer B, Paxton WG, Duff JL, Berk BC, Bernstein KE. 1995. The role of tyrosine phosphorylation in angtiotensin II—mediated intracellur signaling. Cardiovas Res 30:530–536.
18. Ihle JN. 1996. Stats signal transducers and activators of transcription. Cell 84:331–334.
19. Horvath CM, Darnell JE. 1997. The state of the STATS: Recent developments in the study of signal transduction in the nucleu. Curr Opin Cell Biol 9:233–239.
20. Horvath CM, Wen Z, Darnell JE Jr. 1995. A STAT protein domain that determines DNA sequence recognition suggests a novel DNA-binding domain Genes & Development. 9:984–994.
21. Hemmann U, Gerhartz C, Heesel B, Sasse J, Kurapkat G, Grotzinger J, Wollmer A, Zhong Z, Darnell JE Jr. 1996. Graeve L. Heinrich PC. Horn F. Differential activation of acute phase response factor/Stat3 and Stat1 via the cytoplasmic domain of the interleukin 6 signal transducer gp130. II. Src homology SH2 domains define the specificity of stat factor activation. J of Biol Chem 271: 12999–13007.
22. Karin M. 1994. Signal transduction from the cell surface to the nucleus through the phosphorylation of transcription factors. Curr Op in Cell Bio 6:415–424.

23. Gotoh A, Takahira H, Mantel C, Litz-Jackson S, Boswell HS, Broxmeyer HE. 1996. Steel factor induces serine phosphorylation of Stat3 in human growth factor-dependent myeloid cell lines. Blood 88(1):138–145.

24. David M, Petricoin E 3rd, Benjamin C, Pine R, Weber MJ, Larner AC. 1995. Requirement for MAP kinase (ERK2) activity in interferon alpha- and interferon beta-stimulated gene expression through STAT proteins. Science 269:1721–1723.

25. Seidel HM, Milocco LH, Lamb P, Darnell JE, Stein RB, Rosen J. 1995. Spacing of palindromic half sites as a determinant of selective STAT (signal transducers and activators of transcription) DNA binding and transcriptional activity. Proc Natl Acad Sci USA 92:3041–3045.

26. Darnell JE Jr, Kerr IM, Stark GM. 1994. Jak/STAT pathways and transcriptional activation in response to IFNs and other extracellular signaling proteins. Science 264:1415–1421.

27. Fukuzawa J, Booz GW, Hunt RA, Shimizu N, Karoor V, Baker KM, Dostal DE. 2000. Cardiotrophin-1 increases angiotensinogen mRNA in rat cardiac myocytes through STAT3: an autocrine loop for hypertrophy. Hypertension 35(6):1191–1196.

28. Paz Y, Gurevitch J, Frolkis I, et al. 1998. Effects of an angiotensin II antagonist on ischemic and non-ischemic isolated rat heart. Thorac Surg 65:474–479.

29. Mascareno E, El-Shafie M, Maulik N, Sito M, Guo Y, Das DK, Siddiqui MAQ. 2001. JAK/Stat signaling is associated with cardiac dysfunction during ischemia and reperfusion. Circulation 104: 325–329.

30. Kerr JFR, Wyllie AH, Currie AR. 1972. Apoptosis: A basic biological phenomenon with wide ranging implication in tissue connectics. British J Cancer 26:239–257.

31. Yuan J, Shaham S, Ledoux S, Ellis HM, Horvitz HR. 1993. The C. elegans cell death gene cde-3 encodes a protein similar to mammalian interleukin-1 beta converting enzyme. Cell 75:641–652.

32. Yaoita H, Ogawa K, Maelare K, Maruyama Y. 1998. Attenuation of ischemia/reperfusion injury in rats by a caspase inhibitor. Circulation 97:276–281.

33. Ma XL, Kumar S, Gao F, et al. 1999. Inhibition of p38 mitogen activated protein kinase decreases cardiomyocytes apoptosis and improves cardiac function after myocardial ischemia and reperfusion. Circulation 99:1685–1691.

34. Wang Y, Huang S, Sah VP, et al. 1998. Cardiac muscle cell hypertrophy in apoptosis induced by distinct members of the p38 mitogen activated protein kinase family. J Biol Chem 273:2161–2168.

35. Piezetralski P, Reiss K, Cheng W, Sirelli C, Kajstura J, Nitahara JA, Rizk M, Capagrossi MC, Anversa P. 1997. Exp Cell Res 234:57–65.

III. Genetic Approaches to Investigative Cardiac Signal Transduction

Signal Transduction and Cardiac Hypertrophy,
edited by N.S. Dhalla, L.V. Hryshko,
E. Kardami & P.K. Singal
Kluwer Academic Publishers, Boston, 2003

Signaling Pathways Involved in the Stimulation of DNA Synthesis by Tumor Necrosis Factor and Lipopolysaccharide in Chick Embryo Cardiomyocytes

Benedetta Tantini,[1] Carla Pignatti,[1] Flavio Flamigni,[1]
Claudio Stefanelli,[1] Monia Fattori,[1] Annalisa Facchini,[1]
Emanuele Giordano,[1] Carlo Clô,[2] and Claudio Marcello Caldarera[1]

[1] Department of Biochemistry "G. Moruzzi"
School of Medicine, University of Bologna
Italy
[2] Department of Experimental Medicine
School of Medicine, University of Parma
Italy

Summary. Treatment of confluent chick embryo cardiomyocytes (CM) with tumor necrosis factor-α (TNF) and lipopolysaccharide (LPS) increased cell number and [^{3}H]-thymidine incorporation. Addition of TNF and LPS provoked an early increase in active, phosphorylated extracellular-signal regulated kinase (ERK), an induction of ornithine decarboxylase (ODC), and a more delayed enhancement of nitric oxide synthase (NOS) activity, which appeared to be independent on the activation of the ODC/polyamine system. A number of inhibitors of signal transduction pathways involved in mitogenesis inhibited [^{3}H]-thymidine incorporation as well as ODC and/or NOS induction. In particular, PD98059, a specific inhibitor of the ERK pathway, prevented the induction of ODC, but not that of NOS, whereas chelerythine, a protein kinase C inhibitor, reduced NOS, but not ODC activity. TNF and LPS treatment also enhanced the cGMP level in CM and both polyamine and nitric oxide (NO) biosyntheses appeared to be required. Experiments with specific inhibitors of ODC and NOS, as well as with inhibitors of soluble guanylate cyclase (sGC) and cGMP dependent protein kinase (PKG), showed that polyamine-, NO- and cGMP-dependent pathways are required for the mitogenic action of TNF and LPS. In conclusion, the present results suggest that the mitogenic effect of TNF and LPS on CM involves both the induction of

Address for Correspondence: Benedetta Tantini, Department of Biochemistry "G. Moruzzi", University of Bologna, via Irnerio, 48, 40126 Bologna, Italy. Fax: +39 051 2091224, Tel: +39 051 2091225, E-mail: Tantini@biocfarm.unibo.it

ODC, supported by ERK activation, and NOS activity. In turn, polyamine and NO biosyntheses may cooperate to enhance cGMP level, resulting in stimulation of DNA synthesis.

Key words: tumor necrosis factor, nitric oxide synthase, ornithine decarboxylase, cyclic GMP, embryonic cardiomyocytes.

1. INTRODUCTION

Cell proliferation is a tightly controlled event influenced by many intracellular and extracellular factors, in a cell type- and developmental stage-specific manner. Unlike skeletal muscle cells, mammalian cardiac myocytes, differentiated from the very early phases of the embryo, continue to increase in cell number up to the first 2–3 days after birth (1), although the number of DNA synthesizing myocytes begins to decrease during late embryonic development (2). In serum-starved heart cell cultures, the addition of mitogens can rapidly re-induce proliferation of cardiac fibroblasts, but not of cardiomyocytes (CM) (3). Chicken CM continue to proliferate up to 42 days of age and have the ability to re-synthesize DNA also after their withdrawal from the cell cycle. Therefore, confluent chick embryo heart cells, synchronized in the G_0 phase of the cell cycle by serum starvation, represent a useful model to investigate the metabolic pathways leading to the recruitment of CM into the G_1 phase of the cell cycle and their progression into DNA synthesis.

It is known that tumor necrosis factor-α (TNF) and lipopolysaccharide (LPS), important mediators in inflammation, can affect heart function and LPS has been reported to induce TNF expression in CM (4). TNF immunoreactivity has also been shown in chick embryo heart (5). Although the precise biological role for TNF expression within the heart in unknown, TNF has been proposed as an autocrine/paracrine mediator in myocardial remodelling (6). Experimental evidence indicates that TNF and LPS can be cytotoxic, cytostatic or mitogenic, depending on the cell type and the developmental stage (7–9). The pleiotropic nature of the TNF and LPS response in the different systems and conditions may be related to the activation of multiple signalling pathways. In adult CM, which cannot re-enter the cell cycle, treatment with TNF leads to apoptosis, but this effect was not observed in neonatal proliferating CM (10). However, according to a recent report (6), TNF can also stimulate protein synthesis and provoke a hypertrophic growth response in adult CM, in a manner dependent on cell-subsrate interaction.

Recent studies have shown that the generation of nitric oxide (NO) by NO donors or cytokines, such as TNF plus IFN-γ, resulted in suppression of ornithine decarboxylase (ODC) activity in various tumoral or transformed cells (11,12). Increased activity of ODC, the first and key enzyme in polyamine biosynthesis (13), is an early event related to DNA replication and cell proliferation (14). Suppression of ODC with specific inhibitors arrests cells in the G_1 phase and prevents DNA synthesis (13,15). In neonatal CM the increase in ODC activity and polyamine content is involved in the hyperthrophic cell growth (16,17). In many cell types, the ornithine required for polyamine biosynthesis can be derived from arginine, which also represents the substrate for NOS to produce NO (18). In CM the NOS genes may be both constitutively expressed and induced by cytokines or LPS through transcriptional activation (19,20). Recently, a chick inducible isoform (iNOS) has been cloned from LPS-stimulated macrophages (21). Endogenous NO produced by cardiac constitutive or iNOS depresses myocardial contractility and can contribute to heart dysfunction in various pathological conditions (19). Expression of iNOS has been reported to be elevated in failing hearts (22) and the clinical importance of NOS induction is now increasing in cardiovascular research. TNF can induce NOS activity in different cell types, including CM (19). In most cases, the expression of iNOS is enhanced by LPS (20,23). The signalling events transduced by cytokines for the induction of NOS are not completely established and it is not known whether they might be related to the signalling pathways leading to ODC induction and cell proliferation during the hyperplasic phase of cell growth.

We have recently shown that in chick embryo CM cultures TNF and LPS stimulate DNA synthesis via NO and polyamines biosynthesis (24) and that this effect is mediated through a pathway involving NF-κB and ERK activation (25). In the present study we investigated the pathways involved in the observed proliferative effect of TNF and LPS in CM. We report that multiple signal transduction pathways seem to be involved in the inductions of ODC and NOS activities in chick embryo CM cultures treated with TNF and LPS and that the increase of DNA synthesis is related to activation of ERK as well as to an increased intracellular cGMP content.

2. MATERIALS AND METHODS

2.1. Preparation of cardiomyocyte cultures

Preparation of monolayer cultures of spontaneously beating embryo CM from the hearts of 10 day-old chick embryos was carried out by a trypsin disaggregation procedure (26). Myocytes were purified by differential adhesion by a 2 h pre-plating of the initial cell suspension at 37°C. The myocyte-enriched fraction was resuspended in DMEM (GIBCO) containing a high concentration of glucose (25 mM) supplemented with 10% foetal calf serum, 1% streptomycin, 1% penicillin. The cell suspension was diluted to 1×10^6 cells per milliliter, seeded in 35 mm tissue culture dishes (Falcon), incubated at 37°C in a humidified atmosphere containing 5% CO_2 and grown to confluency, with a change in serum-containing medium every 48 h. This method results in preparations containing >95% CM, as assayed by immunofluorescence staining with antibodies against cardiac myosine heavy chain, which began to beat spontaneously after 2 days in culture. Confluent cultures were then serum-starved for 20 h before treatment with the different drugs, as described in the legends.

2.2. Ornithine decarboxylase assay

At the end of the incubations a crude enzyme extract was prepared from cells which were previously washed with phosphate buffered saline (PBS) and scraped in a buffer consisting of 0.1 mM EDTA, 0.02 mM piridoxal phosphate, 2.5 mM dithiothreitol in 10 mM sodium phosphate buffer, pH 7.2. The cells were disrupted by freeze-thawing three times and then centrifuged at 15,000 g for 15 min. The ODC activity was measured by estimation of the release of $^{14}CO_2$ from L-[1-^{14}C]-ornithine, as previously described (27). Data are expressed as pmol/mg protein/min. Proteins were determined according to Bradford (28).

2.3. Nitric oxide synthase assay

NOS activity was tested monitoring L-[^{3}H]-citrulline formation from L-[2,3-^{3}H]-arginine. At the end of the incubation periods, the cells were washed once with HEPES buffer and then incubated for 30 min at 37°C with 1 ml of the same buffer containing 10 mM L-arginine and 1 μCi L-[2,3-^{3}H]-arginine (NEN, 40.5 Ci/mmol specific activity)/plate. The reaction was stopped by washing the cells with cold PBS containing 5 mM L-arginine and 4 mM EDTA. After supernatant removal, 0.5 ml ethanol was added to each monolayer and allowed to evaporate. Two ml of 20 mM HEPES, pH 5.5 were then added. After 5 min, 1 ml of supernatant was mixed with 0.4 ml of slurry Dowex AG50W-X8 Na+ form equilibrated in stop buffer and vortexed for 30 min. Thus, 0.5 ml were collected from the supernatant and counted in a liquid scintillation spectrometer. Proteins were determined after alkaline hydrolysis of the cells. Data are expressed as pmol/mg protein/min.

2.4. cGMP and polyamine determination

At the end of the incubation at 37°C, the medium was aspirated and the cells were rinsed twice with cold 0.85% NaCl, deproteinized with 0.6 M HClO₄, pooled by scraping, frozen and thawed twice and then centrifuged at 15,000 g for 10 min. The pellets were used for protein determination, while the supernatants were neutralized with 5 M K₂CO₃ and then assayed for cGMP content by a radio-immunoassay kit (Amersham).

2.5. [³H]-thymidine incorporation

DNA synthesis was quantified by [³H]-thymidine incorporation of subconfluent CM cultures. The cells, maintained for 20 h in a serum-free DMEM, were then treated with the different drugs, and pulsed during the last 2 h with 3 μCi of [³H]-thymidine per dish (Amersham, 5.0 Ci/mmol specific activity). The cells were then washed twice with ice-cold PBS, collected by scraping in cold 0.6 M HClO₄, frozen and thawed twice and centrifuged at 15,000 g for 10 min. The precipitate, dissolved in 1 M NaOH, was used for radioactivity analysis. Data are expressed as % of the radioactivity measured under basal conditions.

2.6. Western blot analyses of phosphorylated and total ERK

At the end of the incubations the cells were rinsed twice with cold PBS and scraped in 0.2 ml of a lysis buffer consisting of 20 mM Tris-HCl, 100 mM NaCl, 5 mM EDTA, 1 mM EDTA, 1 mM Na₃VO₄, 1 mM benzamidine, 1% Nonidet P40, 1 mM

PMSF, 10 mM *p*-nitrophenylphosphate, 1 mM dithiothreitol, 10 mM β-glycerophosphate, 1 μg/ml aprotinin, leupeptin, pepstatin, pH 8. The cells were disrupted by sonication and then centrifuged. The supernatant was boiled in a loading buffer and an aliquot corresponding to 60 μg of protein was analyzed by SDS/PAGE (12% gel). Separated proteins were transferred to a nitrocellulose membrane (Amersham) for 1 h. The membrane was saturated with 4% powdered milk, 0.05% Tween 20 in 10 mM Tris pH 8, 150 mM NaCl for 1 h, and then incubated with either control anti-ERK antibody or anti-phosphospecific ERK (New England Biolabs) antibody at 4°C overnight. Bands, revealed by the Amersham ECL detection system, were then quantified by the intensitometric software QScan from Biosoft (UK). Data are expressed as % of control.

2.7. Statistical analyses

Values are given as means ± S.D. All experiments were performed with at least three independent cardiomyocyte cultures. Comparison among two groups was performed using t-test. Differences were considered significant for $p < 0.05$.

3. RESULTS

3.1. TNF and LPS induce ODC and NOS activities and increase cGMP content in cardiomyocytes

Figure 1A shows that in confluent and serum-starved chick embryo CM, the treatment with TNF and LPS significantly induced ODC activity, with a peak at 4 h. This induction was followed by the accumulation of polyamines, particularly putrescine and spermidine (not shown). The exposure of CM to TNF and LPS also increased NOS activity with a maximum at 24 h (Figure 1B). NOS induction led to an enhancement of NO levels (not shown). Figure 1B also shows that the presence of α-difluoromethylornithine (DFMO), a specific ODC inhibitor, did not

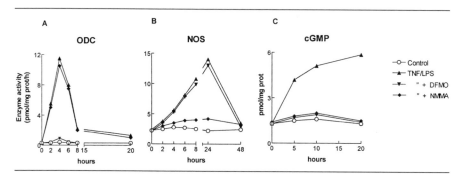

Figure 1. Time course of ODC and NOS inductions and cGMP increase in confluent chick embryo cardiomyocytes treated with TNF and LPS. Effect of DFMO or L-NMMA. Serum starved cardiomyocytes were treated with 500 U/ml TNF and 10 μg/ml LPS. Pretreatments were done for 20 h with 4 mM DFMO or for 1 h with 100 μM L-NMMA. The figure reports data obtained from one experiment representative of 4.

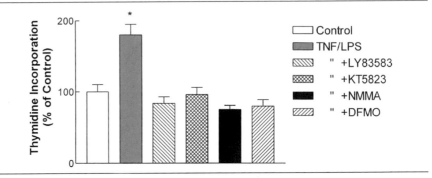

Figure 2. Effect of TNF and LPS on DNA synthesis in confluent chick embryo cardiomyocytes. Serum starved cardiomyocytes were incubated for 20 h with 500 U/ml TNF and 10 μg/ml LPS in the absence or presence of 10 μM LY83583, 1 μM KT5823, 100 μM L-NMMA or 4 mM DFMO. *, P < 0.05 vs untreated cells.

affect the induction of NOS by TNF and LPS, suggesting that the early activation of the ODC/polyamine system is not involved in the more delayed induction of NOS. Conversely, L-monomethylarginine (L-NMMA), a competitive NOS inhibitor, did not influence ODC induction by TNF and LPS (Figure 1A).

The treatment of cells with TNF and LPS was also followed by an increase of cGMP levels up to 20 h (Figure 1C). This effect was dependent on NO generation, since it was abolished by pretreatment with L-NMMA, in accordance with the notion that NO can stimulate sGC (29). In addition, pretreatment with DFMO prevented the effect of TNF and LPS on cGMP accumulation, indicating that endogenous polyamines are also implicated in the increase of intracellular cGMP, as suggested in our previous study (24) where both polyamines and NO resulted to be required for the synthesis of cGMP elicited by NO donors and exogenous polyamines, respectively.

3.2. TNF and LPS stimulate DNA synthesis in cardiomyocytes. Effect of polyamines, NO and cGMP

Figure 2 shows that the treatment of CM cultures with TNF and LPS increased [^{3}H]-thymidine incorporation after 24 h. This mitogenic response was prevented by the presence of the sGC inhibitor LY83583, the specific PKG inhibitor KT5823, the NOS inhibitor L-NMMA or the ODC inhibitor DFMO, suggesting that cGMP-, NO- and polyamine-dependent pathways are all required for the proliferative process in CM. TNF and LPS also stimulate the re-entry of CM into the cell cycle, by increasing cell number from 98×10^4/ml to 197×10^4/ml. Our previous report indicated that in CM cultures the addition of permanent analogous of cGMP increases [H^3]-thymidine incorporation and that exogenous polyamines and/or NO donors stimulate DNA synthesis via an increase of cGMP levels, since their effects were reversed in the presence of inhibitors of sGC or PKG (24). All together these results suggest that not only polyamines and NO are necessary for the mitogenic

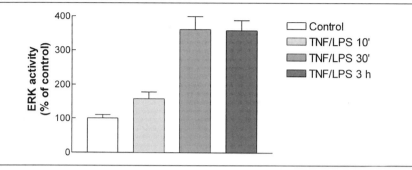

Figure 3. Effect of TNF and LPS on ERK activity in confluent chick embryo cardiomyocytes. Serum starved cardiomyocytes were treated with 500 U/ml TNF and 10 μg/ml LPS for the time indicated. Cell extracts were analyzed by western-blot by using antibodies against total ERK. The intensities of the bands were analyzed and quantified by the intesitometric software.

response of TNF and LPS, but these intracellular mediators may mimic the action of the cytokines.

3.3. Effects of inhibitors of ERK and of other signal transduction pathways

Some signal transduction pathways activated by TNF and/or LPS result in proliferation of certain cell types (8,9). Since the ERK cascade is considered to play an essential role in mitogenesis (30) we investigated the activation/phosphorylation of ERK in our experimental model. Figure 3 shows that phosphorylated ERK increased markedly within 30 min of TNF and LPS treatment and that it was still high after 3 h of treatment. Given the importance of ODC and NOS for the mitogenic effect of TNF and LPS treatment, we investigated the effect of PD98059, a specific MEK inhibitor widely used to dissect the ERK pathway (31), on the inductions of ODC and NOS (Table 1). PD98059, which prevented the TNF and LPS induced ERK activation (not shown), proved to be a potent inhibitor of ODC induction, but did not influence NOS induction. However this was sufficient to prevent the stimulation of DNA synthesis elicited by TNF and LPS (Table 1). The effects of other inhibitors of signaling pathways involved in mitogenesis were tested and reported in Table 1: herbimycin A, a non-receptor tyrosine kinase inhibitor (32), markedly inhibited the increase in ODC, but hardly that in NOS activity; on the contrary, chelerythrine, considered a specific PKC inhibitor (33), was effective in reducing the induction of NOS, but not that of ODC; LY294002 and wortmannin, two structurally unrelated PI3K inhibitors (31), as well as rapamycin, which may inhibit targets downstream of PI3K (31), counteracted the induction of NOS and particularly of ODC. Interestingly DMAP, which has been reported to prevent the activation of ceramide-activated protein kinase and other effects of TNF (34), strongly reduced ODC induction and completely prevented that of NOS. Experiments performed to test the ability of C_6-ceramide, a cell permeant analogue of ceramide, to reproduce the effects of TNF and LPS on ODC and NOS, indicated

Table 1. Effects of various signal transduction inhibitors on ODC activity, NOS activity and [^{3}H]-Thymidine incorporation of quiescent chick embryo cardiomyocytes treated with TNF and LPS

Treatment	Specificity	ODC	NOS	[^{3}H]-Thymidine
			(% of Control)	
TNF + LPS	—	3840 ± 340	526 ± 40	180 ± 20
+ PD98059 (50 μM)	ERK inhibitor	1076 ± 90	531 ± 30	106 ± 17
+ Herbimycin A (1 μM)	cytoplasmic TK inhibitor	1460 ± 175	442 ± 52	108 ± 15
+ Chelerythrine (5 μM)	PKC inhibitor	4320 ± 315	326 ± 35	90 ± 11
+ LY294002 (20 μM)	PI3K inhibitor	800 ± 30	352 ± 47	98 ± 19
+ Wortmannin (100 nM)	PI3K inhibitor	1730 ± 152	378 ± 25	90 ± 9
+ Rapamycin (100 nM)	FRAP Kinase inhibitor	1460 ± 135	330 ± 41	77 ± 7
+ DMAP (1 mM)	Inhibitor of ceramide-activated Protein Kinase	1730 ± 154	105 ± 15	81 ± 15

Serum starved cardiomyocytes were treated with 500 U/ml TNF and 10 μg/ml LPS for 4 h (ODC), 8 h (NOS) or 20 h (^{3}H-Thymidine incorporation). TK, tyrosine kinase. The various inhibitors were added 30 min before TNF and LPS treatment. The results are expressed as percentage with respect to untreated cells (control). Data are depicted as means of three independent experiments ± S.D.

that C_6-ceramide (from 1 to 100 μM) could not increase ODC or NOS activity in CM appreciably, either administered alone or in combination with TNF or LPS (not shown). In summary, all the inhibitors tested, independently of their specific site of action, reduced the induction of ODC and/or NOS by TNF and LPS, which failed to stimulate DNA synthesis (Table 1).

4. DISCUSSION

TNF and LPS act in concert in several experimental systems and may activate multiple signal transduction pathways, but their mode of action is only partially defined (7,9,35). It has been reported that TNF and LPS can be mitogenic or cytotoxic according to the cell type and the developmental stage (7,9). In particular, the cellular receptor for TNF, which is homologous to Fas/Apo-1, can transduce different signals stimulating either apoptosis or proliferation (36). In cardiomyocytes the main effects of TNF observed are those related to cytotoxicity. Induction of NOS activity, leading to cell death, has been observed in adult CM exposed to TNF (37), and more recently evidence has been provided that TNF stimulates apoptosis in adult (10), but not neonatal CM (10,38). This last effect has been related to the absence in neonatal CM of detectable transcript levels for the type I receptor (TNFRI), whose "death domain" has been linked to TNF-induced apoptosis (36). We have recently shown (25) that in chick embryo CM cultures TNF and LPS favour cell survival by reducing both basal and stimulated caspase activities, enzymes closely related to the executive phase of apoptosis.

In the present study we show that the mitogenic effect of TNF and LPS in embryonal CM is mediated by ODC and NOS inductions, increased polyamine and cGMP contents, NO generation and by an involvement of the ERK pathway. NO and cGMP generation has been correlated within mitogenesis in endothelial cells

(39,40), but in other cell types, such as vascular smooth muscle cells, NO and cGMP exert an antiproliferative effect (41,42). On the other hand a positive correlation between polyamine biosynthesis and cellular growth has been widely described (43).

We provide evidence that the addition of TNF and LPS to CM induces ODC and NOS activities independently. In fact, pretreatment with L-NMMA or DFMO did not affect ODC or NOS inductions, respectively. Moreover the exposure of CM to TNF and LPS progressively increases the cellular cGMP level up to 20h. This effect is dependent on both NO generation and polyamine biosynthesis, since it was abrogated by L-NMMA or DFMO.

Some signal transduction pathways activated by TNF and/or LPS result in proliferation of certain cell types. In particular, activations of the transcription factor NF-κB as well as of the ERK cascade may play critical roles in mitogenesis. Our recent report indicated that in CM cultures the induction of ODC and NOS by TNF and LPS is mediated by NF-κB activation (25). Here we show that the mitogenic effect of TNF and LPS, involving polyamines, NO and cGMP, was linked to activation of the ERK cascade. ERK is intimately involved in signal transduction processes that lead to differentiation or proliferation of a wide variety of cell types (44). ERK activation is accompanied by a significant increase in phosphorylation on tyrosine and threonine residues catalyzed by a single type of dual specificity kinase (MEK) (45). In cardiac myocytes, activation of the 42 and 44 Kda isoforms of ERK has been shown to induce the transcriptional response characteristic of hypertrophy (46). TNF treatment induces a rapid and transient increase in ERK phosphorylation and activation in some cells (45). In particular, in the human diploid FS-4 cell line, for which TNF is known to be mitogenic, the 42 and 44 kda ERK were the only proteins whose tyrosine phosphorylation was clearly increased after TNF treatment (45). Analogously, treatment of CM with TNF and LPS leads to a marked and sustained increase (up to 3h) of the active phosphorylated ERK. Evidence has been provided that prolonged activation (1 or 2h) of ERK is a requirement for cell cycle progression (47) and that, in adult CM, ERK activation is probably necessary for NOS induction by cytokines (48). However, in other cells, growth promoting factors known to activate ERK decrease NOS mRNA levels (49).

In chick embryo CM, ERK seems to be involved only in the induction of ODC, since the specific ERK pathway inhibitor PD98059, while reducing the stimulation of ODC activity, was without effect on NOS induction by TNF and LPS. PD98059 also inhibited the stimulation of DNA synthesis by TNF and LPS, suggesting that ERK activation is needed for the mitogenic response of CM. At variance, in endothelial cells, NO and cGMP are considered upstream signals which trigger the activation of ERK involved in the proliferative response to vascular endothelial growth factor (40).

Ceramide, a sphingomyelin metabolite, has been proposed to mediate different responses to TNF, including ERK activation and cell proliferation (35). Furthermore LPS has been shown to possess structural similarity to ceramide and to stimulate ceramide-activated protein kinase in myeloid cells (50). However no evident effect

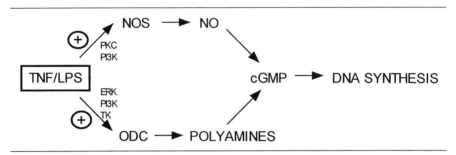

Scheme 1. Pathways involved in the mitogenic effect of TNF and LPS in chick embryo cardiomyocyte cultures.

of a cell permeant ceramide analogue, C_6-ceramide, on ODC or NOS activities was observed in CM, suggesting that ceramide unlikely mediates TNF action in these cells. Therefore, prevention of ODC and NOS inductions by DMAP, an inhibitor of ceramide-activated protein kinase (34), might be due to the impairment of other kinases.

To gain more information on the signal pathways involved in ODC and/or NOS inductions, we tested the effects of other inhibitors with different specificities. The results indicate that, in addition to ERK activation, ODC induction may also involve tyrosine kinases of the Src family, since the inhibitor herbimycin A markedly reduced the increase in ODC activity by TNF and LPS. On the contrary, the NOS induction pathway requires activation of PKC, since it was reduced by about 40% in the presence of chelerythrine, a specific PKC inhibitor. The involvement of PKC in NOS induction was observed in cultured CM treated with LPS or other cytokines (33,48). Besides, the PI3K pathway seems to be involved in NOS and particularly in ODC inductions, as indicated by the negative effects of LY294002 and wortmannin, two structurally unrelated PI3K inhibitors, or of rapamycin, which may inhibit steps downstream of PI3K (31). Recently we found that PI3K and ERK dependent pathways are involved in the expression of ODC in L1210-DR cells stimulated with serum (51).

Various signal transduction pathways appear to be involved in ODC and NOS induction and in the stimulation of DNA synthesis in embryonal CM treated with TNF and LPS (Scheme 1). These pathways may include activation of ERK, tyrosine kinases, PKC and PI3K. Indeed, most of the drugs employed did not show the same efficacy as NOS and ODC inhibitors. We may hypothesize that in our experimental model polyamine and NO biosyntheses, cooperating to enhance intracellular cGMP content, represent steps of two separate pathways correlated with re-entry into the cell cycle and with increased cell proliferation. The ability of TNF and LPS to stimulate proliferation in embryonal CM indicates that in these cells the death signal, normally observed in TNF-treated adult myocytes, is converted into a mitogenic response mediated by polyamines, NO and cGMP. In conclusion we provide evidences for a mitogenic effect of TNF and LPS in embryonal CM that could be of some relevance for the clinical approach to a variety of cardiac disorders related to increased levels of circulating cytokines and/or altered polyamine biosynthesis.

ACKNOWLEDGEMENTS

This research was supported by grants from MURST (ex 40% and 60%), Italy, from Fondazione Banca Del Monte, Bologna, Italy, from University of Bologna (Progetti Pluriennali, e.f. 2000) and from Consorzio Internazionale per la Ricerca Cardiovascolare (CIRC).

REFERENCES

1. Li F, Wang X, Capasso JM, Gerdes AM. 1996. Rapid transition of cardiac myocytes from hyperplasia to hypertrophy during postnatal development. J Mol Cell Cardiol 28:1737–1746.
2. Soonpaa MH, Kim KK, Pajak L, Franklin M, Field LJ. 1996. Cardiomyocyte DNA synthesis and binucleation during murine development. Am J Physiol 271:H2183–H2189.
3. Georgescu SP, Komuro I, Hiroi Y, Mizuno T, Kudoh S, Yamazaki T, Yazaki Y. 1997. Downregulation of polo-like kinase correlates with loss of proliferative ability of cardiac myocytes. J Mol Cell Cardiol 29:929–937.
4. Wagner DR, Combes A, McTiernan C, Sanders VJ, Lemster B, Feldman AM. 1998. Adenosine inhibits lipopolysaccharide-induced cardiac expression of tumor necrosis factor-alpha. Circ Res 82:47–56.
5. Wride MA, Lapchak PH, Sanders EJ. 1994. Distribution of TNF-α-like proteins correlates with some regions of programmed cell death in the chick embryo. Int J Dev Biol 673–682.
6. Yokoyama T, Nakano M, Bednarczyk JL, McIntyre BW, Entman M, Mann DL. 1997 Tumor necrosis factor-α provokes a hypertrophic growth response in adult cardiac myocytes. Circulation 95:1247–1252.
7. Van Lint J, Agostini P, Vandevoorde V, Haegeman G, Fiersi W, Merlevede W, Vandenheede JR. 1992. Tumor necrosis factor stimulates multiple serine/threonine protein kinases in Swiss 3T3 and L929 cells. J Biol Chem 267:25916–25921.
8. Caselles TH, Stutman O. 1993. Immune function of tumor necrosis factor. J Immunol 151:3999–4012.
9. Chow CW, Grinstein S, Rotstein OD. 1995. Signaling events in monocytes and macrophages. New Horiz 3:342–351.
10. Krown KA, Page MT, Nguyen C, Zechner D, Gutierrez V, Comstock KL, Glembotski CC, Quintana PJE, Sabbadini RA. 1996. Tumor necrosis factor alpha-induced apoptosis in cardiac myocytes. J Clin Invest 98:2854–2865.
11. Buga GM, Wei LH, Bauer PM, Fukuto JM, Ignarro LJ. 1998. N^G-hydroxy-L-arginine and nitric oxide inhibit Caco-2 tumor cell proliferation by distinct mechanisms. Am J Physiol 275:R1256–R1264.
12. Satriano J, Ishizuka S, Archer DC, Blantz RC, Kelly CJ. 1999. Regulation of intracellular polyamine biosynthesis and transport by NO and cytokines TNF-α and IFN-γ. Am J Physiol 276:C892–C899.
13. Pegg AE. 1986. Recent advances in the biochemistry of polyamines in eukaryotes. Biochem J 234:249–262.
14. Tabor CW, Tabor H. 1984. Polyamines Annu Rev Biochem 53:749–790.
15. Seidenfeld J, Block AL, Komar KA, Naujokas MF. 1986. Altered cell cycle phase distributions in cultured human carcinoma cells partially depleted of polyamines by treatments with difluoromethylornithine. Cancer Res 46:47–53.
16. Caldarera CM, Flamigni F, Rossoni C, Guarnieri C, Clô C. 1988. Polyamines and heart physiology. In: The Physiology of Polyamines. Eds. U Bachrach and Y Heimes, 1:39–55. New York: CRC Press Inc.
17. Toraason M, Luken ME, Krueger JA. 1990. Cooperative action of insulin and catecholamines on stimulation of ornithine decarboxylase activity in neonatal rat heart cells. J Mol Cell Cardiol 22:637–644.
18. Joshi M. 1997. The importance of L-arginine metabolism in melanoma: an hypothesis for the role of nitric oxide and polyamines in tumor angiogenesis. Free Rad Biol Med 22:573–578.

19. Balligand JL, Cannon PJ. 1997. Nitric oxide synthase and cardiac muscle. Arterioscler Thromb 17:1846–1858.
20. Kinugawa K, Schimizu T, Yao A, Kohmoto O, Serizawa T, Takahashi T. 1997. Transcriptional regulation of inducibile nitric oxide synthase in cultured neonatal rat cardiac myocytes. Circ Res 81:911–921.
21. Lin AW, Chang CC, McCormick CC. 1996. Molecular cloning and expression of an avian macrophage nitric-oxide synthase cDNA and the analysis of the genomic 5′-flanking region. J Biol Chem 271:11911–11919.
22. Haywood GA, Tsao PS, von der Leyen HE, Mann MJ, Keeling PJ, Trindade PT, Lewis NP, Byrne CD, Rickenbacher PR, Bishopric NH, Cooke JP, McKenna WJ, Fowler MB. 1996. Expression of inducible nitric oxide synthase in human heart failure. Circulation 93:1087–1094.
23. Stein B, Frank P, Schmitz W, Scholz H, Thoenes M. 1996. Endotoxin and cytokines induce direct cardiodepressive effects in mammalian cardiomyocytes via induction of nitric oxide synthase. J Mol Cell Cardiol 28:1631–1639.
24. Tantini B, Flamigni F, Pignatti C, Stefanelli C, Fattori M, Facchini A, Giordano E, Clô C, Caldarera CM. 2001. Polyamines, NO and cGMP mediate stimulation of DNA synthesis by tumor necrosis factor and lipopolysaccharide inchick embryo cardiomyocytes. Cardiovascular Res 49:408–416.
25. Tantini B, Pignatti C, Fattori M, Flamingi F, Stefanelli C, Giordano E, Menegazzi M, Clô C, Caldarera CM. 2002. NF-κB and ERK cooperate to stimulate DNA synthesis by inducing ornithine decarboxylase and nitric oxide synthase in cardiomyocytes treated with TNF and LPS. FEBS Lett 512:75–79.
26. Pignatti C, Tantini B, Stefanelli C, Giordano E, Bonavita F, Clô C, Caldarera CM. 1998. Nitric Oxide mediates eithr proliferation or cell death in cardiomyocytes. Involvement of polyamines. Amino Acids 6:181–190.
27. Pignatti C, Stanic' I, Stefanelli C, Tantini B, Rossoni C, Flamingi F. 1998. Modulation of the induction of ornithine decarboxylase by some opioid receptor agonists in immune cells and cardiomyocytes. Mol Cell Biochem 185:47–53.
28. Bradford MH. 1976. A rapid and sensitive method for quantitation of microgram quantities of protein utilizing the principle of protein-dye-binding. Anal Biochem 72:248–254.
29. Schmidt HHHV, Lohmann SM, Walter U. 1993. The nitric oxide and cGMP signal transduction system: regulation and mechanism of action. Biochim. Biophys. Acta 1178:153–175.
30. Chang L, Karin M. 2001. Mammalian MAK kinase signaling cascades. Nature 410:649–683.
31. Proud CG, Denton RM. 1997. Molecular mechanisms for the control of translation by insulin. Biochem J 328:329–341.
32. Fukazawa H, Li PM, Yamamoto C, Murakami Y, Mizuno S, Uehara Y. Specific inhibition of cytoplasmic protein tyrosine kinases by herbimycin A in vitro. Biochem Pharmacol 42:1661–1671.
33. McKenna TM, Li S, Tao S. 1995. PKC mediates LPS-and phorbol-induced cardiac cell nitric oxide synthase activity and hypocontractility. Am J Physiol 269:H1891–H1898.
34. Marino MW, Dunbar JD, Wu LW, Ngaiza JR, Han HM, Guo D, Matsushita M, Nairn AC, Zhang Y, Kolesnick R, Jaffe EA, Donner DB. 1996. Inhibition of tumor necrosis factor signal transduction in endothelial cells by dimethylaminopurine. J Biol Chem 271:28624–28629.
35. Testi R. 1996. Sphingomyelin breakdown and cell fate. Trends Biol Sci 21:468–471.
36. Vanderabeele P, Declercq W, Beyaert R, Fiers W. 1995. Two tumor necrosis factor receptors: structure and function. Trends Cell Biol 5:392–399.
37. Pinsky DJ, Cai B, Yang K, Rodriguez C, Sciacca RR, Cannon PJJ. 1995. The lethal effects of cytokine-induced nitric oxide on cardiac myocytes are blocked by nitric oxide synthase antagonism or transforming growth factor β. J Clin Invest 95:677–685.
38. Ing DJ, Zang J, Dzau VJ, Webster KA, Bishopric NH. 1999. Modulation of cytokine-induced cardiac apoptosis by nitric oxide, Bak, and Bcl-x. Circ Res 84:21–33.
39. Morbidelli L, Chang CH, Douglas JG, Granger HJ, Ledda F, Ziche M. 1996. Nitric oxide mediates mitogenic effect of VEGF on coronary venular endothelium. Am J Physiol 270:H411–H415.
40. Parenti A, Morbidelli L, Cui XL, Douglas JG, Hood JD, Granger HJ, Ledda F, ZicheM. 1998. Nitric oxide is an upstream signal of vascular endothelial growth factor-induced extracellular signal-regulated kinase$_{1/2}$ activation in postcapillary endothelium. J Biol Chem 273:4220–4226.
41. Koyama H, Bornfeldt KE, Fukumoto S, Nishizawa Y. 2001. Molecular pathways of cyclic nucleotide-induced inhibition of arterial smooth muscle cell proliferation. J Cell Physiol 186:1–10.
42. Tanner FC, Meier P, Greutert H, Champion C, Nabel EG, Luscher TF. 2000. Nitric oxide modulates expresson of cell cycle regulatory proteins: a cytostatic strategy fro inhibition of human vascular smooth muscle cell proliferation. Circulation 101:1982–1989.

43. Thomas T, Thomas TJ. 2001. Polyamines in cell growth and cell death: molecular mechanisms and therapeutic applications. Cell Mol Life Sci 58:244–258.
44. Blumer KJ, Johnson GL. 1994. Diversity in function and regulation of MAP kinase pathways. Trends Biochem Sci 19:236–240.
45. Vietor I, Schwenger P, Li W, Schlessinger J, Vilcek J. 1993. Tumor necrosis factor-induced activation and increased tyrosine phosphorylation of mitogen-activated protein (MAP) kinase in human fibroblasts. J Biol Chem 268:18994–18999.
46. Fuller SJ, Davies EL, Gillespie-Brown J, Sun H, Tonks NK. 1997. Mitogen-activated protein kinase phosphatase 1 inhibits the stimulation of gene expression by hypertrophic agonists in cardiac myocytes. Biochem J 323:313–319.
47. Meloche S, Seuwen K, Pages G, Pouyssegur J. 1992. Biphasic and synergistic activation of p44mapk (ERK1) by growth factors: correlation between late phase activation and mitogenicity. Mol Endocrinol 6:845–854.
48. Singh K, Balligand JL, Fischer TA, Smith TW, Kelly RA. 1996. Regulation of cytokine-inducible nitric oxide sinthase in cardiac myocytes and microvascular endothelial cells. J Biol Chem 271:1111–1117.
49. Nakayama I, Kawahara Y, Tsuda T, Okuda M, Yokoyama M. 1994. Angiotensin II inhibits cytokine-stimulated inducible nitric oxide synthase expression in vascular smooth muscle cells. J Biol Chem 269:11628–11633.
50. Joseph CK, Wright SD, Bornmann WG, Randolph JT, Kumar E, Bittman R, Liu J, Kolesnick RN. 1994. Bacterial lipopolysaccharide has structural similarity to ceramide and stimulates ceramide-activated protein kinase in myeloid cells. J Biol Chem 269:17606–17610.
51. Flamigni F, Facchini A, Capanni C, Stefanelli C, Tantini B, Caldarera CM. 1999. p44/42 Mitogen-activated protein kinase is involved in the expression of ornithine decarboxylase in leukemia L1210 cells. Biochem J 341:363–369.

Signal Transduction and Cardiac Hypertrophy,
edited by N.S. Dhalla, L.V. Hryshko,
E. Kardami & P.K. Singal
Kluwer Academic Publishers, Boston, 2003

The Application of Genetic Mouse Models to Elucidate a Role for Fibroblast Growth Factor-2 in the Mammalian Cardiovascular System

Karen A. Detillieux, Sarah K. Jimenez, David P. Sontag,
Elissavet Kardami,[1] Peter W. Nickerson,[2] and Peter A. Cattini

Departments of Anatomy[1]
Immunology[2] *and Physiology*
University of Manitoba
730 William Avenue, Winnipeg
Manitoba R3E 3J7, Canada

Summary. Fibroblast growth factor (FGF)-2 is a polypeptide growth factor which plays multiple roles in the mammalian cardiovascular system, having direct proliferative, migratory and differentiation effects on cardiac myocytes, fibroblasts, smooth muscle and endothelial cells. To date, a number of genetic approaches in mice have been used to further our understanding of these roles and effects. The three main approaches used so far have been overexpression, gene disruption ("knockout"), and the use of a reporter gene for the study of transcriptional regulation *in vivo*. The application of genetic models offers the advantage of endogenous production, depletion or regulation as opposed to exogenously added growth factor or regulation studied *ex vivo*. The variety of approaches available has resulted in the publication of two overexpression models, four separate "knockout" models and one reporter gene system in transgenic mice. These models have been summarized in this review and will be discussed collectively in the context of the many roles for FGF-2 in the cardiovascular system, including development, cardioprotection, angiogenesis, blood pressure regulation, and hypertrophy. The reporter gene system will be highlighted in terms of the study of gene regulation *in vivo*. Finally, various means for fine-tuning transgenic systems will be considered with respect to the ability to control endogenous FGF-2 production more precisely.

Address for Correspondence: Dr. Peter A. Cattini, Dept. of Physiology, University of Manitoba, 730 William Avenue, Winnipeg, MB R3E 3J7, Canada. Phone: (204) 789-3735, Fax: (204) 789-3934, E-mail: <Peter_Cattini@UManitoba.CA>

Keywords: fibroblast growth factor-2, transgenic mice, cardioprotection, angiogenesis, hypertrophy.

INTRODUCTION: GENETIC APPROACHES TO THE STUDY OF FGF-2 ROLE AND REGULATION

Fibroblast growth factor (FGF)-2 has many effects on many tissues throughout embryonic development and into adulthood. It is a potent mesoderm inducer and during cardiac development, FGF-2 along with activin-A mimics and may mediate the effect of the anterior endoderm on mesodermal precardiac cells (1). Later, FGF-2 also mediates the transformation of epithelial cells to mesenchyme during the formation of the cardiac cushions (2), a process involving loss of cell-cell interactions and increased migratory potential. FGF-2 also promotes cell survival during organogenesis, demonstrated in many tissues such as neurons (3), endothelial cells (4), and vascular smooth muscle cells (5).

The effects of FGF-2 on DNA synthesis and cell proliferation are also evident in most, if not all, cardiovascular cell types. FGF-2 is a potent angiogen, stimulating the proliferation of both endothelial and vascular smooth muscle cells (reviewed in 6). The potentially beneficial angiogenic properties of FGF-2 are balanced against an atherosclerotic potential, demonstrated by its role in vascular remodeling (including hyperplasia) and lumen narrowing in response to altered blood flow or vascular injury (7). However, in clinical trials angiogenic agents have not displayed any accelerated atherosclerosis (8), suggesting the balance of effects is tipped in favor of angiogenesis. In addition to this growth and remodeling effect, FGF-2 appears to directly affect vascular function, having both vasodilatory (9) and negative inotropic (10) properties.

FGF-2 has also been shown to have multiple effects on cardiac myocytes. These effects are endpoints of at least two signal transduction pathways initiated by the binding of FGF-2 to its high affinity tyrosine receptor, FGFR1, followed by receptor dimerization and autophophorylation (reviewed in 11). The Ras/Raf/MAP kinase cascade is linked to effects on cell growth (including hypertrophy) and proliferation. A second signaling pathway mediated by FGF-2 through FGFR1 is the activation of phospholipases β and γ_1, leading eventually to translocation and activation of protein kinase C (PKC) isoforms (12). This activity of FGF-2 induces changes to cardiac gap junctions (13) and mediates its cardioprotective effects (10).

FGF-2 exists in high and low molecular weight isoforms as a result of alternative translation start sites on the same messenger RNA. Although the exact size of these isoforms varies among species, low molecular weight (LMW) FGF-2 is the result of translation from a single AUG (methionine) start codon, while multiple high molecular weight (HMW) isoforms orginate from upstream CUG (leucine) start codons. It is generally accepted that LMW FGF-2 is preferentially exported from the cell or localized to the cytoplasm, and HMW FGF-2 is directed to the nucleus. In embryonic chicken and neonatal rat cardiac myocytes, both high and low molecular weight species increase cell cycle entry, but only HMW FGF-2 seemed to have an effect on nuclear and/or chromatin morphology (14,15). Overexpression of the HMW isoforms was associated with an increase in neonatal rat cardiac myocyte binucleation (15). In terms of chromatin, DNA "clumping" was observed with rat or human HMW FGF-2 overexpression (14–16), but could not be shown to be associated with either mitosis or apoptosis (16). Recently, however, with more efficient gene transfer using adenoviral vectors, a dose-dependent effect of HMW FGF-2 was identified (17). A lower dose and early time points were associated with a proliferative phenotype, while a higher dose and later time points promoted chromatin compaction, a loss of the proliferative effect, and apoptotic-like cell death.

Given the complexity of FGF-2 functions in the cardiovascular system, the application of genetic models offers two major advantages to the scientific community. First, it allows the study of the effects of endogenous growth factor as opposed to exogenously added protein. Secondly, the variety of genetic approaches available allows for the study of both gene product overexpression and depletion, in addition to gene regulation using reporter gene systems. In this review we will present an overview of the applications of these various techniques in the study of FGF-2 function and regulation with special emphasis on the cardiovascular system.

A summary of published works involving genetic models for the study of FGF-2 in the cardiovascular system is given in Table 1. Generally, the three main approaches have been (1) overexpression, (2) gene disruption or "knockout", and (3) a reporter gene system for the study of transcriptional regulation *in vivo*. In the first approach, two separate groups have introduced modified FGF-2 genes, under the control of a strong promoter, into murine pronuclei to produce transgenic mice overexpressing one or more isoforms or FGF-2 (18,19). Such models have given insight into roles for FGF-2 in development, angiogenesis, vascular smooth muscle cell proliferation, cardioprotection and isoproterenol-induced injury. The second approach involves disruption of the endogenous FGF-2 gene in embryonic stem (ES) cells by homologous recombination, followed by the incorporation of the engineered ES cells into host blastocysts and the ultimate generation of mice lacking any endogenous FGF-2 at any point during development. Four such models have been produced by independent groups (20–23), with a plethora of results pertaining to neuronal defects, blood pressure regulation, wound healing, vascular smooth muscle cell proliferation, hypertrophy and cardiac function. Finally, a luciferase reporter gene driven by rat FGF-2 promoter sequences was used to generate transgenic mouse lines by pronuclear injection (24). This model has given insight into the regulation of endogenous gene expression by catecholamines via adrenergic stimulation. These models will be collectively discussed in relation to particular functions of FGF-2 in the cardiovascular system.

FGF-2 IN CARDIOVASCULAR DEVELOPMENT

Given the known developmental roles for FGF-2 from *in vitro* studies discussed in the introduction to this chapter, there are two genetic approaches from which we can gain important information about the role for FGF-2 in development *in vivo*. The first is overexpression, in which the amount of FGF-2 in tissues is increased endogenously. The second is gene disruption or "knockout", in which all endogenous production of FGF-2 is eliminated. Each of these will be discussed in turn.

Two transgenic models overexpressing FGF-2 in the heart have been published (see Table 1). Coffin and colleagues (18) reported constitutive expression of the human full-length FGF-2 cDNA under the control of the phosphoglycerate kinase (PGK) promoter. The most obvious phenotype initially characterized was a series of skeletal defects, including shortened longbones and an enlarged skull. No defects in the myocardium were reported, although overexpression of FGF-2 in the heart did occur. Cultured vascular smooth muscle cells from these animals showed hypertrophy but no unrestricted growth. These results will be discussed in more detail in the section on *"FGF-2 and Angiogenesis"*.

The second overexpression model was produced in our laboratory (19). A modified rat FGF-2 cDNA under the control of a Rous Sarcoma Virus (RSV) promoter (RSVmetFGF) was used to produce three transgenic mouse lines by microinjection. The modified cDNA was designed to exclude the upstream CUG codons and thus specifically produce LMW FGF-2. Unlike the PGK promoter used by Coffin and colleagues (18), which directed transgene expression in a variety of tissues, RSV promoter activity was restricted to striated muscle, specifically skeletal and cardiac muscle, consistent with previous reports (25,26). The RSVmetFGF mice showed no skeletal anomalies, consistent with this restricted transgene expression. In addition, no change in heart-to-body weight ratio was observed. Upon closer examination, a significant increase in capillary density in transgenic versus control animals could be detected, suggesting that angiogenesis during development was upregulated. Overexpression of FGF-2 in the heart was associated with activation of downstream targets of FGF-2 signaling: increased phosphorylation of the stress-activated MAP kinases JNK and p38 was observed; there was also an increase in membrane translocation of PKC-α. The physiological consequences of this seemed not to involve development but instead were related to other cardiovascular effects, which will be addressed in the section *"FGF-2 and Cardioprotection"*.

Thus, in both cases overexpression of FGF-2 in cardiac cells during development failed to produce any gross abnormalities in cardiac development. Interestingly, in other studies, implantation of FGF-2-soaked beads in the cardiac region of the developing chick embryo resulted in teratogenic effects on cardiac development (27,28). Overexpression studies using transgenic models in development are limited by the promoters used to direct transgene expression. Promoter activity is often insufficient to mimic effects seen with exogenous addition of a gene product *in vitro* or *in vivo*. Instead, gene disruption is an alternate approach that can be used to "tie the hands" of a factor thought to be involved in development. Disruption of the FGF signaling pathway interferes with precardiac mesoderm development (29,30). Antisense oligonucleotides complimentary to FGF-2 inhibited precardiac mesoderm cell proliferation in chick embryos (31) and disrupted cardiovascular development in mouse embryos in culture (32).

Given these results *in vitro* that point to a critical role for FGF-2 in mesoderm induction and cardiovascular development, it was fully expected in the scientific

Table 1. Summary of genetic mouse models of FGF-2 expression and regulation

Model	Construction	Major Findings	Ref.
FGF-2 overexpression (Coffin)	PGK promoter human FGF-2 cDNA (full length)	Skeletal abnormalities (chondrodysplasia, macrocephaly) VSMC hypertrophy	(18)
		$\uparrow$ angiogenesis (with stimulus)	(43)
	human FGF2 cDNAs (isoform-specific)	VSMC hypertrophy (autocrine and paracrine effects)	(42)
FGF-2 overexpression (Cattini)	RSV promoter modified rat FGF-2 cDNA	$\uparrow$ FGF-2 release $\uparrow$ FGF-2 in ECM $\uparrow$ capillary density $\uparrow$ JNK, p38, PKCα activation $\uparrow$ myocyte viability following IR injury	(19)
		After Isp-induced injury, $\uparrow$ hypertrophy $\uparrow$ myocardial damage $\uparrow$ T-cell infiltration	(41)
FGF-2 knockout (Doetschman)	1st exon (0.5 kb) replaced with HPRT minigene	Hypotensive at baseline $\downarrow$ cardiac function in vivo Normal cardiac function in isolated working heart $\downarrow$ VSMC contractility	(20)
		$\downarrow$ hypertrophy after AC	(48)
FGF-2 knockout (Basilico)	1st exon replaced with *neo* selection gene	Defects in neocortex Delayed wound healing	(21)
		Impaired hematopoiesis No compensation by FGF-1	(44)
FGF-2 knockout (Dono)	1st exon replaced with *neo* selection gene	Hypotensive at baseline Neuronal deficiencies; Autonomic NS dysfunction Impaired baroreceptor reflex Normal AngII-induced hypertension	(22)
	Wnt-1-directed FGF-2 overexpressing transgenic crossed with KO	Phenotype rescued with FGF2 expression exclusively in developing NS	(45)
FGF-2 knockout (Pedrazzini)	deletion of 2nd exon	2K1C model of renovascular hypertension Normal resting BP Impaired compensatory hypertrophy $\downarrow$ JNK and ERK activation	(23)
FGF-2 regulation (Cattini)	luciferase reporter gene directed by 1.1 kb of 5'-flanking region of rat FGF-2 gene	FGF-2 promoter activity in heart $\uparrow$ by α-adrenergic stimulation (PE injection)	(24)

Abbreviations: AC; aortic coarctation; BP, blood pressure; ECM, extracellular matrix; FGF-2, fibroblast growth factor 2; IR, ischemia-reperfusion; Isp, isoproterenol; KO, knockout; NS, nervous system; PE, phenylephrine; PGK, phospho-glycerate kinase; RSV, Rous sarcoma virus; VSMC, vascular smooth muscle cell.

community that mice lacking FGF-2 might not be viable. It was thus surprising when three independent groups produced, in the same year, a genetic model in which mice completely lacking any endogenous FGF-2 gene expression from conception onward were born alive and with functional cardiovascular systems (20,21,22). A fourth model appeared two years later (23). In all four cases, perfectly healthy, viable and fertile mice were born which lacked any endogenous FGF-2. At first, this might have been interpreted to mean that FGF-2 is redundant *in vivo*. Such a view would ignore previous results *in vitro* (31,32), which suggest that once a developmental pathway has been committed to "using" FGF-2, loss of this factor would disrupt development, as seen with the dramatic vascular effects in mouse embryos (32). Furthermore, upon closer examination, all four groups discovered "hidden" phenotypes in adult animals that often required some sort of stimulus to be seen. Overall, two things are surprising: first, that a "null" genotype that is viable and generally morphologically "normal" could generate such a volume of genuinely interesting results; secondly, the consistency of the results from group to group indicates reproducibility and together support several key hypotheses with respect to the biological importance of FGF-2 in the cardiovascular system and elsewhere. These results will be discussed in relation to the specific functions or roles of FGF-2 they represent.

FGF-2 AND CARDIOPROTECTION

In isolated perfused rat hearts, exogenous addition of FGF-2 resulted in improved functional (contractile) recovery following global ischemia-reperfusion injury (33), an effect associated with the activation of the novel PKC isoform ε (10). Using a transient coronary ligation protocol, addition of FGF-2 also improved functional recovery following ischemia-reperfusion injury *in vivo* in the rat (34). Improved myocardial function with FGF-2 treatment was also observed in a porcine model of chronic myocardial ischemia (35). The healing effect of FGF-2 has been associated with its angiogenic potential. In the heart, FGF-2 promotes angiogenesis in animal models of chronic myocardial ischemia (35–37). In fact, clinical trials are underway in which the angiogenic nature of FGF-2 is exploited in human patients suffering from chronic myocardial ischemia (38,39). However, the cardioprotective nature of FGF-2 does not seem entirely dependent on its ability to revascularize an area, since FGF-2 lends direct protection to the cardiac myocyte in culture (40) and in isolated hearts during ischemia and reperfusion through a PKC-mediated pathway (10).

The RSVmetFGF overexpressing model produced by our laboratory was used to assess the effect of increased endogenous production of FGF-2 on cardioprotection (19). Overexpression of FGF-2 in the heart was associated with an increase in membrane translocation of PKC-α, a potential mediator of the cardioprotective effect of FGF-2 (11). Isolated, Langendorff-perfused transgenic hearts showed an increase in FGF-2 release relative to control hearts as measured in perfusates. In addition, these isolated hearts showed strong FGF-2 staining in the cytoplasm and extracellular spaces of cardiac myocytes when subjected to cryosectioning and immunohisto-

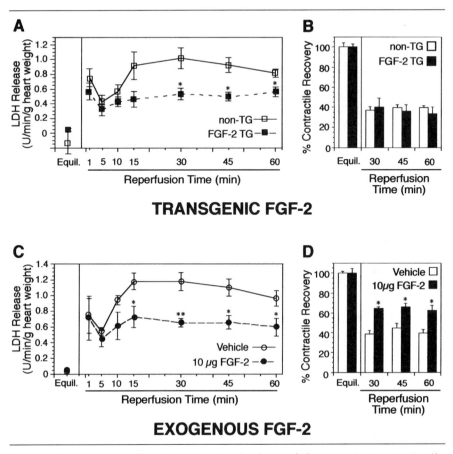

Figure 1. Cardioprotective effects of FGF-2 produced endogenously by transgenic overexpression (A and B) or added exogenously (C and D). Isolated perfused mouse hearts were subjected to 30 minutes global ischemia followed by reperfusion. Myocyte integrity was assessed by LDH activity in collected perfusates (A and C). Contractile recovery is based on developed pressure in the left ventricle expressed as a percentage of the corresponding value for the same heart obtained prior to ischemia (B and D). Adapted from (19).

chemistry after 30 minutes of perfusion. This intensified "presence" and activity of FGF-2 translated to increased myocyte viability following ischemia-reperfusion injury, indicated by decreased lactate dehydrogenase (LDH) release in transgenic relative to control animals (Figure 1A). Interestingly, the decreased LDH release in transgenic hearts was not accompanied by an improvement in contractile recovery, even though such an observation was made when FGF-2 was added exogenously (Figure 1, B and D). Again, this may represent a limitation of the RSV promoter directing FGF-2 expression in transgenic animals. Unlike a bolus delivery of a known amount of exogenous growth factor, endogenous expression is constitutive and in an unmeasured "dose". Furthermore, the mode of delivery itself is different

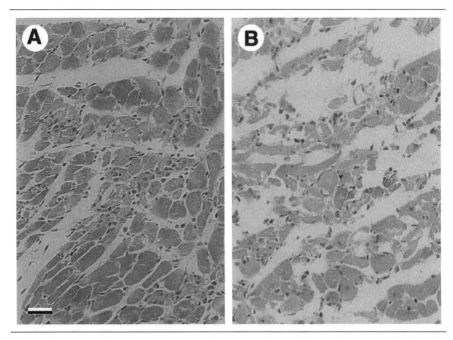

Figure 2. Examination of myocyte disarray and myocardial lesions following isoproterenol-induced injury in non-transgenic (A) and transgenic mice overexpressing FGF-2 (B). Mice were injected intraperitoneally with 160 mg/kg isoproterenol and euthanized 1 day later. Paraffin-embedded ventricular sections were stained for nuclei and cytoplasm with hematoxylin and eosin, respectively. Bar = 50 μm.

between the two systems. While exogenously added FGF-2 must travel from the vessels to the myocardium, the FGF-2 produced in transgenic mouse hearts comes from the myocytes themselves. Only when released from the myocytes on contraction or with loss of membrane integrity through damage would FGF-2 be free to enter the blood vessels.

An *in vivo* injury model, in which the β-adrenergic agonist isoproterenol was injected intraperitoneally in these same RSVmetFGF transgenic mice, demonstrated that the cardioprotective effect of endogenously and chronically produced FGF-2 may well be balanced by other more adverse cellular effects (41). In this study myocardial injury was induced by intraperitoneal injection of isoproterenol and damage to hearts was assessed 1 day and 4 days following injection. Surprisingly, transgenic hearts showed an exacerbated amount of damage compared to control animals (Figure 2). This was observed as increased myocardial disarray, increased lesion size and number, and increased left ventricular pathology scores in transgenic animals (41). In addition, transgenic hearts showed increased hypertrophy as measured by heart-to-body weight ratios. The increased damage was attributed to an exacerbated immune response. At 1 day following injury, T-cell infiltration was apparent in all areas of cardiac myocyte damage. Treatment of animals with immunosuppressive drugs 4 days before and 4 days after injury abolished the exacerbation of injury in transgenic animals. This raises the possibility that the excess FGF-2 contributed to the exacerbated inflammatory response following injury. Thus, while exogenous addition of FGF-2 has been shown to be cardioprotective both *in vitro* and *in vivo*, it is possible that chronically high levels of FGF-2 in the myocardium may result in the masking of the cardioprotective effect by other more adverse cellular effects of FGF-2. However, the functional significance of this inflammatory response is not yet known. Time course experiments in which cardiac function is recorded *in vivo* over an extended period may reveal, for example, that a protective effect will be uncovered once the inflammatory response has passed.

FGF-2 AND ANGIOGENESIS

As mentioned above, RSVmetFGF mice overexpressing FGF-2 in the heart showed a slight but significant increase in capillary density (19). Whether this was due to direct action of FGF-2 on vascular cells was not explored. However, PGK-directed overexpression of FGF-2 resulted in increased isolated aortal vascular smooth muscle cell hypertrophy but not unrestricted growth (18). Subsequently, additional transgenic models were constructed by this group (42), which specifically express different isoforms of FGF-2. In addition to the original that expressed all four human isoforms (24, 22, 21 and 18 kDa), three other transgenics were generated expressing: (1) only 24 kDa FGF-2, (2) all three nuclear-targeted isoforms (24, 22 and 21 kDa) and (3) only the lowest molecular weight, secreted isoform (18 kDa) (42). From each of these four models, cultured vascular smooth muscle cell lines were generated. Initial characterization using the original model expressing all four isoforms showed no unrestricted growth of vascular smooth muscle cells, but an increased rate of DNA and protein synthesis prior to growth arrest. No down regulation of FGF receptor signaling was observed since transgenic cells had similar growth response curves to control cells after the addition of exogenous FGF-2. Overexpression of any isoform increased the proliferative response of vascular smooth muscle cells as measured by tritiated thymidine incorporation; however, nuclear-targeted HMW isoforms had a much greater effect relative to the LMW, secreted isoform. Furthermore, HMW FGF-2 mediates its growth-stimulatory effects in these cells independently of cell-surface signaling, as neutralizing antibodies against FGF-2 failed to abolish the observed effect (42). Overexpression of HMW FGF-2 by gene transfer in cultured cardiac myocytes resulted in a nuclear phenotype in which the chromatin aggregated or "clumped" together (14–16). This phenotype is dependent on both time and FGF-2 dose (17). It was not reported whether this nuclear phenotype occurs in cultured transgenic vascular smooth muscle cells (42). It would be of interest to know if such a phenotype does occur, to perhaps link the phenotype with the intracrine effects of HMW FGF-2 that were observed in these cells.

A third study using the PGK-directed FGF-2 overexpression model reported a previously unobserved phenotype, in which an enhanced response to an angiogenic stimulus was observed (43). Subcutaneous injection of extracellular matrix was used as an angiogenic assay. Transgenic animals overexpressing all four FGF-2 isoforms developed vascularized cysts, while cysts in control animals were avascular. Heparin amplified the angiogenic reaction in transgenic animals. Thus, while no spontaneous angiogenesis or vascular defects were observed in this model, the provision of an angiogenic substrate or stimulus resulted in an amplified response.

The FGF-2 knockout models have also given us some insight, although indirect, into the role of FGF-2 in angiogenesis. While developmental angiogenesis appeared to be intact in these animals, one group reported delayed wound healing in mice lacking FGF-2 (21). Assessment of skin wound healing revealed a temporary delay, about 3 days duration, in the complete closure of wounds in FGF-2 null mice. However, relating more to the question of the role of FGF-2 in atherosclerosis, another group reported that early phase vascular hyperplasia following injury of the carotid artery appeared unaffected by the absence of FGF-2 (20). Such vascular effects of FGF-2 were not explored in the overexpressing models.

As an aside, impaired hematopoiesis was also reported in FGF-2 null mice, as assessed by counting colony-forming units in long-term bone marrow cultures (44). By irradiating and seeding these cultures, this defect was determined to be in the stromal layer and not in the hematopoietic progenitors themselves. Of great interest to the question of redundancy in FGF signaling is the fact that this second study included an FGF-1 knockout and a double knockout lacking both FGF-1 and FGF-2. The double knockout appeared similar in every way to mice lacking FGF-2 alone, and the FGF-1 null mice showed no detectable phenotype whatsoever, thus eliminating compensation by FGF-1 as a possibility for redundancy in the absence of FGF-2.

FGF-2 AND BLOOD PRESSURE REGULATION

As mentioned above, developmental angiogenesis also seemed to be unaffected by the lack of FGF-2 in mice. Two groups reported decreased mean arterial blood pressure (20,22), while one group reported normotensive mice at baseline (23). In at least one group hypotension was associated with decreased left ventricular developed pressure, and decreased rates of contraction and relaxation compared to control mice, whereas heart rate was normal (20). In this model, isolated work performing hearts revealed uncompromised cardiac Starling function, so extra-cardiac factors were deemed to be responsible for the depressed cardiac function *in vivo*. Isolated aorta and portal vein were tested for vascular smooth muscle contractility, and while no change in function was detected in aortic muscle, the portal vein showed significantly reduced spontaneous contractile activity.

In the other model where hypotension was reported (22), the results point not to intrinsic problems with vascular smooth muscle cell contractility, but rather implicate autonomic nervous system dysfunction and an impaired baroreceptor reflex. The results are compelling: Angiotensin II (AngII), when added exogenously as a vasoconstrictor, induced hypertension in FGF-2 null mice, with an exaggerated increase that brought blood pressure to levels comparable to control animals stimulated with AngII. However, when the baroreceptor reflex was provoked via the intravenous infusion of isoproterenol (acting as an acute peripheral vasodilator), FGF-2 null mice showed a drop in blood pressure and no change in heart rate, while control animals had increased heart rate and no change in blood pressure. The hypotensive response of these mice lacking any endogenous FGF-2 is a hallmark indicator of autonomic dysfunction. Given that FGF-2 itself has been reported in the past to have a hypotensive effect (9), this left the authors with the need to reconcile their results with this known activity of FGF-2. The argument was made that signaling by endogenous FGF-2 may not affect blood pressure directly under normal physiological conditions. Only under pathophysiological conditions, such as with increased mechanical strain in hypertension, would FGF-2 release from vascular smooth muscle cells (VSMC) be sufficient to lower blood pressure. In contrast, autonomic nervous dysfunction is characteristically associated with hypotension, as is observed in these FGF-2 null mice. The observations (1) that the AngII-induced increase in blood pressure is exaggerated in FGF-2 null mice, (2) that isoproterenol infusion results in decreased blood pressure in null mice, indicating a defective baroreceptor reflex, and (3) that neuronal deficiencies evident in the cerebral cortex at birth, all point to autonomic nervous system dysfunction as the root of the anomalies in blood pressure regulation observed in these mice.

These same authors went on to modify their genetic model further by crossing their knockout model with a previously generated transgenic expressing a chicken FGF-2 cDNA under the control of the *Wnt-1* promoter, thus restricting FGF-2 expression to the developing nervous system between embryonic days 9.5 and 14.5 (45). This selective re-introduction of FGF-2 into otherwise null embryos resulted in reversal of the hypotensive phenotype in adult animals. Significantly, this rescue occurred in the absence of any FGF-2 expression in the developing heart or vasculature. Thus, the role for FGF-2 in blood pressure regulation appears to take place both indirectly through effects on neuronal development, as well as directly through vasodilatory effects in the adult.

FGF-2 AND HYPERTROPHY

A fourth model of FGF-2 deficiency, published recently, is unique in that it was generated by the replacement of the second exon, not the first, resulting in the deletion of sequences encoding amino acids 82–93 (23). Confirmation of a null phenotype was not given in this publication, but rather was reported as unpublished results. The specific purpose of this study was to examine the effect of FGF-2 or its absence in a surgical model of AngII-dependent renovascular hypertension, in which one renal artery is clipped to restrict blood flow. This is known as the 2-kidney-1-clip (2K1C) model. This group reports dilated cardiac myopathy and depressed cardiac function as a basal phenotype for FGF-2 null mice, as assessed by echocardiography in anesthetized mice. Unlike Zhou and colleagues (20), this group did not find a significant decrease in resting blood pressure. However, in accordance with the results of Dono and colleagues (22), the AngII-dependent hypertensive response is intact in FGF-2 null mice, although mean blood pressure levels did not rise as high as in control mice. Four to six weeks after renal artery clipping, control mice showed an increase in cardiac mass accompanied by an increase in left ventricular wall thickness, evidence of compensatory hypertrophy. In contrast, hypertensive FGF-2 null mice showed no increase in heart mass or in left ventricular wall thickness, and likewise no compensatory increase in cardiac function. This lack of hypertrophy was accompanied by decreased MAP kinase activation (JNK, ERK and p38) compared to control animals. This group then went on to generate primary cultures, from neonatal hearts, of cardiac myocytes and non-myocytes from either control or FGF-2 null mice. When cardiac myocytes were directly stimulated by AngII or FGF-2, direct activation of MAP kinase was observed independently of the cells' ability to produce FGF-2 endogenously. Thus the lack of hypertrophic response in FGF-2 null mice did not appear to be the direct result of defects in myocyte response to stimuli. Instead, it was postulated that the lack of FGF-2 as a paracrine factor produced by neighbouring non-myocytes may be the source of the altered hypertrophic signal. MAP kinase activation (measured by JNK, ERK and p38 phosphorylation) was triggered in wild-type cardiac myocytes by supernatants from wild-type non-myocyte cultures that had been conditioned with AngII. Conditioning with AngII was essential for any activation to take place. Activation was maximized when conditioned supernatant was combined with AngII added directly to the myocytes. The activation was blocked, but only partially, by the addition of antibodies against FGF-2. Supernatants from conditioned FGF-2 null non-myocytes also resulted in partial but not complete blockage of MAP kinase activation. This would imply that FGF-2 and AngII are not the sole players in cardiac myocyte hypertrophy, which is not surprising given the recent attention given to calcineurin in pressure overload-induced hypertrophy (46,47).

Indeed, a follow-up study with the FGF-2 knockout mouse from Doetschman's group (48) indicated that FGF-2 does play a significant, although not exclusive, role in the hypertrophic response. In this study mice were subjected to transverse aortic coarctation and evaluated by echocardiography over a period of ten weeks. Interestingly, these particular FGF-2 null mice subjected to this kind of pressure overload did develop some degree of hypertrophy, but to a lesser degree than wild-type mice subjected to the same procedure. It was apparent that the lesser degree of hypertrophy was compensatory, as it was associated with a slight preservation of function relative to wild-type coarcted mice. Furthermore, responsiveness to dobutamine was intact following coarctation in FGF-2 null mice, suggesting that β-adrenergic receptors are not downregulated as they are in wild-type animals. A hallmark of pressure overload hypertrophy is the upregulation of fetal cardiac genes at the expense of adult isoforms. This study addressed levels of myosin heavy chain (MHC) message in coarcted and control animals with and without endogenous FGF-2. It was found that relative to wild-type mice, FGF-2 null mice had exceptionally high baseline (non-coarcted) levels of both α and β MHC, suggesting that FGF-2 functions to regulate levels of MHC genes in the absence of hypertrophic stimuli. With coarctation, however, levels of α-MHC (the "adult" isoform) in FGF-2 null mice were dramatically reduced compared to non-coarcted controls, suggesting that factors other than FGF-2 are responsible for these changes in this particular kind of hypertrophy. It is important to note that in this model of pressure overload, hypertrophy occurs independently of the renin-angiotensin system. In fact, at least two studies have indicated that hypertrophy does occur in murine hearts lacking the angiotensin II type 1a receptor in situations of pressure overload (49,50). Therefore, from these studies we can ascertain that FGF-2 plays an essential role in one form of hypertrophy and a significant but not essential role in another. Only with the ablation of endogenous levels of FGF-2 could such insight be obtained.

FGF-2 GENE REGULATION IN VIVO

As we have already seen, an increase in the "endogenous" levels of FGF-2 in the murine heart via overexpression of an FGF-2 transgene stimulated cardiac myocyte survival in an isolated heart model of ischemia-reperfusion injury (19). While the reasons behind the exacerbation of isoproterenol-induced injury in these same mice (41) still remains to be explored, the clear cardioprotective and angiogenic nature of FGF-2 when added exogenously (19,33–39) leads us to hypothesize that the ability to control levels of endogenous FGF-2 in the heart, and specifically cardiac myocytes, could potentially limit the extent of damage and improve recovery from an ischemic episode. Progress in understanding of the regulation of endogenous FGF-2 gene expression has been limited by the relative difficulty of assessing FGF-2 gene versus protein expression in quiescent cells, particularly in adult tissues using conventional RNA blotting methodology (24,51). Presumably, this is because of the low levels of transcription and/or rapid degradation of FGF-2 RNA. Also, results from RNA blotting, RNase protection and reverse transcriptase-PCR reflect steady state production and as such FGF-2 RNA degradation as well as synthesis. Because of the low levels of accumulation, poly-adenylated RNA-enriched samples are invariably used for these measurements, and this may require the pooling of samples if the amount of tissue is in short supply.

As an alternative, the use of a hybrid reporter gene to monitor promoter activity as a measure of synthesis offers many advantages for the study of FGF-2 gene regulation. The approach can be applied *in vitro* (culture) and, more importantly, *in vivo* through the generation of transgenic mice. This approach has been used successfully by us to investigate adrenergic regulation of FGF-2 synthesis *in vivo*. We constructed a hybrid firefly luciferase gene (−1058FGFp.*luc*) using a 1112 base pair promoter region from the rat FGF-2 gene corresponding to nucleotides −1058/+54 (52), and used it to generate transgenic mice (24). The use of the luciferase reporter avoids the problems associated with the relative instability of the FGF-2 RNA. The sensitivity of the reporter assay allows low promoter activity to be measured and, perhaps more importantly when applied to genetic mouse models, smaller or individual tissue samples to be assessed. The main disadvantage of using hybrid reporter genes relates to the question of how much flanking and promoter sequences are sufficient to reflect the pattern of expression normally observed with the endogenous gene. We first tested the −1058FGFp.*luc* gene for regulation by catecholamines in primary rat neonatal cardiac myocytes (24). Both endogenous FGF-2 RNA levels

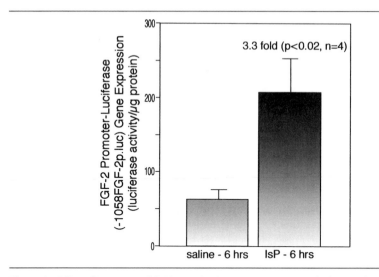

Figure 3. Effect of isoproterenol (IsP) on FGF-2 promoter activity in the hearts of −1058FGF-2p.luc transgenic mice. Mice were injected intraperitoneally with 80 mg/kg isoproterenol or an equivalent volume of saline and euthanized after 6 hours. Supernatants from heart homogenates were assayed for luciferase activity and the values were expressed relative to protein content in the sample.

and transfected FGF-2 promoter activity (−1058FGFp.*luc*) were increased by α_1-adrenergic stimulation. With regard to α-adrenergic stimulation *in vivo*, a significant 3–7 fold stimulation of FGF-2 promoter activity was detected in the hearts of two independent −1058FGFp.*luc* transgenic mouse lines six hours after intraperitoneal administration of the α_1-adrenergic agonist phenylephrine (24). An increase in endogenous FGF-2 transcript levels was also seen. These data suggest a role for this regulatory pathway *in vivo*, and the transcription factor Egr-1 has, more recently, been implicated in this response (53). Also, the *in vitro* transfection and transgenic mouse data suggest that the −1058/+54 region of the rat FGF-2 gene contains sufficient information to allow α-adrenergic regulation of the FGF-2 promoter *in vitro* and *in vivo* (24).

In contrast to the results with α-adrenergic stimulation, no significant β-adrenergic stimulation of FGF-2 promoter activity was observed in isolated neonatal rat cardiac myocytes transfected with −1058FGFp.*luc* (24). Nonetheless, preliminary studies suggest that β-adrenergic stimulation for six hours via the β-agonist isoproterenol will increase FGF-2 promoter activity in −1058FGFp.*luc* transgenic mice (Figure 3). These results could be explained by autocrine regulation of FGF-2 production which has been reported in other systems (54–56). FGF-2 has been reported to be released from cardiac myocytes on contraction through a transient remodeling (or wounding) of the plasma membrane, a process that is increased significantly with isoproterenol treatment (57,58). Indeed, isoproterenol infusion was associated with the activation of the baroreceptor reflex, the activation of which results in increased heart rate in normal mice (22). Furthermore, FGF-2 was shown to signal its own synthesis at the transcriptional level in human hepatocellular carcinoma (Hep3B) cells via, interestingly, Egr-1 (59). Thus, a possible mechanism for the increase in FGF-2 promoter activity observed in the −1058FGFp.*luc* transgenic mice, is that β-adrenergic stimulation increases heart rate and force of contraction, and thus FGF-2 release from cardiac myocytes. This in turn feeds back on the cardiac myocytes, signaling an increase in FGF-2 synthesis. The reason for the blunted response in culture may reflect disruption of the feedback mechanism during the isolation and culturing of cardiac myocytes.

FUTURE DIRECTIONS: FINE-TUNING THE SYSTEM

To date, the existing models of genetically altered FGF-2 expression have been limited mainly by the "global" nature of the genetic alterations. Looking back over the various sections of this review, it becomes clear that the ability to target the increase in or knockout of FGF-2 expression to particular tissues at particular times would clearly enhance the usefulness of such approaches to further our understanding of the role of FGF-2 in the cardiovascular system. While the developmental effects in the knockout models were for the most part subtle, they are definitely present, especially in the case of neural defects in the FGF-2 knockout and their consequences in blood pressure regulation (22,45). However, the developmental effects were mild in comparison to those observed with other approaches, such as antisense oligonucleotides (31,32). One hypothesis is that "commitment" to a particular signal for a developmental pathway may occur depending on the factors present, such that in the absence of FGF-2, a different signal is chosen leading to a viable phenotype. However, if commitment to a particular signal like FGF-2 has been established, the loss of FGF-2 later in development may result in a more severe phenotype as observed *in vitro* (32). The use of conditional systems to control the timing of either gene disruption or the overexpression of an antisense messenger RNA would allow such a hypothesis to be tested. Targeted gene disruption has been achieved in transgenic mice through the use of Cre recombinase in the so-called Cre-lox system (60,61). Targeted overexpression in a temporal manner has until recently been at the mercy of available promoters. The recent rise in popularity of drug-inducible systems allows us to combine tissue-specificity with temporal control. Such systems are commercially available and have been reviewed elsewhere (62,63).

Chronic overexpression of FGF-2 also had subtle but significant effects on capillary density (19), presumably developmental effects on angiogenesis, as well as more obvious consequences on bone development (18). The isolation and culture of vascular smooth muscle cells was one approach used to eliminate extraneous factors (42). Alternatively, targeting transgene expression using a tissue-specific promoter to a particular cell type such as cardiac myocytes, vascular smooth muscle or endothelial cells would allow for more specific questions to be addressed. For example, what is the relative influence of FGF-2 release specifically from cardiac myocytes or nonmyocytes with respect to cardioprotection? Temporal control is especially attractive when studying pathophysiological conditions in the adult. The developmental effects that were observed in the various models to date, although subtle, are clearly carried into adulthood and it is not known what effects they may be having when additional stimuli are introduced. With conditional transgene expression, the time-course dependency on the presence of FGF-2 in relation to cardioprotection, hypertrophy, angiogenesis and even atherosclerosis could be studied in various *in vivo* settings in adult animals. What are the differences in acute versus chronic effects? Is a long-term abundance of FGF-2 really beneficial or is controlled short-term expression more therapeutic?

Confining FGF-2 gene disruption both spatially and temporally would also allow us to answer lingering questions in *in vivo* settings. Pellieux and colleagues (23) showed that FGF-2 from non-myocytes is important in cardiac myocyte hypertrophy. However, these experiments were done using cultured cells taken from genetically modified animals. Specific gene disruption in myocytes or other cardiovascular cells may allow these same questions to be addressed in the whole animal. For example, if we take away FGF-2 expression specifically in adult cardiac myocytes, does hypertrophy still occur in response to AngII or pressure overload? The Cre-lox system of tissue-specific gene disruption has also been used in combination with drug inducibility (64) to exert both spatial and temporal control. Alternatively, the use of anti-sense RNA to bind and interfere with messenger RNA processing and translation has been used in transgenic animals in other systems. Such anti-sense approaches could be combined with drug inducibility to create a model in which FGF-2 gene expression could be switched off and on in a particular cell type according to the needs of a particular experiment. Temporal control is most attractive when there is a need to circumvent developmental effects. For example, the neuronal effects of FGF-2 in development clearly resulted in defective blood pressure regulation in the adult. Such indirect effects may mask other more direct effect on cardiovascular cells. Restricting the loss of FGF-2 activity to particular cardiovascular cell types specifically in the adult would allow us to relate FGF-2 function more directly to particular pathophysiological conditions.

CONCLUSION

To date, a number of genetic approaches have led to significant progress in our understanding of the roles of FGF-2 in the mammalian heart and vasculature. As we have seen, a single model can give information pertaining to several different biological functions of FGF-2. Clearly FGF-2 is an important player, directly or indirectly, alone or in combination with other factors, in many aspects of cardiovascular physiology, including development, angiogenesis, cardioprotection, hypertrophy, and blood pressure regulation. Studies with a reporter gene system have increased our understanding of how the transcriptional regulation of FGF-2 is connected to its biological activity. Fine-tuning our approaches to increase the precision of the changes in FGF-2 levels we wish to exert will allow us to further increase our understanding of the contribution this growth factor makes to significant physiological or pathophysiological events in the cardiovascular system.

REFERENCES

1. Sugi Y, Lough J. 1995. Activin-A and FGF-2 mimic the inductive effects of anterior endoderm on terminal cardiac myogenesis in vitro. Dev Biol 168:567–574.
2. Markwald R, Eisenberg C, Eisenberg L, Trusk T, Sugi Y. 1996. Epithelial-mesenchymal transformations in early avian heart development. Acta Anat (Basel) 156:173–186.
3. Grothe C, Wewetzer K. 1996. Fibroblast growth factor and its implications for developing and regenerating neurons. Int J Dev Biol 40:403–410.
4. Miao JY, Araki S, Kaji K, Hayashi H. 1997. Integrin beta-4 is involved in apoptotic signal transduction in endothelial cells. Biochem Biophys Res Comm 233:182–186.
5. Fox JC, Shanely JR. 1996. Antisense inhibition of basic fibroblast growth factor induces apoptosis in vascular smooth muscle cells. J Biol Chem 271:12578–12584.
6. Poole TJ, Finkelstein EB, Cox CM. 2001. The role of FGF and VEGF in angioblast induction and migration during vascular development. Dev Dyn 220:1–17.
7. Bryant SR, Bjerke RJ, Erichsen DA, Rege A, Lindner V. 1999. Vascular remodeling in response to altered blood flow is mediated by fibroblast growth factor-2. Circ Res 84:323–328.
8. Isner JM. 2002. Myocardial gene therapy. Nature 415:234–238.
9. Cuevas P, Carceller F, Ortega S, Zazo M, Nietol I, Gimenez-Gallego G. 1991. Hypotensive activity of fibroblast growth factor. Science 254:1208–1210.
10. Padua RR, Merle PL, Doble BW, Yu CH, Zaradka P, Pierce GN, Panagia V, Kardami E. 1998. FGF-2-induced negative inotropism and cardioprotection are inhibited by chelerythrine: Involvement of sarcolemmal calcium-independent protein kinase C. J Mol Cell Cardiol 30:2695–2709.
11. Kardami E, Padua RR, Doble BW, Sheikh F, Cattini PA. 2002. Signaling cascades mediating the pleiotropic actions of FGF-2 on cardiac myocytes. In: Fibroblast Growth Factor in the Cardiovascular System. Ed. P Cuevas, in press.
12. Tappia PS, Padua RR, Panagia V, Kardami E. 1999. Fibroblast growth factor-2 stimulates phospholipase Cβ in adult cardiomyocytes. Biochem Cell Biol 77:569–575.
13. Doble BW, Chen Y, Bosc DG, Litchfield DW, Kardami E. 1996. Fibroblast growth factor-2 decreases metabolic coupling and stimulates phosphorylation as well as masking of connexin-43 epitopes in cardiac myocytes. Circ Res 79:647–658.
14. Pasumarthi KBS, Doble BW, Kardami E, Cattini PA. 1994. Over-expression of CUG-or AUG-initiated forms of basic fibroblast growth factor in cardiac myocytes results in similar effects on mitosis and protein synthesis but distinct nuclear morphologies. J Mol Cell Cardiol 26:1045–1060.
15. Pasumarthi KBS, Kardami E, Cattini PA. 1996. High and low molecular weight fibroblast growth factor-2 increase proliferation of neonatal rat cardiac myocytes but have differential effects on binucleation and nuclear morphology. Evidence for both paracrine and intracrine actions of fibroblast growth factor-2. Circ Res 78:126–136.
16. Sun G, Doble BW, Sun JM, Fandrich RR, Florkiewicz R, Kirshenbaum L, Davie JR, Cattini PA, Kardami E. 2001. CUG-initiated FGF-2 induces chromatin compaction in cultured cardiac myocytes and in vitro. J Cell Physiol 186:457–467.
17. Hirst C, Herlyn M, Cattini PA, Kardami E. 2002. High levels of CUG-initiated FGF-2 expression cause chromatin compaction, decreased cardiomyocyte mitosis, and cell death. Mol Cell Biochem in press.
18. Coffin JD, Florkiewicz RZ, Neumann J, Mort-Hopkins T, Dorn GW II, Lightfoot P, German R, Howles PN, Kier A, O'Toole BA, Sasse J, Gonzalez AM, Baird A, Doetschman T. 1995. Abnormal bone growth and selective translational regulation in basic fibroblast growth factor (FGF-2) transgenic mice. Mol Biol Cell 6:1861–1873.
19. Sheikh F, Sontag DP, Fandrich RR, Kardami E, Cattini PA. 2001. Overexpression of FGF-2 increases cardiac myocyte viability after injury in isolated mouse hearts. Am J Physiol Heart Circ Physiol 280:H1039–H1050.
20. Zhou M, Sutliff RL, Paul RJ, Lorenz JN, Hoying JB, Haudenschild CC, Yin M, Coffin JD, Kong L, Kranias EG, Luo W, Boivin GP, Duffy JJ, Pawlowski SA, Doetschman T. 1998. Fibroblast growth factor 2 control of vascular tone. Nat Med 4:201–207.
21. Ortega S, Ittmann M, Tsang SH, Ehrlich M, Basilico C. 1998. Neuronal defects and delayed wound healing in mice lacking fibroblast growth factor 2. Proc Natl Acad Sci USA 95:5672–5677.
22. Dono R, Texido G, Dussel R, Ehmke H, Zeller R. 1998. Impaired cerebral cortex development and blood pressure regulation in FGF-2 deficient mice. EMBO J 17:4213–4225.
23. Pellieux C, Foletti A, Peduto G, Aubert JF, Nussberger J, Beerman F, Brunner HR, Pedrazzini T.

2001. Dilated cardiomyopathy and impaired cardiac hypertrophic response to angiotensin II in mice lacking FGF-2. J Clin Invest 108:1843–1851.

24. Detillieux KA, Meij JTA, Kardami E, Cattini PA. 1999. α_1-Adrenergic stimulation of FGF-2 promoter in cardiac myocytes and in adult transgenic mouse hearts. Am J Physiol 276 (Heart Circ Physiol 45):H826–H833.

25. Conti FG, Powell R, Pozzi L, Zezze G, Faraggiana T, Gannon F, Fabbrini A. 1995. A novel line of transgenic mice (RSV/LTR-bGH) expressing growth hormone in cardiac and striated muscle. Growth Regul 5:101–108.

26. Jackson T, Allard MF, Sreenan CM, Doss LK, Bishop SP, Swain JL. 1990. The c-myc proto-oncogene regulates cardiac development in transgenic mice. Mol Cell Biol 10:3709–3716.

27. Watkins BP, Bolender DL, Lough J, Kolesari GL. 1998. Teratogenic effects of implanting fibroblast growth factor-2-soaked beads in the cardiac region on the stage 24 chick embryo. Teratology 57:140–145.

28. Franciosi JP, Bolender DL, Lough J, Kolesari GL. 2000. FGF-2-induced imbalance in early embryonic heart cell proliferation: A potential cause of late cardiovascular anomalies. Teratology 62:189–194.

29. Amaya E, Musci TJ, Kirschner MW. 1991. Expression of a dominant negative mutant of the FGF receptor disrupts mesoderm formation in Xenopus embryos. Cell 66:257–270.

30. Zhu X, Sasse J, Lough J. 1999. Evidence the FGF receptor signaling is necessary for endoderm-regulated development of precardiac mesoderm. Mech Ageing Dev 108:77–85.

31. Sugi Y, Sasse J, Lough J. 1993. Inhibition of precardiac mesoderm cell proliferation by antisense oligodeoxynucleotide complementary to fibroblast growth factor-2 (FGF-2). Dev Biol 157:28–37.

32. Leconte I, Fox JC, Baldwin HS, Buck CA, Swain JL. 1998. Adenoviral-mediated expression of antisense RNA to fibroblast growth factors disrupts murine vascular development. Dev Dyn 213:421–430.

33. Padua RR, Sethi R, Dhalla NS, Kardami E. 1995. Basic fibroblast growth factor is cardioprotective in ischemia-reperfusion injury. Mol Cell Biochem 143:129–135.

34. Cuevas P, Carcellar F, Lozano RM, Crespo A, Zazo M, Gimenez-Gallego G. 1997. Protection of rat myocardium by mitogenic and non-mitogenic fibroblast growth factor during post-ischemic reperfusion. Growth Factors 15:29–40.

35. Harada K, Grossman W, Friedman M, Edelman ER, Prasad PV, Keighly CS, Manning WL, Sellke FW, Simons M. 1994. Basic fibroblast growth factor improves myocardial function in chronically ischemic porcine hearts. J Clin Invest 94:623–630.

36. Lazarous DF, Scheinowitz M, Shou M, Hodge E, Rajanayaram S, Hunsberger S, Robison WG Jr, Stiber JA, Correa R, Epstein SE, Unger EF. 1995. Effects of chronic systemic administration of basic fibroblast growth factor on collateral development in the canine heart. Circulation 91:145–153.

37. Yanagisawa-Miwa A, Uchida Y, Nakamura F, Tomaru T, Kido H, Kamijo T, Sugimoto T, Kaji K, Utsuyama M, Kurashima C, Ito H. 1992. Salvage of infarcted myocardium by angiogenic action of basic fibroblast growth factor. Science 257:1401–1403.

38. Epstein SE, Fuchs S, Zhou YF, Baffour R, Kornowski R. 2001. Therapeutic interventions for enhancing collateral development by administration of growth factors: basic principles, early results and potential hazards. Cardiovasc Res 49:532–542.

39. Simons M, Annex BH, Laham RJ, Kleiman N, Henry T, Dauerman H, Udelson JE, Gervino EV, Pike M, Whitehouse MJ, Moon T, Chronos NA. 2002. Pharmacological treatment of coronary artery disease with recombinant fibroblast growth factor-2. Circulation 105:788–793.

40. Kardami E, Padua RR, Pasumarthi KBS, Liu L, Doble BW, Davey SE, Cattini PA. 1993. Expression, localization, and effects of basic fibroblast growth factor on cardiac myocytes. In: Growth Factors and the Cardiovascular System. Ed. P Cummins, 55–76. Kluwer Academic Publishers.

41. Meij JTA, Sheikh F, Jimenez SK, Nickerson PW, Kardami E, Cattini PA. 2002. Exacerbation of myocardial injury in transgenic mice overexpressing FGF-2 is T-cell dependent. Am J Physiol Heart Circ Physiol 282:H547–H555.

42. Davis MG, Zhou M, Safdar A, Coffin JD, Doetschman T, Dorn GW II. 1997. Intracrine and autocrine effects of basic fibroblast growth factor in vascular smooth muscle cells. J Mol Cell Cardiol 29:1061–1072.

43. Fulgham DL, Widhalm SR, Martin S, Coffin JD. 1999. FGF-2-dependent angiogenesis is a latent phenotype in basic fibroblast growth factor transgenic mice. Endothelium 6:185–195.

44. Miller DL, Ortega S, Bashayan O, Basch R, Basilico C. 2000. Compensation by fibroblast growth factor 1 does not account for mild phenotypic defects observed in FGF2 null mice. Mol Cell Biol 20:2260–2268.

45. Dono R, Faulhaber J, Galli A, Zuniga A, Volk T, Texido G, Zeller R, Ehmke H. 2002. FGF-2 signaling is required for the development of neuronal circuits regulating blood pressure. Circ Res 90:e5–e10.
46. Murat A, Pellieux C, Brunner HR, Pedrazzini T. 2000. Calcineurin blockade prevents cardiac mitogen-activated protein kinase activation and hypertrophy in renovascular hypertension. J Biol Chem 275:40867–40873.
47. Zou Y, Hiroi Y, Uozumi H, Takimoto E, Toko H, Zhu W, Kudoh S, Mizukami M, Shimoyama M, Shibasaki F, Nagai R, Yazaki Y, Komuro I. 2001. Calcineurin plays a critical role in the development of pressure overload-induced cardiac hypertrophy. Circulation 104:97–101.
48. Schultz JJ, Witt SA, Niemann ML, Reiser PJ, Engle SJ, Zhou SJ, Zhou M, Pawlowski SA, Lorenz JN, Kimball TR, Doetschman T. 1999. Fibroblast growth factor-2 mediates pressure-induced hypertrophic response. J Clin Invest 104:709–719.
49. Kudoh S, Komuro I, Hiroi Y, Zou Y, Harada K, Sugaya T, Takekoshi N, Murakami K, Kadowaki T, Yazaki Y. 1998. Mechanical stretch induces hypertrophic responses in cardiac myocytes of angiotensin II type 1a receptor knockout mice. J Biol Chem 273:24037–24043.
50. Harada K, Komuro I, Zou Y, Kudoh S, Kijima K, Matsubara H, Sugaya T, Murakami K, Yazaki Y. 1998. Acute pressure overload could induce hypertrophic responses in the heart of angiotensin II type 1a knockout mice. Circ Res 82:779–785.
51. Cattini PA, Jin Y, Sheikh F. 1998. Detection of 28S RNA with the FGF-2 cDNA at high stringency through related G/C-rich sequences. Mol Cell Biochem 189:33–39.
52. Pasumarthi KBS, Jin Y, Cattini PA. 1998. Cloning of the rat fibroblast growth factor-2 promoter region and its response to mitogenic stimuli in glioma C6 cells. J Neurochem 68:898–908.
53. Jin Y, Sheikh F, Detillieux KA, Cattini PA. 2000. Role for early growth response-1 protein in α_1-adrenergic stimulation of fibroblast growth factor-2 promoter activity in cardiac myocytes. Mol Pharmacol 57:984–990.
54. Fisher TA, Ungureanu-Longrois D, Singh K, de Zengotita J, deUgarte D, Alali A, Gadbut AP, Lee MA, Balligand JL, Kifor I, Smith TW, Kelly RA. 1997. Regulation of bFGF expression and ANG II secretion in cardiac myocytes and microvascular endothelial cells. Am J Physiol 272 (Heart Circ Physiol 41):H958–H968.
55. Weich HA, Iberg N, Klagsbrun M, Folkman J. 1991. Transcriptional regulation of basic fibroblast growth factor gene expression in capillary endothelial cells. J Cell Biochem 47:158–164.
56. Alberts GF, Hsu DKW, Peifley KA, Winkles JA. 1994. Differential regulation of acidic and basic fibroblast growth factor gene expression in fibroblast growth factor-treated rat aortic smooth muscle cells. Circ Res 75:261–267.
57. Clarke MS, Caldwell RW, Chiao H, Miyake K, McNeil PL. 1995. Contraction-induced cell wounding and release of fibroblast growth factor in the heart. Circ Res 76:927–934.
58. Kaye D, Pimental D, Prasad S, Maki T, Berger HJ, McNeil PL, Smith TW, Kelly RA. 1996. Role of transiently altered sarcolemmal membrane permeability and basic fibroblast growth factor release in the hypertrophic response of adult rat ventricular myocytes to increased mechanical activity in vitro. J Clin Invest 97:281–291.
59. Wang D, Mayo MW, Baldwin AS Jr. 1997. Basic fibroblast growth factor transcriptional autoregulation requires EGR-1. Oncogene 14:2291–2299.
60. Rossant J, McMahon A. 1999. "Cre"-ating mouse mutants—a meeting review on conditional mouse genetics. Genes Dev 13:142–145.
61. Gaussin V, Van De Putte T, Mishina Y, Hanks MC, Zwijsen A, Huylebroeck D, Behringer RR, Schneider MD. 2002. Endocardial cushion and myocardial defects after cardiac myocyte-specific conditional deletion of the bone morphogenetic protein receptor ALK3. Proc Natl Acad Sci USA 99:2878–2883
62. Fishman GI. 1998. Timing is everything in life: Conditional transgene expression in the cardiovascular system. Circ Res 82:837–844.
63. Zhu Z, Ma B, Homer RJ, Zheng T, Elias JA. 2001. Use of tetracycline-controlled transcriptional silencer (tTS) to eliminate transgene leak in inducible overexpression transgenic mice. J Biol Chem 276:25222–25229.
64. Sohal DS, Ngheim M, Crackower MA, Witt SA, Kimball TR, Tymitz KM, Penninger JM, Molkentin JD. 2001. Temporally regulated and tissue-specific gene manipulations in the adult and embryonic heart using a tamoxifen-inducible Cre protein. Circ Res 89:20–25.

Signal Transduction and Cardiac Hypertrophy,
edited by N.S. Dhalla, L.V. Hryshko,
E. Kardami & P.K. Singal
Kluwer Academic Publishers, Boston, 2003

Interaction of COUP-TF II with the Rat Carnitine Palmitoyltransferase I β Promoter in Neonatal Rat Cardiac Myocytes

Guo-Li Wang, Meredith Moore, and Jeanie B. McMillin

The Department of Pathology and Laboratory Medicine
The University of Texas Medical School at Houston
The University of Texas Health Science Center
The Texas Medical Center
6431 Fannin, Houston
TX 77030 U.S.A.

Summary. The rat muscle isoform of carnitine palmitoyltransferase I β (CPT-I β) demonstrates a modest (three-fold) up-regulation of transcriptional activity when neonatal rat cardiac myocytes are co-transfected with the CPT-I β luciferase reporter gene and Peroxisomal Proliferator-Activated Receptor-α (PPAR-α). Neonatal cardiac myocytes contain undetectable levels of PPAR-α protein by immunoblotting. Cotransfection of CPT-I β luciferase with Retinoid X Receptor-α (RXR-α) alone fails to increase promoter gene expression, consistent with the low amounts of PPAR-α in neonatal rat heart. COUP-TF II, but not COUP-TF I, inhibits the activation of the CPT-I β luciferase reporter gene expression, indicating that the repressor effects are isoform specific. Anti-sense COUP-TF II transfection augments CPT-I β reporter gene expression by 80%. Mutation of the PPAR-α/RXR-α site increases CPT-I β gene expression in neonatal cardiac myocytes. Luciferase expression of both the wild type and mutant promoters is significantly inhibited by co-transfection of COUP-TF II. The data suggest that COUP-TF II represses CPT-I β activation in neonatal heart myocytes by occupying the PPAR-α/RXR-α binding site within the wild type promoter. The data also support mediation by COUP-TF II of promoter repression by interacting with other trans-acting factors on the CPT-I β promoter in neonatal heart.

Address for Correspondence: Jeanie B. McMillin, The Department of Pathology and Laboratory Medicine, The University of Texas Medical School at Houston, 6431 Fannin, Houston, TX 77030; Telephone: 713-500-5335; Fax: 713-500-0730.

Key words: Carnitine Palmitoyltransferase I β promoter, Peroxisomal Proliferator-Activated Receptor-α, COUP-TF II, neonatal rat cardiac myocytes.

INTRODUCTION

Carnitine palmitoyltransferase I β (CPT-I β) represents the muscle- and cardiac-specific isoform of CPT-I. This isoform is believed to represent the flux-generating step in β oxidation in the heart (1). The ability of CPT-I β to regulate long chain fatty acid oxidation depends on tissue concentrations of the CPT-I inhibitor, malonyl-CoA (1). CPT-I β transcription/translation increases with cardiac development until adulthood when CPT-I β constitutes the predominant isoform in adult heart (2). Recent studies from our laboratory on the transcriptional regulation of rat CPT-I β in neonatal rat cardiac myocytes demonstrate that Serum Response Factor (SRF) and the tissue-restricted isoform, GATA-4, synergistically drive robust expression of CPT-I β (3). A *Fatty Acid Response Element* (designated as FARE by Kelly and co-workers (4)) was also identified in the rat gene at −303 to −289 (3). This element is composed of a Nuclear Hormone Receptor Response Element (NRRE) complex of binding sites containing binding sequences for members of the nuclear hormone superfamily (RXR-α, PPAR-α, COUP-TF) as well as AP-1, and NFAT-3. This site binds PPAR-α/RXR-α as a heterodimer where these transcriptional activators interact with specific ligands as co-activators (for Review, see (5)). Oleic acid up-regulates hCPT-I β expression as co-activator of PPAR-α transfected into neonatal rat cardiomyocytes (4). A physiological role for fatty acid-mediated upregulation of CPT-I β in heart (4,6) is controversial as no changes in either PPAR-α or CPT-I β mRNA or CPT-I activity can be demonstrated during fasting or diabetes in adult rat heart (7–9).

Evidence for a role of PPAR-α in partial transcriptional control of CPT-I β is the coordinate regulation of PPAR-α and the enzymes of β-oxidation during development (10). Recent work has focused on down- regulation of enzymes of β-oxidation, including CPT-I β, during hypertrophy and failure of the adult heart (5,11). Levels of the nuclear receptor, COUP-TF, increase in pressure-overload hypertrophic growth (12). COUP-TF antagonizes PPAR-α binding at the NRRE (FARE) sites located in the promoter regions of genes encoding for enzymes of fatty acid oxidation. These observations are consistent with the reported compensatory shift in substrate metabolism in the failing heart to glucose (5).

COUP-TF II is critical to cardiac development and is generally present at high levels in internal organs such as heart (for review, see 13). In contrast, COUP-TF I is differentially expressed in the nervous system (13). Although striking sequence identities exist in the DNA binding and ligand-binding domains between COUP-TF I and COUP-TF II, there is significant divergence in the N-terminal activation domains, having only 45% identity (13). This finding suggests distinct function for these two proteins, with null mutants of COUP-TF II producing embryonic lethality while COUP-TF I null mice die perinatally (13).

We examined the role of COUP-TF in the regulation of the rat CPT-I β expression and the potential tissue-specific role of COUP-TF II and PPAR-α in neonatal cardiac gene expression. Our findings suggest that COUP-TF II may serve to suppress CPT-I β gene expression during early neonatal life, not only by binding to FARE but also by potential interaction with other transcriptional regulators. Repression of CPT-I β transcription in neonatal heart favors utilization of the liver-specific isoform, CPT-I α, which exhibits a low Km for its substrate, carnitine. Repression of the high Km, muscle –specific isoform (CPT-I β) would be compensatory during an early period of cardiac growth when tissue concentrations of carnitine are low (2).

MATERIALS AND METHODS

Cell culture and transfections

Neonatal rat (1–2 day old) cardiac myocytes were isolated as described previously by this laboratory (14), and plated in 6-well plates at a density of 6×10^5 cells/well in complete Dulbecco's modified Eagle's medium (DMEM) containing 10% Hyclone bovine calf serum, 500 units/ml penicillin/streptomycin. The cells were incubated at 37°C in 95% air-5% CO_2 for 24–36h before transfection. In the transient transfections, 1 μg CPT-I β firefly luciferase reporter gene construct (p-391/+80) and a series of expression vectors: 0.2 μg pSG5-hPPAR-α, 0.2 μg pSG5-mRXR-α, 0.2–0.8 μg pCR3.1-mCOUP-TF II, 0.2–0.8 μg pCR3.1-mCOUP-TF I, 0.2–0.8 μg pcDNA3.1(-)-Rev.mCOUP-TF II, were co-transfected into myocytes using LipofectAMINE Plus reagent system (Invitrogen Living Science, Carlsbad, CA) in serum-free medium as described previously (15). Total DNA of each transfection was corrected to a final concentration of 2 μg by adding empty vector pcDNA3.1. To normalize each experiment for transfection efficiency, 0.2 μg of Renilla luciferase (construct pRL-CMV) and 1.8 μg of pcDNA3.1 were co-transfected. Total protein in each well was measured using the BCA protein assay reagent kit (Pierce, Rockford, Il). CPT-I β luciferase activity was measured using the dual-luciferase reporter assay system (Promega Life Science, Madison, WI, USA). The relative luciferase activity was corrected for protein content and normalized to Renilla luciferase expression.

Plasmids and constructs

Rat CPT-I β promoter luciferase reporter construct, p-391/+80, has been reported previously (15). The promoter fragment, −391/+80, was inserted into the multiple cloning site of the promoter-less firefly luciferase vector, pGL3 basic (Promega Life Science, Madison, WI). Constructs of pSG5-hPPAR-α and pSG5-mRXR-α were kindly provided by Dr. Bart Staels (INSERM, Institut Pasteur, Lille, France). The expression vectors of pCR3.1-mCOUP-TF II and pCR3.1-mCOUP-TF I were obtained from Drs. Ming-Jer Tsai and Sophia Y. Tsai (Department of Cell Biology, Baylor College of Medicine). The construct, pcDNA3.1(-)-Rev.mCOUP-TF II, was cloned by directly inserting the 1.5 kb mCOUP-TF II cDNA fragment, cut from pCR3.1-mCOUP-TF II BamHI/XhoI sites, into the corresponding restriction sites in the pcDNA3.1(-) vector. The pcDNA3.1(-) vector and pRL-CMV construct were purchased from Invitrogen Living Science (Carlsbad, CA) and Promega Life Science (Madison, WI), respectively.

Western blotting

To identify the products of immunoblots, 1 μg PPAR-α + 1 μg pcDNA3.1 or 1 μg RXR-α + 1 μg pcDNA3.1 were transfected into neonatal heart cells. After transfection, the cells were cultured in complete DMEM for another 36 h. Both non-transfected and transfected neonatal rat heart cells were lysed with 200 μl per well of 1× sample buffer (1.5% SDS/60 mM Tris-Cl (pH 6.8)/11% Glycerol in PBS). Samples were sonicated for 15 min and boiled for 10 min. Sample protein (20 μg) was separated on 10% SDS–Polyacrylamide "Ready Gels" (Bio-Rad Laboratories, Hercules, CA) and electrophoretically transferred on ice to PVDF membranes (NEN Life Science Products, Inc., Boston, MA). The hPPAR-α and mRXR-α proteins were translated *in vitro* from their expression constructs using TNT-coupled reticulocyte lysate systems (Promega Life Science, Madison, WI), and 2 μl of each TNT product was loaded on the same gel to provide positive controls. Immunoblotting was performed with 1 : 1000 diluted polyclonal antibodies (Santa Cruz Biotechnology, Inc., Santa Cruz, CA) against PPAR-α (H-98), RXR-α (D-20), and/or actin (I-19). The immuno-reactive proteins were detected by enhanced chemiluminescence according to the manufacturer's instructions (PerkinElmer Life Sciences, Inc., Boston, MA).

Statistics

Each transfection experiment was performed using at least three different cultures of neonatal rat heart cells, with each experiment carried out in triplicate. The reported values represent the mean of the three experiments ± standard deviation. The significance of the differences was determined using Student's t test for non-paired and paired variates (SigmaPlot statistics software, Chicago, IL).

RESULTS

Immunoblot analysis of the neonatal rat cardiac myocyte content of the nuclear hormone receptors, PPAR-α and RXR-α, demonstrate no detectible levels of PPAR-α in control, non-transfected cells (Figure 1, lane 1). In contrast, RXR-α is clearly present in control myocytes (Figure 1, lane 1). Over-expression of PPAR-α and/or RXR-α by liposomal transfection produces elevated levels of both proteins (Figure 1, lanes 2 and 3). The cellular proteins migrate according to their respective translation products and both are identified by antibody staining (Figure 1, lanes 4 and 5) and compared to the actin content of the myocyte preparations.

Co-transfection of the CPT-Iβ p-391/80 promoter/luciferase reporter gene with expression vectors for either PPAR-α or RXR-α (0.2 μg each, see Materials and Methods) produces a 3.5-fold enhancement in CPT-I β gene expression in the presence of PPAR-α, but not RXR-α (Figure 2). This enhancement suggests that sufficient endogenous RXR-α is available to form heterodimers with transfected

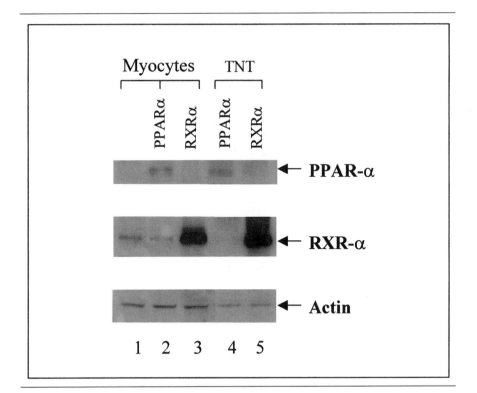

Figure 1. PPAR-α and RXR-α expression in transfected and non-transfected neonatal rat cardiac myocytes. 20 μg total protein isolated from non-transfected and PPAR-α or RXR-α transfected neonatal cardiac myocytes were separated on 10% SDS-polyacrylamide "Ready Gels" for Western blot analysis. As positive controls, 2 μl each of the hPPAR-α and mRXR-α TNT products were loaded on the same gel. PPAR-α and RXR-α expression was detected using specific antibodies, i.e. PPAR-α(H-98) and RXR-α(D-20), respectively. Actin served as the loading control.

PPAR-α. In contrast, strong over-expression of RXR-α results in an insignificant change in CPT-I β/luciferase activity, consistent with the very low levels of endogenous PPAR-α available to form activation complexes with RXR-α. The data also suggest that potential formation of RXR-α homodimers, and transcriptional activation by 1,25 dihydroxy vitamin D3 (16) does not occur in the context of the myocyte cell culture.

COUP-TF I and COUP-TF II share DNA binding sequence homology. Therefore, they should both compete with PPAR-α/RXR-α binding to the FARE site (17). The effects of the two isoforms of COUP on the PPAR-α-mediated increase in CPT-I β reporter gene expression was studied in neonatal cardiac myocytes co-transfected with CPT-I β, PPAR-α, and varying concentrations of COUP-TF (Figure 3A and 3B). COUP-TF II produces significant inhibition of CPT-I β reporter gene expression at DNA concentrations greater than 0.2 μg with almost complete suppression of the inductive effect at 0.8 μg COUP-TF II DNA (Figure

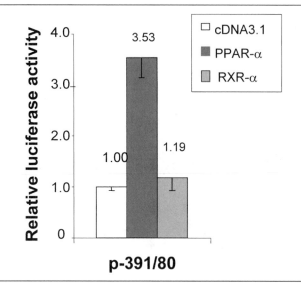

Figure 2. Increased CPT-I β promoter activation by PPAR-α. 0.2 μg of PPAR-α, RXR-α and 1 μg of p-391/+80 CPT-I β promoter luciferase construct were co-transfected into neonatal rat cardiac myocytes. The firefly luciferase activity ± PPAR-α or RXR-α was compared with the p-391/+80 transfected alone (normalized as 1.0) after correction for protein and *Renilla* luciferase expression. Bars represent means ± S.D. from three independent experiments each performed in triplicate.

3A). In contrast, COUP-TF I at any concentration fails to inhibit the induction of CPT-I β by PPAR-α/RXR-α (Figure 3B).

To study the role of COUP-TF II to repress CPT-I β transcriptional activation in the cardiac myocyte *in situ*, anti-sense COUP-TF II cDNA was transfected into cells and CPT-I β reporter gene expression compared to control transfections of empty vector. Anti-sense mRNA stimulated CPT-I β luciferase expression in a concentration-dependent manner with an 80% increase at 1 μg reverse (REV) COUP-TFII transfected (Figure 4). These data provide strong evidence that CPT-I β is transcriptionally repressed by COUP-TF II in the neonatal rat cardiac myocyte.

To examine whether COUP-TF II acts primarily to inhibit PPAR-α-mediated induction of CPT-I β, the FARE site was mutated and COUP-TF II was co-transfected with both the wildtype and mutated CPT-I β reporter gene constructs in the absence of exogenous PPAR-α (Table 1). Surprisingly, 0.5 μg of COUP-TF II suppressed by 50 to 60% reporter gene expression of both wildtype CPT-I β and the FARE mutant. The data suggest that COUP-TF II may down-regulate CPT-I β expression in the neonatal heart via interaction with other transcriptional regulators at sites distinct from the NRRE (FARE).

DISCUSSION

COUP-TF proteins are orphan (i.e. ligands unknown) members of the nuclear receptor superfamily and have been demonstrated to play roles in repression as well

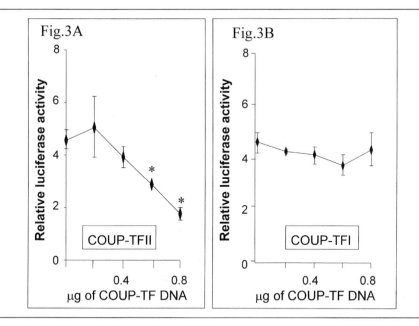

Figure 3. Inhibition of PPAR-α-mediated CPT-Iβ promoter activation by COUP-TF II. 0.2 to 0.8 μg of COUP-TF II (A) or COUP-TFI (B) constructs were co-transfected with 1 μg of p-391/ +80 CPT-Iβ construct, 0.2 μg of PPAR-α and 0.2 μg of RXR-α into neonatal rat cardiac myocytes. Firefly luciferase activity was normalized to protein and Renilla luciferase expression. Symbols represent means ± S.D. from three independent experiments each performed in triplicate. (*, p < 0.01)

as activation of gene transcription (for review, see 13). A prominent role for this family of transacting proteins has been demonstrated in control of enzymes of fatty acid oxidation in the heart during hypertrophy and failure (5). The level of CPT-I β mRNA expression has been suggested to increase with cardiac development in parallel with up regulation of PPAR-α and PGC-1 genes, the latter factor identified as a critical regulatory molecule of mitochondrial number (10). In contrast, other investigators have reported high expression of CPT-I β throughout fetal and post-natal development (9). The low level of CPT-I β *activity* was originally proposed to be a function of the low carnitine concentrations in neonatal heart (2) so that the liver CPT-I α isoform is differentially activated (Km for carnitine is six-fold lower than the muscle isoform).

Regulation of CPT-I β at the NRRE (FARE) in the adult heart with potential physiological relevance during fasting and diabetes is mediated by fatty acid activation of PPAR-α (5). Although liver CPT-I α is subject to long-term regulation by fasting- feeding cycles (9,18), others have reported that there are no changes in the activity of CPT-I β or its sensitivity to malonyl-CoA under these conditions or in response to diabetes (8,9). The sensitivity of cardiac levels of malonyl-CoA to fasting (levels decreased, 19) and insulin (levels increased, 20) suggests instead that the primary regulator of long chain fatty acid oxidation in heart is the production of

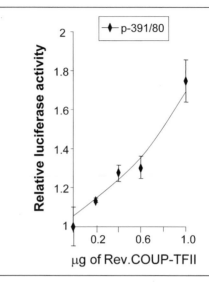

Figure 4. Blockade of endogenous COUP-TF II mRNA production and activation of CPT-I β reporter gene expression. COUP-TF II anti-sense construct [pcDNA3.1(-)-Rev.mCOUP-TF II] (0.2 to 1 μg) and 1 μg of CPT-I β promoter luciferase construct, p-391/+80, were co-transfected into neonatal rat cardiac myocytes. Firefly luciferase activity was compared with the p-391/+80 transfected alone (normalized as 1.0) after correction for protein and Renilla luciferase expression. Symbols represent means ± S.D. from three independent experiments each performed in triplicate.

Table 1. COUP-TFII suppresses wild type and FARE mutant CPT-1β

	Construct		
CMV-COUP-TFII	−	+	Percent Suppression
Wild-Type	1.0 ± 0.06	0.48 ± 0.1[‡]	50%
FARE mutation	2.6 ± 0.3[*]	0.92 ± 0.2[‡]	60%

Neonatal cardiac myocytes were transfected with 1.0 μg of Wild-Type or FARE mutant luciferase reporter construct with 0.5 μg either empty pcDNA3.1 or CMV-COUP-TF II using the Lipofectamine transfection system. Data are expressed as mean ± SEM for three separate cultures in triplicate. [*]p < 10⁻⁴ vs. Wild-Type. [‡]p < 0.001 vs. pcDNA3.1.

malonyl-CoA via acetyl CoA carboxylase (ACC-280). The cardiac ACC is a muscle-specific isoform (280 kD) and is affected by fasting/feeding cycles and hormones, e.g., epinephrine and insulin.

The transcriptional control of nuclear-encoded mitochondrial genes involved in energy metabolism is less well understood with respect to tissue specificity and in response to increasing energy demand, growth and/or hypertrophy and failure. Studies from our laboratory have demonstrated that muscle CPT-I β contains the same pattern of cardiac specific regulatory elements as do several proteins involved in excitation-contraction coupling (3). Serum response factor and the tissue restricted isoform GATA-4 drive robust transcriptional activation of CPT-I β (3).

Kelly and co-workers have recently identified important interactions of the co-activator PGC-1 with PPAR-α to increase expression of mitochondrial genes, including CPT-I β and genes of mitochondrial energy transduction and electron transport (10). Deactivation of PPAR-α with increased tissue levels of COUP-TF II, has been proposed to antagonize this up-regulation and repress CPT-I β gene transcription.

COUP-TF I and COUP-TF II have high sequence homology in the putative ligand-binding (96%) and DNA-binding (98%) domains (13). Using electrophoretic mobility shift analysis of neonatal rat myocyte nuclear protein binding to the FARE site in the rat CPT-I β gene, we have previously reported competition of a FARE oligonucleotide: protein retardation band by COUP-TF II antibody (3). No super-shifts could be demonstrated with PPAR-α, RXR-α, AP-1 or NFAT3 (data not shown). The preference for COUP-TF binding to FARE, rather than PPAR-α, is likely a consequence of concentration-dependent protein competition for the DNA binding site. The repression of PPAR-α-mediated CPT-I β transcriptional activation by COUP-TF II occurs over a concentration range of DNA comparable to trans-fected PPAR-α, confirming physiological competition for this site. Another example of dose-dependent regulation of gene transcription by COUP-TF is repression of the OCT3/4 gene by COUP-TF binding to the Retinoic Acid Receptor Element oct site. COUP-TF binds with much higher affinity than the RAR/RXR heterodimer (21). It has been proposed that gene regulation can occur by varying the ratios of repressor to inducer and by the relative affinity of each factor for the DNA binding site (17).

Absence of ligand can lead to an orphan receptor complex on the DNA where binding of a co-repressor recruits histone deacetylase to depress target gene expression (22). The finding that COUP-TF II can suppress CPT-I β gene activation independent of the FARE, or DNA binding site is novel. This finding indicates that the NRRE site for PPAR-α/RXR-α and COUP-TF II binding, i.e. the DR1, is not the sole requirement for COUP-TF II repression of CPT-I β gene expression. COUP-TF is an orphan receptor that forms either monomers or homodimers (22). Identification of ligands for this class of orphan receptors has proven difficult. The site of action of COUP-TF II independent of the DR1 (FARE) binding site is a subject of future study.

ACKNOWLEDGEMENTS

The authors thank Mr. Chad E. Jones for assistance in the preparation of the neo-natal rat cardiac myocyte cultures. This work was supported by NHLBI Grant RO1 HL38863 to JBM.

REFERENCES

1. McGarry JD, Mannaerts GP, Foster DW. 1977. A possible role for malonyl-CoA in the regulation of hepatic fatty acid oxidation and ketogenesis. J Clin Invest 60:265–270.
2. Weis BC, Cowan AT, Brown, N, Foster DW, McGarry JD. 1995. Mitochondrial carnitine palmi-toyltransferase I isoform switching in the developing rat heart. J Biol Chem 270:8952–8957.

3. Moore ML, Wang GL, McMillin JB. 2001. GATA-4 and serum response factor regulate transcription of the muscle-specific carnitine palmitoyltransferase I β in rat heart. J Biol Chem 276:1026–1033.
4. Brandt JM, Djouadi F, Kelly DP. 1998. Fatty acids activate transcription of the muscle carnitine palmitoyltransferase I gene in cardiac myocytes via the peroxisome proliferator-activated receptor α. J Biol Chem 273:23786–23792.
5. Barger PM, Kelly DP. 2000. PPAR signaling in the control of cardiac energy metabolism. Trends Cardiovasc Med 10:238–245.
6. Mascaro C, Acosta E, Ortiz JA, Marrero PF, Hegardt FG, Haro D. 1998. Control of human muscle-type carnitine palmitoyltransferase I gene transcription by peroxisome proliferator-activated receptor. J Biol Chem 273:8560–8563.
7. Escher P, Braissant O, Basu-Modak S, Michalik L, Wahli W, Desvergne B. 2001. Rat PPARs: quantitative analysis in adult rat tissues and regulation in fasting and feeding. Endocrinol 142:4195–4202.
8. Mynatt, RL, Lappi MD, Cook GA 1992. Myocardial carnitine palmitoyltransferase of the mitochondrial outer membrane is not altered by fasting. Biochim Biophys Acta 1128:105–111.
9. Cook GA, Edwards TL, Jansen MS, Bahouth SW, Wilcox HG, Park EA. 2001. Differential regulation of carnitine palmitoyltransferase-I gene isoforms (CPT-I alpha and CPT-I beta) in the rat heart. J Mol Cell Cardiol 33:317–329.
10. Lehman JJ, Barger PM, Kovacs A, Saffitz JE, Medeiros DM, Kelly DP. 2000. Peroxisome proliferator-activated receptor γ coactivator-1 promotes cardiac mitochondrial biogenesis. J Clin Invest 106:847–856.
11. Barger PM, Brandt JM, Leone TC, Weinheimer CJ, Kelly DK. 2000. Deactivation of peroxisome proliferator-activated receptor-α during cardiac hypertrophic growth. J Clin Invest 105:1723–1730.
12. Barger PM, Kelly DP. 1999. Fatty acid utilization in the hypertrophied and failing heart: molecular regulatory mechanisms. Am J Med Sciences 318:36–42.
13. Zhou, C, Tsai SY, Tsai M-J. 2000. From apoptosis to angiogenesis: new insights into the roles of nuclear orphan receptors, chicken ovalbumin upstream promoter-transcription factors, during development. Biochim Biophys Acta 1470:M63–M68.
14. McMillin JB, Hudson EK, Buja LM. 1993. Long-chain acyl-CoA metabolism by mitochondrial carnitine palmitoyltransferase: A cell model for pathological studies. Methods Toxicol 2:301–309.
15. Wang DC, Harrison W, Buja LM, Elder FFB, McMillin JB. (1998). Genomic DNA sequence, promoter expression, and chromosomal mapping of rat muscle carnitine palmitoyltransferase I. Genomics 48:314–323.
16. Thompson PD, Remus LS, Hsieh JC, Jurtka PW, Whitfield GK, Galligan MA, Encinas Dominguez C, Haussler CA, Haussler MR. 2001. Distinct retinoid X receptor activation function-2 residues mediate transactivation in homodimeric and vitamin D receptor heterodimeric contexts. J Mol Endocrinol 27:211–27.
17. Lee Y-F, Young W-J, Burbach JPH, Chang C. 1998. Negative feedback control of the retinoid-retinoic acid/retinoid X receptor pathway by the human TR4 orphan receptor, a member of the steroid receptor superfamily. J Biol Chem 272:13437–13443.
18. McGarry JD, Woeltje KF, Kuwajima M, Foster DW. 1989. Regulation of ketogenesis and the renaissance of carnitine palmitoyltransferase. In: Diabetes/Metabolism Reviews Vol.5, No.3, 271–284. John Wiley & Sons, Inc.
19. McGarry JD, Mills SE, Long CS, Foster DW. 1983. Observations on the affinity for carnitine, and malonyl-CoA sensitivity of carnitine palmitoyltransferase I in animal and human tissues. Biochem J 214:21–28.
20. Awan MM, Saggerson ED. 1993. Malonyl-CoA metabolism in cardiac myocytes and its relevance to the control of fatty acid oxidation. Biochem J 295:61–66.
21. Ben-Shushan E, Sharir H, Pikarsky E, Bergman Y. 1995. A dynamic balance between ARP-1/COUP-TFII, EAR-3/COUP-TFI, and retinoic acid receptor:retinoid X receptor heterodimers regulates Oct-3/4 expression in embryonal carcinoma cells. Mol Cell Biol 15:1034–1048.
22. Cooney AJ, Lee CT, Lin S-C, Tsai SY, Tsai M-J. 2001. Physiological function of the orphans GCNF and COUP-TF. Trends in Endocrinology & Metabolism 12:247–251.

Signal Transduction and Cardiac Hypertrophy,
edited by N.S. Dhalla, L.V. Hryshko,
E. Kardami & P.K. Singal
Kluwer Academic Publishers, Boston, 2003

Altered Expression of Conventional Calpains Influences Apoptosis

Ronald L. Mellgren, Tao Lu, and Ying Xu

The Department of Pharmacology and Therapeutics
The Medical College of Ohio
Toledo, Ohio 43614-5804 USA

Summary. Calpains are non-lysosomal, cysteine proteases ubiquitously expressed in animal cells. Most cells also express an inhibitor protein, calpastatin, that is highly specific for calpains. Among many proposed functions, calpains are thought to participate in apoptosis signaling through various pathways. Most studies of calpain function in apoptosis have relied on methodologies that cannot separate the influence of the conventional calpains (μ- and m-calpains) from other calpain family members, or non-calpain proteases in some cases. The present investigation addresses this issue by unambiguously altering the abundance of conventional calpains in cultured cells, and determining the effect on various models of apoptosis. Overexpression of μ-calpain enhanced apoptosis of Chinese hamster ovary (CHO) cells in response to the calcium ionophore A23187, the sarcolemma Ca^{2+}-pump inhibitor, thapsigargin, or serum deprivation. Overexpression of calpastatin had the opposite effect. Altered expression of calpain or calpastatin had no detectable influence on apoptosis caused by exposure to H_2O_2, ultraviolet light, or the protein kinase inhibitor, staurosporine. Increased expression of μ-calpain protected against TNF-alpha triggered apoptosis. These results demonstrate that calpain/calpastatin balance is important in some forms of apoptosis in CHO cells, but not in others. Moreover, in the TNF-alpha apoptosis pathway calpains had a protective effect, as previously proposed (Han, Y., et al. *J. Biol. Chem.* 274:787, 1999).

Key words: calpain, calpastatin, apoptosis, IGF-1, CHO cells.

Address for Correspondence: Ronald L. Mellgren, Department of Pharmacology, Medical College of Ohio, 3035 Arlington Avenue, Toledo, OH 43614-5804 USA. Telephone: 419-383-5307, Fax: 419-383-2871, E-mail: rmellgren@mco.edu

INTRODUCTION

The discovery that cells can undergo a regulated form of suicide, called apoptosis or programmed cell death (PCD), has led to the hope that myocardial damage produced in ischemia and heart failure, may be limited by subverting defined pathways to death (reviewed in refs. 1–3). While much has been discovered about the signal pathways leading from different apoptosis triggering events to ultimate cell destruction, there is still a great deal of information to learn before rational approaches to limiting apoptosis can be generated. A key issue to be resolved is the interplay of the many components thought to act in multiple apoptosis pathways.

Proteolytic events are now recognized to be of paramount importance in programmed death, with caspases, cysteine proteases cleaving after aspartic acid residues, being the major players (reviewed in refs. 4,5). The calpain family of cysteine proteases are also thought to be important in some forms of apoptosis (6–10). The focus has been on the conventional calpains, μ- and m-calpain, that require Ca^{2+} for activity. In the present study, evidence is presented linking conventional calpains to several different apoptotic pathways in our model Chinese hamster ovary (CHO) cell system. Other apoptosis signals did not appear to involve calpains. The results point to pathways in heart that might have a calpain component, and therefore may be responsive to treatment with pharmacologic agents directed against these proteases.

MATERIALS AND METHODS

Materials

SHI cells were selected from a CHO cell line by challenging with the calpain inhibitor, ZLLY-DMK, as previously described (11). The pIND (SP1)/V5-His C vector for ecdysone-inducible expression from EcR–CHO cells was purchased from Invitrogen. Calpain small subunit cDNA was a gift from Dr. John S. Elce at Queen's University, Kingston, Ontario, Canada. The full-length human calpastatin cDNA was a gift from Dr. Masatoshi Maki, Nagoya University, Japan. Mouse anti-spectrin (nonerythroid) monoclonal antibody was obtained from Chemicon. Mouse anti-β-spectrin monoclonal antibody and the calpain inhibitor SJA6017 were gifts from Dr. Kevin K.W. Wang at Pfizer Inc., Ann Arbor Laboratories, USA. IκB-α polyclonal antibody was obtained from Santa Cruz. Mouse anti-human μ-calpain large subunit monoclonal antibody, 1A–11; mouse anti-human calpastatin monoclonal antibody 5–8A; mouse anti–calpain small subunit monoclonal antibody, P-1; and a rabbit immune serum against bovine m-calpain, which also recognized the hamster antigen, were made in-house. Fibroblasts derived from calpain small subunit knockout [*Capn4* (–/–)] mouse embryos, or from wild-type littermates (12), were kindly provided by Dr. John S. Elce

Human calpain overexpressing clones

Human μ-Calpain large subunit cDNA, and rat p21 truncated calpain small subunit cDNA (13), were separately inserted into pSBC-B and pSBC-A plasmids, respectively. These plasmids were cut and ligated (14), to form a dicistronic construct, pSBC-S/L, allowing co-expression of calpain large and small subunit in equal amounts. SHI cells were co-transfected with pSBC-S/L and NEO vectors, and G418 was used for selection. Several human calpain producing cell lines were established. Twenty cell lines with no detectable human μ-calpain expression by western blot were pooled together randomly, and early passages of this cell pool were used as mock-transfected cells, SHI-NEO.

Human full-length calpastatin overexpressing clones

The full-length human calpastatin cDNA was inserted into the polylinker EcoRI site of pIND (SP1)/V5-His C vector. EcR-CHO cells which already constitutively express ecdysone receptor, were transfected with the calpastatin construct using electroporation, and selected in the presence of G418 (1.4 mg/ml) and zeocin (0.25 mg/ml). We identified two stable cell lines, clone 83 and 106, which overexpressed human calpastatin when induced with ponasterone. Mock-transfected cells were obtained by transfecting the EcR-CHO cells with empty vector.

Calpain and calpastatin assays

CHO cells or clones were lysed in a hypotonic buffer: 50 mM imidazole-HCl, 1 mM EGTA, 1 mM dithiothreitol, 70 mM NaCl, 0.1% Triton X-100, pH 7.4. A 10,000 X g supernatant was prepared and assayed for calpain activity by hydrolysis of ^{14}C-methylcasein, as previously described (15). Calpastatin activity was determined by its ability to inhibit 1 ng/ml purified human erythrocyte μ-calpain in the standard ^{14}C-caseinolytic assay.

Cell culture and treatments

S/L clone cells were cultured in 5% CO_2 and 95% humidified air atmosphere at 37°C in complete IMDM medium supplemented with heat-inactivated 10% bovine serum, 100 units/ml penicillin, and 100 μg/ml streptomycin. Calpastatin overexpressing clones were cultured in complete Ham's F12 medium containing 10% heat-inactivated fetal bovine serum and the same antibiotics. For induction of calpastatin expression, cells transfected with human calpastatin cDNA were cultured until 95–100% confluent, and pre-treated for three days with 5 μM ponasterone A before any other treatments. Mock transfected EcR-CHO cells were subjected to the same pre-treatment protocol. Cells were treated with 100 nM thapsigargin for 3 days, 5 μM A23187 for 2 days, 1 μM staurosporine for 24 hours, 3 mM EGTA for 24 hrs, or 3 mM–10 mM H_2O_2 for 2 hrs. They were then changed back to normal medium for another 24 hrs before harvest.

Cell survival assay

Cell viability after various treatments was estimated by using the MTT assay method (16).

UV light irradiation

Experiments were performed as described (17). Briefly, culture medium was exchanged for a PBS/Mg^{2+} solution, and the cells were exposed to 254 nm radiation at 5 mJ/cm^2 for different times. The cells were then transferred to the usual growth medium, and further cultured for another two days before performing MTT assays. Irradiation was carried out by using the Stratagene Corp. product Stratalinker® UV crosslinker.

DNA fragmentation assay

Cells were lysed in DNA extraction solution (50 mM Tris.HCl, 10 mM EDTA, 0.5% Triton, and 100 μg/ml proteinase K, pH 8.0). After incubating overnight, Dnase-free Rnase A was added to 100 μg/ml. The samples were incubated at 37°C for 2 hrs, extracted with an equal volume of phenol/chloroform (1 : 1 v/v), and centrifugated at 20,000×g for 10 mins at 4°C. The aqueous phase was re-extracted with chloroform. DNA was collected by precipitating the aqueous supernatant with 2 volumes of cold absolute ethanol in the presence of 1/10 volume of 3 M NaAc. After washing with 70% ethanol, the DNA pellet was dissolved in 40 μl of 10 mM Tris-HCl and 1 mM EDTA, pH 8.0. DNA was separated on 1.8% agarose gel containing 0.5 μg/ml ethidium bromide, and DNA fragments were visualized by exposing the gels to UV light.

Statistical analysis

Where indicated, samples were analysed by Students unpaired T-test, and the results are expressed as mean plus or minus the standard deviation. A P value less than 0.05 was considered to be statistically significant.

RESULTS

Characterization of calpain and calpastatin overexpressing CHO clones

After transfection with the dicistronic calpain vector as described in the Materials and Methods section, several clones overexpressing μ-calpain were isolated. Of these, the S/L18 and S/L225 clones consistently demonstrated intermediate and high levels of m–calpain expression, respectively (Figure 1). Unlike several of the other clones, they did not possess anomalies in chromatin content, cell size and shape, cell cycle kinetics, or growth rates in standard culture medium. Therefore, they were chosen for further investigation. Transfection of EcR–CHO cells with calpastatin vector produced two stable clones that overexpressed human calpastatin, as revealed by immunoblot analysis and calpastatin assay of cell lysates (Figure 2). Both clones displayed significant expression of human calpastatin in the absence of the inducer, ponasterone (panel A), but levels of expression were clearly much higher after induction (Figure 2, panel B). To determine if the expressed human calpastatin could inhibit endogenous hamster calpains, the experiment depicted in Figure 3 was performed. Activation of calpains in cells is often accompanied by their autoproteolysis. Therefore, calpastatin function in cells can be detected by protection of calpains

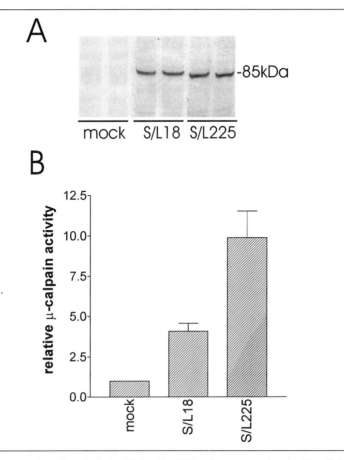

Figure 1. Overexpression of μ-calpain in CHO cells. CHO cells were transfected with a dicistronic vector containing inserts for human μ-calpain and rat calpain small subunit cDNAs, and clones were isolated as described in the Materials and Methods section. Panel A: immunoblot of mock transfected cells, clone S/L18, and clone S/L225 for human μ-calpain. Panel B: calpain activity in mock transfected, S/L18 and S/L225 cell lysates, measured at low Ca^{2+} (μ-calpain activity).

from auto-degradation. Overexpression of calpastatin greatly reduced the proteolysis of m-calpain large subunit in response to exposure to thapsigargin, indicating that the overexpressed calpastatin could bind to calpain and inhibit its proteolytic function.

Effect of altered calpain and calpastatin balance on response to typical apoptotic stimuli

To initiate our studies, the various clones and mock transfected cells were exposed to apoptotic stimuli, and cell survival was estimated by the MTT reductase assay, as described in the Materials and Methods section. As indicated in Table 1, several

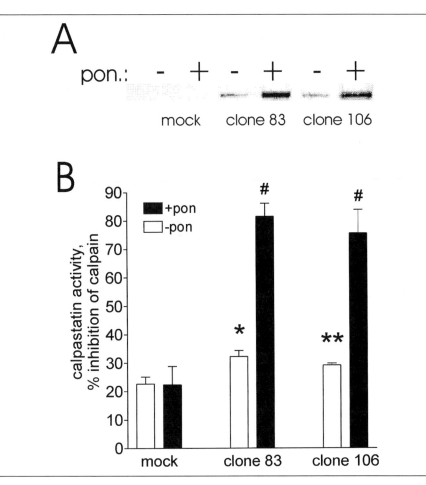

Figure 2. Induced overexpression of calpastatin in CHO cells. Ecr-CHO cells were transfected with a vector containing human calpastatin cDNA, and stable clones isolated as described in the Materials and Methods section. Panel A: immunoblot for human calpastatin. Cell lysates from mock transfected cells or clone 83 and clone 106 cells were blotted and probed with anti–human calpastatin antibody. Pon = cells were incubated with 5 μM ponasterone for 3 days prior to lysis. Panel B: calpastatin activity in lysates from mock transfected, clone 83 and clone 106 cells ± induction with ponasterone A (pon). P = 0.029 relative to mock transfected –pon (*). P = 0.042 relative to mock transfected –pon (**). P < 0.001 relative to mock transfected +pon (#).

apoptotic conditions were found to respond to alterations in calpain/calpastatin balance. In response to A23187, thapsigargin, or serum deprivation, cell survival was increased by overexpression of calpastatin, and decreased by overexpression of μ-calpain. Because the MTT reductase method cannot distinguish between apoptosis and necrosis, other methods were employed to verify the mechanism of cell death. Cell morphology studies and DNA ladder formation verified that all of the agents listed in Table I, except H_2O_2 treatment, resulted in apoptosis. Results for A23187

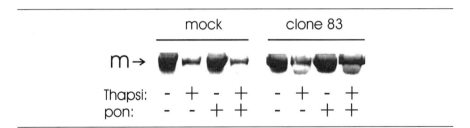

Figure 3. Inhibition of m-calpain proteolysis in CHO cells by calpastatin overexpression. Cells were cultured plus or minus 5 μM ponasterone. After 3 days, 100 nM thapsigargin were added, as indicated. After a further 3 days, cell lysates were prepared and immunoblotted for m-calpain large subunit. The arrow indicates the migration of purified bovine m-calpain large subunit, on the same gel.

Table 1. The effects of different stimuli on the cell death of calpastatin overexpressing clone #83 and calpain overexpressing S/L clones

	Percent Cell Survival						
	Calpastatin overexpressing				Calpain overexpressing		
	Mock		Clone #83				
Treatment[@]	−Pon.	+Pon.	−Pon.	+Pon.	Mock	S/L18	S/L225
−Serum	62.1 ± 2.5	58.3 ± 3.7	60.0 ± 3.1	78.1 ± 5.4★	53.1 ± 1.4	50.7 ± 2.1	29.4 ± 1.8[#]
A23187	26.6 ± 1.4	25.0 ± 0.8	23.6 ± 1.5	37.9 ± 2.4★	51.9 ± 1.4	50.8 ± 2.5	41.3 ± 0.7[#]
Thapsigargin	66.2 ± 2.4	68.0 ± 2.4	65.0 ± 2.6	86.9 ± 3.3★	49.9 ± 2.0	42.0 ± 0.8[#]	40.6 ± 1.1[#]
Staurosporine	35.7 ± 4.4	37.0 ± 1.3	35.3 ± 6.8	39.9 ± 1.5	36.2 ± 1.1	34.2 ± 1.0	37.0 ± 0.3
EGTA	66.0 ± 1.7	65.4 ± 1.4	68.0 ± 1.6	66.8 ± 2.5	64.2 ± 1.7	65.5 ± 0.8	64.6 ± 1.7
H_2O_2	30.3 ± 6.7	29.9 ± 4.4	31.3 ± 3.3	30.2 ± 4.0	47.4 ± 1.5	47.1 ± 3.3	43.7 ± 1.7
UV	54.7 ± 2.7	53.6 ± 2.0	56.1 ± 2.6	53.1 ± 2.3	46.6 ± 0.6	44.7 ± 0.9	45.4 ± 2.0

★P < 0.001 compared with −pon. samples.
[#]P < 0.001 compared with mock transfected cells.
[@]Conditions: −Serum, 24 hours culture in the absence of serum; A23187, 3 μM for 2 days; Thapsigargin, 100 nM for 3 days; Staurosporine, 1 μM for 24 hours; EGTA, 3 mM for 24 hours; H_2O_2, 3 mM for 2 hours; uv light, as described in the Methods section.
Reproduced from [26], with permission.

and thapsigargin experiments are presented in Figures 4 and 5. Other studies showed that β-spectrin breakdown was specifically accelerated by all of the stimuli except H_2O_2. The latter produced necrotic cell death at several concentrations tested, as evidenced by DNA "smearing" instead of ladder formation, and global degradation of proteins, instead of selective cleavage of spectrin.

Calpain protected against apoptosis following exposure to TNF-α

Exposure of CHO cells to TNF-α resulted in cell death (Figure 6). Contrasting with the pro-apoptotic effect of calpains in the other systems we explored, increasing calpain expression increased survival of cells exposed to TNF-α (Figure 6, S/L18 and S/L225 samples). This paradoxic protective effect is predictable from the previously postulated proteolysis of IκB-α by calpains in TNF-α stimulated HepG2 liver cells (18). Proteolysis of IκB-α would release the transcription factor NF-κB,

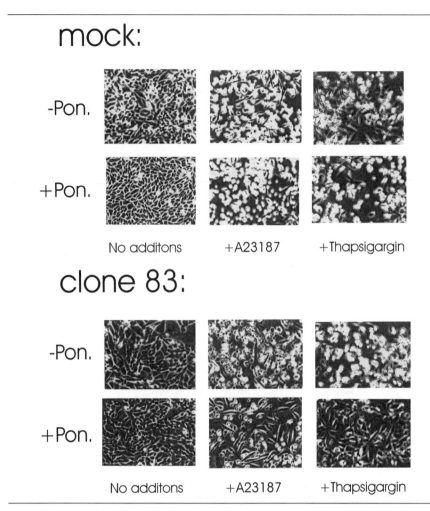

Figure 4. Calpastatin overexpression protects against thapsigargin- or A23187-induced apoptosis. Cells were cultured plus or minus ponasterone for 3 days, where indicated, and then exposed to 100nM thapsigargin or 3μM A23187 for 3 days or 2 days, respectively. Cells were observed for damage, as assessed by rounding and lifting from the culture dish, by phase contrast microscopy at 100× magnification. Reproduced from (26), with permission.

and allow it to transcribe inhibitors of apoptosis (19). However, we found no evidence that calpains are involved in the TNF-α stimulated proteolysis of IκB-α in CHO cells (data not shown). Therefore, the protective effect of calpain in CHO cells must be through another mechanism.

Apoptosis in mouse *Capn4* knockout fibroblasts

While these studies were in progress, fibroblasts from calpain small subunit knockout mice became available (12), allowing a second model to test the apoptotic effects of calpain depletion. In studies done so far, it has been possible to demonstrate the

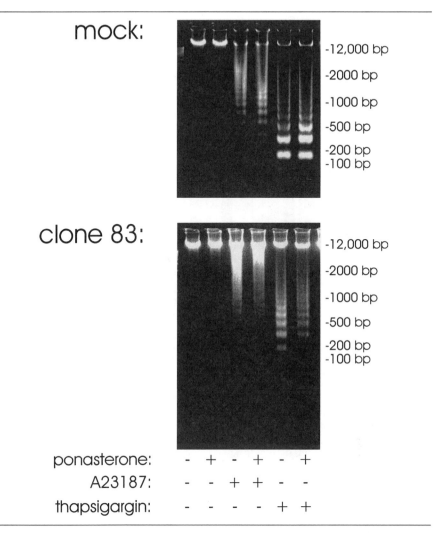

Figure 5. Decreased DNA ladder formation in A23187 or thapsigargin-treated clone 83 cells. Clone 83 or mock-transfected cells were exposed to A23187 or thapsigargin under the same conditions as in Figure 4. DNA was prepared and analyzed for apoptotic ladder formation as described in the Materials and Methods section. Reproduced from (26), with permission.

pro-apoptotic effect of conventional calpains following exposure of fibroblasts to A23187, and in serum-deprivation (Figure 7). The anti-apoptotic effect in TNF-α treated fibroblasts was also demonstrable.

IGF-1 can prevent apoptosis triggered by serum deprivation

Because IGF-1 is an important mediator of the serum-survival pathway (20,21), we decided to study its ability to counteract the CHO cell death upon serum withdrawal. As shown in Figure 8, addition of 1 µg IGF-1/ml completely protected

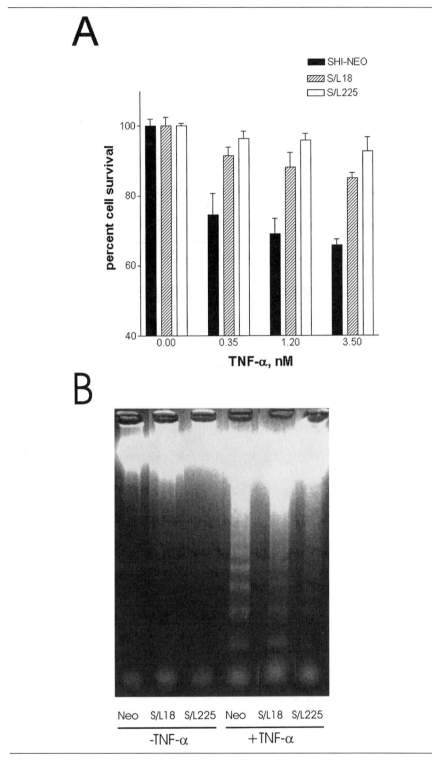

Figure 6. Calpain overexpression protected against TNF-α-induced apoptosis. Panel A: mock-transfected cells (SHI-NEO), S/L18, or S/L225 cells were cultured in the presence of the indicated concentration of TNF-a for 20 hours, and then assayed for cell survival using the MTT reductase method. Panel B: DNA ladder of cells cultured for 20 hours ± 3.5 nM TNF-α. Reproduced from (26), with permission.

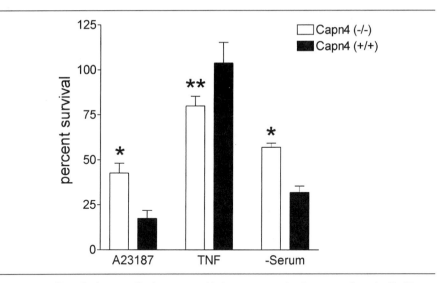

Figure 7. Effect of calpain small subunit gene ablation on apoptosis of mouse embryonic fibroblasts. Fibroblasts derived from Capn4(−/−) or Capn4(+/+) mouse embryos were exposed to various apoptotic agents, and assessed for cell viability, as described in the Materials and Methods section. Reproduced from (26), with permission.

against cell death of either mock-transfected, or S/L225 calpain overexpressing CHO cells.

DISCUSSION

It seems likely that the calpains are important components of at least some signal transduction mechanisms leading to apoptosis (6,10,22,23). The benefit of calpain inhibitors in combating apoptosis in some scenarios, for instance in myocyte death following ischemia or in congestive heart failure, will depend on the pathways involved. The present investigation clearly showed that in a given cell type, calpains may be involved in one or more apoptosis signaling pathways, but not at all in others. Even though CHO cells and mouse embryonic fibroblasts were utilized, it is not far-fetched to extrapolate to heart cells and posit that calpain influences on apoptosis may well depend on the pathway(s) involved in the particular insult or disease state producing cell death.

Of the pathways studied, the calpain influences in TNF-α and serum-deprivation induced apoptosis deserve special consideration, because they involve signaling events that might be altered in myocardial insult. Both have a calpain component, but the directions are opposite: apoptosis by serum deprivation was enhanced by calpain, while calpain appeared to protect against TNF-α apoptosis signaling. It has been suggested that the TNF-α signaling component may be most important in autoimmune cardiomyopathies, while the mitochondrial pathway is paramount in most other forms of heart failure (1). Thus, one might want to spare calpain activity or

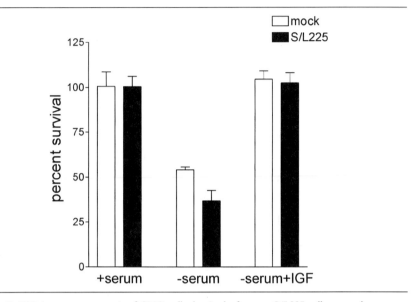

Figure 8. IGF-1 prevents apoptosis of CHO cells deprived of serum. S/L225 cells or mock-transfected cells were cultured for 20 hours plus 10% fetal bovine serum, minus serum, or minus serum plus 1 µg IGF-1/ml. Viability was assessed by MTT reductase activity, as described in the Materials and Methods section.

somehow enhance it in the former condition, but inhibit calpains to combat most cardiac insults. It is important that the calpain effect associated with serum-deprivation can be completely reversed by IGF-1 (Figure 8), which has been shown to be beneficial in limiting apoptosis in infarction (24) and in dilated cardio-myopathy (25).

ACKNOWLEDGMENTS

The authors wish to thank Dr. John Elce for providing Capn4 (−/−) and (+/+) fibroblasts, and Dr. Masatoshi Maki for the gift of human calpastatin cDNA. We acknowledge Dr. Kevin K.W. Wang for kindly providing SJA6017 inhibitor, and for his valuable advice. We thank Maura Mericle for her excellent technical assistance. This work was supported in part by NIH grant HL36573.

REFERENCES

1. Kang PM, Izumo S. 2000. *Apoptosis and heart failure: A critical review of the literature.* Circ Res 86:1107–1113.
2. Elsasser A, Suzuki K, Schaper J. 2000. *Unresolved issues regarding the role of apoptosis in the pathogenesis of ischemic injury and heart failure.* J Mol Cell Cardiol 32:711–724.
3. Dispersyn GD, Borgers M. 2001. *Apoptosis in the heart: about programmed cell death and survival.* News Physiol Sci 16:41–47.
4. Villa P, Kaufmann SH, Earnshaw WC. 1997. *Caspases and caspase inhibitors.* Trends Biochem Sci 22:388–393.

5. Colussi PA, Kumar S. 1999. *Targeted disruption of caspase genes in mice: what they tell us about the functions of individual caspases in apoptosis.* Immunol Cell Biol 77:58–63.

6. Squier MK, Miller AC, Malkinson AM, Cohen JJ. 1994. *Calpain activation in apoptosis.* J Cell Physiol 159:229–237.

7. Lu Q, Mellgren RL. 1996. *Calpain inhibitors and serine protease inhibitors can produce apoptosis in HL-60 cells.* Arch Biochem Biophys 334:175–181.

8. Nath R, Raser KJ, McGinnis K, Nadimpalli R, Stafford D, Wang KK. 1996. *Effects of ICE-like protease and calpain inhibitors on neuronal apoptosis.* Neuroreport 8:249–255.

9. Baghdiguian S, Martin M, Richard I, Pons F, Astier C, Bourg N, Hay RT, Chemaly R, Halaby G, Loiselet J, Anderson LV, Lopez de Munain A, Fardeau M, Mangeat P, Beckmann JS, Lefranc G. 1999. *Calpain 3 deficiency is associated with myonuclear apoptosis and profound perturbation of the IkappaB alpha/NF-kappaB pathway in limb-girdle muscular dystrophy type 2A.* Nat Med 5:503–511.

10. Wang KK. 2000. *Calpain and caspase: can you tell the difference?* Trends Neurosci 23:20–26.

11. Mellgren RL, Lu Q, Zhang W, Lakkis M, Shaw E, Mericle MT. 1996. *Isolation of a Chinese hamster ovary cell clone possessing decreased mu-calpain content and a reduced proliferative growth rate.* J Biol Chem 271:15568–15574.

12. Dourdin N, Bhatt AK, Dutt P, Greer PA, Arthur JS, Elce JS, Huttenlocher A. 2001. *Reduced cell migration and disruption of the actin cytoskeleton in calpain-deficient embryonic fibroblasts.* J Biol Chem 276:48382–48388.

13. Elce JS, Davies PL, Hegadorn C, Maurice DH, Arthur JS. 1997. *The effects of truncations of the small subunit on m-calpain activity and heterodimer formation.* Biochem J 326:31–38.

14. Dirks W, Wirth M, Hauser H. 1993. *Dicistronic transcription units for gene expression in mammalian cells.* Gene 128:247–249.

15. Mellgren RL, Repetti A, Muck TC, Easly J. 1992. *Rabbit skeletal muscle calcium-dependent protease requiring millimolar CA2+. Purification, subunit structure, and Ca2+-dependent autoproteolysis.* J Biol Chem 257:7203–7209.

16. Mosmann T. 1983. *Rapid colorimetric assay for cellular growth and survival: application to proliferation and cytotoxicity assays.* J Immunol Meth 65:55–63.

17. Waterhouse NJ, Finucane DM, Green DR, Elce JS, Kumar S, Alnemri ES, Litwack G, Khanna K, Lavin MF, Watters DJ. 1998. *Calpain activation is upstream of caspases in radiation-induced apoptosis.* Cell Death Differ 5:1051–1061.

18. Han Y, Weinman S, Boldogh I, Walker RK, Brasier AR. 1999. *Tumor necrosis factor-alpha-inducible IkappaBalpha proteolysis mediated by cytosolic m-calpain. A mechanism parallel to the ubiquitin-proteasome pathway for nuclear factor-kappab activation.* J Biol Chem 274:787–794.

19. Sonenshein GE. 1997. *Rel/NF-kappa B transcription factors and the control of apoptosis.* Semin Cancer Biol 8:113–119.

20. Tamm I, Kikuchi T. 1990. *Insulin-like growth factor-1 (IGF-1), insulin, and epidermal growth factor (EGF) are survival factors for density-inhibited, quiescent Balb/c-3T3 murine fibroblasts.* J Cell Physiol 143:494–500.

21. Prisco M, Romano G, Peruzzi F, Valentinis B, Baserga R. 1999. *Insulin and IGF-I receptors signaling in protection from apoptosis.* Horm Metab Res 31:80–89.

22. Roberts-Lewis JM, Marcy VR, Zhao Y, Vaught JL, Siman R, Lewis ME. 1993. *Aurintricarboxylic acid protects hippocampal neurons from NMDA- and ischemia-induced toxicity in vivo.* J Neurochem 61:378–381.

23. Sarin A, Adams DH, Henkart PA. 1993. *Protease inhibitors selectively block T cell receptor-triggered programmed cell death in a murine T cell hybridoma and activated peripheral T cells.* J Exp Med 178:1693–1700.

24. Li Q, Li B, Wang X, Leri A, Jana KP, Liu Y, Kajstura J, Baserga R, Anversa P. 1997. *Overexpression of insulin-like growth factor-1 in mice protects from myocyte death after infarction, attenuating ventricular dilation, wall stress, and cardiac hypertrophy.* J Clin Invest 100:1991–1999.

25. Lee WL, Chen JW, Ting CT, Ishiwata T, Lin SJ, Korc M, Wang PH. 1999. *Insulin-like growth factor I improves cardiovascular function and suppresses apoptosis of cardiomyocytes in dilated cardiomyopathy.* Endocrinology 140:4831–4840.

26. Lu T, Xu Y, Mericle MT, Mellgren RL. 2002. *Participation of the conventional calpains in apoptosis.* Biochim Biophys Acta, in press.

Signal Transduction and Cardiac Hypertrophy,
edited by N.S. Dhalla, L.V. Hryshko,
E. Kardami & P.K. Singal
Kluwer Academic Publishers, Boston, 2003

KLF5/BTEB2, a Krüppel-like Transcription Factor, Regulates Smooth Muscle Phenotypic Modulation

Ryozo Nagai, Takayuki Shindo, Ichiro Manabe,
Toru Suzuki, Kennichi Aizawa, Saku Miyamoto, Shinsuke Muto,
Keiko Kawai-Kowase, and Masahiko Kurabayashi

Department of Cardiovascular Medicine
University of Tokyo, Tokyo
2nd Department of Internal Medicine
University of Gunnma, Maebashi

Summary. KLF5/BTEB2 is a Krüppel-like zinc-finger type transcription factor of a non-muscle type myosin heavy chain gene SMemb, which is markedly induced in phenotypically modulated smooth muscle (SMC). KLF5/BTEB2 expression in SMC is downregulated with vascular development *in vivo* but upregulated in neointima that is produced in response to vascular injury. KLF5/BTEB2 activates the promoter of not only SMemb gene, but also of other genes which are actvated in synthetic SMC, including plasminogen activator inhibitor-1 (PAI-1), iNOS, PDGF-A, Egr-1 and VEGF receptors. Mitogenic stimulation activates KLF5/BTEB2 gene expression through MEK1 and Egr-1. KLF5/BTEB2 +/− mice showed a marked reduction in neointimal formation, angiogenesis and cardiac fibrosis induced by various kinds of stress. We suggest that KLF5/BTEB2 is a crucial transcription factor involved in smooth muscle phenotypic modulation as well as mesenchymal cell activation in cardio-vascular disease.

Key words: KLF5/BTEB2; SMC; smooth muscle; phenotypic modulation.

Address for Correspondence: Ryozo Nagai, M.D., Ph.D., Department of Cardiovascular Medicine, University of Tokyo, 7-3-1 Hongo, Bunkyo, Tokyo, Japan. Tel: +81-3-5800-6526, Fax: +81-3-3815-2087, E-mail: nagai-tky@umin.ac.jp

INTRODUCTION

Phenotypic modulation of vascular smooth muscle cells is a key event occuring during development of atherosclerosis and restenosis after balloon angioplasty (1). Phenotypic modulation of SMC is characterized by the loss of expression of the SMC-specific genes as well as a selective up-regulation of fetal/neonatal isoforms of the contractile proteins, extracellular matrix proteins, growth factors and their receptors (2–6). Alteration of the phenotype from adult type to embryonic/fetal type should require a change in expression levels of a member of this transcription factor subset (3,7,8). However, the intracellular signaling pathways and the transcriptional mechanisms for phenotypic modulation in vascular SMCs are poorly understood. We previously demonstrated that the expression of SMemb/NMHC-B, an embryonic isoform of myosin heavy chain, is induced in the neointima resulting from vascular injury (2), suggesting that SMemb gene serves as an excellent molecular marker for identifying the signaling pathways as well as transcriptional factors involved in phenotypic modulation of SMCs.

We previously isolated a zinc finger transcription factor KLF5/BTEB2 as a binding protein to the promoter region of the SMemb gene (3,9,10). KLF5/BTEB2 belongs to a family of Krüppel-like zinc finger factors such as Sp1, GKLF and LKLF, which contain three C2H2 zinc finger domains (Figure 1). Although KLF5/BTEB2 seems to be involved in activation of the SMemb gene in response to growth stimuli, the upstream intracellular signals as well as involvement of other transcription factors are not well known. We here demonstrate that the MEK-1 pathway positively regulates the KLF5/BTEB2 gene and that KLF5/BTEB2 plays a crucial role in development of cardiovascular remodeling that occurs in response to external stress.

KLF5/BTEB2 REGULATES EXPRESSION OF THE SMEMB GENE

We previously isolated cDNA clones encoding transcription factors that control the expression of the SMemb gene through binding to a *cis*-regulatory element, SE1(3,9) located at −105 bp. Sequence analysis revealed that one of the cDNA clones corresponds to the rabbit homologue of KLF5/BTEB2 (Basic Transcriptional Element Binding protein-2), which has previously been identified as a Krüppel-like transcription factor. Gel mobility shift assays and antibody supershift analyses with nuclear extract from SMC indicate that KLF5/BTEB2 is a major component of the DNA-binding complex of the promoter sequence of SMemb. In support of the functional interaction of KLF5/BTEB2 binding, basal promoter activity and KLF5/BTEB2-induced transcriptional activation were markedly attenuated by the disruption of SE1. In adult rabbit tissues, KLF5/BTEB2 mRNA was most highly expressed in intestine, urinary bladder and uterus. KLF5/BTEB2 mRNA levels were down-regulated in the rabbit aorta during normal development. Moreover, immunohistochemical analysis showed marked induction of KLF5/BTEB2 protein in neointimal SMCs after balloon injury in the rat aorta (Figure 2). These results suggest that KLF5/BTEB2 mediates transcriptional regulation of the SMemb/NMHC-B gene, and possibly plays a role in regulating gene expression during phenotypic modulation of vascular SMCs.

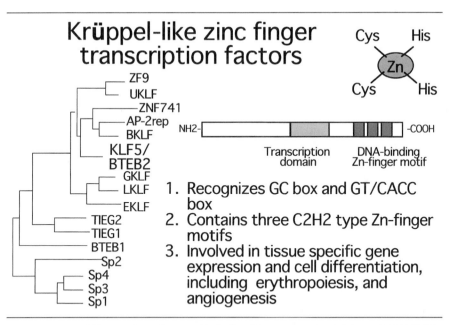

Figure 1. Krüppel-like zinc finger factors. This family of factors recognize GC box and GT/CACC box, contain three C2H2 type Zn-finger motifs and are suggested to be involved in tissue specific gene expression and cell differentiation, including erythropoiesis, and angiogenesis.

TRANSCRIPTIONAL ACTIVATION OF KLF5/BTEB2 GENE IS MEDIATED BY EGR-1 THROUGH MITOGEN-ACTIVATED PROTEIN KINASE (MAPK) PATHWAYS

We next investigated the molecular mechanisms regulating KLF5/BTEB2 expression in vascular SMCs in vitro. KLF5/BTEB2 mRNA expression is rapidly and persistently induced in SMCs by phorbol 12-myristate 13-acetate (PMA) and bFGF. We have isolated and characterized the promoter region of the human KLF5/BTEB2 gene to determine the regulatory network controlling expression of this gene in vascular SMCs (10). Cotransfection reporter assay studies with the KLF5/BTEB2 promoter coupled to a luciferase reporter gene demonstrated activation of the promoter by PMA and bFGF. Deletion analysis of the KLF5/BTEB2 gene defined a 268 bp fragment between positions −32 bp and +236 bp as a PMA-responsive region. Mutation analysis and supershift assays indicated that a GC-rich sequence between −32 bp and −12 bp, referred to as GC-1, interacts with the two zinc finger proteins Egr-1 and KLF5/BTEB2. Forced expression of Egr-1 markedly activated the minimal KLF5/BTEB2 promoter in a GC-1-dependent manner. In addition, we showed that GC-1 mediates inducible expression through the mitogen-activated protein (MAP) kinase pathways. These results indicate that KLF5/BTEB2 is a target of the early response gene Egr-1, and that the MAP kinase pathways directly or indirectly activates KLF5/BTEB2 expression. We further analyzed basal and PMA-stimulated Egr-1 expression in C2/2 cells by Northern blot analysis.

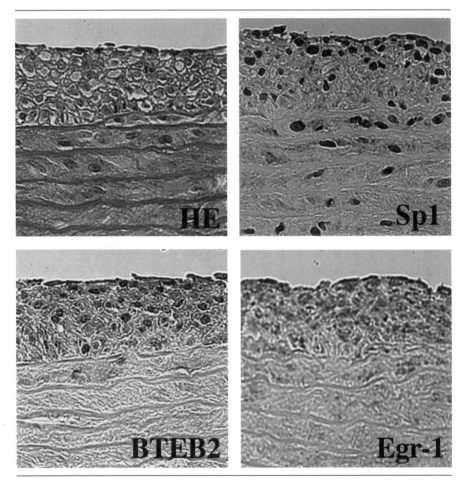

Figure 2. Induction of KLF5/BTEB2, Sp1 and Egr-1 in neointima of rat aorta after ballooning injury.

Egr-1 mRNA showed noticeable basal levels which was induced by PMA stimulation. As described in a variety of cell types, Egr-1 mRNA is rapidly and transiently induced by PMA in SMCs. In contrast, KLF5/BTEB2 mRNA levels were gradually increased with a peak at 4 hours after stimulation which remained elevated for more than 12 hrs (Figure 3).

DISRUPTION OF KLF5/BTEB2 GENE RESULTS IN REDUCED CARDIOVASCULAR RESPONSE TO STRESS

To better understand the involvement of KLF5/BTEB2 in cardiovascular remodeling, we generated KLF5/BTEB2 knockout mice (Figure 4). Homozygous mice (KLF5/BTEB2 −/−) always died *in utero* before E8.5 (11). Heterozygotes (KLF5/

PMA induces sustained KLF5/BTEB2 mRNA levels

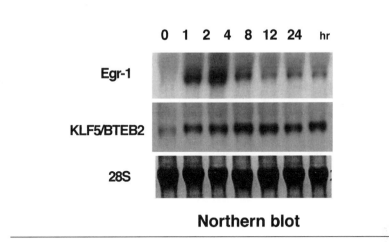

Figure 3. Time-course of the induction of Egr-1 and BTEB2 mRNAs by PMA. SMCs were incubated with 100 ng/ml PMA for the indicated times (for 0, 1, 2, 4, 8, 12, or 24 hours) and steady sate mRNA levels for BTEB2 and Egr-1 were assessed by Northern blot analysis. 28S ribosomal RNA stained by methylene blue indicates that similar amounts of total RNA were blotted onto the membrane.

BTEB2 +/−), on the other hand, survived until adulthood and were apparently normal and fertile. However, when a polyethylene tube was placed around the femoral artery of mice, we found that KLF5/BTEB2 +/− mice developed markedly reduced response in terms of formation of granulomatous tissue formation, accumulation of inflammatory cells, deposition of extracellular matrices, angiogenesis and neointimal cell proliferation (data not shown). Moreover, angiotensin II, a potent growth factor known to play a central role in both cardiac hypertrophy and vascular remodeling, was continuously infused for 14 days from an osmotic pump placed subcutaneously, the hearts of wild-type mice were significantly heavier than those of heterozygous mice, and showed much more prominent perivascular and interstitial fibrosis (data not shown).

TRANSCRIPTIONAL COFACTORS BIND TO KLF5/BTEB2

To understand the transcriptional regulatory and activation mechanisms of KLF5/BTEB2, we have begun a systematic approach to understand the protein-protein interactions which define the regulatory network governing KLF5/BTEB2's actions. Our objective is to isolate the necessary components to understand the key components and combination necessary for phenotypic modulation of smooth muscle cells at the transcription level. Affinity purification using purified recombinant subjected to a binding assay with nuclear extract from smooth muscle cells is a biochemically defined reaction but done in a cell-free environment. Use of TOF-

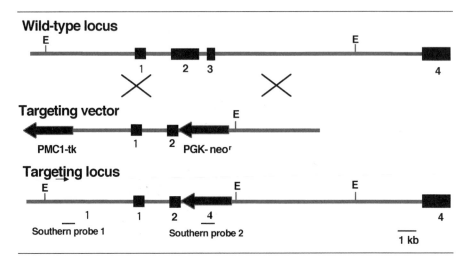

Figure 4. Targeted disruption of the mouse KLF5/BTEB2 gene. Targeting vector (PGK-neo) was inserted to cover the exon 2, intron 2 and exon 3.

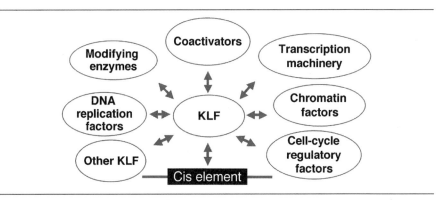

Figure 5. Cofactors that can associate with KLF.

MAS technology for the affinity purification procedure will be advantageous in identifying proteins. We envision that transcriptional cofactors, chromatin remodeling factors, modifying enzymes, cell-cycle regulatory factors, DNA-replication factors, and others will be among the factors isolated (Figure 5). Preliminary analysis suggests that such factors are among the interacting proteins identified to date.

It is of importance to mention that transcription studies should be now extended to the level of chromatin DNA and not only the naked DNA state that was addressed in the past. Recent studies in this field have isolated numerous chromatin remodeling factors and complexes as well as identified known cofactors to actually be acetyltransferases which by acetylating histones and non-histones result in activation of transcription. Interaction and regulation among these factors likely allows for modulation of the chromatin state allowing for the DNA-binding transcription factors to access DNA. An understanding of the mechanisms of chromatin modulation is essential in understanding biologically relevant transcriptional processes as eukaryotic DNA is packaged into chromatin (Figure 5).

Through our above mentioned studies on the KLF5/BTEB2 factor, notably its protein-protein interactions, we expect to isolate and identify factors which are necessary to modulate its actions, and ultimately to understand the molecular mechanisms underlying the actions of KLF5/BTEB2 which will allow for development of new molecular targeted therapies against pathogenic smooth muscle phenotypic modulation.

REFERENCES

1. Ross R. 1995. Growth regulatory mechanisms and formation of the lesions of atherosclerosis. Ann N Y Acad Sci 748:1–4.
2. Kuro-o M, Nagai R, Nakahara K, Katoh H, Tsai RC, Tsuchimochi H, Yazaki Y, Ohkubo A, Takaku F. 1991. cDNA cloning of a myosin heavy chain isoform in embryonic smooth muscle and its expression during vascular development and in arteriosclerosis. J Biol Chem 266:3768–3773.
3. Watanabe N, Kurabayashi M, Shimomura Y, Kawai-Kowase K, Hoshino Y, Manabe I, Watanabe M, Aikawa M, Kuro-o M, Suzuki T, Yazaki Y, Nagai R. 1999. BTEB2, a Krüppel-like transcription factor, regulates expression of the SMemb/nonmuscle myosin heavy chain B (SMemb/NMHC-B) gene. Circ Res 85:182–191.
4. White SL, Low RB. 1996. Identification of promoter elements involved in cell-specific regulation of rat smooth muscle myosin heavy chain gene transcription. J Biol Chem 271:15008–15017.
5. Madsen CS, Hershey JC, Hautmann MB, White SL, Owens GK. 1997. Expression of the smooth muscle myosin heavy chain gene is regulated by a negative-acting GC-rich element located between two positive-acting serum response factor-binding elements. J Biol Chem 272:6332–6340.
6. Solway J, Seltzer J, Samaha FF, Kim S, Alger LE, Niu Q, Morrisey EE, Ip HS, Parmacek MS. 1995. Structure and expression of a smooth muscle cell-specific gene, SM22 alpha. J Biol Chem 270:13460–13469.
7. Shimizu RT, Blank RS, Jervis R, Lawrenz SS, Owens GK. 1995. The smooth muscle alpha-actin gene promoter is differentially regulated in smooth muscle versus non-smooth muscle cells. J Biol Chem 270:7631–7643.
8. Kim S, Ip HS, Lu MM, Clendenin C, Parmacek MS. 1997. A serum response factor-dependent transcriptional regulatory program identifies distinct smooth muscle cell sublineages. Mol Cell Biol 17:2266–2278.
9. Manabe I, Kurabayashi M, Simomura Y, Kuro-o M, Watanabe N, Watanabe M, Aikawa M, Suzuki T, Yazaki Y, Nagai R. 1997. Isolation of the embryonic form of smooth muscle myosin heavy chain (SMemb/NMHC-B)gene and characterization of its 5′-flanking region. Biochem Biophy Res Commun 239:598–605.
10. Kawai-Kowase K, Kurabayashi M, Hoshino Y, Ohyama Y, Nagai R. 1999. Transcriptional activation of the zinc finger transcription factor BTEB2 gene by Egr-1 through mitogen-activated protein kinase pathways in vascular smooth muscle cells. Circ Res 85:787–795.
11. Shindo T, Manabe I, Fukushima Y, Tobe K, Aizawa K, Miyamoto S, Kawai-Kowase K, Moriyama N, Imai Y, Kawakami H, Nishimatsu H, Ishikawa T, Suzuki T, Morita H, Maemura K, Sata M, Hirata Y, Komukai M, Kagechika H, Kadowaki T, Kurabayashi M, Nagai R. 2002. Krüppel-like transcription factor KLF5/BTEB2 is a target for angiotensin II signaling and an essential regulator of cardiovascular remodeling. Nature Med 8:856–863.

Signal Transduction and Cardiac Hypertrophy,
edited by N.S. Dhalla, L.V. Hryshko,
E. Kardami & P.K. Singal
Kluwer Academic Publishers, Boston, 2003

Transgenic Manipulation of SERCA and PLB Levels and their Effect on Cardiac Contractility

Kalpana J. Nattamai and Muthu Periasamy

Department of Physiology and Cell Biology
Ohio State University College of Medicine and Public Health
Columbus, Ohio, 43210

Summary. Myocardial contractility is determined by the regulated release and removal of Ca^{2+}. Altered calcium handling is a common feature observed both in cardiac hypertrophy and heart failure. Especially a defective calcium transport into the SR due to decreased expression and activity of SERCA pump seems to be responsible for impaired function of the failing heart. There have been also studies showing a decreased phosphorylation status of PLB and defective Ca^{2+} transport in human heart failure. Advances in genetic technology over the past decade have significantly improved our knowledge and understanding of the role of SERCA and PLB in myocardial contractility. This review highlights recent data from transgenic animal models, where the SERCA and PLB protein expression and activity are altered. In particular we discuss how changes in SR Ca^{2+} transport through SERCA and PLB, affect myocardial function in mouse models.

Key words: SR Ca^{2+}ATPase, Phospholamban, Transgenic mouse.

INTRODUCTION

The sarcoplasmic reticulum (SR) is an intracellular membranous Ca^{2+} storage system, which plays an essential role in the beat-to-beat function of the heart, by virtue of its ability to tightly regulate the release and removal of Ca^{2+} from the cytosol. Muscle

Address for Correspondence: Muthu Periasamy, Department of Physiology and Cell Biology, Ohio State University College of Medicine and Public Health, 302, Hamilton Hall, 1645, Neil Ave, Columbus, OH—43210. Tel: (614) 292 2310, Fax: (614) 292 4888, E-mail: *periasamy.1@osu.edu*

contraction is initiated when Ca^{2+} enters the cell via L-type Ca^{2+} channel and triggers the release of a much larger amount of Ca^{2+} from the SR via the SR Ca^{2+} release channels (RYR). The Ca^{2+} released from the SR initiates the cross bridge cycling and hence the contraction of the muscle and subsequent Ca^{2+} reuptake from the cytosol causes muscle relaxation. Sequestration of Ca^{2+} into the SR is mediated by the Sarco-endoplasmic Reticulum Ca^{2+} ATPase (SERCA) pump and its integral partner Phospholamban (PLB). A small amount of Ca^{2+} is also pumped out of the cell by the plasma membrane Ca^{2+} ATPase (PMCA) and Sodium Ca^{2+} Exchanger (NCX) (1).

The cardiac SR Ca^{2+} ATPase is a trans-membrane protein of 110 KDa and belongs to a family of highly conserved proteins. SERCA2 gene encodes two isoforms SERCA2a and 2b, SERCA2a is the one predominantly expressed in the heart. Alterations both in the rate and amount of Ca^{2+} transport by SERCA, plays an important role in regulating both contraction and relaxation of the muscle. SR Ca^{2+} load or content is one of the important physiological regulators of Ca^{2+} release from the SR. Decreased SR Ca^{2+} content due to slow SERCA pump activity has negative inotropic effect (2). Moreover a decrease in Ca^{2+} uptake capacity can also delay the muscle relaxation and can affect subsequent contraction relaxation cycles.

SERCA2a pump is regulated by a 52-aminoacid/6 KDa phosphoprotein called Phospholamban (1). PLB is co-expressed with SERCA 2a and its regulatory role has been well characterized in the cardiac muscle. Under basal conditions, PLB inhibits the transport of Ca^{2+} by physically interacting with SERCA and decreasing its affinity for Ca^{2+}. Such inhibition increases the EC_{50} of the enzyme for Ca^{2+}, resulting in decreased Ca^{2+} uptake into the SR and ultimately prolonging muscle relaxation (3). In-vitro studies, using purified cardiac SR membranes, have shown that PLB can be phosphorylated at three distinct sites, which are associated with the stimulation of apparent affinity of the SERCA for Ca^{2+} (4). β adrenergic stimulation reverses the inhibition on SERCA by phosphorylating PLB and increasing the rate of Ca^{2+} uptake hence accelerates muscle relaxation (5). By increasing Ca^{2+} stores, PLB phosphorylation also increases contractility. The key regulatory portions of PLB that lies within the cytosol are, a serine residue at position 16 (Ser16) and a threonine residue at position 17 (Thr17) both of which are phosphorylated by cAMP dependent protein kinase and Ca^{2+}/Calmodulin dependent protein kinase respectively (4). PLB has been shown to exist primarily as a pentamer in equilibrium with a small fraction of monomers by SDS-PAGE- and fluorescence energy transfer studies (6,7). Also studies based on electron paramagnetic spectroscopy and fluorescence energy transfer showed that SERCA2 preferentially binds to the monomeric form of PLB and phosphorylation of PLB promotes oligomerization of PLB, consistent with reduced inhibition (7,8). Thus PLB is a key regulator of cardiac function and a prominent mediator of β adrenergic effects in the myocardium.

Advances in genetic technology have greatly helped us to improve our understanding of the functional role of the various Ca^{2+} handling proteins in cardiac physiology and pathology. In this review we discuss the key aspects of transgenic manipulation of SERCA and PLB-the two major determinants of SR Ca^{2+} transport.

EXPRESSION AND REGULATION OF SERCA AND PLB IN THE HEART

Molecular cloning analyses have identified a family of SERCA pumps encoded by three highly homologous genes namely SERCA1, SERCA2 and SERCA3. The SERCA2 gene is alternatively spliced and encodes SERCA2a and SERCA2b isoforms (9). Although, SERCA2a is the primary isoform expressed in the heart, the expression level of SERCA2a pump is highly variable during the life of an animal. There are also naturally occurring regional differences, developmental changes and aging related effects as well as alterations due to variations in thyroid hormone levels (9). In the developing rat heart, SERCA2 mRNA is abundantly present in the cardiogenic plate of the 9th day old presomite embryo, even before the occurrence of the first contraction (10). It was also shown that in mouse, rat and rabbit the expression of SERCA pump increases several fold during heart development and the expression is highest in the inflow tract and atrium (10,11). The expression level of SERCA is found to be two fold higher in the atria than in ventricles in mouse, rat, rabbit and in humans (12). Further, The SERCA2 expression levels increase several-fold post-natally coinciding with increases in thyroid hormone levels (13). Hearts from rats and mice with increased thyroxin levels showed increased SERCA expression with significantly increased contractility, whereas hypothyroid hearts displayed decreased SERCA levels together with reduced contractility (14). In the past three decades a decrease in SERCA gene expression and activity has been observed in a wide variety of pathological conditions. In addition, studies with animal models of heart disease and heart failure have shown decrease in SERCA expression similar to the observation seen in human heart failure (15,16). These studies implicate the importance of SERCA protein level and activity for cardiac function.

PLB gene is expressed in cardiac, slow twitch skeletal and smooth muscles. The amino acid sequence of PLB is highly conserved across all species and currently no isoform of PLB is known (17). In the rat embryo, PLB mRNA is first detected at 12th day embryo and the expression remains highest in the ventricle and outflow tract, which is virtually opposite to the expression pattern of SERCA (10). Like SERCA, the expression of PLB is not fixed. Thyroid hormone mediated changes in PLB expression is inversely related to the alterations in the SERCA expression pattern. Hyperthyroidism is associated with decreases in PLB protein levels, while hypothyroidism is associated with increases in PLB protein expression (13). Recent studies in failing human hearts revealed reduced levels of PLB phosphorylation and increased mRNA expression and activity of a type-1 protein phosphatase suggesting that a higher fraction of PLB is in the dephosphorylated state and contributes to greater inhibition of SERCA hence impaired cardiac function (18,19).

IMPORTANCE OF PLB/SERCA RATIO IN CARDIAC CONTRACTILITY

Changes in the expression of SERCA and PLB protein levels have been reported during pathological conditions. Also, there are naturally occurring variations in the expression of these proteins in different chambers of the heart. SERCA2 mRNA is expressed at highest levels in the upstream part of the cardiac tube and PLB prevailing in the down stream in the developing rat heart (10). This observation is also held true in the adult myocardium of mouse, rat, rabbit, guinea pig and human beings where the SERCA2 RNA and protein levels are higher in the atrium than in the ventricle, whereas PLB RNA and protein levels are higher in the ventricle than in the atrium (12). Particularly in mouse, the atrial SERCA2 mRNA is 2 fold above that of the ventricular muscle, while atrial PLB mRNA is three fold lower than the ventricular muscle (20). The duration of contraction in isolated electrically driven preparations from atrium and ventricle of mouse, rat, rabbit, guinea pig, dog and human was consistently shorter in atria compared to ventricular preparations (20,21). In mouse it has been shown that the atrial muscles exhibit on average a three-fold faster rate of contraction relaxation parameters than did the ventricular muscle and this relationship is also maintained in isoproterenol stimulated muscles (20). The potential implication of the observed molecular pattern is that the relative levels of PLB/SERCA2 in the cardiac muscle plays an important role in the cardiac muscle's overall contractility status. Ventricle has higher relative ratio of PLB to SERCA, which may reflect a greater portion of SERCA in the inhibited state at low Ca^{2+} concentration. Where as, atrium has lower relative PLB/SERCA ratio and has greater capacity to clear Ca^{2+}. This indicates that there is a specific PLB/SERCA ratio maintained for different chambers of the heart. Lower the ratio, faster is the rates of muscle contraction and relaxation and higher ratio has the opposite effect. The ratio of PLB/SERCA is also altered during hyper and hypothyroidism. During hyperthyroidism the ratio is decreased further due to the up regulation of SERCA and down regulation of PLB whereas in hypothyroidism the opposite effect is seen (21). Studies with cardiomyocytes treated with thyroid hormone in primary culture for 48h, exhibited decreases in the PLB/SERCA2 ratio, as well as increases in both myocyte contractile function and Ca^{2+} parameters (22). Studies using animal models of heart failure and in end stage human heart failure have shown that the expression level of SR Ca^{2+} ATPase was decreased both at the mRNA level and protein level (23–25). This alters the relative PLB/SERCA ratio and hence the normal function. These observations indicate that the ratio of PLB/SERCA has an essential role to play in determining cardiac contractility. However, the difference in the ratio of PLB: SERCA is not the only explanation for differences in the contractile and Ca^{2+} handling properties of atrial *vs* ventricular muscle and failing *vs* non-failing myocardium (12).

GENETICALLY ENGINEERED MOUSE MODELS WITH ALTERED PLB/SERCA2 RATIO

The functional relevance of alteration in SERCA and PLB level has been defined using genetically engineered mice in which either SERCA or PLB is overexpressed in the cardiac chamber or decreased by gene disruption methods. These mouse models have been very valuable to study the importance of PLB/SERCA ratio in cardiac contractility.

Table 1. Mouse Models with alterations in SERCA and PLB levels

Mouse Model	SERCA Protein Level	PLB Protein Level	SERCA Affinity for Ca^{2+}	Ca^{2+} uptake rate	Cardiac function	Cardiac pathology Yes/No
SERCA2a OE	1.3 & 1.5 fold ↑	Not altered	No change	37% ↑	Enhanced	No
SERCA1a OE	2.5 fold ↑	40% ↓	No change	1.9 fold ↑	Enhanced	No
SERCA2b OE	8–10 fold ↑	Not altered	↑	No change	Enhanced	No
SERCA2 KO (+/−)	35% ↓	40% ↓	No change	35% ↓	Depressed	No
PLB OE	Not altered	2 fold ↑	↓	↓	Depressed	No
PLB OE	Not altered	4 fold ↑	↓	↓	Depressed	Yes
PLB KO (−/−)	Not altered	Absent	↑	No change	Enhanced	No

The data shown in the table are obtained from TG mouse models for SERCA (Periasamy Laboratory) and PLB (Kranias Laboratory).
OE—Overexpression.
KO—Knock out.

Transgenic mice overexpressing SERCA in the heart

Transgenic animals with increased SERCA pump levels were generated by a number of investigators (26–29). In our laboratory, mouse models overexpressing different SERCA isoforms 1) the cardiac isoform SERCA2a, 2) fast twitch skeletal muscle isoform SERCA1a and 3) the housekeeping SERCA2b isoform were generated. Two independent mouse lines overexpressing SERCA2a protein 1.2 fold and 1.5 fold were studied (27). Transgenic hearts showed 37% increase in the Ca^{2+} uptake rates over the non-transgenic hearts (Table 1). However the apparent affinity for Ca^{2+} was not altered in transgenic hearts despite of an increase in the pump level. Isolated work performing hearts showed a significantly higher myocardial contractile function, as indicated by increased maximal rates of pressure development for contraction (+dP/dt) and relaxation (−dP/dt) together with the shortening of time to peak pressure and time to half relaxation (27).

We additionally tested whether SERCA1a the skeletal muscle isoform can substitute for the cardiac isoform. Transgenic mice expressing the SERCA1a isoform in the mouse heart are healthy and reproduce well (28). Overexpression of this pump increased total SERCA levels to 2.5 fold and Ca^{2+} uptake rates to 1.9 fold without changing the apparent affinity of the pump for Ca^{2+} (Figure 1 & Table 1). The measured functional parameters of these hearts were clearly enhanced. Interestingly, the expression of SERCA1a led to a 50% down regulation of the

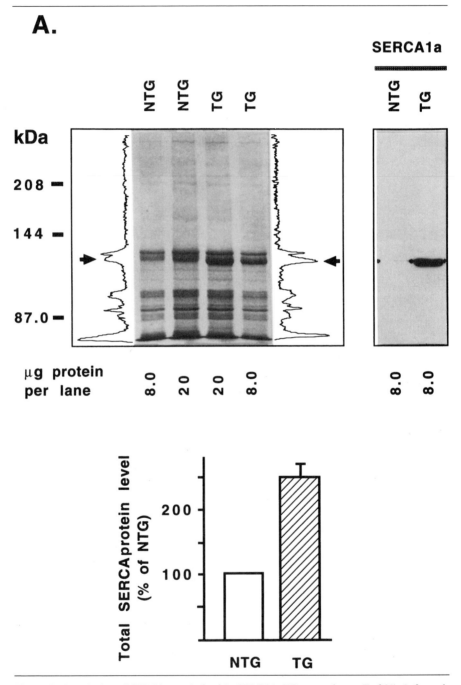

Figure 1. Quantitation of SERCA protein level in SERCA1a TG mouse hearts (Ref 28). Left panel shows Coomassie blue staining of SR proteins from SERCA1a TG and NTG hearts (6% SDS-PAGE). Right panel shows immuno-blotting with SERCA1a antibody. Bottom, Bar graph shows the total SERCA protein level in TG hearts.

endogenous SERCA2a pump as detected by isoform specific antibodies. This mouse model clearly demonstrates that SERCA1a can functionally substitute for SERCA2a in the heart (28).

Whereas, overexpression of the ubiquitous isoform that has higher affinity for Ca^{2+} did not alter the Ca^{2+} uptake rate but increased the apparent affinity for Ca^{2+} (Table 1). The SERCA2b showed enhanced contractility and did not show any pathology or hypertrophy (29). In a recent study, Verheyen et al. generated mice that altogether lacked SERCA2a isoform but expressed the alternate SERCA2b isoform. These mice while managed to survive, developed cardiac hypertrophy and heart failure (30).

SERCA2 (+/−) heterozygous mice

Using gene-targeting approach, the SERCA2 gene was disrupted. Homozygous SERCA2 null mutants were not observed, indicating that deletion of both copies result in embryonic lethality, whereas heterozygous mice with a single functional allele are alive and reproduce well (31). Biochemical analysis of heart samples showed that SERCA2 mRNA was reduced by ~45% and that SERCA2 protein and maximal velocity of Ca^{2+} uptake into the sarcoplasmic reticulum were reduced by ~35% (Table 1). However, EC_{50} value of the Ca^{2+} uptake was unchanged. The rates of myocyte shortening and relengthening were decreased by ~40% in the heterozygous myocytes. Measurements of cardiovascular performance via transducers in the left ventricle and right femoral artery revealed reductions in mean arterial pressure, systolic ventricular pressure and the absolute values of both positive and negative dP/dt in heterozygous mice (31). In spite of these deficits no cardiac pathology or hypertrophy is observed in this model. These findings led us to believe that the Ca2+ transport function might be compensated by alterations in other Ca^{2+} transport proteins and their activity. We found that (a) The PLB level is decreased by ~40% in the heterozygous hearts which is comparable to the decrease in the SERCA2 level (Figure 1 & Table 1) (b) The basal phosphorylation of PLB at Ser16 and Thr 17, which relieves the inhibition, was increased ~2 and ~2.1 fold (Figure 2) (c) Also the ratio of pentameric PLB to monomeric PLB increased ~1.4 fold (Figure 2) (d) In addition there were alterations in NCX expression and function; both the forward and reverse mode NCX currents were increased in these hearts (32).

Transgenic mice overexpressing PLB in the heart

Transgenic mice expressing two-fold higher level of PLB in the heart were generated in the laboratory of Kranias (33) (Table 1). Functional analyses on cardiac myocytes revealed diminished shortening fraction (63%) and decreased rates of shortening (64%) and relengthening (55%) compared with wild type cardiomyocytes. The decreases in contractile parameters of transgenic cardiomyocytes reflected decreases in the amplitude (83%) of the Ca^{2+} signal, which was associated with a decrease in the apparent affinity of the SERCA for Ca^{2+} (56%) compared to wild type myocytes. In vivo analysis of left ventricular systolic function revealed decreases in fractional

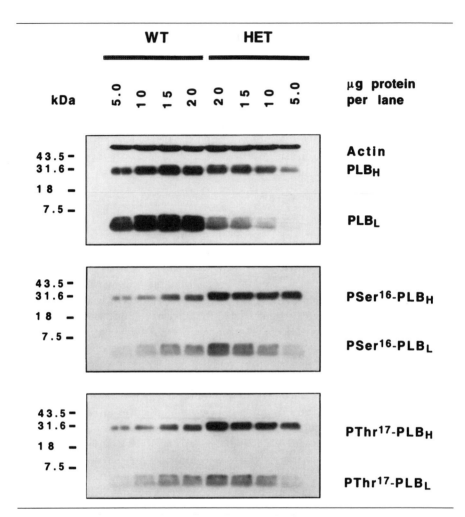

Figure 2. SERCA2 heterozygous hearts show decreased Phospholamban protein level and increased phosphorylation status (Ref 32). Top panel shows PLB monomer and pentamer levels in wild-type (*WT*) and heterozygous (*HET*) hearts. α-Sarcomeric actin was used as an internal control. *PLB$_H$*, pentameric form of PLB; *PLB$_L$*, monomeric form of PLB. The basal phosphorylation at PLB Ser-16 and Thr-17 residues was detected using polyclonal PLB site-specific phosphorylation antibodies that specifically recognize either phosphoserine 16 (*PSer^{16}-PLB$_H$* and *PSer^{16}-PLB$_L$*) or phosphothreonine 17 (*PThr^{17}-PLB$_H$* and *PThr^{17}-PLB$_L$*).

shortening (79%) and the normalized mean velocity of circumferential shortening (67%) in transgenic mice compared to wild type. The differences in contractile parameters and Ca^{2+} kinetics in transgenic mice were abolished upon isoproterenol stimulation. The inhibition of contractile parameters is also seen in the atrial muscle where the PLB level is threefold higher in the atria when compared with their isogenic wild types. These findings indicate that 1) a fraction of the SERCA in native

SR is not regulated by PLB, 2) an increase in PLB protein can have negative effect on Ca^{2+} transport and cardiac function (33).

PLB knockout mice

Using gene knock out technique, homozygous and heterozygous mice for PLB gene ablation were generated in the lab of Dr. Kranias. The PLB heterozygous mice expressed 40% of the PLB protein levels present in wild type hearts, whereas the PLB homozygous mice expressed no PLB mRNA or protein (34,35) (Table 1). Reduction or ablation of PLB was not associated with any phenotypic alterations at the gross morphology or ultra structural levels of the heart (36). However there were increases in the affinity of the SR Ca^{2+}ATPase for Ca^{2+}. Furthermore, an apparent linear correlation between the levels of PLB and the Ca^{2+} affinity of the SR Ca^{2+}ATPase was observed. Reduction or ablation of PLB, results in increases in the extent of myocyte cell shortening, rate of contraction and rate of relengthening (37). These alterations in the dynamics of cardiac myocyte mechanics are associated with parallel alterations in cardiac contractile parameters, assessed in work performing heart preparations. The rates of contraction (+dP/dt) and relaxation (−dP/dt) are significantly higher in PLB heterozygous hearts compared with wild types and even higher in PLB deficient hearts compared with PLB heterozygous (38). No alteration in other major Ca^{2+} handling proteins associated with the hyper dynamic contractile function is reported, except for 25% decrease in RYR protein levels (39). Direct measurement of ventricular pressure and contractile parameters in wild type, PLB hetero and homozygous hearts revealed no differences in heart rate or left ventricular end-diastolic pressure. However, the basal parameters for contraction and relaxation were higher in PLB heterozygous and even more in PLB deficient mice compared with wild types (40). The elevated contractile parameters of the PLB deficient hearts could not be further stimulated by β agonist or by thyroxin induced increases in SERCA2 expression (40,41).

DISCUSSION

A change in, either in the level of SERCA or PLB affects the relative ratio of PLB/SERCA. Increases in SERCA pump level shifts the equilibrium of PLB/SERCA ratio in favor of more free pumps and likewise decreases in PLB can lead to less inhibition of the existing pumps. These approaches differ in that decrease in PLB increases the pump affinity for Ca^{2+} whereas increase in the SERCA pump level doesn't necessarily increase its affinity for Ca^{2+}. But the resultant effect is increase in Ca^{2+} transport rate and enhancement in cardiac contraction relaxation parameters. These two studies clearly show that there is a direct correlation between the levels of SERCA, PLB and the contractile status of the heart. Furthermore, the SERCA overexpression studies indicate that it is possible to increase the SERCA pump levels in vivo and it results in a gain of function without producing cardiac pathology (27–29).

PLB overexpression studies elegantly show higher PLB/SERCA ratio results in depressed cardiac function. These studies can be interpreted that a fraction of the SERCA pump in the SR is not regulated by PLB and the functional stoichiometric ratio of PLB/SERCA in vivo is not exactly $1:1$. Moreover, a close linear correlation was observed between the levels of PLB expression and the EC_{50} of SR Ca^{2+} transport in PLB overexpression, WT, PLB heterozygous and PLB deficient hearts. Furthermore, these studies also suggest that free pumps in the SR are inhibited by the overexpression of PLB in transgenic hearts and the functional stoichiometric ratio of PLB/SERCA is estimated to be less than $0.5/1.0$ (42).

Studies with SERCA2 heterozygous mice clearly indicate that 2 functional copies of SERCA2 gene are required to maintain normal function. We also made an interesting observation that chronic alterations in SERCA2a pump levels modify the PLB protein levels. We found that PLB protein level decreased to ~40% of control, corresponding to the decrease in SERCA2 level (~35%) in this mouse model. This finding may suggest that a cross talk exists between these two proteins to maintain an optimal PLB/SERCA ratio (32). Even though the PLB/SERCA ratio is optimized along with other compensatory changes in this model, the net effect is still a deficit in cardiac function. These studies suggest that there exists an optimum PLB/SERCA ratio for different tissues and it may be further adjusted depending on the patho-physiological status of the heart.

SERCA AND PLB AS THERAPEUTIC DRUG TARGETS

In recent years gene therapy for heart diseases has become a promising area of research. In particular abnormalities in Ca^{2+} handling during hypertrophy and heart failure has received much attention. A decrease in SERCA expression and activity seems to be a major defect responsible for impaired function of the failing heart. Thus a potential therapeutic strategy for heart failure is to enhance the calcium handling ability of the failing myocardium. The beneficial effect of increased SERCA levels in terms of enhanced contractile function and decrease in mortality has been demonstrated in transgenic mice and animal models of heart failure (43). Therefore, a number of recent studies were focused on restoring SERCA pump activity by adenoviral mediated gene transfer. Hajjar et al., and Giordano et al. have elegantly demonstrated that the overexpression of SERCA2a in isolated myocytes through adenoviral mediated gene transfer results in increased contractility and a faster decay of the cytosolic Ca^{2+} transient (44,45). In addition, Hajjar and colleagues have used a catheter-based technique of adenoviral gene transfer to achieve global myocardial transduction of SERCA2a in vivo (46). In their attempt to restore the dysfunction induced by pressure overload, SERCA2a overexpression by gene transfer in vivo restored both systolic and diastolic dysfunction to normal levels. SERCA overexpression decreased left ventricular size and restored the slope of the end diastolic pressure-dimension relationship to control levels (47). These studies provide strong evidence that increased SERCA expression can be used to restore Ca^{2+} transport and contractility. The other strategy may be to alter the PLB expression level. Introduction of antisense PLB cDNA or RNA into rat neonatal cardiomyocytes to decrease PLB levels was also associated with increased rates of decay in Ca^{2+} transients (48,49). These data suggest the feasibility of cardiac gene transfer into failing hearts as a therapeutic intervention.

SUMMARY AND CONCLUSIONS

These transgenic mouse models have been a very valuable tool to explain how alteration in SERCA and PLB levels can affect Ca^{2+} transport and cardiac function. Since mouse models have a higher metabolic and heart rate, it is difficult to predict whether these findings can be extrapolated to human in its entirety. However, We have also learnt a number of valuable lessons; some were unexpected from these models. These include:

1) SERCA1a can functionally substitute for SERCA2a (50,51).
2) A 30–40% decrease in SERCA pump is not sufficient by itself to induce cardiac pathology (31,32).
3) A number of compensatory mechanisms are induced to maintain normal Ca^{2+} transport and cardiac function. Both the expression and function of the NCX, RYR receptor and L type calcium channel are adjusted to changes in SR Ca2+ load (32,41,50,51).
4) Cardiac function in isolated TG hearts does not correlate with *in vivo* function, suggesting additional *in vivo* compensation (52).
5) From the PLB mouse models we learned that loss of PLB does not cause cardiac hypertrophy or pathology (35–42).
6) On the other hand, a significant increase in PLB/SERCA ratio by overexpression of PLB can lead to cardiac pathology (53).
7) A change in PLB/SERCA ratio modifies the Ca^{2+} entry, Ca^{2+} release, Ca^{2+} uptake and SR Ca^{2+} load, thus altering EC coupling process and cardiac function.

REFERENCE

1. Katz AM. 2001. Physiology of the Heart. In: Excitation Contraction Coupling, pp. 189–239. Lippincott Williams & Wilkins.
2. Katz AM. 2001. Physiology of the Heart. In: Regulation of Myocardial Contractility and relaxation, pp. 368–397. Lippincott Williams & Wilkins.
3. Kranias EG, Garvey JL, Srivastava RD, Solaro RJ. 1985. Phosphorylation and functional modifications of sarcoplasmic reticulum and myofibrils in isolated rabbit hearts stimulated with isoprenaline. Biochem J 226:113–121.
4. Simmerman HK, Collins JH, Theibert JL, Wegener AD, Jones LR. 1986. Protein Sequence analysis of phospholamban. Identification of phosphorylation sites and two major structural domains. J Biol Chem 261:13333–13341.
5. Talosi L, Edes I, Kranias EG. 1993. Intracellular mechanisms mediating reversal of beta-adrenergic stimulation in intact beating hearts. Am J Physiol 264:H791–H797.
6. Wegener AD, Jones LR. 1984. Phosphorylation-induced mobility shift in phospholamban in sodium dodecyl sulfate-polyacrylamide gels. Evidence for a protein structure consisting of multiple identical phosphorylatable subunits. J Biol Chem 259:1834–1841.
7. Reddy LG, Jones LR, Thomas DD. 1999. Depolymerization of phospholamban in the presence of calcium pump: a fluorescence energy transfer study. Biochemistry 38:3954–3962.
8. Cornea RL, Jones LR, Autry JM, Thomas DD. 1997. Mutation and phosphorylation change the oligomeric structure of phospholamban in lipid bilayers. Biochemistry 36:2960–2967.
9. Loukianov E, Ji Y, Baker DL, Reed T, Babu J, Loukianova T, Greene A, Shull G, Periasamy M. 1998.

Sarco(endo)plasmic reticulum Ca2+ ATPase isoforms and their role in muscle physiology and pathology. Ann N Y Acad Sci 853:251–259.

10. Moorman AF, Vermeulen JL, Koban MU, Schwartz K, Lamers WH, Boheler KR. 1995. Patterns of expression of sarcoplasmic reticulum Ca^{2+}-ATPase and Phospholamban mRNAs during rat heart development. Circ Res 76:616–625.

11. Arai M, Otsu K, MacLennan DH, Periasamy M. 1992. Regulation of sarcoplasmic reticulum gene expression during cardiac and skeletal muscle development. Am J Physiol 262:C614–C620.

12. Luss I, Boknik P, Jones LR, Kirchhefer U, Knapp J, Linck B, Luss H, Meissner A, Muller FU, Schmitz W, Vahlensieck U, Neumann J. 1999. Expression of cardiac calcium regulatory proteins in atrium v ventricle in different species. J Mol Cell Cardiol 31:1299–1314.

13. Reed TD, Babu GJ, Ji Y, Zilberman A, Ver Heyen M, Wuytack F, Periasamy M. 2000. The expression of SR calcium transport ATPase and the Na(+)/Ca(2+) Exchanger are antithetically regulated during mouse cardiac development and in Hypo/hyperthyroidism. J Mol Cell Cardiol 32:453–464.

14. Kimura Y, Otsu K, Nishida K, Kuzuya T, Tada M. 1994. Thyroid hormone enhances Ca2+ pumping activity of the cardiac sarcoplasmic reticulum by increasing Ca2+ ATPase and decreasing phospholamban expression. J Mol Cell Cardiol 26:1145–1154.

15. Arai M, Matsui H, Periasamy M. 1994. Sarcoplasmic reticulum gene expression in cardiac hypertrophy and heart failure. Circ Res 74:555–564.

16. Hasenfuss G, Reinecke H, Studer R, Meyer M, Pieske B, Holtz J, Holubarsch C, Posival H, Just H, Drexler H. 1994. Relation between myocardial function and expression of sarcoplasmic reticulum Ca(2+)-ATPase in failing and nonfailing human myocardium. Circ Res 75:434–442.

17. Kadambi VJ, Kranias EG. 1997. Phospholamban: a protein coming of age. Biochem Biophys Res Commun 239:1–5.

18. Schmidt U, Hajjar RJ, Kim CS, Lebeche D, Doye AA, Gwathmey JK. 1999. Human heart failure: cAMP stimulation of SR Ca(2+)-ATPase activity and phosphorylation level of phospholamban. Am J Physiol 277:H474–H480.

19. Neumann J, Eschenhagen T, Jones LR, Linck B, Schmitz W, Scholz H, Zimmermann N. 1997. Increased expression of cardiac phosphatases in patients with end-stage heart failure. J Mol Cell Cardiol 29:265–272.

20. Koss KL, Grupp IL, Kranias EG. 1997. The relative phospholamban and SERCA2 ratio: a critical determinant of myocardial contractility. Basic Res Cardiol 92(Suppl 1):17–24.

21. Kiss E, Jakab G, Kranias EG, Edes I. 1994. Thyroid hormone-induced alterations in phospholamban protein expression. Regulatory effects on sarcoplasmic reticulum Ca2+ transport and myocardial relaxation. Circ Res 75:245–251.

22. Holt E, Sjaastad I, Lunde PK, Christensen G, Sejersted OM. 1999. Thyroid hormone control of contraction and the Ca(2+)-ATPase/phospholamban complex in adult rat ventricular myocytes. J Mol Cell Cardiol 31:645–656.

23. Matsui H, MacLennan DH, Alpert NR, Periasamy M. 1995. Sarcoplasmic reticulum gene expression in pressure overload-induced cardiac hypertrophy in rabbit. Am J Physiol 268:C252–C258.

24. Nagai R, Zarain-Herzberg A, Brandl CJ, Fujii J, Tada M, MacLennan DH, Alpert NR, Periasamy M. 1989. Regulation of myocardial Ca2+-ATPase and phospholamban mRNA expression in response to pressure overload and thyroid hormone. Proc Natl Acad Sci USA 86:2966–2970.

25. Mercadier JJ, Lompre AM, Duc P, Boheler KR, Fraysse JB, Wisnewsky C, Allen PD, Komajda M, Schwartz K. 1990. Altered sarcoplasmic reticulum Ca2(+)-ATPase gene expression in the human ventricle during end-stage heart failure. J Clin Invest 85:305–309.

26. He H, Giordano FJ, Hilal-Dandan R, Choi DJ, Rockman HA, McDonough PM, Bluhm WF, Meyer M, Sayen MR, Swanson E, Dillmann WH. 1997. Overexpression of the rat sarcoplasmic reticulum Ca2+ ATPase gene in the heart of transgenic mice accelerates calcium transients and cardiac relaxation. J Clin Invest 100:380–389.

27. Baker DL, Hashimoto K, Grupp IL, Ji Y, Reed T, Loukianov E, Grupp G, Bhagwhat A, Hoit B, Walsh R, Marban E, Periasamy M. 1998. Targeted overexpression of the sarcoplasmic reticulum Ca2+-ATPase increases cardiac contractility in transgenic mouse hearts. Circ Res 83:1205–2514.

28. Loukianov E, Ji Y, Grupp IL, Kirkpatrick DL, Baker DL, Loukianova T, Grupp G, Lytton J, Walsh RA, Periasamy M. 1998. Enhanced myocardial contractility and increased Ca2+ transport function in transgenic hearts expressing the fast-twitch skeletal muscle sarcoplasmic reticulum Ca2+-ATPase. Circ Res 83:889–897.

29. Greene AL, Lalli MJ, Ji Y, Babu GJ, Grupp I, Sussman M, Periasamy M. 2000. Overexpression of SERCA2b in the heart leads to an increase in sarcoplasmic reticulum calcium transport function and increased cardiac contractility. J Biol Chem 275:24722–24727.

30. Ver Heyen M, Heymans S, Antoons G, Reed T, Periasamy M, Awede B, Lebacq J, Vangheluwe P, Dewerchin M, Collen D, Sipido K, Carmeliet P, Wuytack F. 2001. Replacement of the muscle-specific sarcoplasmic reticulum Ca(2+)-ATPase isoform SERCA2a by the nonmuscle SERCA2b homologue causes mild concentric hypertrophy and impairs contraction-relaxation of the heart. Circ Res 89:838–846.
31. Periasamy M, Reed TD, Liu LH, Ji Y, Loukianov E, Paul RJ, Nieman ML, Riddle T, Duffy JJ, Doetschman T, Lorenz JN, Shull GE. 1999. Impaired cardiac performance in heterozygous mice with a null mutation in the sarco(endo) plasmic reticulum Ca2+-ATPase isoform 2 (SERCA2) gene. J Biol Chem 274:2556–2562.
32. Ji Y, Lalli MJ, Babu GJ, Xu Y, Kirkpatrick DL, Liu LH, Chiamvimonvat N, Walsh RA, Shull GE, Periasamy M. 2000. Disruption of a single copy of the SERCA2 gene results in altered Ca2+ home-ostasis and cardiomyocyte function. J Biol Chem 275:38073–38080.
33. Kadambi VJ, Ponniah S, Harrer JM, Hoit BD, Dorn GW 2nd, Walsh RA, Kranias EG. 1996. Cardiac-specific overexpression of phospholamban alters calcium kinetics and resultant cardiomyocyte mechanics in transgenic mice. J Clin Invest 97:533–539.
34. Luo W, Wolska BM, Grupp IL, Harrer JM, Haghighi K, Ferguson DG, Slack JP, Grupp G, Doetschman T, Solaro RJ, Kranias EG. 1996. Phospholamban gene dosage effects in the mammalian heart. Circ Res 78:839–847.
35. Luo W, Grupp IL, Harrer J, Ponniah S, Grupp G, Duffy JJ, Doetschman T, Kranias EG. 1994. Targeted ablation of the phospholamban gene is associated with markedly enhanced myocardial contractility and loss of beta-agonist stimulation. Circ Res 75:401–409.
36. Chu G, Luo W, Slack JP, Tilgmann C, Sweet WE, Spindler M, Saupe KW, Boivin GP, Moravec CS, Matlib MA, Grupp IL, Ingwall JS, Kranias EG. 1996. Compensatory mechanisms associated with the hyperdynamic function of phospholamban-deficient mouse hearts. Circ Res 79:1064–1076.
37. Wolska BM, Stojanovic MO, Luo W, Kranias EG, Solaro RJ. 1996. Effect of ablation of phospho-lamban on dynamics of cardiac myocyte contraction and intracellular Ca2+. Am J Physiol 271:C391–C397.
38. Lorenz JN, Kranias EG. 1997. Regulatory effects of phospholamban on cardiac function in intact mice. Am J Physiol 273:H2826–H2831.
39. Masaki H, Sato Y, Luo W, Kranias EG, Yatani A. 1997. Phospholamban deficiency alters inactivation kinetics of L-type Ca2+ channels in mouse ventricular myocytes. Am J Physiol Feb;272:H606–H612.
40. Hoit BD, Khoury SF, Kranias EG, Ball N, Walsh RA. 1995. In vivo echocardiographic detection of enhanced left ventricular function in gene-targeted mice with phospholamban deficiency. Circ Res 77:632–637.
41. Kiss E, Brittsan AG, Edes I, Grupp IL, Grupp G, Kranias EG. 1998. Thyroid hormone-induced alter-ations in phospholamban-deficient mouse hearts. Circ Res 83:608–613.
42. Brittsan AG, Kranias EG. 2000. Phospholamban and cardiac contractile function. J Mol Cell Cardiol 32:2131–2139.
43. Ito K, Yan X, Feng X, Manning WJ, Dillmann WH, Lorell BH. 2001. Transgenic expression of sarcoplasmic reticulum Ca(2+) atpase modifies the transition from hypertrophy to early heart failure. Circ Res 89:422–429.
44. Hajjar RJ, Kang JX, Gwathmey JK, Rosenzweig A. 1997. Physiological effects of adenoviral gene transfer of sarcoplasmic reticulum calcium ATPase in isolated rat myocytes. Circulation 95:423–429.
45. Giordano FJ, He H, McDonough P, Meyer M, Sayen MR, Dillmann WH. 1997. Adenovirus-mediated gene transfer reconstitutes depressed sarcoplasmic reticulum Ca2+-ATPase levels and shortens prolonged cardiac myocyte Ca2+ transients. Circulation 96:400–403.
46. Hajjar RJ, Schmidt U, Matsui T, Guerrero JL, Lee KH, Gwathmey JK, Dec GW, Semigran MJ, Rosenzweig A. 1998. Modulation of ventricular function through gene transfer in vivo. Proc Natl Acad Sci U S A 95:5251–5256.
47. Miyamoto MI, del Monte F, Schmidt U, DiSalvo TS, Kang ZB, Matsui T, Guerrero JL, Gwathmey JK, Rosenzweig A, Hajjar RJ. 2000. Adenoviral gene transfer of SERCA2a improves left-ventricular function in aortic-banded rats in transition to heart failure. Proc Natl Acad Sci USA 97:793–798.
48. He H, Meyer M, Martin JL, McDonough PM, Ho P, Lou X, Lew WY, Hilal-Dandan R, Dillmann WH. 1999. Effects of mutant and antisense RNA of phospholamban on SR Ca(2+)-ATPase activ-ity and cardiac myocyte contractility. Circulation 100:974–980.
49. Eizema K, Fechner H, Bezstarosti K, Schneider-Rasp S, van der Laarse A, Wang H, Schultheiss HP, Poller WC, Lamers JM. 2000. Adenovirus-based phospholamban antisense expression as a novel approach to improve cardiac contractile dysfunction: comparison of a constitutive viral versus an endothelin-1-responsive cardiac promoter. Circulation 101:2193–2199.

50. Ji Y, Loukianov E, Loukianova T, Jones LR, Periasamy M. 1999. SERCA1a can functionally substitute for SERCA2a in the heart. Am J Physiol 276:H89–H97.
51. Jane Lalli M, Yong J, Prasad V, Hashimoto K, Plank D, Babu GJ, Kirkpatrick D, Walsh RA, Sussman M, Yatani A, Marban E, Periasamy M. 2001. Sarcoplasmic reticulum Ca(2+) atpase (SERCA) 1a structurally substitutes for SERCA2a in the cardiac sarcoplasmic reticulum and increases cardiac Ca(2+) handling capacity. Circ Res 89:160–167.
52. Huke S, Prasad V, Nieman M, Kalpana Nattamai J, Grupp IL, Lorenz JN, Periasamy M. 2002. Altered dose-response to B-agonists in SERCA1a expressing hearts *ex* and *iv vivo*. Am J Physiol (in press).
53. Dash R, Kadambi V, Schmidt AG, Tepe NM, Biniakiewicz D, Gerst MJ, Canning AM, Abraham WT, Hoit BD, Liggett SB, Lorenz JN, Dorn GW 2nd, Kranias EG. 2001. Interactions between phospholamban and beta-adrenergic drive may lead to cardiomyopathy and early mortality. Circulation 103:889–896.

Signal Transduction and Cardiac Hypertrophy,
edited by N.S. Dhalla, L.V. Hryshko,
E. Kardami & P.K. Singal
Kluwer Academic Publishers, Boston, 2003

Expression of Vascular Endothelial Growth Factor and Hypoxia-Inducible Factor 1α in the Myocardium

Toshiyuki Takahashi, Yasuyuki Sugishita, Tatsuya Shimizu, Atsushi Yao, Kazumasa Harada, and Ryozo Nagai

Department of Cardiovascular Medicine
Graduate School of Medicine
University of Tokyo
Tokyo, Japan

Summary. Expression of vascular endothelial growth factor (VEGF) and hypoxia-inducible factor 1α (HIF-1α), a transcription factor involved in the VEGF induction, was examined in the myocardium. In the 10-day-old chick embryonic hearts and ventricular myocytes, the mRNA species encoding VEGF and HIF-1α were abundantly expressed even at the basal conditions. The steady-state levels of the VEGF mRNA were regulated by various protein kinases. In the cultured neonatal rat ventricular myocytes, VEGF expression was upregulated by lipopolysaccharide. These data suggest that VEGF and HIF-1α expressed in cardiac myocytes may play significant roles in cardiovascular development. Furthermore, the cardiac myocyte-derived VEGF may also contribute to the pathogenesis of systemic inflammatory response syndrome, including myocardial interstitial edema.

Key words: myocardium, vascular endothelial growth factor, hypoxia-inducible factor 1α.

INTRODUCTION

Vascular endothelial growth factor (VEGF) is a specific mitogen for endothelial cells, and plays essential roles in endothelial proliferation, angiogenesis, and development of cardiovascular systems during embryonic stages (1–8). In addition, VEGF is also

Address for Correspondence: Toshiyuki Takahashi, MD, Department of Cardiovascular Medicine, Graduate School of Medicine, University of Tokyo, 7-3-1 Hongo, Bunkyo-ku, Tokyo 113-8655, Japan. Tel: +81-3-3815-5411 ext. 33076, Fax: +81-3-3814-0021, E-mail: toshitak-tky@umin.ac.jp

known as vascular permeability factor that can induce capillary hyperpermeability (4,9,10). Cardiac myocyte is one of the important cell types producing and secreting VEGF, and the secreted VEGF is suggested to contribute to collateral vessel formation in the ischemic myocardium (11–15).

On the other hand, hypoxia-inducible factor 1 (HIF-1) has been implicated to play essential roles in oxygen homeostasis of various tissues (16). HIF-1 is a heterodimer consisting of two subunits, HIF-1α and arylhydrocarbon receptor nuclear translocator (ARNT) (17,18). HIF-1α and ARNT belong to the basic helix-loop-helix-Per/ARNT/Sim (bHLH-PAS) family of transcription factors (16–18). HIF-1 can bind consensus DNA sequences named as hypoxia responsive elements, which have been found in the 3′- or 5′-flanking regions of various genes, including VEGF (19). HIF-1 is also suggested to play indispensable roles in embryonic cardiovascular development by stimulating vasculogenesis as well as angiogenesis (20–23).

In this manuscript, we will review the results of our recent work concerning expression of VEGF and HIF-1α in the myocardium (24–26). First, the data suggesting possible roles of these proteins in embryonic cardiovascular development will be introduced (24,25). Second, those implicating a significance of VEGF in the pathogenesis of systemic inflammatory response syndrome (SIRS) will be shown.

Molecular cloning and expression patterns of the VEGF cDNAs in the chick embryonic ventricular myocytes and tissues

First, we have cloned VEGF cDNAs from the 10-day-old chick embryonic ventricular myocytes with the reverse transcription-polymerase chain reaction (RT-PCR) method (24). Similar to the quail VEGF cDNAs (27), the RT-PCR produced at least 4 different bands in the chick embryonic ventricular myocytes (Figure 1A). The longest (702 bp) isoform (cVEGF190) showed 99.6% homology at the nucleic acid level and 100% identity at the deduced amino acid level to the quail embryonic VEGF cDNA isoform, qVEGF190 (28). At the deduced amino acid level, the cVEGF190 cDNA also showed more than 70% homology to the human, rat and mouse VEGF cDNAs.

Sequencing data suggested that these isoforms might be generated by alternative mRNA splicing as in the VEGF isoforms of other species (Figure 1B). In the chick embryonic ventricular myocytes, the cVEGF166 and cVEGF122 isoforms were dominantly expressed. This finding may be different from that obtained in the embryonic quail heart, in which the qVEGF190 and qVEGF166 isoforms were major isoforms (27).

The RT-PCR showed that the expression pattern of the VEGF isoforms was similar in both in the 10-day-old chick embryonic heart and cultured ventricular myocytes (Figure 1C). In contrast, in the 10-day-old chick embryonic brain, liver, or skeletal muscles, relative expression levels of individual isoforms were different from those in the ventricular myocytes (Figure 1C). By Northern blot analysis, VEGF mRNA was detected abundantly in the 10-day-old chick embryonic liver as well as heart, and much less in the embryonic brain and skeletal muscle. This mRNA

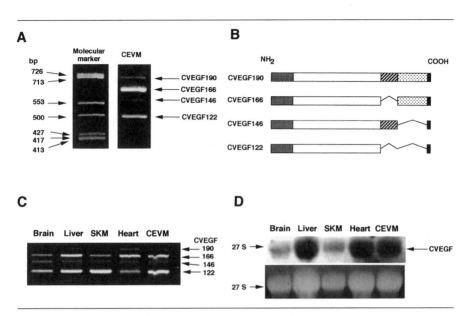

Figure 1. Expression of the chick VEGF mRNA species in embryonic ventricular myocytes and tissues. **Panel A**, a representative result of RT-PCR performed with the oligonucleotide primers specific for the quail VEGF cDNA. The chick VEGF cDNAs amplified from CEVM (chick embryonic ventricular myocytes) consisted of at least four different species, corresponding to the isoforms of 190, 166, 146 and 122 amino acids (named as cVEGF190, cVEGF166, cVEGF146 and cVEGF122, respectively). **Panel B**, a schema illustrating generation of the chick VEGF isoforms by alternative mRNA splicing. **Panel C**, a representative result of RT-PCR using RNA samples obtained from various 10-day-old chick embryonic tissues and the specific oligonucleotide primers. **Panel D**, a representative result of Northern blot analysis using the ^{32}P-labeled cVEGF166 probe. A picture of ethidium bromide-stained 27S rRNAs is shown as an internal control. SKM, skeletal muscle; CEVM, chick embryonic ventricular myocytes. (Reproduced from Sugishita et al. (24) by written permission of Academic Press, Ltd.)

species was also detected abundantly in the chick embryonic ventricular myocytes even at the basal, aerobic culture condition (room air plus 5% CO_2) (Figure 1D), suggesting that these myocytes may be one of the major production sites of VEGF during embryonic stages.

Activation of protein kinase A with forskolin (100 μM) or protein kinase C with phorbol 12-myristate, 13-acetate (200 nM) for 6h augmented the levels of mRNA encoding VEGF (Figure 2). These findings are in agreement with those observed in other types of cells (28,29) as well as neonatal rat cardiac myocytes (15). Treatment with bisindolylmaleimide (75 nM), an inhibitor of protein kinase C, for 6h did not affect the basal levels of VEGF mRNA. Interestingly, treatment with H89 (100 μM), an inhibitor of protein kinase A, modestly (~30%) but significantly increased the VEGF mRNA level. In contrast, genistein (100 μM) significantly decreased the basal expression of VEGF mRNA within 6h, suggesting that protein tyrosine kinases may

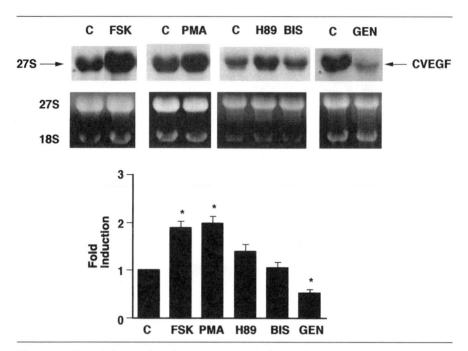

Figure 2. Effects of pharmacological interventions on the levels of VEGF mRNA in chick embryonic ventricular myocytes. The ventricular myocytes were treated for 6 h with one of the following
drugs: forskolin (FSK, 100 μM), a stimulator of protein kinase A; phorbol 12-myristate, 13-acetate
(PMA, 200 nM), a stimulator of protein kinase C; H89 (100 μM), an inhibitor of protein kinase A;
bisindolylmaleimide (BIS, 75 nM), an inhibitor of protein kinase C; genistein (100 μM), an inhibitor of
protein tyrosine kinases. The upper panels show representative results of Northern blot analysis using
the ^{32}P-labeled cVEGF166 probe and pictures of ethidium bromide-stained 27 S and 18 S rRNAs as
internal controls. The lower panels are bar graphs representing the mean + S.E. of relative radioactivity counts of the VEGF signals, which were determined directly with InstantImager™ Electronic
Autoradiography System (Packard Instrument, Meriden, CT). The relative radioactivity counts of the
control samples (treated with vehicles) were set as 1.0 for individual experiments. Results are obtained
from 6–8 independent experiments. *P < 0.05 vs. the controls. †P < 0.01 vs. the controls. (Reproduced from Sugishita et al. (24) by written permission of Academic Press, Ltd.)

be involved in maintaining the steady-state levels of VEGF mRNA in the chick
embryonic ventricular myocytes (Figure 2).

Molecular cloning and expression patterns of the HIF-1α cDNAs in the chick embryonic ventricular myocytes and tissues

Next, we have cloned the chick HIF-1α cDNAs from 10-day-old embryonic
ventricular myocytes with 5′- and 3′-RACE (rapid amplification of cDNA ends)
methods as previously described (26). The deduced amino acid sequence of the
chick HIF-1α showed high identities with the mammalian HIF-1α cDNAs. In contrast, sequence homology of the amino acid sequences between the chick HIF-1α

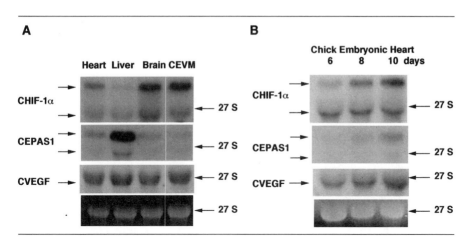

Figure 3. Expression of HIF-1α, EPAS1 and VEGF mRNA species in chick embryonic tissues and ventricular myocytes. **Panel A**, expression of the HIF-1α, EPAS1 and VEGF mRNA species in the heart, liver, brain and cultured ventricular myocytes (CEVM) obtained from 10-day-old chick embryos. **Panel B**, Expression of the HIF-1α, EPAS1 and VEGF mRNA species in the hearts from 6-, 8- and 10-day-old chick embryos. Northern blot analyses were performed with ^{32}P-labeled specific cDNA probes. Pictures of ethidium bromide-stained 27 S rRNA are shown as internal controls. (Reproduced from Takahashi et al. (26) by written permission of Academic Press, Ltd.)

and endothelial PAS domain protein 1 (EPAS1) cDNAs, another member of the bHLH-PAS family, was much lower (49%) (26).

Northern blot analysis detected two major transcripts (approximately 6.8 and 3.8 kb) of the HIF-1α mRNA in various 10-day-old chick embryonic tissues (Figure 3A). The levels of the longer transcript were high in the chick embryonic heart, brain and ventricular myocytes, while much less in the embryonic liver. The shorter transcript was less abundant than the longer one in the embryonic tissues except the liver, in which the levels of these two transcripts were comparable. The EPAS1 mRNA also consisted of two transcripts (5.2 and 3.8 kb) (Figure 3A). In contrast to the HIF-1α mRNA, the EPAS1 mRNA was highly expressed in the embryonic liver, as reported earlier (30), and much less in the other tissues. Particularly, this mRNA species was scarcely detected in the ventricular myocytes. Thereby, expression of these two bHLH-PAS proteins may be regulated in a reciprocal fashion at mRNA level.

We have also analyzed expression of the chick HIF-1α, EPAS1 and VEGF mRNA species in developing chick hearts (Figure 3B). The levels of the VEGF mRNA were gradually increased in the hearts obtained from the 6-, 8- and 10-day old chick embryos. During these stages, the levels of the longer transcript of the chick HIF-1α mRNA were dramatically augmented, while those of the shorter transcript remained almost unchanged. In contrast, expression of the chick EPAS1 mRNA was low in these embryonic hearts, though its levels tended to be increased. The low levels of EPAS1 expression in the embryonic hearts may be related to the findings of the EPAS1 gene inactivation study (31), in which vasculogenesis, angiogenesis or cardiac development was not impaired in the EPAS1-/-mice. Thus, HIF-1α may play more important roles than EPAS1 in development of the 6- to 10-day-old chick embryonic hearts.

**Effects of lipopolysaccharide (LPS) on the VEGF
expression in rat ventricular myocytes**

LPS is known to cause SIRS, in which vascular hyperpermeability is responsible for the characteristic pathophysiological changes, including myocardial interstitial edema (32–34). On the other hand, VEGF is known as a potent vascular permeability factor (4,9,10). Accordingly, we examined effects of LPS on the VEGF expression in cultured neonatal rat ventricular myocytes (25).

Northern blot analysis revealed that the stimulation with LPS (10 μg/ml) rapidly augmented the levels of VEGF mRNA within only 1 h (Figure 4A and 4B). The levels of the VEGF mRNA remained significantly high for 1–6 h after the LPS stimulation, and then decreased to the control levels at 12 hr later. In agreement with our previous studies (35,36), LPS also strongly induced the iNOS mRNA within 6 h, but its induction took place significantly later than the LPS-induced increases in the levels of VEGF mRNA (Figure 4A and 4B).

As shown in Figure 4C and 4D, inhibition of nuclear factor-κB (NF-κB) activation with pyrrolidinedithiocarbamate (PDTC, 100 μM), or tyrosine kinases with genistein (100 μM) failed to suppress the LPS-induced augmentation of the VEGF mRNA expression. In contrast, both of the inhibitors markedly suppressed the LPS-induced expression of iNOS mRNA as shown in our previous study (35). These data suggest that LPS may affect expression of VEGF and iNOS mRNA species through distinct signaling pathways in the ventricular myocytes.

Figure 4D shows the results of ELISA for VEGF. The VEGF concentrations in the conditioned media were actually increased at 6–12 hr after the LPS stimulation as compared with the controls (Figure 4D). Interestingly, this time course of the VEGF secretion from the ventricular myocytes was similar to that of myocardial interstitial edema caused by LPS administration in the *in vivo* animal models (32–34). Thus, the VEGF secreted from ventricular myocytes may contribute to development of SIRS, by provoking not only myocardial interstitial edema by a paracrine action, but also systemic edema by an endocrine action.

CONCLUSION

Our recent data have shown that VEGF is highly expressed in cardiac myocytes during embryonic development and inflammatory responses such as SIRS. Thus, VEGF and possibly HIF-1α, one of its important regulator, may be involved in the pathogenesis of various cardiovascular diseases, including congenital heart diseases, myocarditis and heart failure in general. In this regard, these molecules may become new targets also in treatment of these diseases, though their pathophysiological roles remain to be clarified.

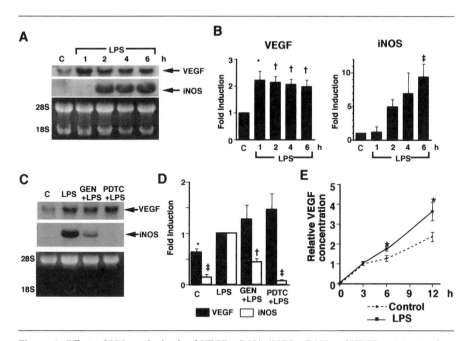

Figure 4. Effects of LPS on the levels of VEGF mRNA, iNOS mRNA and VEGF protein in cultured neonatal rat ventricular myocytes. **Panel A**, representative results of Northern blot analyses of the VEGF and iNOS mRNA expression in cultured neonatal rat ventricular myocytes. The cells were treated with LPS (10 μg/ml) for predetermined periods. A picture of ethidium bromide-stained 28 S and 18 S ribosomal RNAs is shown as an internal control. **Panel B**, the levels of VEGF and iNOS mRNA expression determined with the InstantImager™ (Packard Instrument). Data were obtained from six independent experiments. The levels of VEGF or iNOS mRNA in the controls were arbitrarily set as 1.0 for each mRNA species and each individual experiment. ★P < 0.05, †P < 0.01 vs. the controls. **Panel C**, representative results of Northern blot analyses of the VEGF and iNOS mRNA expression at 6 h after LPS stimulation, under pretreatment for 2 h with pyrrolidinedithiocarbamate (PDTC, 100 μM), an NF-κB inhibitor, or genistein (GEN, 100 μM), a tyrosine kinase blocker. A picture of ethidium bromide-stained 28 S and 18 S ribosomal RNAs is shown as an internal control. **Panel D**, the levels of VEGF and iNOS mRNA expression determined with the InstantImager™ (Packard Instrument). Data were obtained from four independent experiments. The levels of VEGF or iNOS mRNA at 6 h after the LPS treatment were arbitrarily set as 1.0 for each mRNA species and each individual experiment. ★P < 0.05, †P < 0.01 vs. the cells stimulated with LPS for 6 hr. **Panel E**, the effects of LPS on VEGF concentrations in the conditioned media. The VEGF concentrations in the conditioned media were measured with a mouse VEGF ELISA kit (R&D SYSTEMS). To calculate relative concentrations, the VEGF concentrations in the conditioned media of the control cells at 3 h after the media change were arbitrarily set as 1.0 for each independent experiment. Graphs represent mean ± SEM of five independent experiments. ★P < 0.05 vs. the controls at each time point. (Reproduced from Sugishita et al. (25) by written permission of Academic Press, Ltd.)

REFERENCES

1. Levy AP, Tamargo, R, Brem, H, Nathans, D. 1989. An endothelial growth factor from the mouse neuroblastoma cell line NB 41. Growth Factors 2:9–19.
2. Ferrara N, Houck K, Jakeman L, Leung DW. 1992. Molecular and biological properties of the vascular endothelial growth factor family of proteins. Endocr Rev 13:18–32.
3. Senger DR, Van de Water L, Brown LF, Nagy JA, Yeo KT, Yeo TK, Berse B, Jackman RW, Dvorak AM, Dvorak HF. 1993. Vascular permeability factor (VPF,VEGF) in tumor biology. Cancer Metastasis Rev 12:303–324.
4. Connolly DT, Heuvelman DM, Nelson R, Olander JV, Eppley BL, Delfino JJ, Siegel NR, Leimgruber RM, Feder J. 1989. Tumor vascular permeability factor stimulates endothelial cell growth and angiogenesis. J Clin Invest 84:1470–1478.
5. Leung DW, Cachianes G, Kuang WJ, Goeddel DV, Ferrara N. 1989. Vascular endothelial growth factor is a secreted angiogenic mitogen. Science 246:1306–1309.
6. Keck PJ, Hauser SD, Krivi G, Sanzo K, Warren T, Feder J, Connolly DT. 1989. Vascular permeability factor, an endothelial cell migration related to PDGF. Science 246:1309–1312.
7. Carmeliet P, Ferreira V, Breier G, Pollefeyt S, Kieckens L, Gertsenstein M, Fahrig M, Vandenhoeck A, Harpal K, Eberhardt C, Declercq C, Pawling J, Moons L, Collen D, Risau W, Nagy A. 1996. Abnormal blood vessel development and lethality in embryos lacking a single VEGF allele. Nature 380:435–439.
8. Ferrara N, Carver-Moore K, Chen H, Dowd M, Lu L, O'Shea KS, Powell-Braxton L, Hillan KJ, Moore MW. 1996. Heterozygous embryonic lethality induced by targeted inactivation of the VEGF gene. Nature 380:439–442.
9. Connolly DT, Olander JV, Heuvelman D, Nelson R, Monsell R, Siegel N, Haymore BL, Leimgruber R, Feder J. 1989. Human vascular permeability factor. isolation from U937 cells. J Biol Chem 264: 20017–20024.
10. Connolly DT. 1991. Vascular permeability factor: a unique regulator of blood vessel formation. J Cell Biochem 47:219–223.
11. Ladoux A, Frelin C. 1993. Hypoxia id a strong inducer of vascular endothelial growth factor mRNA expression in the heart. Biochem Biophys Res Commun 195:1005–1010.
12. Ladoux A, Frelin C. 1994. Cobalt stimulates the expression of vascular endothelial growth factor mRNA in rat cardiac cells. Biochem Biophys Res Commun 204:794–798.
13. Banai S, Shweiki D, Pinson A, Chandra M, Lazarovici G, Keshet E. 1994. Upregulation of vascular endothelial growth factor expression induced by myocardial ischaemia: implications for coronary angiogenesis. Cardiovasc Res 28:1176–1179.
14. Hashimoto E, Ogita T, Nakaoka T, Matsuoka R, Takao A, Kira Y. 1994. Rapid induction of vascular endothelial growth factor by ischemia in rat heart. Am J Physiol 267:H1948–H1954.
15. Levy AP, Levy NS, Loscalzo J, Calderone A, Takahashi N, Yeo K-T, Koren G, Colucci WS, Goldberg MA. 1995. Regulation of vascular endothelial growth factor in cardiac myocytes. Circ Res 76:758–766.
16. Semenza GL. 1999. Regulation of mammalian O_2 homeostasis by hypoxia-inducible factor 1. Annu Rev Cell Dev Biol 15:551–578.
17. Wang GL, Jian B-H, Rue EA, Semenza GL. 1995. Hypoxia-inducible factor 1 is a basic-helix-loop-helix-PAS heterodimer regulated by cellular O_2 tension. Proc Natl Acad Sci USA 92:5510–5514.
18. Gradin K, McGuire J, Wenger RH, Kvietikova I, Whitelaw ML, Toftgård R, Tora L, Gassman M, Poellinger L. 1996. Functional interference between hypoxia and dioxin signal transduction pathways: competition for recruitment of the Arnt transcription factor. Mol Cell Biol 16:5221–5231.
19. Forsythe JA, Jiang BH, Iyer NV, Agani F, Leung SW, Koos RD, Semenza GL. 1996. Activation of vascular endothelial growth factor gene transcription by hypoxia-inducible factor 1. Mol Cell Biol 16:4604–4613.
20. Iyer NV, Kotch LE, Agani F, Leung SW, Laughner E, Wenger RH, Gassmann M, Gearhart JD, Lawler AM, Yu AY, Semenza GL. 1998. Cellular and developmental control of O_2 homeostasis by hypoxia-inducible factor 1α. Genes Dev 12:149–162.
21. Ryan HE, Lo J, Johnson RS. 1998. HIF-1α is required for solid tumor formation and embryonic vascularization. EMBO J 17:3005–3015.
22. Kotch LE, Iyer NV, Laughner E, Semenza GL. 1999. Defective vascularization of HIF-1α-null embryo is not associated with VEGF deficiency but with mesenchymal cell death. Dev Biol 209:254–267.
23. Maltepe E, Schmidt JV, Baunoch D, Bradfield CA, Simon MC. 1997. Abnormal angiogenesis and

responses to glucose and oxygen deprivation in mice lacking the protein ARNT. Nature 386:403–407.

24. Sugishita Y, Takahashi T, Shimizu T, Yao A, Kinugawa K, Sugishita K, Harada K, Matsui H, Nagai R. 2000. Expression of genes encoding vascular endothelial growth factor and its Flk-a receptor in the chick embryonic heart. J Mol Cell Cardiol 32:1039–1051.

25. Sugishita Y, Shimizu T, Yao A, Kinugawa K, Nojiri T, Harada K, Matsui H, Nagai R, Takahashi T. 2000. Lipopolysaccharide augments expression and secretion of vascular endothelial growth factor in rat ventricular myocytes. Biochem Biophys Res Commun 268:657–662.

26. Takahashi T, Sugishita Y, Nojiri T, Shimizu T, Yao A, Kinugawa K, Harada K, Nagai R. 2001. Cloning of hypoxia-inducible factor 1α cDNA from chick embryonic ventricular myocytes. Biochem Biophys Res Commun 281:1057–1062.

27. Flamme I, von Reutern M, Drexler HC, Syed-Ali S, Risau W. 1995. Overexpression of vascular endothelial growth factor in the avian embryo induces hypervascularization and increased vascular permeability without alterations of embryonic pattern formation. Dev Biol 171:399–414.

28. Tischer E, Mitchell R, Hartman T, Silva M, Gospodarowicz D, Fiddes JC, Abraham JA. The human gene for vascular endothelial growth factor. 1991. Multiple protein forms are encoded through alternative exon splicing. J Biol Chem 266:11947–11954.

29. Shima DT, Kuroki M, Deutsch U, Ng Y-S, Adamis AP, D'Amore PA. The mouse gene for vascular endothelial growth factor. 1996. Genomic structure, definition of the transcriptional unit, and characterization of transcriptional and post-transcriptional regulatory sequences. J Biol Chem 271:3877–3883.

30. Favier J, Kempf H, Corvol P, Gasc J-M. 1999. Cloning and expression pattern of EPAS1 in the chicken embryo. Colocalization with tyrosine hydroxylase. FEBS Lett 462:19–24.

31. Tian H, Hammer RE, Matsumoto AM, Russel DW, McKnight SL. 1998. The hypoxia-responsive transcription factor EPAS1 is essential for catecholamine homeostasis and protection against heart failure during embryonic development. Genes Dev 12:3320–3324.

32. Gotloib L, Shostak A, Galdi P, Jaichenko J, Fudin R. 1992. Loss of microvascular negative charges accompanied by interstitial edema in septic rats' heart. Circ Shock 36:45–56.

33. Fukui M, Qiao Y, Guo F, Asano G. 1995. Cell damage and liberation of nitric oxide synthase in rat heart by endotoxin administration. J Nippon Med Sch 62:469–481.

34. Goddard CM, Allard MF, Hogg JC, Walley KR. 1996. Myocardial morphometric changes related to decreased contractility after endotoxin. Am J Physiol 270:H1446–H1452.

35. Kinugawa K, Kohmoto O, Yao A, Serizawa T, Takahashi T. 1997. Cardiac inducible nitric oxide synthase negatively modulates myocardial function in cultured rat myocytes. Am J Physiol 272:H35–H47.

36. Kinugawa K, Shimizu T, Yao, A, Kohmoto O, Serizawa T, Takahashi T. 1997. Transcriptional regulation of inducible nitric oxide synthase in cultured neonatal rat cardiac myocytes. Circ Res 81:911–921.

Signal Transduction and Cardiac Hypertrophy,
edited by N.S. Dhalla, L.V. Hryshko,
E. Kardami & P.K. Singal
Kluwer Academic Publishers, Boston, 2003

Gene-Based Therapy of Advanced Heart Failure Secondary to the Disruption of Dystrophin-Related Proteom

Teruhiko Toyo-oka and Tomie Kawada*

Department of Organ Pathophysiology and Internal Medicine
The University of Tokyo and
* Division of Pharmacy
Niigata University Medical Hospital
Japan

Summary. The first proof-of-concept studies demonstrated the feasibility of gene transfer into the heart and vasculature of experimental animals about 10 years before. There has been a dramatic increase in the nature and sophistication of gene transfer techniques and also in the number of cardiovascular diseases that are potential targets for several gene-based therapies. This review covers only the articles on cardiomyocyte-specific gene therapy, excluding another significant area in cardiology, vascular medicine. We addressed to the current methodology of gene delivery to myocardial cells *in vivo* and have a notion that gene for the transfection might be one of the most specific agents, when the responsible or causative gene is precisely corrected. Therapeutic gene may also be potent to prevent transition of heart failure to the advanced stage, even when pharmaceutical agents developed so far are less effective. The authors also present here their tentative scheme for the progression of heart failure *via* disruption of dystrophin-related proteins in sarcolemma secondary to congenital or acquired origins. Then also present a new strategy using rAAV vectors for the treatment of the intractable cardiac dysfunction for which gene therapy shows a great promise.

Key words: advanced heart failure, dilated cardiomyopathy, human genome, invivo gene transfer, dystrophin-related proteins, rAAV vector.

Address for Correspondence: Dr. Teruhiko Toyo-oka, Prof. of Med., The Second Department of Internal Medicine, University of Tokyo, Hongo 7-3-1, Tokyo 113-0033, Japan. Tel: +81-3-5841-2570, Fax: +81-3-3813-2009, E-mail: toyooka-2im@h.u-tokyo.ac.jp

INTRODUCTION

Cardiac transplantation is an ultimate treatment of advanced heart failure, but this therapy includes a variety of socioeconomic problems in addition to medical short-comings. Particularly, the infantile or juvenile cases may be not appropriate for heart transplantation, because of difficulties for the transplanted heart to adopt the patient's growth and/or the repeated cardiac transplantation. The hereditary origin of dilated cardiomyopathy (DCM) is estimated to comprise about 1/5 in patients (1). In addition DCM shares most of the cases in advanced heart failure in Japan, different from the U.S. and European countries where ischemic cardiomyopathy is predominant. These clinical settings require development of a novel treatment in addition to pharmaceutical treatment.

With the recent completion of human genome sequencing program, gene transfer technology is useful for studying the biologic function of novel genes (Table 1). On the gene therapy in cardiovascular systems in general, there have been lots of sophisticated reviews (2–5) including the recent one by the late Jeff Isner (4). He described phase 1 clinical trials indicating high levels of safety and clinical benefits with gene therapy using several angiogenic growth factors (VEGF, BFGF, HGF) in myocardial or limb ischemia, though gene therapy for heart failure is still at the pre-clinical stage (4). Heart failure represents an attractive clinical challenge requiring effective therapeutic approaches. At present, gene therapy for cardiac dysfunction deserves the consideration because of improvements in vector development, gene delivery, and most importantly, insight of the molecular pathogenesis of heart failure (2).

Then, we present a new scheme for the progression of cardiac dysfunction to the advanced heart failure by the disruption of dystrophin or dystrophin-related proteins (DRP), irrespective of the hereditary (6–8) or acquired origins (9,10). We also introduce the first success in rescuing the gene-deficient DCM with supplementing normal gene in vivo for short- and long-terms (11,12). Furthermore, bridging the basic studies and clinical gene therapy still remains a formidable task. Early experiments in rodents should be extended to large animals or humans with using clinical-grade vector and delivery system to assess both the efficacy and safety. A growing understanding on the pathogenesis of heart failure may allow reason for cautious optimism for the future.

Table 1. Characteristics of cardiomyocyte-specific gene therapy *in vivo*

Gene	Vector	Gene delivery	Target index	Duration	Species	Reference
β_2AR	adeno-V/EBV	intramyocardial	echo, IS, NB	2–4 dyas	rat/hamster	15
		transcoronary	HD	7–21 days	rabbit/rat	13,14
Modified β_2AR						16
SERCA2a	adeno-V	catheter-based			rat	23,24
Phospholamban	adeno-V	catheter-based	LVP	7 days	rat	25
Paralbumin	adeno-V					26
δ-SG	rAAV	intramyocardial	HD, IS, NB	70–140 dyas	TO-2 hamster	11
			HD, IS, Prognosis	250 days	TO-2 hamster	12

CANDIDATE GENES OR TARGETING SYSTEMS

1. β₂-adrenergic receptor (β₂-AR) and G-protein-coupled receptor (GPCR) signaling

Exogenous gene delivery to alter the function of the heart is a potential novel therapeutic strategy for treatment of heart failure. Lefkowitz's group has tested the hypothesis that genetic manipulation of the myocardial β_2-AR system can enhance cardiac function, delivering adenoviral transgenes, including the human β_2-AR, to the rabbit myocardium. Catheter-mediated β_2-AR gene delivery produced diffuse multichamber myocardial expression, peaking 1 week after gene transfer. A total of 5×10^{11} viral particles of β_2-AR reproducibly produced 5- to 10-fold β_2-AR over-expression in the heart, which, at 7 and 21 days after delivery, resulted in increased *in vivo* hemodynamic function (13). Focusing on the feasibility of restoring β-adrenergic signaling deficiencies that are a characteristic of chronic CHF, the same group has studied isolated ventricular myocytes from rabbits that have been chronically paced to produce hemodynamic failure and documented molecular defects including down-regulation of myocardial β-adrenergic receptors (β-ARs), functional β-AR uncoupling, and an up-regulation of the β-AR kinase (BARK1). Adenoviral-mediated gene transfer of the human β_2-AR or an inhibitor of BARK1 to these failing myocytes led to the restoration of β-AR signaling (14).

Another group has injected the Epstein-Barr virus-based plasmid vector carrying human β_2-AR gene was into the left ventricular muscle of Bio14.6 cardiomyopathy hamsters. The echocardiographic examinations revealed that stroke volume and cardiac output were significantly elevated at a few days after the β_2-AR gene transfer, indicating that the adrenergic response was augmented by the genetic transduction. Immunohistological examinations and RT-PCR demonstrated both transcript and transgene in failing heart, but not in the liver, spleen, or kidney (15).

Because native GPCRs are disadvantageous for ectopic therapeutic expression, Small et al. utilized the β_2AR as a scaffold to construct 19 kinds of a highly modified therapeutic receptor-effecter complex (TREC) for the gene therapy. The ligand-binding site of β_2AR in addition to critical sites for agonist-promoted down-regulation and for phosphorylation by the corresponding kinases was re-engineered to promote the efficacy of β-agonist bindings. These TREC modifications of the receptor resulted in a depressed agonist-stimulated adenylate cyclase activity and were not activated by β-agonists but rather by a nonbiogenic amine. The TREC did not display tachyphylaxis to prolonged agonist exposure. Thus, β_2AR can be tailored to have optimal signaling characteristics for gene therapy (16).

As a fundamental criticism on these studies, is it reasonable to increase cardiac contractility and output for the purpose to improve the prognosis of patients with advanced heart failure? Past pharmaceutical evidence that long-acting Ca^{2+} entry blocker of the third generation (17,18) or some, but not all, β-adrenoblockers distinctly indicated the improvement of both mortality and morbidity of the patients with heart failure (19,20), as was the case in angiotensin converting enzyme inhibitor or vasodilator therapy (21,22). These mass studies together with the adverse effect of β-agonists in long-term treatment suggest that not positive but negative inotropic or chronotropic agents are beneficial for the therapy of heart failure. It might be more effective to reduce myocardial burden even when gene therapy is employed.

2. Sarcoplasmic/endoplasmic reticulum Ca^{2+} ATPase (SERCA2a) or Ca^{2+} handling system

In human and experimental models of heart failure, SERCA2a activity is decreased. Hajjar's group has reported that overexpression of SERCA2a in human heart muscle resulted in an increase in both protein expression and pump activity and induced a faster contraction velocity and enhanced relaxation velocity. Diastolic Ca^{2+} was decreased in failing cardiomyocytes overexpressing SERCA2a, whereas systolic Ca^{2+} was increased (23). The same group also demonstrated that heart failure due to aortic constriction in rats received an adenovirus with the SERCA2a gene by using a catheter-based technique. The failing hearts were characterized by decreased amount and activity of SERCA2a compared with nonfailing rats. In addition, these failing hearts had reduced left-ventricular systolic pressure, dP/dt_{max}, dP/dt_{min}, and rate of isovolumic relaxation (tau). Overexpression of SERCA2a restored both SERCA2a expression and ATPase activity. Furthermore, animals infected with SERCA2a had significant improvement in these physiological parameters (24).

Prior to these works, they used a catheter-based technique to achieve generalized cardiac gene transfer *in vivo* and to alter cardiac function by overexpressing phospholamban (PL), which regulates the activity of the SERCA2a. Rat hearts were transduced *in vivo* with recombinant adenoviral vectors carrying cDNA for PL. Western blot analysis of ventricles transduced by PL showed a 2.8-fold increase. Two days after infection, rat hearts transduced with PL had lower peak left ventricular pressure. Both peak rate of pressure rise and pressure fall decreased in hearts overexpressing PL compared with hearts infected with the reporter gene. The time constant of left ventricular relaxation increased significantly in hearts overexpressing PL compared with uninfected hearts or hearts infected reporter gene. These differences in ventricular function were maintained 7 days after infection (24,25).

Heart failure frequently involves diastolic dysfunction characterized by a prolonged relaxation that is typically the result of a decreased rate of intracellular Ca^{2+} sequestration. As an approach to possibly correct the diastolic dysfunction, cardiac myocytes expression of the Ca^{2+} binding protein, parvalbumin that is normally present in fast skeletal muscle, might be beneficial for the Ca^{2+} sink in isolated adult cardiac myocytes. Wahr et al. have shown that expression of parvalbumin dramatically increases the rate of Ca^{2+} sequestration and the relaxation rate in both normal and diseased cardiac myocytes (26).

RECONSTRUCTION OF DRP, USING RECOMBINANT ADENO-ASSOCIATED VIRUS (rAAV) VECTORS

Cardiac muscle is destined to repeat contraction and relaxation throughout life and sarcolemma should be more resistant to the expansion-shrinkage cycling in the heartbeat than skeletal muscle. DRP form a complex connecting dystrophin at sub-

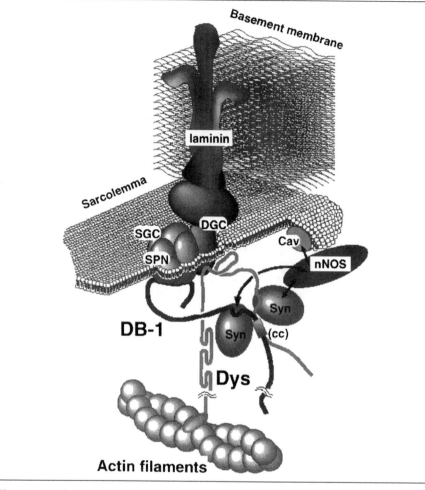

Figure 1. A scheme of dystrophin-related proteins (DRP). DRP is made of protein complex consisting of α- and β-dysroglycans (DGC), α-, β-, γ- and δ-sarcoglycans (SGC), sarcospan (SPN), and syntrophin (Syn). Note that the complex connect with intracellular contractile machinery actin *via* dystrophin (Dys) and basement membrane at the extracellular matrix *via* laminin α-2 in addition to neuronal nitric oxide synthase (nNOS) and caveolin (Cav). This illustration was kindly presented by Dr. M. Yoshida, Department of Cell biology, National Institute of Neuroscience, National Center of Neurology and Psychiatry, Japan.

sarcolemma with laminin α-2 at the extracellular matrix (Figure 1). The DRP complex may work to stabilize the elastic sarcolemma. Vectors for the gene therapy of the degenerative diseases including DCM should be efficient in the transfection potency and long-lasting to cover whole life, if possible. First of all, the authors would like to present their own experience of DCM therapy that have already been described (11,12). Normal and TO-2 strain hamsters lacking δ-SG gene with DCM from the onset (7,11,12) were 5 weeks old at the gene transduction. TO-2 strain hamsters were divided to the following subgroups; (i) totally untreated animals, (ii) transfected by the reporter gene, Lac Z, alone and (iii) cotransfected by Lac Z and δ-SG gene with normal sequence. Polyclonal, site-directed antibody to δ-SG was prepared in high titer, using synthetic peptide as a specific epitope of which amino acid sequence was deduced from the cloned cDNA (7).

The rAAVs containing a reporter gene, Lac Z, or δ-SG gene both of which were driven by cytomegalovirus (CMV) promoter were prepared as described previously (11). Under open chest surgery, rAAV-reporter gene alone or the mixture of rAAV-Lac Z and rAAV-δ-SG gene was intramurally administered the cardiac apex and the left ventricular free wall (30 μl each, 8.4×10^{10} and 6×10^{10} copies for Lac Z and δ-SG gene in total, respectively). Then, animals were cared for 10 or 35 weeks after the transduction.

Northern and Western blottings of samples after the transfection revealed appreciable expression of both transcript and transgene. Immunostaining of δ-SG protein also indicated that the transgene expression was not restricted to the injected sites, but distant region was also transfected (11). Wall thickness of the left ventricle of TO-2 heart revealed that the *in vivo* cotransduction of reporter and δ-SG genes increased the thickness by (p < 0.05), compared with the heart transfected by the reporter gene alone (12).

High-frequency (13 MHz) echocardiography and its digital recording have made it possible to exactly evaluate the mechanical performances *in vivo*. Operation procedure at 30 weeks before did not disturb visualization of the ventricular cavity. The *in vivo* cotransduction of reporter gene and δ-SG gene to TO-2 strain reduced the enlarged left ventricular systolic dimension (LVDs). In contrast, the left ventricular diastolic dimension (LVDd) did not change even after the gene therapy in both groups. These results were reflected to the improvement of both % fractional shortening (FS) and the left ventricular ejection fraction (EF) after the transfer of δ-SG gene. The hemodynamic parameters in both ventricles were recorded after A/D transduction (11,12). Open chest surgery for the gene transduction did not hamper the exact measurement of the hemodynamics at 10 or 35 weeks after the gene transduction (Figure 2). Cotransduction of both the reporter and δ-SG genes significantly improved the dP/dt_{min}, the LVEDP and the CVP. The gene therapy did not modify the LVP, the dP/dt_{max}, or the HR.

To evaluate the rAAV-δ-SG treatment, sarcolemmal integrity was analyzed by *i.v.* injection of Evans blue dye at 3 hours before sacrificing the animals. The dye excluded cardiomyocytes that preserved normal sarcolemmal permeability, but is taken up by the cardiomyocytes with leaky cell membrane (27). The immunostaining of δ-SG and Evans blue were visualized under double fluorescence. Actually, present results demonstrate that the exogenously applied Evans blue dye permeated plasma membrane of cardiomyocytes that did not possess δ-SG when TO-2 hamsters started to die of the heart failure (Figure 3). In contrast, myocardial cells expressing δ-SG after the gene transduction did not take up the dye at the same age. After the transduction, cardiac tissue examined by the double fluorescence

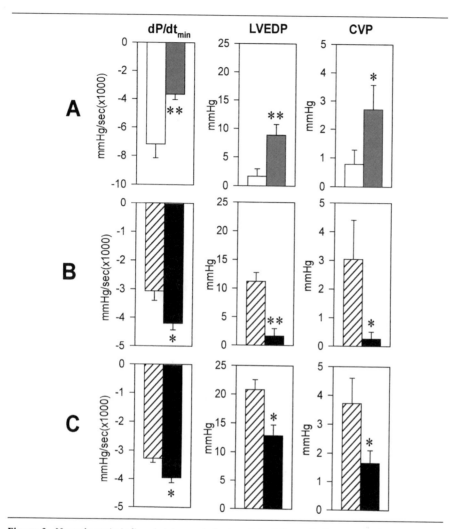

Figure 2. Hemodynamic indices (minimum derivative of the left ventricular pressure, dP/dt$_{min}$; left ventricular end-diastolic pressure, LVEDP; and central venous pressure, CVP) of the control hamsters (F1B strain, while open bar in A) and DCM hamsters (TO-2 strain, meshed bars) at 15 weeks old. Note that these parameters were improved after the co-transduction of reporter gene (Lac Z) plus δ-SG gene using rAAV vector (11,12) for 15 weeks (closed bar in B) or 40 weeks (closed bar in C). * and **denote a significant difference compared with normal strain or TO-2 hearts transfected by the reporter gene alone (hatched bar in B and C) in rAAV vectors.

microscopy distinctly showed the mutual cell-exclusivity of δ-SG expression and the dye uptake (12). It should be intensified that the rAAV-δ-SG treatment of TO-2 muscle achieved the protection of cardiomyocytes from sarcolemmal leakage as late as 40 weeks old, when some TO-2 hamsters died of heart failure. In the distant myocardium where β-Gal or δ-SG was not detected, Evans Blue was strongly

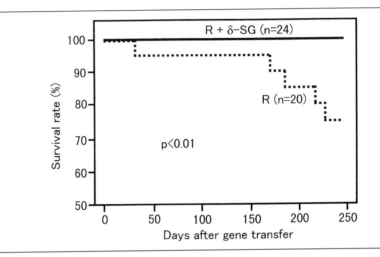

Figure 3. Kaplan-Meier's analysis of the survival rate of TO-2 strain DCM hamsters transduced by the reporter gene alone (R) or co-transduced by plus δ-SG gene driven by the same CMV promoter in rAAV vectors.

stained. Quantitative assessment of the relationship between δ-SG staining and Evans blue uptake demonstrate that Evans blue-positivity conferred 6 folds protective effect of the gene therapy.

Final effect of the gene therapy was evaluated by the life-saving action in the TO-2 animals (n = 24) with cotransduction of δ-SG plus reporter genes, comparing with another animal group transfected by the reporter gene alone (n = 20). All animals were operated at 5 weeks old, randomly allocated for each treatment and kept housed for 40 weeks, exceeding the mean life span of TO-2 strain hamsters. The survival rate was evaluated by Kaplan-Meier's analysis. The group treated by reporter gene alone started to die at 34 days old and the number of deceased animals gradually increased from 171 to 228 days after the gene transfer (Figure 3). The death timing supports the previous data of the same strain without the gene manipulation. In contrast, all animals in another group cotransfected by the reporter plus δ-SG genes survived and remained active (p < 0.01). Thus, we concluded that present gene therapy prolonged the survival rate, when the responsible gene to cause DCM was supplemented *in vivo*.

Though the rAAV type 2 vectors are potent for the widespread and long-lasting gene transduction *in vivo*, the efficacy was still low and confirms our previous results of the gene therapy for short or mid-term (11). More efficient gene transfer *via* coronary circulation, as succeeded in heterotopically transplanted heart after the isolated perfusion, would completely restore these pathological alterations before the progression to irreversible degeneration. The apparent discrepancy between the reduced LVDs by echocardiography, and no effect on the LVP or dP/dt$_{max}$ might be explained by the insufficient gene delivery to cover whole heart. Escape of both atria from the gene transduction and their reduced contractility may decrease the preload of both ventricles and would not be reflected to the increment of LVP or dP/dt_{max}. We have reported that transduction of 30 to 40% cells and 12% protein amount were sufficient for improving hemodynamics, as was verified by immuno-histology and Western blotting, respectively, for the level of δ-SG to rescue the animals (11).

Missing of a component in DRP is not lethal (11,12), but its full set may be needed to keep both the membrane integrity and normal life span. Gradual leakage of sarcolemma to Ca^{2+} in addition to the Ca^{2+} entry during slow inward current would elevate the intracellular Ca^{2+} level because of the depletion of high-energy phosphates (28) and activate endogenous protease, calpain (Ca^{2+}-activated neutral protease). On the precise mechanism of DCM progression or coronary spasm, more detailed study would be required on sarcolemmal fluidity (28). Present results distinctly indicate that somatic gene therapy with using potent vector is promising for human DCM treatment, if the rAAV vector is available for the clinical use.

Several phase I/II clinical trials are currently ongoing in gene therapy of cardiovascular disease. These trials are mostly based on the use of adenoviral vectors and nonviral vectors. Novel vectors to improve the efficacy and safety of gene delivery in target organs, such as heart, skeletal muscle, vasculature, and liver, have been recently generated. The rAAV has already been successfully validated in preclinical models of several diseases (29,30) and transferable in both mitotic and non-mitotic cells (30,31). In addition, the rAAV transfectant is long surviving and does not cause pathogenicity in cardiac muscle of Syrian hamsters with DCM (11,12).

Although the rAAV-based vector system has gained attention as a potentially useful alternative to the more commonly used retroviral and adenoviral vectors for human gene therapy, the single-stranded (ss) nature of the viral genome, and consequently the rate-limiting step for second-strand viral DNA synthesis significantly affect its transduction efficiency. In contrast, the phosphorylated form of ssD-binding protein (BP) in human hematopoietic progenitor cells, the efficiencies of AAV-mediated transgene expression were significantly lower than in murine corresponding cells because of the dephosphorylated form of the ssD-BP and an efficient transduction by the rAAV vectors (31). Accordingly, to enhance the efficacy of rAAV transfection in humans, an additional maneuver may be needed to shift phosphorylated D-BP to the dephosphorylated state.

CONCLUSION

Successful application of the 'one size fits all' treatment is encouraging with respect to people with heart failure without further molecular distinction. But the ultimate evolution of these experimental studies in combination with genomic and proteomic studies may potentially useful for the gene transfer that customized to target the individual molecular defect. The novel strategy may provide an actual tailored medicine or specific treatment based on patient's background at the responsible gene level.

ACKNOWLEDGEMENTS

Present study was financially supported by the Ministry of Education, Science and Culture; the Ministry for Welfare and Labor, Japan; Uehara Memorial Foundation and Motor Vehicle Foundation. The authors appreciate Dr. Setsuro Ebashi and Dr. Tomoh Masaki, their encouragement throughout the study and Dr. Jutta Schapar, Department of Experimental Cardiology, Max Planck Institute in Bad Nauheim, Germany, for her kind and fruitful discussion on the results.

REFERENCES

1. Michels VV, Moll PP, Miller FA, Tajik AJ, Chu JS, Driscoll DJ, Burnett JC, Rodeheffer RJ, Chesebro JH, Tazelaar HD. 1992. The frequency of familial dilated cardiomyopathy in a series of patients with idiopathic dilated cardiomyopathy. N Engl J Med 326:77–82.
2. Seidman JG, Seidman C. 2000. The gene basis for cardiomyopathy: from mutation identification to molecular paradigms. Cell 104:557–567.
3. Dzau VJ, Mann MJ, Ehsan A, Griese DP. 2001. Gene therapy and genomic strategies for cardiovascular surgery: The emerging field of surgiomics. J Thorac Cardiovasc Surg 121:206–216.
4. Isner JM. 2002. Myocardial gene therapy. Nature 415:234–239.
5. Ross J Jr. 2002. Dilated cardiomyopathy-Concepts derived from gene deficient and transgenic animal models. Circ J 66:219–224.
6. Cox GF, Kunkel LM. 1997. Dystrophies and heart disease. Curr Opin Cardiol 12:329–343.
7. Sakamoto A, Ono K, Abe M, Jasmin G, Eki T, Murakami Y, Masaki T, Toyo-oka T, Hanaoka F. 1997. Both hypertrophic and dilated cardiomyopathies are caused by mutation of the same gene, δ-sarcoglycan, in hamster: A model of dystrophin-associated glycoprotein complex. Proc Natl Acad Sci USA 94:13873–13878.
8. Tsubata S, Bowles KR, Vatta M, Zintz C, Titus J, Muhonen L, Bowles NE, Towbin JA. 2000. Mutations in the human delta-sarcoglycan gene in familial and sporadic dilated cardiomyopathy. J Clin Invest 106:655–662.
9. Badorff C, Lee G-H, Lamphear BJ, Martone ME, Campbell KP, Rhoads RE, Knowlton KU. 1999. Enteroviral protease 2A cleaves dystrophin: evidence of cytoskeletal disruption in an acquired cardiomyopathy. Nature Med 5:320–326.
10. Xi H, Shin WS, Suzuki J, Nakajima T, Kawada T, Uehara Y, Nakazawa M, Toyo-oka T. 2000. Dystrophin disruption might be related to myocardial cell apoptosis caused by isoproterenol. J Cardiovasc Pharmacol 36(Suppl.2):S25–S29.
11. Kawada T, Sakamoto A, Nakazawa M, Urabe M, Masui F, Hemmi C, Wang Y, Shin WS, Nakatsuru Y, Sato H, Ozawa K, Toyo-oka T. 2001. Morphological and physiological restorations of hereditary form of dilated cardiomyopathy by somatic gene therapy. Biochem Biophys Res Commun 284:431–435.
12. Kawada T, Nakazawa M, Nakauchi S, Yamazaki K, Shimamoto R, Urabe M, Nakata J, Hemmi C, Masui F, Nakajima T, Suzuki J-i, Monahan J, Sato H, Masaki T, Ozawa K, Toyo-oka T. 2002. Rescue of hereditary form of dilated cardiomyopathy by rAAV-mediated somatic gene therapy. Proc Natl Acad Sci USA 99:901–906.
13. Akhter SA, Skaer CA, Kypson AP, McDonald PH, Peppel KC, Glower DD, Lefkowitz RJ, Koch WJ. 1997. Restoration of β-adrenergic signaling in failing cardiac ventricular myocytes via adenoviral-mediated gene transfer. Proc Natl Acad Sci USA 94:12100–12105.
14. Maurice JP, Hata JA, Shah AS, White DC, McDonald PH, Dolber PC, Wilson KH, Lefkowitz RJ, Glower DD, Koch WJ. 1999. Enhancement of cardiac function after adenoviral-mediated in vivo intracoronary beta2-adrenergic receptor gene delivery. J Clin Invest 104:21–29.
15. Tomiyasu K, Oda Y, Nomura M, Satoh E, Fushiki S, Imanishi J, Kondo M, Mazda O. 2000. Direct intra-cardiomuscular transfer of β$_2$-adrenergic receptor gene augments cardiac output in cardiomyopathic hamsters. Gene Ther 7:2087–2093.
16. Small KM, Brown KM, Forbes SL, Liggett SB. 2001. Modification of the β$_2$-adrenergic receptor to engineer a receptor-effector complex for gene therapy. J Biol Chem 276:31596–31601.
17. Packer M, Bristow MR, Cohn JN, Colucci WS, Fowler MB, Gilbert EM, Shusterman NH. 1996. The effect of carvedilol on morbidity and mortality in patients with chronic heart failure. U.S. Carvedilol Heart Failure Study Group. N Engl J Med 334:1349–1355.

18. Toyo-oka T, Naylor WG. 1996. Third generation calcium entry blockers. Blood Pressure 5:206–208.

19. Packer M, Colucci WS, Sackner-Bernstein JD, Liang CS, Goldscher DA, Freeman I, Kukin ML, Kinhal V, Udelson JE, Klapholz M, Gottlieb SS, Pearle D, Cody RJ, Gregory JJ, Kantrowitz NE, LeJemtel TH, Young ST, Lukas MA, Usterman NH. 1996. Double-blind, placebo-controlled study of the effects of carvedilol in patients with moderate to severe heart failure. The PRECISE Trial. Prospective Randomized valuation of Carvedilol on Symptoms and Exercise. N Engl J Med 335:1107–1114.

20. Multicenter Study. Effect of metoprolol CR/XL in chronic heart failure (MERIT-HF). 1999. Lancet 353:2001–2007.

21. The CONSENSUS Trial Study Group. 1987. Effects of enalapril on mortality in severe congestive heart failure. Results of he Cooperative North Scandinavian Enalapril Survival Study (CONSENSUS). N Engl J Med 316:1429–1435.

22. Cohn JN, Franciosa JA. 1977. Vsodilator therapy of cardiac failure. N Engl J Med 97:27–31.

23. del Monte F, Harding SE, Schmidt U, Matsui T, Kang ZB, Dec GW, Gwathmey JK, Rosenzweig A, Hajjar RJ. 1999. Restoration of contractile function in isolated cardiomyocytes from failing human hearts by gene transfer of SERCA2a. Circulation 100:2308–2311.

24. Miyamoto MI, del Monte F, Schmidt U, DiSalvo TS, Kang ZB, Matsui T, Guerrero JL, Gwathmey JK, Rosenzweig A, Hajjar RJ. 2000. Adenoviral gene transfer of SERCA2α improves left-ventricular function in aortic-banded rats in transition to heart failure. Proc Natl Acad Sci USA 97:793–798.

25. Hajjar RJ, Schmidt U, Matsui T, Guerrero JL, Lee KH, Gwathmey JK, Dec GW, Semigran MJ, Rosenzweig A. 1998. Modulation of ventricular function through gene transfer *in vivo*. Proc Natl Acad Sci USA 95:5251–5256.

26. Wahr PA, Michele DE, Metzger JM. 1999. Parvalbumin gene transfer corrects diastolic dysfunction in diseased cardiac myocytes. Proc Natl Acad Sci USA 96:11982–11985.

27. Greelish JP, Su LT, Lankford EB, Burkman JM, Chien H, Koenig SK, Mercier IM, Desjardins PR, Mitchell MA, Zheng XG, Leferovich J, Gao GP, Balice-Gordon RJ, Wilson JM, Stedman HH. 1999. Stable restoration of the sarcoglycan complex in dystrophic muscle perfused with histamine and a recombinant adeno-associated viral vector. Nature Med 5:439–443.

28. Toyo-oka T, Nagayama K, Suzuki J-i, Sugimoto T. 1992. Noninvasive assessment of cardiomyopathy development with simultaneous measurement of topical ^{1}H- and ^{31}P-magnetic resonance spectroscopy. Circulation 86:295–301.

29. Wagner JA, Reynolds T, Moran ML, Moss RB, Wine JJ, Flotte TR, Gardner P. 1998. Efficient and persistent gene transfer of AAV-CFTR in maxillary sinus. Lancet 351:1702–1703.

30. Kay MA, Manno CS, Ragni MV, Larson PJ, Couto LB, McClelland A, Glader B, Chew AJ, Tai SJ, Herzog RW, Arruda V, Johnson F, Scallan C, Skarsgard E, Flake AW, High KA. 2000. Evidence for gene transfer and expression of factor IX in haemophilia B patients treated with an AAV vector. Nature Genet 24:257–261.

31. Qing K, Khuntirat B, Mah C, Kube DM, Wang XS, Ponnazhagan S, Zhou S, Dwarki VJ, Yoder MC, Srivastava A. 1998. Adeno-associated virus type 2-mediated gene transfer: Correlation of tyrosine phosphorylation of the cellular single-stranded D sequence-binding protein with transgene expression in human cells in vitro and murine tissues *in vivo*. J Virol 72:1593–1599.

32. Hajjar RJ, Schmidt U, Matsui T, Guerrero JL, Lee KH, Gwathmey JK, Dec GW, Semigran MJ, Rosenzweig A. 1998. Modulation of ventricular function through gene transfer in vivo. Proc Natl Acad Sci USA. 95:5251–5256.

33. Hoshijima M, Ikeda Y, Iwanaga Y, Minamisawa S, Date MO, Gu Y, Iwatate M, Li M, Wang L, Wilson JM, Wang Y, Ross J Jr, Chien KR. 2002. Chronic suppression of heart-failure progression by a pseudophosphorylated mutant of phospholamban via in vivo cardiac rAAV gene delivery. Nature Med. 8:864–871.

ABBREVIATION USED IN THIS ARTICLE

β_2-AR, β_2-adrenergic receptor,

BARK, β-adrenoreceptor kinase,

β-Gal, β-galactosidase,

CANP, Ca^{2+}-activated neutral protease,

CVP, central venous pressure,

dP/dt_{max}, the maximum derivative of left ventricular pressure,

dP/dt_{min}, the minimum derivative of left ventricular pressure,

δ-SG, delta-sarcoglycan,

DCM, dilated cardiomyopathy,

DRP, dystrophin-related proteins,

EF, left ventricular ejection fraction,

FS, fractional shortening,

GPCR, G-protein-coupled receptor,

HR, heart rate,

LVDs, left ventricular systolic dimension,

LVDd, left ventricular diastolic dimension,

LVEDP, left ventricular end-diastolic pressure,

LVP, left ventricular pressure,

PL, phospholamban,

rAAV, recombinant adeno-associated virus,

RT-PCR, reverse transcriptase-polymerase chain reaction,

SERCA, sarcoplasmic/endoplasmic reticulum Ca^{2+} ATPase, and

TREC, therapeutic receptor-effector complex.

Signal Transduction and Cardiac Hypertrophy,
edited by N.S. Dhalla, L.V. Hryshko,
E. Kardami & P.K. Singal
Kluwer Academic Publishers, Boston, 2003

Adaptation to Ischemia by in vivo Exposure to Hyperoxia—Signalling Through Mitogen Activated Protein Kinases and Nuclear Factor Kappa B

Guro Valen,[1,2] Peeter Tähepôld,[1] Joel Starkopf,[3]
Arno Ruusalepp,[1] and Jarle Vaage[2]

[1] Crafoord Laboratory of Experimental Surgery
[2] Department of Thoracic Surgery
Karolinska Hospital, Stockholm, Sweden
[3] Clinic of Anesthesiology and Intensive Care
University of Tartu, Tartu
Estonia

Summary. We have established a model of adaptation to ischemia by breathing a hyperoxic gas mixture, which may be directly employed in clinical practice. Hyperoxia improves postischemic function and reduces myocardial necrosis in globally and regionally ischemic rat and mouse hearts, protects hearts of animals with severe atherosclerosis, and modulates in vitro reactivity of isolated aortic rings. Hyperoxic preconditioning is most efficient when the inspired oxygen fraction is >80% oxygen, with different exposure times in rats and mice. In rats the protection is both immediate and delayed, while in mice only immediate protection can be evoked. Exposure to hyperoxia causes an oxidative stress evident as increased serum lipid peroxidation products and reduced antioxidant defence. When breathing hyperoxic gas a rapid nuclear translocation of nuclear factor kappa B (NFκB) in the lungs is followed by a cardiac NFκB activation. In conjunction with hyperoxia the mitogen activated protein kinases (MAPK) p38, ERK1/2, and JNK are phosphorylated in the heart. Pharmacological inhibition of NFκB activation abolished the beneficial effects of hyperoxia. During

Address for Correspondence: Guro Valen, MD, PhD., Crafoord Laboratory L6:00, Karolinska Hospital, 17176 Stockholm, Sweden. Tel: +46-8-51774846, Fax: +46-8-51773557, E-mail: *Guro.Valen@cmm.ki.se*

Langendorff-perfusion with induced global ischemia, phosphorylation of MAPK as well as translocation of NFκB is reduced in animals subjected to hyperoxia prior to the experiments, the latter perhaps due to increased formation of the NFκB inhibitor IκBα. A posssible role for the NFκB-regulated gene inducible nitric oxide synthase (iNOS) in the hyperoxia response was investigated in knock out mice, who had no functional or antiinfarct protection of preconditioning by either hyperoxia or classic ischemic preconditioning. However, neither cardiac iNOS nor contents of antioxidants, heat shock protein 70, or endothelial NOS in the heart increased after hyperoxia. Thus, the signal transduction pathways and organ effectors of hyperoxic protection are not fully determined, but appear to involve MAPK and NFκB. Hyperoxia may have a large potential in the pretreatment of patients undergoing not only open heart procedures, but also in front of any major surgery.

Key words: Nuclear factor kappa B, mitogen activated protein kinases, endogenous myocardial protection, hyperoxia.

BACKGROUND

Clinical relevance

Ischemic heart disease is a major cause of morbidity and mortality in the Western world. In 1994 approximately 23,000 individuals died from coronary artery disease in Sweden. Annually about 40,000 myocardial infarctions occur, and approximately 7000 operations with coronary artery bypass grafting are performed (the population of Sweden is 8.8 million). Revascularization of the ischemic myocardium is essential for its survival, and thrombolysis, percutanous transluminal coronary angioplasty, stenting, and coronary artery bypass grafting are everyday clinical procedures. Paradoxically, the ischemia-reperfusion of these interventions represents an additional injury, and the patients would benefit from an improved myocardial protection in these situations. Activation of endogenous cell defense by preconditioning or preconditioning-like responses would be a clinical advantage if such methods were available.

Ischemic preconditioning

Short episodes of ischemia and reperfusion prior to a sustained ischemic event, termed ischemic preconditioning, reduces infarct size and improves cardiac function (1). Preconditioning is the most powerful experimental cardioprotective method discovered, and is protective either when the preconditioning takes place less than two hours before the sustained ischemia (termed classic preconditioning), or when the sustained ischemia is 24–72 hours after the preconditioning episode (termed delayed preconditioning). In the last years it has become apparent that preconditioning of other organs will protect both the organ itself and the heart (remote preconditioning). The perspective of preconditioning research is to find the underlying mechanism of action which could be exploited pharmacologically in patients for increased myocardial protection, as occlusion and reperfusion of the coronary vasculature—ischemic preconditioning itself—is not an acceptable way of evoking the response in a large scale treatment.

An overview of possible mechanisms of preconditioning

Despite more than a decade of research trying to determine the mechanisms of pre-conditioning, there is still a lot left to be discovered before the signal transduction pathways are unravelled. A summary of the most acknowleged underlying mecha-nisms are shown in Figure 1. During the preconditioning episodes, intracellular triggering of the response may be due to release of nitric oxide (NO), low doses of reactive oxygen intermediates (ROS), adenosine, bradykinin, and/or prostacyclin (2–4). Either through G-protein coupled membrane receptors or directly, the trigger substances may cause activation of kinase cascades. Protein kinase C, tyrosine kinase, as well as members of the mitogen activated protein kinase families (MAPK) have been identified as important mediators in different models (5,6). Which kinase is upstream or downstream to which is currently an issue of debate, and may depend on the trigger in the specific model selected. Adenosine signaling has been linked to protein kinase C-dependent opening of mitochondrial ATP-sensitive potassium channals (7), which may also be end-effectors of myocardial protection (8). The adenosine A_1 receptor may also signal to the K_{ATP} channel through tyrosine kinases and MAPK (9). Additionally, the importance of the K_{ATP} channel may actually be signalling to something else through generation of ROS upon activation (10). A possible component in the signal transduction pathway is activation of transcription factors by phosphorylated protein kinases, ROS, or NO, of which particularly the transcription factor nuclear factor kappa-B (NFκB) has been investigated in both classic and delayed models (11,12). Activation of transcription factors may induce transcription of cardioprotective mediators. The endogenous cardioprotective sub-stances which are suggested upregulated and protective during preconditioning are heat shock proteins of the 70 kDA (13) or 27 kDa (14) families, antioxidants (15), inducible nitric oxide synthase (16), and inducible cyclooxygenase (17). Heat shock proteins are not regulated by NFκB but have their own transcription factors, however, they do modulate NFκB activation. Another mechanism by which pre-conditioning protects the heart may be through reducing apoptosis, which may be linked to a NFκB-dependent increase of cardiac Bcl-2 (11,18) (Figure 1).

NFκB in ischemic preconditioning

The role of NFκB in vascular and cardiac biology has recently been revewied by us (19). NFκB regulates more than 160 genes involved in innate and adaptive immu-nity, most of which are associated with proinflammatory effects such as leukocyte adhesion molecules, cytokines, and chemokines, and has been indicated as impor-tant for initiation and progression of pathogenesis of inflammatory disease such as in atherosclerosis, inflammatory bowel disease, autoimmune arthritis, glomeru-lonephritis, asthma, and myocardial ischemia-reperfusion injury (19). However, also beneficial effects of NFκB through reduction of apoptosis, promotion of ischemic preconditioning, and in resolving inflammation is becoming apparent (19,20). A schematic presentation of NFκB regulation is presented in Figure 2. Transactivation of NFκB can be induced by preconditioning-relevant stimuli such as ROS,

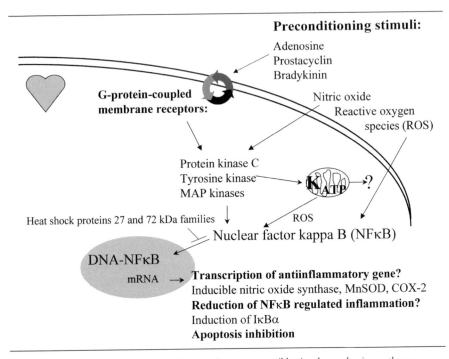

Preconditioning stimuli:

Figure 1. A schematic overview over the most important possible signal transduction pathways underlying the mechanisms of ischemic preconditioning. During preconditioning trigger substances are released, which may be adenosine, prostacyclin, bradykinin, nitric oxide, and/or reactive oxygen species (ROS). Either through G-protein coupled membrane receptors, or directly, phosphorylation of protein kinases may occur. The ATP-dependent potassium channel may be downstream to this, and may through an unknown mechanism be the end-effector of protection. It is also possible that ROS released through activation of the ion channel may contribute, along with the other factors depicted, to activation of the transcription factor nuclear factor kappaB (NFκB). NFκB translocates to the cell nucleus during preconditioning, binds to DNA promoter regions, and may start transcription of an antiinflammatory gene such as inducible nitric oxide synthase, manganese superoxide dismutase (MnSOD), or inducible cycloxygenase (COX-2) which may be the end-effector(s) of heart protection. It is also possible that the role NFκB activation in preconditioning is through reducing its own activation during sustained ischemia by induction of the inhibitory protein IκB, as most genes regulated by NFκB are proinflammatory and associated with increased infarctions. A third, possible way of protection afforded by NFκB is through inhibition of apoptosis. Preconditioning may be mediated by genes not regulated by NFκB, of which heat shock proteins are included in the figure, as they have properties modulating NFκB activation and DNA binding.

hypoxia/anoxia, cytokines, protein kinase C, MAPkinases, and NO (2,5,6,19). The NFκB family consists of the members p50, p52, p65 (RelA), c-Rel, and RelB which form various homo- and heterodimers, where the most common active form is the p50 or p52/RelA heterodimer. NFκB dimers in resting cells reside in the cytoplasm in an inactive form bound to inhibitory proteins known as IκB. At least six IκB proteins are involved in controlling the activity of the NFκB dimer. IκBα and IκBβ are the two stimulus–regulatory proteins of NFκB which may play a role for preconditioning, and are phosphorylated by stimuli activating the IκB kinase. The

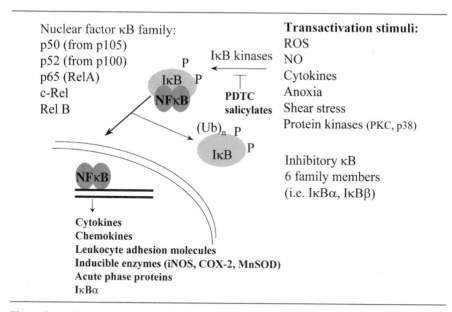

Figure 2. Nuclear factor kappa B (NFκB) consists of 5 family members with or without precursors as shown, which form various hetero- or homodimers. The most usual is the p50/p65 heterodimer. In the cytoplasm of the resting cell the dimer is held inactive by inhibitory proteins known as IκB. There are at least 6 IκB family members, of which IκBα and IκBβ are the stimulus-specific relevant to ischemic preconditioning. During preconditioning, stimuli such as reactive oxygen species (ROS), nitric oxide (NO), etc, may activate the IκB-kinase complex, leading to phosphorylation of IκB. IκB then dissociates from NFκB, is ubiquitinated and rapidly degraded, while NFκB translocates to the nuclei and starts transcription of the genes it regulates as shown. IκB-kinase may be inhibited by several drugs, among them PDTC and salisylates.

phosphorylated IκBs are then ubiquitinated and proteolytically degraded. This process activates NFκB, which translocates to the nucleus and binds to promoter or enhancer regions of specific genes, initiating transcription (19) (Figure 2).

Evidence for involvement of NFκB in ischemic preconditioning is partially indirect: activation of protein kinase C, tyrosine kinase and p38 MAP kinase appear to be crucial for the preconditioning response, and these kinases can also activate NFκB (5,6,9,11,12,21). NFκB translocates to the nuclei during the preconditioning episodes, and pharmacological inhibition of NFκB abolishes the cardioprotection in both classic and delayed models (11,12,21,22,23). ROS are suggested to be trigger substances for preconditioning, and they induce NFκB activation (6,15). Adenosine har been indicated as another trigger of the preconditioning response. Purines may induce activation of NFκB (24,25), although this is controversial (26). Preconditioning or adenosine protected a human cardiomyocyte cell line via a p38MAPK pathway (27), while adenosine A1 receptor stimulation could evoke delayed preconditioning in the intact rabbit via upregulation of the NFκB-regulated manganese superoxide dismutase (28). In mice, adenosine A1 stimulation involves signalling through p38MAPK, tyrosine kinase, the KATP channel, and NFκB, employing inducible nitric oxide synthase as organ-effector of protection (9,22,23).

Myocardial protection by NFκB activation may be caused by preischemic induction of a NFκB-regulated protein such as manganese superoxide disumutase, inducible cyclo-oxygenase, and inducible nitric oxide synthase (iNOS). All these enzymes are associated with modulation and resolution of the inflammatory response, and are suggested as end-effectors of the preconditioning response (16,17,20,22,27,28). Down-regulation of the inflammatory response during reperfusion may also an important consequence of preischemic NFκB activation. Morgan et al. (21) found a reduced activation of NFκB after sustained ischemia in hearts which had been subjected to preconditioning. In HUVECs preconditioned by hydrogen peroxide, reduced upregulation of cytokines and leukocyte adhesion molecules after subsequent stimulation with TNFα was found (29). A similar reduction of mRNA for NFκB regulated genes was observed during reperfusion of preconditioned rat hearts (30). Heat shock proteins of the 70 kDa family, which are upregulated during preconditioning (13), modulate AP-1 and NFκB DNA binding activity (31,32), and might reduce NFκB activation and thereby reduce inflammation during reperfusion. A last possible route of NFκB mediated cardioprotection is through the antiapoptotic effect of preconditioning. NFκB regulates several antiapoptotic molecules, such as Bcl-2 (11,18), survivin (33), inhibitor of apoptosis protein-1 (34), as well as X-linked inhibitor of apoptosis protein-1 (35).

Preconditioning by hyperoxia

Rationale

ROS have been suggested to trigger ischemic preconditioning, signalling through MAPK and NFκB activation (6,15,36,37). Experimental studies in cell cultures and organs show that hyperoxia generates reactive oxygen species and induces lipid peroxidation (38,39). Although long-lasting hyperoxia is injurious, a short exposure inducing a low-graded oxidative stress may potentially be a clinically acceptable way to elicit myocardial protection analogous to ischemic preconditioning. Normobaric hyperoxia induces oxidative stress and induces NFκB activation in cell cultures (38,40). Increasing the oxygen content in inspiratory gas is a general, potentially lifesaving principle in the treatment of patients with respiratory insufficiency. If hyperoxic treatment could induce a preconditioning-like myocardial protection, it is a method potentially directly clinical available for treatment of a large number of patients.

Basic physiology of the model

Awake animals (rats or mice) are kept in a hyperoxic environment (41–45). We have studied the impact of the inspired oxygen fraction on the function and infarct development in the later isolated and Langendorff-perfused heart of rats or mice (41). Rats were confined in a cage, and exposed to 95%, 80%, 60, or 40% oxygen or air for 60 minutes prior to heart isolation and Langendorff-perfusion with 25 minutes of induced global ischemia followed by 60 minutes of reperfusion. A concentration-dependent protection of heart function and infarct size was observed, with a maximal effect after 80 and 95% oxygen in inspired air. Different durations of exposure to 95% oxygen (ranging from 15 minutes to 3 hours) was attempted in rats and mice (41). In rats a preconditioning-like effect could be evoked by exposure to 60 or 180 minutes of hyperoxia, but neither shorter times nor two hours exposure had any effect. The protection was present when hearts were isolated immediately after the hyperoxic exposure, and also protected when hearts were isolated 24 hours later and subjected to ischemia and reperfusion (41,42). In the mouse heart functional and infarct-limiting effects could be induced by pretreatment for 15 or 30, but not by 60 minutes of ≥95% oxygen (41). The exception to this was the apolipoprotein E/low density lipoprotein receptor double knockout mice subjected to hyperoxic exposure before global ischemia. The mice had a severe atherosclerosis at the time of the experiments, and reduced function as well as increased infarctions compared with wild type mice (43). In those mice 60 minutes hyperoxic exposure protected function and infarction before global ischemia, and the effect was as profound as that of classic preconditioning (43). There have been some discussions about the efficacy of preconditioning in atherosclerotic humans as clinical studies have not always found that preconditioning protects; however, our findings in atherosclerotic mice clarify that this may not be due to atherosclerosis per se, but rather to other factors in the selection of patients, mode of surgical myocardial protection, and end points of the study (43). The protective effect of hyperoxia in wild type mice could only be evoked for immediate protection (41). Since >95% oxygen gave optimal protection, this was employed for all further studies.

Signalling of protection

Evidence of oxidant stress

Blood was sampled after 60 or 120 minutes of hyperoxia or normoxia from rats to investigate indices of systemic oxidative stress. Serum levels of conjugated dienes were significantly increased after 60 minutes of hyperoxic exposure, indicating that oxidative stress with lipid peroxidation occurred (42). After 180 minutes of hyperoxic exposure the total antioxidative capacity in serum was reduced (42). We sampled pulmonary and cardiac tissues from rats serially in conjunction with hyperoxic breathing to study any possible translocation of NFκB by electromobility shift assay (Figure 3a, ref 44). In lungs, increased NFκB DNA-binding was apparent already 2 minutes after start of hyperoxic breathing, then gradually normalized in a 60 min observation period. In the heart, a small translocation of NFκB could be observed 5 minutes after start of hyperoxic breathing. 20 and 60 minutes later the NFκB DNA-binding in hearts was clearly increased (Figure 3a). The bands were abolished by cold probe competition and supershiftet with a p50 antibody, verifying the band identity as NFκB (Figure 3a). Activation of cardiac NFκB in conjunction with preconditioning is also observed in models of classic preconditioning in rats and rabbits (11,21), or in delayed preconditioning of the rabbit and mouse (12,16,17).

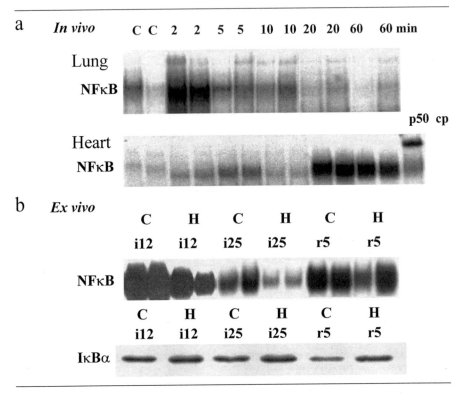

Figure 3. a. Rats were kept in a hyperoxic (>95% oxygen) environment, and hearts and lungs were biopsied serially after 0–60 min hyperoxia (n = 2 at each time point). C are unstimulated animals. Nuclear proteins were extracted, and electrophoresed after incubation with a radiolabelled NFκB probe (electromobility shift assay). NFκB-DNA binding increased already after 2 min in the lungs, thereafter gradually decreased. In cardiac protein extracts, a small increase of NFκB-DNA binding was apparent already after 5 min, with a large increase 20–60 min after start of hyperoxic treatment. The band was supershifted when an anti-p50 antibody was added (p50), and abolished by cold probe competition (cp), verifying the band identity as NFκB. Look into reference 44 for details. **b.** After 60 min hyperoxic exposure (H) or corresponding normoxia (C) hearts were isolated and Langendorff-perfused with 25 min global ischemia. The upper panel shows an electromobilty shift assay of cardiac nuclear protein extracts with a radiolabelled NFκB probe taken after 12 and 25 min global ischemia, as well as 5 min reperfusion. Note that hearts subjected to hyperoxia in vivo consistently had less NFκB translocation than hearts of normoxic rats (reference 44). The lower panel shows an immunoblot of cytoplasmatic protein extracts from the same hearts as above, with an antibody against the inhibitory IκBα. IκBα was consistently higher in hearts of animals exposed to in vivo hyperoxia.

Phosphorylation of mitogen activated protein kinases (MAPK)

To further characterize the signalling cascades involved in adaptation to ischemia by hyperoxic breathing, mice hearts were sampled after 30 minutes exposure to >95% oxygen, or after normoxic breathing in the same cage. Additional hearts were sampled after 25 minutes of stabilization during modified Langendorff perfusion (the procedures described in detail in ref 43) or after 30 minutes of reperfusion after 40 minutes global ischemia from animals exposed to hyperoxia or normoxia in vivo

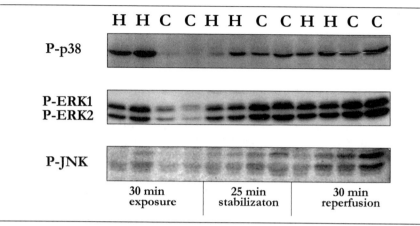

Figure 4. Experiments were performed in mice subjected to 30 minutes exposure to hyperoxic (>95% oxygen, H) or normoxic breathing (C), where hearts were isolated, Langendorff-perfused, and subjected to 25 minutes stabilization followed by 40 minutes global ischemia and 30 minutes reperfusion (n = 2 at each time point). Proteins were extracted from the hearts and subjected to immunoblotting with phosphospecific antibodies to the mitogen activated protein kinases p38, ERK1/2, and JNK. Immediateley after the hyperoxic preconditioning increased phosphorylations of MAPK were seen (30 min exposure). During Langendorff stabilization and reperfusion MAPK were phosphorylated in all hearts. Hearts from animals pretreated with hyperoxia had reduced phosphorylation reactions.

prior to heart isolation. Proteins were extracted, and electrophoresed under reducing conditions. The gels were transferred to nitrocellulose membranes, and incubated with rabbit polyclonal antibodies detecting phosphorylated p38 MAPK, ERK1/2, and JNK. Enhanced chemiluminescence was used for visualization. A clear phosphorylation of p38 and ERK1/2 were observed in conjunction with hyperoxic exposure in vivo, while only small changes were observed in the phosphorylation of JNK (Figure 3). Heart isolation and Langendorff-perfusion induced phosphorylations of all three MAPKs, but less in the hearts of animals with previous exposure to hyperoxia. The increased phosphorylations observed during reperfusion after global ischemia were less pronounced in hearts of animals with a prior exposure to hyperoxia (Figure 4). Thus, although MAPK activation was observed during hyperoxic exposure, it was reduced during Langendorff-perfusion with induced ischemia and reperfusion. Activation of MAPKs during classic ischemic preconditioning has been found by a number of researchers, although the principal MAPK appears to differ between preconditioning model, laboratory and species (5,46–49). In agrement with the present findings, Marais et al. (46) found that preconditioned hearts had a reduced MAPK phosphorylation during sustained ischemia. This would in theory lead to a reduced NFκB activation during sustained ischemia.

Activation of NFκB

Translocation of NFκB was detected early after start of hyperoxic exposure, indicating that oxidative stress was a component of the triggering of the effect. When rats were treated with the NFκB inhibitors SN50 or PDTC prior to hyperoxia, the beneficial effects of hyperoxia on heart function and infarct size disappeared (44). NFκB translocation after hyperoxia was reduced when SN50 was used compared with hyperoxia alone, confirming that SN50 inhibited NFκB activation (44). When hearts were sampled serially during ischemia and reperfusion after either hyperoxic or normoxic exposure, a consistant reduction of NFκB activation was observed in hearts of hyperoxic animals compared with normoxic controls (Figure 3b). This may be due to hyperoxia increasing cardiac contents of the NFκB inhibitor IκBα as evaluated by immunoblot (Figure 3b). A reduced NFκB activation during sustained ischemia, but translocation during preconditioning, has previously been observed in classic preconditioning of rabbit hearts (21). Furthermore, preconditioning reduced expression of NFκB-regulated proinflammatory genes in rat hearts (30) and cell cultures (29). Cardiac NFκB is been associated with proinflammatory effects, and inhibiting NFκB during reperfusion in models without any adaptation is beneficial for reduction of infarct size and improvement of cardiac function (50,51). In our studies Langendorff-perfused rat hearts subjected to global ischemia without any preceeding adaptation benefited from inhibition of NFκB transactivation during reperfusion (44). Thus the role of NFκB in the heart appears to be dual and confer both protection during preconditioning and hyperoxic exposure, and inflammation during sustained ischemia (19). A full clarification of this issue is warranted. It is possible that the benefit of NFκB during preconditioning and hyperoxia is to induce its own inhibition during sustained ischemia due to IκBα upregulation, secondarily reducing NFκB activation and inflammation. Perhaps the benefit can partially be due to induction of genes associated with resorption of inflammation, i.e. the inducible enzymes cyclooxygenase 2, manganese superoxide dismutase, or iNOS (19,20).

Organ effectors of protection

In order to elucidate the tissue mediators of protection in both the delayed and immediate models of hyperoxic adaptation to ischemia, rat hearts were sampled for analysis of contents of the antioxidants catalase, superoxide dismutase (all isoforms), glutathione peroxidase, as well as total antioxidant capacity corresponding to time to start of Langendorff-perfusion (42). Hyperoxic exposure immediately or 24 hours earlier did not influence cardiac contents of antioxidants. Neither were cardiac indices of lipid peroxidation (lipid peroxides, conjugated dienes, lipid hydroperoxides, oxidized/reduced glutathione ratio) different between groups. A small increase of glutathione reductase activity immediately after 60 min hyperoxia was detected, but is not sufficient to explain the profound functional and infarct-limiting effect found in the study (42). In the delayed model of hyperoxia, we also studied cardiac contents of endothelial nitric oxide synthase and heat shock protein 72 by immunoblotting. Neither of these were influenced by hyperoxia in vivo 24 hours earlier (42).

A role for iNOS in organ protection?

INOS has been suggested as an important organ mediator of pharmacologic as well as delayed preconditioning (16,22,23). We wanted to investigate a possible role of

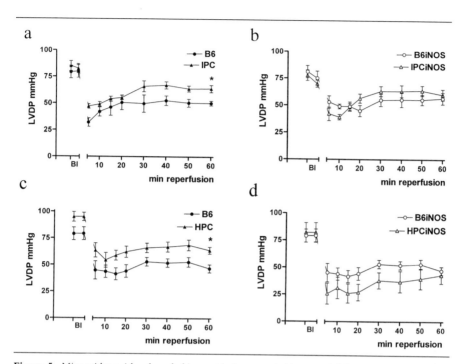

Figure 5. Mice without (closed symbols) or with (open symbols) targeted deletion of the inducible nitric oxide synthase (iNOS) gene were subjected to hyperoxia for 30 min (HPC) or normoxic controls (B6 in the lower panels). In another set of experiments, classic ischemic preconditioning (IPC) were compared with time-matched controls (B6 in the lower panels). After Langendorff stabilization or stabilization/IPC (BI), 40 min global ischemia was induced and followed by 60 min reperfusion. The ischemia-induced depression of left ventricular developed pressure (LVDP) was attenuated by HPC or IPC in wild type mice, but not in hearts of iNOS knock out animals. The graph shows mean ± SEM of n = 5–8 in each group. *denotes $p < 0.05$.

iNOS in the immediate model of hyperoxia in mice. iNOS knock out and wild type mice were subjected to 30 min exposure to >95% hyperoxia, and thereafter their hearts were excised and Langendorff-perfused in a constant pressure model as previously described (43). In addition normoxic hearts of the same strains of mice were isolated and subjected to a preconditioning protocol of 2 episodes of 2 minutes of global ischemia followed by reperfusion for 5 minutes, before 40 minutes of global ischemia and 60 minutes reperfusion (n = 5–8 in each group). Left ventricular developed pressure was reduced during reperfusion of wild type mice, and this was attenuated by either classic ischemic preconditioning or by hyperoxia (Figure 5a and c). However, when the experiments were performed in iNOS deficient mice, this protection was abolished (Figure 5b and d). Left ventricular end-diastolic pressure increased during reperfusion of wild types, and this was attenuated by both classic and hyperoxic preconditioning (Figure 6a and c). In iNOS knockout animals this effect disappeared (Figure 6b and d). Infarct size was evaluated by triphenyl tetrazolium chloride solution as described elswhere (41), and was reduced by classic

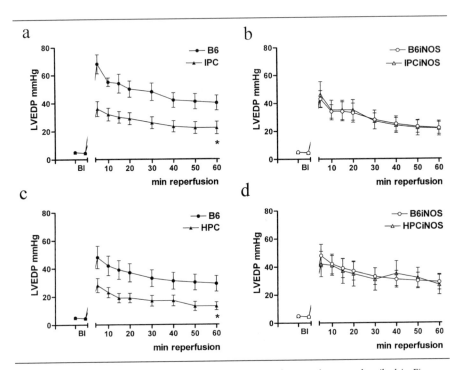

Figure 6. Left ventricular end-diastolic pressure (LVEDP) in the same hearts as described in Figure 5. The ischemia-induced increased of LVEDP was attenuated by HPC or IPC in wild type mice, but not in hearts of iNOS knock out animals. The graph shows mean ± SEM of n = 5–8 in each group. *denotes p < 0.05.

preconditioning and tended to be reduced by hyperoxia (Figure 7a and b). This effect was not apparent in hearts from iNOS knockout mice (Figure 7). The time frame of observation between preconditioning stimuli and functional protection was approximately 1½ hour in the hyperoxia model (30 minutes hyperoxia in vivo, 25 minutes stabilization in Langendorff, 40 minutes of global ishemia), and 1 hour in the classic preconditioning. Although this is at the shorter border to allow for transcription and translation for iNOS, we collected hearts for analysis of iNOS protein by immunoblotting during hyperoxia and Langendorff-perfusion. INOS was not influenced by hyperoxic adaptation (Figure 7), or by classic preconditioning (not shown). Thus, iNOS does play a role for hyperoxic preconditioning, but probably not as an organ effector.

OTHER APPLICATIONS

We have also investigated protection by hyperoxia in other models, i.e. whether hyperoxia influences vasomotor function of aortic rings in vitro, and if it has a role against injury induced by regional ischemia of the heart (45). Isolated rings of the thoracic aorta were obtained from rats immediately or 24 hours after in vivo

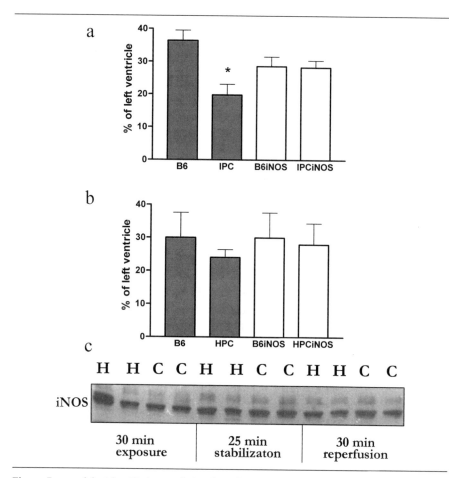

Figure 7. a and b. After 60 min reperfusion the infarct size in the hearts shown in Figures 5 and 6 was determined by triphenyl tetrazolium chloride. In wild type mice, IPC reduced infarct size, while HPC tended to reduce it. This effect of preconditioning was abolished in iNOS KO animals. **c** Mice were subjected to 30 minutes exposure to hyperoxic (>95% oxygen, H) or normoxic breathing (C). Thereafter hearts were Langendorff-perfused with 25 minutes stabilization followed by 40 minutes global ischemia and 30 minutes reperfusion (n = 2 at each time point). Proteins were extracted from the hearts and subjected to immunoblotting with a rabbit polyclonal antibody to inducible nitric oxide synthase (iNOS). No differences in the expression of iNOS were observed after hyperoxia per se, hyperoxia followed by Langendorff-perfusion, or hyperoxia followed by global ischemia and reperfusion compared with normoxic controls.

exposure to 60 minutes of hyperoxia, and the in vitro dose-response to phenylephrine, prostaglandin $F_{2\alpha}$, endothelin-1, acetylcholine and sodium nitroprusside was assessed. Hyperoxia in vivo increased the relaxation of aortic rings to acetylcholine and sodium nitroprusside, while it delayed contraction to phenylephrine (45). Preconditioning of the vasculature against loss of vasomotor function following local ischaemia-reperfusion injury has been demonstrated in several studies (52–54). These studies concentrate on the function of the coronary vasculature in Langendorff preparations or in vivo models, and found that local ischemic preconditioning in particular preserves endothelium-dependent vasodilatory function. We have previously investigated vasomotor function after remote, delayed preconditioning in mice, and found that aortic rings harvested from mice with induced brain ischemia 24–36 hours before the experiments enhanced in vitro relaxation to acetylcholine, attenuated contractions to prostaglandin $F_{2\alpha}$, and induced iNOS in the vessel wall (55). When the experiments were performed in the presence of the iNOS inhibitor aminoguanidine or vessels from iNOS deficient animals, the beneficial effects of brain ischemia were abolished. An impaired response to prostaglandin $F_{2\alpha}$ was found in aortic rings from Apolipoprotein E/low density lipoprotein mice with severe atherosclerosis and in vivo spontaneous ischemic events, while relaxations to acetylcholine were unchanged (55). Laude et al. (56,57) induced regional cardiac ischemia in rats 24 hours after in vivo preconditioning or sham operation, and mounted isolated coronary segments from the ischemic-reperfused area in a myograph. The endothelium dependent relaxation was reduced by ischemia/reperfusion, and in accordance with the present finding, the impaired vessel reactivity could be protected by ischemic preconditioning (56,57). Interestingly, hyperoxia also reduced infarct size in isolated, Langendorff-perfused rat hearts subjected to 30 minutes of regional ischemia and reperfused for 120 minutes (45). So far we have not elucidated whether the cardiac effects are primary due to myocyte influences, or secondary to changes in vascular tone and function. Systemic oxidative stress evoked by hyperoxia induces not only cardiac protection against global or regional ischemia, but also induces a general protection of vascular function.

FUTURE CONSIDERATIONS

We have established a model of adaptation to ischemia through breathing a hyperoxic gas mixture, which protects isolated hearts of rats and mice against global and regional ischemia, and influences the in vitro vessel reactivity. In theory, the model can be used directly in patients regardless of mechanisms of actions, and as such may be of great clinical importance for treatment of a large range of patients. However, unravelling the signalling pathways of protection are of considerable academic interest, as understanding this model and comparing with other models of cardioprotection may help pinpoint universal factors underlying endogenous protection. So far we have determined that hyperoxia causes a systemic oxidative stress, and signals through MAPK, NFκB, and IκBα. Neither iNOS, eNOS, heat shock protein 72, or antioxidants are organ effectors, but NO does appear involved as iNOS knock out mice could not be preconditioned. We want to further pinpoint the cascades involved in the signalling and protection and how they interact, as well as discover new application fields for the model.

ACKNOWLEDGEMENTS

Allan Sirsjö is gratefully acknowledged for providing iNOS knockout mice, and Theres Jägerbrink is acknowledged for excellent technical assistance. The work has been supported by grants from the Swedish Medical Research Council (11235 and 12665), the Swedish Heart-Lung Foundation, Gösta Franckels Foundation, Jeanssonska Stiftelserna, Fredrik and Ingrid Thuring Foundation, King Gustav V:s and Queen Victorias Foundation, and the Karolinska Institute.

REFERENCES

1. Murry CE, Jennings RB, Reimer KA. 1986. Preconditioning with ischemia: A delay in lethal injury in ischemic myocardium. Circulation 74:1124–1136.
2. Bolli R, Manchikalapudi S, Tang X-L, Takano H, Qiu Y, Guo Y, Zhang Q, Jadon AK. 1997. The protective effect of late preconditioning against myocardial stunning in conscious rabbits is mediated by nitric oxide synthase. Circ Res 81:1094–1107.
3. Takano H, Tang XL, Qiu Y, French BA, Bolli R. 1998. Nitric oxide donors induce late preconditioning against myocardial stunning and infarction in conscious rabbits via an antioxidant sensitive mechanism. Circ Res 83:73–84.
4. Parrat JR, Vegh A. 1999. Coronary vascular endothelium-myocyte interactions in protection of the heart by ischemic preconditioning. J Physiol Pharmacol 50:509–524.
5. Cohen MV, Baines CP, Downey JM. 2000. Ischemic preconditioning: From adenosine receptor to KATP channel. Ann Rev Physiol 62:79–109.
6. Das DK, Engelman RM, Maulik N. 1999. Oxygen free radical signalling in ischemic preconditioning. In: Heart in stress. Ed DK Das, 49–65. New York: Ann NY Acad Sci.
7. Sato T, Sasaki N, O'Rourke B, Marban E. 2000. Adenosine primes the opening of mitochindrial ATP-sensitive potassium channals: a key step in ischemic preconditioning? Circulation 102:800–805.
8. de Jong JW, de Jonge R, Keijzer E, Bradamante S. 2000. The role of adenosine in preconditioning. Pharmacol Ther 87:141–149.
9. Zhao TC, Hines DS, Kukreja RC. 2001. Adenosine-induced late preconditioning in mouse hearts: role of p38 MAP kinase and mitochondrial K_{ATP} channels. Am J Physiol 280:H1278–H1285.
10. Pain T, Yang XM, Critz SD, Yue Y, Nakano A, Liu GS, Heusch G, Cohen MV, Downey JM. 2000. Opening of mitochondrial K(ATP) channels triggers the preconditioned state by generating free radicals. Circ Res 87:431–433.
11. Maulik N, Sato M, Price BD, Das DK. 1998. An essential role of NFkB in tyrosine kinase signalling of p38 MAP kinase regulation of myocardial adaption to ischemia. FEBS letters 429:365–369.
12. Xuan Y-T, Tang X-L, Banerjee S, Takano H, Li RCX, Han H, Qiu Y, Li J-J, Bolli R. 1999. Nuclear factor-kB plays an essential role in the late phase of ischemic preconditioning in conscious rabbits. Circ Res 84:1095–1109.
13. Marber MS, Latchman DS, Walker JM, Yellon DM. 1993. Cardiac stress protein elevation 24 hours after brief ischaemia or heat stress is associated with resistance to myocardial infarction. Circulation 88:1264–1272.
14. Dana A, Skarli M, Papakrivopoulou J, Yellon DM. 2000. Adenosine A(1) receptor indiced delayed preconditioning in rabbits: induction of p38 mitogen-activated protein kinase activation and HSP27 phosphorylation via tyrosine kinase and protein kinase C dependent mechanism. Circ Res 86:989–997.
15. Steeves G, Singh N, Singal PK. 1994. Ischemic preconditioning and antioxidant defence against reperfusion injury. In: Cellular, biochemical, and molecular aspects of reperfusion injury. Ed DK Das, 116–127. New York Acad Sci.
16. Guo Y, Jones WK, Xuan YT, Tang XL, Bao W, Wu WJ, Han H, Laubach VE, Ping P, Yang Z, Qiu Y, Bolli R. 1999. The late phase of ischemic preconditioning is abrogated by targeted disruption of the inducible NO synthase gene. Proc Natl Acad Sci U S A 96:11507–11512.
17. Shinmura K, Tang XL, Wang Y, Liu SQ, Takano H, Bhatnagar A, Bolli R. 2000. Cyclooxygenase-2 mediates the cardioprotective effects of the late phase of ischemic preconditioning in conscious rabbits. Proc Natl Acad Sci 97:10197–10202.
18. Maulik N, Goswami S, Galang N, Das DK. 1999. Differential regulation of Bcl-2, AP-1, and NFkB on cardiomyocyte apoptosis during myocardial ischemic stress adaption. FEBS letters 443:331–336.
19. Valen G, Yan Z-Q, Hansson GK. 2001. Nuclear Factor kappa-B and the heart. Journal of American College of Cardiology 38:307–314.
20. Lawrence T, Gilroy DW, Colville-Nash PR, Willoughby DA. 2001. Possible role for NF-kB in the resolution of inflammation. Nature Medicine 7:1291–1297.

21. Morgan EN, Boyle EM, Yun W, Griscavage-Ennis JM, Farr A, Canty TG, Pohlman TH, Verrier ED. 1999. An essential role for NFkB in the cardioadaptive response to ischemia. Ann Thorac Surg 68:377–382.

22. Zhao T, Chelliah J, Levasseur JE, Kukreja RC. 2000. Inducible nitric oxide synthase mediates delayed myocardial protection induced by activation of adenosine A(1) receptors: Evidence from gene-knockout animals. Circulation 102:902–907.

23. Zhao TC, Taher MM, Valerie KC, Kukreja RC. 2001. P38 triggers late preconditioning elicited by anisomycin in heart. Involvement of NFkB and iNOS. Circ Res 89:915–922.

24. von Albertini M, Palmetshofer A, Kaczmarek E, Koziak K, Stroka D, Grey ST, Stuhmeier KM, Robson SC. 1998. Extracellular ATP and ADP activate transcription factor NF-kappaB and induce endothelial cell apoptosis. Biochem Biophys Res Commun 248:822–829.

25. Nie Z, Mei Y, Ford M, Rybak L, Marcuzzi A, Ren H, Stiles GL, Ramkumar V. 1998. Oxidative stress increases adenosine A1 receptor expression by activating nuclear factor kappa B. Mol Pharmacol 53:663–669.

26. Li C, Tuanzhu T, Liu L, Browder W, Kao RL. 2000. Adenosine prevents activation of transcription factor NF-kB and enhances activator protein-1 binding activity in ischemic rat heart. Surgery 127:161–169.

27. Carroll R, Yellon DM. 2000. Delayed cardioprotection in a human cardiomyocyte-derived cell line: the role of adenosine, p38MAP kinase and mitochondrial KATP. Basic Res Cardiol 95:243–249.

28. Dana A, Jonassen AK, Yamashita N, Yellon DM. 2000. Adenosine A(1) receptor activation induces delayed preconditioning in rats mediated by manganese superoxide dismutase. Circulation 101:2841–2848.

29. Zahler S, Kupatt C, Becker BF. 2000. Endothelial preconditioning by transient oxidative stress reduces inflammatory responses of cultured endothelial cells to TNF-alpha. FASEB J 14:555–564.

30. Hiasa G, Hamada M, Ikeda S, Hiwada K. 2001. Ischemic preconditioning and lipopolysaccharide attenuate nuclear factor kappa-B activation and gene expression of inflammatory cytokines in the ischemic-reperfused rat heart. Jpn Circ J 65:984–990.

31. Carter DA. 1997. Modulation of cellular AP-1 DNA binding activity by heat shock proteins. FEBS Lett 416:81–85.

32. Vayssier M, Favatier F, Pinot F, Bachelet M, Polla BS. 1998. Tobacco smoke induces coordinate activation of HSF and inhibition of NFkappaB in human monocytes: effects on TNFalpha release. Biochem Biophys Res Commun 252:249–256.

33. Zhu L, Fukuda S, Cordis G, Das DK, Maulik N. 2001. Anti-apoptotic protein survivin plays a significant role in tubular morphogenesis of human coronary arteliolar endothelial cells by hypoxic preconditioning. FEBS letters 508:369–374.

34. Erl W, Hansson GK, de Martin R, Draude G, Weber KS, Weber C. 1999. Nuclear factor-kappa B regulates induction of apoptosis and inhibitor of apoptosis protein-1 expression in vascular smooth muscle cells. Circ Res 84:668–677.

35. Liston P, Roy N, Tamai K, Lefebvre C, Baird S, Cherton-Horvat G, Farahani R, McLean M, Ikeda JE, MacKenzie A, et al. 1996. Suppression of apoptosis in mammalian cells by NAIP and a related family of IAP genes. Nature 379:349–353.

36. Valen G, Starkopf J, Takeshima S, Kullisaar T, Vihalemm T, Kengsepp AT, Vaage, J. 1998. Preconditioning with hydrogen peroxide (H_2O_2) or ischemia in H_2O_2-induced cardiac dysfunction. Free Radic Res 29:235–245.

37. Tritto I, D'Andrea D, Eramo N, Scognamiglio A, De Simone C, Violante A, et al. 1997. Oxygen radicals can induce preconditioning in rabbit hearts. Circ Res 80:743–748.

38. Gille JJ, Joenje H. 1992. Cell culture models for oxidative stress: superoxide and hydrogen peroxide versus normobaric hyperoxia. Mutat Res 275:405–414.

39. Ahotupa M, Mäntylä E, Peltola V, Puntala A, Toivonen H. 1992. Pro-oxidant effects of normobaric hyperoxia in rat tissues. Acta Physiol Scand 145:151–157.

40. Li Y, Zhang W, Mantell LL, Kazzaz JA, Fein AM, Horowitz S. 1997. Nuclear factor-kappaB is activated by hyperoxia but does not protect from cell death. J Biol Chem 272:20646–20649.

41. Tähepôld P, Ruusalepp A, Li G, Vaage J, Starkopf J, Valen G. 2002. Cardioprotection by breathing hyperoxic gas—relation to oxygen concentration and exposure time in rats and mice. Eur J cardio-Thor Surg, 21:987–994.

42. Tähepôld P, Valen G, Starkopf J, Karaine C, Zilmer M, Löwbeer C, Dumitrescu A, Vaage J. 2001. Pretreating rats with hyperoxia attenuates ischaemia-reperfusion injury of the heart. Life Sciences 68:1629–1640.

43. Li G, Tokuno S, Tähepôld P, Vaage J, Löwbeer C, Valen G. 2001. Ischemic and hyperoxic

preconditioning improve myocardial function and reduce infarct size in the severely atherosclerotic mouse heart. Ann Thorac Surg 71:1296–1303.

44. Tähepôld P, Starkopf J, Vaage J, Valen G. 2002. Hyperoxia elicits preconditioning through a NFkB-dependent mechanism in the rat heart. J Thorac Cardiovasc Surg, in press.

45. Tähepôld P, Elfström P, Eha I, Kals J, Taal G, Taalonpoika A, Valen G, Vaage J, Starkopf J. 2002. Exposure of rats to hyperoxia enhances the relaxation of isolated aortic rings and reduces the infarct size of isolated hearts. Acta Physiol Scand, 175:271–277.

46. Marais E, Genade S, Strijdom H, Moolman JA, Lochner A. 2001. P38 MAPK activation triggers pharmacologically induced beta-adrenergic preconditioning, but not ischemic preconditioning. J Mol Cell Cardiol 33:2157–2177.

47. Takeishi Y, Huang Q, Wang T, Glassman M, Yoshizumi M, Baines CP, Lee JD, Kawakatsu H, Che W, Lerner-Marmorosh N, Zhang C, Yan C, Ohta S, Walsh RA, Berk BC, Abe J. 2001. Src family kinase and adenosine differentially regulate multiple MAP kinases in ischemic myocardium: modulation of MAP kinase activation by ischemic preconditioning. J Mol Cell Cardiol 33:1989–2005.

48. Fryer RM, Patel HH, Hsu AK, Gross GJ. 2001. Stress-activated protein kinase phosphorylation during cardioprotection in the ischemic myocardium. Am J Physiol 281:H1184–H1192.

49. Saurin AT, Martin JL, Heads RJ, Foley C, Mockridge JW, Wright MJ, Wang Y, Marber MS. 2000. The role of differential activation of p38 mitogen activated protein kinases in preconditioned ventricular myocytes. FASEB J 14:2237–2246.

50. Morishita R, Sugimoto T, Aoki M, Kida I, Tomita N, Moriguchi A, Maeda K, Sawa Y, Kaneda Y, Higaki J, Ogihara T. 1997. In vivo transfection of cis element "decoy" against nuclear factor-kB binding site prevents myocardial infarction. Nature Med 3:894–899.

51. Sawa Y, Morishita R, Suzuki K, Kagisaki K, Kaneda Y, Maeda K, Kadoba K, Matsuda H. 1997. A novel strategy for myocardial protection using in vivo transfection of cis element "decoy" against NFkB binding site. Circulation 96 (suppl. II), II-280–II-285.

52. Maczewski M, Beresewicz A. 1998. The role of adenosine and ATP-sensitive potassium channels in the protection afforded by ischemic preconditioning against the post-ischemic endothelial dysfunction in guinea-pig hearts. J Mol Cell Cardiol 30:1735–1747.

53. Merkus D. Stepp DW, Jones DW, Nishikawa Y, Chilian WM. 2000. Adenosine preconditions against endothelin-induced constriction of coronary arterioles. Am J Physiol 279:H2593–2597.

54. Giannella E, Mochmann HC, Levi R. 1997. Ischemic preconditioning prevents the impairment of hypoxic coronary vasodilatation caused by ischemia/reperfusion: role of adenosine A1/A3 and bradykinin B2 receptor activation. Circ Res 81:415–422.

55. Tokuno S, Chen F, Jiang J, Pernow J, Valen G. 2002. Effects of spontaneous or induced brain infarctions on vessel reactivity: The role of iNOS. Life Sciences, 71:679–692.

56. Laude K, Thuillez C, Richard V. 2001. Coronary endothelial dysfunction after ischemia and reperfusion: A new therapeutic target? Braz J Med Biol Res 34:1–7.

57. Laude K, Richard V, Henry JP, Lallemand F, Thuillez C. 2000. Evidence against a role of inducible nitric oxide synthase in the endothelial protective effects of delayed preconditioning. Br J Pharmacol 130:1547–1552.

Signal Transduction and Cardiac Hypertrophy,
edited by N.S. Dhalla, L.V. Hryshko,
E. Kardami & P.K. Singal
Kluwer Academic Publishers, Boston, 2003

The SERCA2 gene: genomic organization and promoter characterization

Angel Zarain-Herzberg* and Georgina Alvarez-Fernández

*Laboratorio de Biología Molecular
Departamento de Bioquímica, Facultad de Medicina
Universidad Nacional Autónoma de México
México, D.F. 04510*

Summary. The sarco(endo)plasmic reticulum Ca^{2+}-ATPases belong to a family of active calcium transport enzymes encoded by SERCA1, 2 and 3 genes. In this study, we describe the complete structure of the human SERCA2 gene and its 5'-regulatory region. The hSERCA2 gene is located in chromosome 12 position q24.1 in Contig NT_009770.8, spans 70 kb and is organized in 21 exons intervened by 20 introns. The last two exons of the pre-mRNA produce by alternative splicing the cardiac/slow-twitch muscle specific SERCA2a isoform and the ubiquitous SERCA2b isoform. The sequence of the proximal 225 bp region of the SERCA2 genes is 80% G+C-rich, is highly conserved among human, rabbit, rat and mouse species, and contains a TATA-like-box, an E-box/USF sequence, a CAAT-box, four Sp1 binding sites, and a thyroid hormone responsive element (TRE). There are other two conserved regulatory regions located between positions −410 to −661 bp and from −919 to −1410 bp. Among the DNA cis-elements present in these two regulatory regions are potential binding sites for: GATA-4, -5, -6, Nkx-2.5/Csx, OTF-1, USF, MEF-2, SRF, PPAR/RXR, AP-2 and TREs. Upstream from position −1.5 kb there is no significant homology among the SERCA2 genes cloned. In addition, the human gene has several repeated sequences mainly of the Alu and L2 type located upstream from position −1.7 kb spanning in a continuous fashion for more than 40 kb. In this study we report the cloning of 2.4 kb of 5'-regulatory region and demonstrate that the proximal promoter region is sufficient for expression in cardiac myocytes and that the region from −225 to −1232 bp contains regulatory DNA elements which modulate negatively the expression of the SERCA2 in neonatal cardiomyocytes, suggesting that this region might be important during cardiac hypertrophy and

Address for Correspondence: Departamento de Bioquímica, Facultad de Medicina, UNAM, Apartado Postal 70-159, México, D.F. 04510. Tel: (5255) 5623-2258, Fax: (5255) 5616-2419, E-mail: angelz@bq.unam.mx.

479

in response to hormonal and metabolic signals. Taken together, these findings suggest that the entire functional 5′-regulatory region of the SERCA2 gene is confined within 1.5 kb of upstream from the transcription initiation site.

Key words: Heart, sarcoplasmic, reticulum, SERCA2, calcium, ATPase, transcription, splicing human, gene, structure.

INTRODUCTION

The sarcoplasmic reticulum (SR) Ca^{2+} transport ATPase activity determines the rate of contraction and relaxation of cardiac, skeletal and smooth muscle. Three types of sarco(endo)plasmic reticulum Ca^{2+}-ATPase genes (SERCA1, SERCA2 and SERCA3) have been cloned which encode at least seven isoforms (1–5). The SERCA1 gene is expressed in fast-twitch skeletal muscle and encodes two isoforms that are developmentally regulated, named SERCA1a (adult) and SERCA1b (neonatal) (1,2). The SERCA2 gene encodes two isoforms produced by alternative splicing (SERCA2a and SERCA2b) which are expressed in a tissue specific fashion (3,4). The SERCA2a isoform is predominantly expressed in cardiac and slow-twitch skeletal muscle, although it is also expressed at lower levels in smooth muscle and non-muscle tissues (4). The SERCA2b isoform is expressed ubiquitously in most cell types including smooth muscle and non-muscle cells (4). It is noteworthy that the level of SERCA2a mRNA and protein in cardiac muscle and slow-twitch skeletal muscle is 10- to 50-fold higher compared to smooth muscle and non-muscle cells (4). The SERCA3 gene encodes three isoforms and is expressed in many cell types but predominantly in epithelial and vascular endothelial cells (5).

In order to understand the transcriptional mechanisms that regulate the human SERCA2 gene expression in the normal and hypertrophic heart, the 5′-flanking region of rabbit, rat, human and mouse SERCA2 genes have been cloned and some functional analyses of the regulatory regions have been reported (6–9). Using a stable cell line containing a −254 bp promoter SERCA2/CAT fusion construct of the rabbit gene, it has been demonstrated that the proximal 5′-flanking region is sufficient to regulate the expression of the SERCA2 gene during myogenic differentiation of the mouse skeletal cell line C_2C_{12} (6). The rat SERCA2 gene has three functional TREs within the first 500 bp of promoter region (7,10–12). One binding site for the THRα1 receptor is located within the proximal promoter region (−72 to −284 bp) of the SERCA2 gene (TRE-3) (7,10–12). Transient co-transfection studies have demonstrated transactivation by thyroid hormone receptor (TR) alpha-1 isoform of rat and rabbit SERCA2promoter/CAT constructs containing the proximal promoter region (10–12). However, to date, the transcriptional mechanisms involved in SERCA2 tissue specific gene expression during cell differentiation, development and growth are not fully understood.

In this study, we have elucidated the complete genomic organization of the human SERCA2 gene, identified the precise location of exon/intron junctions and mapped the gene to chromosome position 12q24.1 according to its Contig localization. We have cloned a 2.9 kb fragment containing −2.5 kb of the hSERCA2 promoter region and engineered several deletion constructs. Sequence analysis of the cloned region revealed the presence of various potential transcription factor response elements. Functional analysis of SERCA2/Luc constructs demonstrates that the proximal −259 bp of regulatory region is sufficient to confer strong transcriptional activity in cardiac myocytes. In contrast, constructs containing at least 1.2 kb of regulatory sequences showed 3- to 5-fold lower transcriptional activity suggesting the presence of DNA cis-elements down regulating the transcription of the gene in neonatal rat cardiomyocytes in culture.

MATERIALS AND METHODS

Restriction endonucleases, modifying enzymes, Lipofectamine, tissue culture reagents and fetal bovine serum (FBS) were from Invitrogen. The human PAC clone RPC 13-305I20 was purchased from Children's Hospital Oakland BACPAC resources, Oakland, CA, USA. The pGL3-promoter, pGL3-basic and pRL-CMV and Dual Luciferase assay System were purchased from Promega Co. All other chemical and reagents were Molecular Biology grade or the highest purity available.

Neonatal rat cardiomyocyte cultures

One or two day old rat cardiac myocytes were isolated by a modification of the procedure previously described (10). Briefly, the rat hearts were surgically removed, ventricles were dissected, minced in 1 × ADS buffer [final concentration: 116 mM NaCl, 20 mM Hepes (pH 7.4), 1 mM NaH2PO4, 5.5 mM Glucose, 5.4 mM KCl, 0.8 mM MgSO4], and washed to remove erythrocytes, followed by dissociation with 0.3% collagenase type I (Invitrogen), 0.6% pancreatin from porcine pancreas (Sigma) and DNAase I, 1 μg/mL (Sigma). Enzymatic activities were stopped by adding cold DMEM (glutamine free and glucose 4.5 g/L) containing 100 U/mL of penicillin, streptomycin, 110 μg/mL, amphotericin B 0.25 μg/mL, nystatin 10 U/mL and supplemented with 50% FBS. Cells were pelleted by low speed centrifugation and resuspended in DMEM plus 10% FBS. The dissociated cells were pooled and plated in 12-well culture dishes coated with 1% gelatin at a density of 1–3 × 105 cells per well in DMEM supplemented with 10% FBS and antibiotic/antimycotic cocktail. Cultures were maintained at 37°C in a humidified incubator under atmosphere of 5% CO_2 and 95% air during 48 h before transfection.

Cloning of the human SERCA2 promoter

The DNA from the PAC clone RPC 13-305I20 containing the entire human SERCA2 gene was digested with Sst1 and separated in 1% agarose gel. The 2.9 kb Sst1 fragment contained 2,579 bp of promoter region and 323 bp of 5′-nontranslated sequence of exon 1. The fragment was isolated and purified using Geneclean II kit, and subcloned into the unique Sst1 site located in polylinker of the promoterless pGL3-basic. The orientation of the 2.9 kb Sst1 insert was confirmed by restriction enzyme analysis. Three deletion constructs were generated from the sense Sst1-pGL3 construct using the restriction enzymes BglII, PvuII, and KpnI. The resulting deletion constructs contained 1741, 1232, 259 bp of 5'-flanking sequence, respectively. Plasmid constructs were amplified and purified using the Qiagen kit and protocol, and then used for DNA transfection experiments as described below.

Transient DNA transfections and luciferase assays

Plasmid constructs were transfected into primary cardiomyocytes cultures following a modification of the Lipofectamine procedure (Invitrogen). Briefly, 1 µg of the purified recombinant chimeric hSERCA2/Luc plasmids were mixed with 0.2 µg of pRL-CMV. After 4 h of incubation at 37°C, 5% CO_2 the transfected cells were supplemented with DMEM containing 5% FCS and incubated at 37°C, 5% CO_2 for 60 h. Transfected cells were harvested in 1 × PLB (Promega), incubated for 1 h at RT under agitation, frozen at −80°C and thawed at RT. Cell extracts were prepared by centrifugation at 11,000 × g, for 2 min. The supernatant was collected and used to measure the Firefly and Renilla luciferase enzymatic activities using the Dual Luciferase assay system from Promega and the Victor-2 multi-well plate luminometer (Wallac). Protein was measured using the micro-BCA kit (Sigma).

DNA sequence analysis

The sequence from the genomic insert in the clone RPC 13-305I20 is in Genebank with accession number AC006088. Identification of exon/intron boundaries, transcription regulatory sites and homology with other sequences were performed using MacVector 6.0.1 (Kodak), BLAST (NCBI), and GEMS (Genomatix) analysis packages.

RESULTS

Structural organization of the human SERCA2 gene

Search for the SERCA2 gene in the human genome using BLAST analysis software from NCBI of the human SERCA2a and 2b mRNA sequences revealed that the entire gene is located within a fragment of 122,605 bp long in the PAC clone RPC 13-305I20. The nucleotide sequence of the clone was used to performed extensive nucleotide analysis to identify the precise location of exons within the genomic clone. From the 2354 genes present in human chromosome 12, the SERCA2 gene is located in bands 12q23–q24.1 according to cytogenetic analysis. The SERCA2 gene is located between positions 115,916,977 and 116,017,977 of chromosome 12 in Contig NT_009770.8, making possible to locate the SERCA2 gene more precisely to position 12q24.1 (Figure 1). The genomic clone contains 41,909 bp of 5'-flanking sequence upstream of the transcription initiation site, including the promoter region. The transcribed genomic sequence of the hSERCA2 gene spans 70 kb from position 41,910 to 111,737 of the genomic clone. The gene is organized in 21 exons intervened by 20 introns (Figure 2). Introns 3, 4, 7, 8, 10, 11, 12, 13, 14, 17 and 19 are in phase 0; introns 1,2,5,6,16 and 20 are in phase 1; and introns 9, 15 and 18 are in phase 2 (Table 1). Nineteen out of 20 introns contain the conserved GT and AG dinucleotides at the donor and acceptor sites,

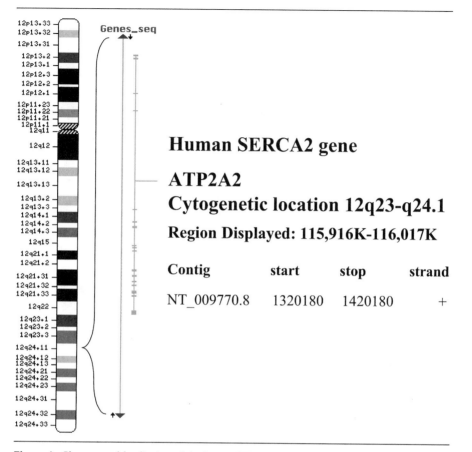

Figure 1. Chromosomal localization of the human SERCA2 gene. The ideogram shows the localization of the SERCA2 gene in human chromosome 12. The schematic representation of exons of the SERCA2 gene in the 132 to 142K region of Contig NT_009770.8 in strand + is shown in gray.

respectively, and only intron 12 starts with the GC sequence. The first exon is 646 bp long and contains 528 bp of non-coding sequence and 118 bp of coding sequence. The second exon is only 18 bp and is in phase with exons 1 and 3. The longest intron is number 5 and is 26,255 bp long.

Figure 3A shows the location of the last three exons of the gene. By a mechanism of alternatively splicing the last two exons of the pre-mRNA produce two different mRNAs that encode the SERCA2a and SERCA2b isoforms. Therefore, the SERCA2 pre-mRNA undergoes alternative splicing in a tissue or cell type specific fashion. To produce the SERCA2b mRNA isoform the pre-mRNA sequence of exon 20 is transcribed entirely. Exon 20 encodes the carboxyl terminal 89 amino acids of SERCA2b and contains at least 845 bp of 3′-nontranslated sequence. Exon

Table 1. Organization of the human SERCA2 gene

Exon	Exon Size bp	Exon 3' Sequence	5' Junction	Intron	Intron Size kb	3' Junction	Exon 5' Sequence	Spliced aa	Type
1	121	TCC AAC G	aggt	1	0.7	ctac ag	AG TTA CCG	Glu-40	1
2	18	GAA GAA G	aatc	2	0.09	ttac ag	GA AAA ACC	Gly-46	1
3	83	ATA TCT TTT	aagt	3	9.22	ttct ag	GTT TTG GCT	Val-74	0
4	105	GTA TGG CAG	aagc	4	4.47	atac ag	GAA AGA AAT	Glu-109	0
5	139	ATT GCT G	gagt	5	26.25	aatt ag	TT GGT GAC	Val-155	1
6	81	CTC ACA G	aaat	6	3.32	gctt ag	GT GAA TCT	Gly-182	1
7	86	CTG TTT TCT	aagt	7	1.08	tcct ag	GGT ACA AAC	Gly-211	0
8	465	GTC TGC AGG	aaga	8	4.58	ctac ag	ATG TTC ATT	Met-366	0
9	89	GGA GAA GT	gagt	9	0.5	gggc ag	G CAT AAA	Val-395	2
10	103	TAC AAT GAG	aagt	10	0.73	atac ag	GCA AAG GGT	Ala-430	0
11	132	TGC AAC TCA	gagt	11	5.14	ttgt ag	GTC ATT AAA	Val-474	0
12	124	TTT GTG AAG	aagt	12	0.10	ttcc ag	GGT GCT CCT	Gly-515	0
13	219	AAA TAT GAG	tagc	13	0.94	tttt ag	ACC AAT CTG	Thr-588	0
14	336	ACA GCT ATG	gagc	14	1.23	tttc ag	ACT GGC GAT	Thr-700	0
15	221	GTT GTC TG	aggt	15	0.78	aaac ag	T ATT TTC	Cys-773	2
16	203	ATT GGC T	gagt	16	1.45	tccc ag	GT TAC GTC	Cys-841	1
17	86	TAC CAG CTG	actc	17	0.28	ttgc ag	AGT CAT TTC	Ser-870	0
18	134	CTC AAC AG	tagt	18	0.62	ctgc ag	C TTG TCC	Ser-914	2
19	118	CCC TTG CCA	aagt	19	0.08	tgtc ag	CTC ATC TTC	Leu-954	0
20	121	GAA CCT G	aaag	20	3.97	tttc ag	CA ATA CTG	Ala-994	1
20*	+1109	CAT TTT AAA							
21	+798	TTC TAT GAT							

Exon sequences are indicated by uppercase letters and intron sequences by lowercase letters. Only the 3' end of exon 1 and the 3' ef exons 20* and 21 are shown. See text for details.

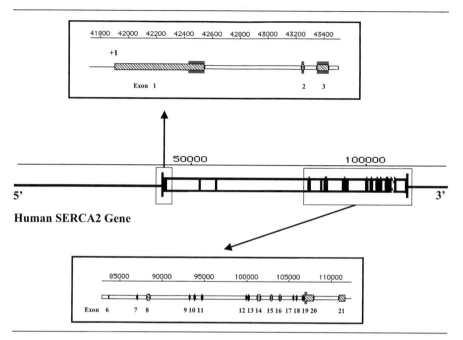

Figure 2. Genomic structure of the human SERCA2 gene. Schematic representation of the SERCA2 gene in clone RPC 13-305I20 is shown. The upper box shows the location of exons of the 5'-end region of the gene. Translated region is indicated with gray bars. The lower box indicates the position of exons 6 to 21.

20 contains an internal intron donor site (GT) within its coding sequence immediately after the 40th amino acid that encodes (Figure 3A). This donor site is preferentially used in cardiac and slow-twitch muscle by the splicing machinery to include exon 21 in the SERCA2a mRNA. As a result, the SERCA2a mRNA isoform lacks the sequence that encodes for the last 49 amino acids present in SERCA2b isoform, and instead it contains the four amino acids encoded by exon 21 (AILE), followed by a TAA stop codon and at least 788 bp of 3'-nontranslated sequence.

Analysis of the regulatory region of SERCA2 gene

The 5'-regulatory regions of the mouse, rat, rabbit and human SERCA2 genes have been cloned and sequenced (6–9). Alignment analysis of the genomic DNA sequences of the 5'-flanking regions of these genes reveals important observations (Figure 4). The first observation is that the 5'-regulatory sequence of the SERCA2 genes is organized in regions of homology containing cis-acting DNA regulatory elements. The first region includes 225 bp of proximal promoter region and contains a TATA-like-box (5'-GATAAA-3'), an E-box/USF consensus sequence (5'-CACATG-3'), a CAAT-box (5'-GCCAAT-3'), four consensus Sp1 binding sites

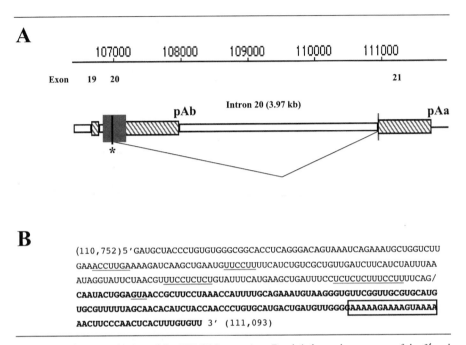

Figure 3. Splicing mechanism of the SERCA2 transcripts. *Panel A* shows the structure of the 3′-end region of the gene and the line indicates the splicing mechanism of the primary transcript to produce the alternate isoforms. The asterisk (★) indicates the position of internal donor site of splicing located in exon 20. pAa and pAb indicate the polyadenylation sites for the SERCA2a and SERCA2b mRNAs, respectively. *Panel B* shows the nucleotide sequence of the junction region of intron 20 and exon 21 of the human SERCA2 pre-mRNA. The consensus intronic splicing suppressor (ISS) sequences within intron 20 and the stop codon in exon 21 are *underlined*. The intron/exon junction acceptor site is indicated by a (/) line. The exon 21 sequences are in **bold** letters. The exonic splicing enhancer (ESE) consensus sequence is *boxed*.

(5′-GGGCGG-3′ and 5′-CCGCCC-3′) and four 5′-GGGAGG-3′ sequences that can also bind Sp1 and possibly other transcription factors, and a thyroid hormone responsive element (TRE) (5′-GGCCTCGATCCGGGTTC/ACTG/A-3′). The second region of homology is located between position −410 to −661 bp of the human gene and contains TRE-1, one serum response element (SRE), one muscle M-CAT, one activator protein-2 (AP-2) and one E-box/USF consensus sequences. Between position −662 to −992 bp there are only two short regions of homology, one between position −875 to −905 bp and contains and E-box element, another from position −944 to −975 bp that contains a T/A-rich sequence with homology to the muscle specific SRE/CArG-box element. The third region of homology starts at position −919 and ends at position −1410 and contains one putative TRE, one E-box, and consensus M-CAT, MEF-2, N-FAT, OTF-1, and GATA elements. The second important observation is that upstream from this region there is no homology among all the SERCA2 genes cloned. In addition, in the human gene, several

```
-1580      CCTTCTCCTGCCTGCAGTGCTTCTATCGGTCCTGAAAGAGACAGAGGAGGTAAGGGAGAAG
(40332)


AATTGGTACGAAATGGTGCAGAGCTGGTCTCAGAGGGCAACAACAGCCAGCCCTCCATGACCACACTCCC   Human

                                                  TRE               E-box
                                              -1410
ACCGTGCACTCACGTGCCCCTCTTGAAGCGGCTCTGATCCTGTGACCTAACCAGTTTCCACCTGGCTTCT-  Human
                                          |||||||||||||||||||||||| ||||||
RAT      (1)  -1581  GGATCCTCCAGAAGAGGCTGTGACCTAACCAGTTTCCACCTtGCTTCTA
                    **************||||||||||||||||||||||||*||||||*
MOUSE           CAGGCAGTCACCTGATCCTCCAGAAGAGGCTGTGACCTAACCAGTTTCCACCTtGCTTCTA
         (1962) -1605


RABBIT  (700) -1114 cAaAtgaaTTcGcTTGTTTGTTTCGTGTAGGGTTcTcTcGGTcCTTTTCC
                    | |       || | ||||||||||||||||||||| | | ||| ||*||||
CTCAGTGCGTTGCCATATAGTATAATTTTTTGTTTGTTTGTTTCGTGTAGGGTTTTGTTGGTTCTTTTCC   Human
|||||| |||| ||| |||| || ||||||||||||||||||||||||||||| |||||| || ||||
ggCAGTGCaTTGCtATAcAGTAgAA-TTTTTGTTTGTTTGTTTCGTGTAGGGTTcTGTTGGTcCTaTTCC   Rat
**||||||*||||*|||*||||*|| ||||||||||||||||||||||||||||||||||||||*||||
ggCAGTGCaTTGCtATAcAGTAgAA-TTTTTGTTTGTTTGTTTCGTGTAGGGTTcTGTTGGTcCTgTTCC   Mouse


          M-CAT          M-CAT/MEF-2/N-FAT
AAGTATCAATCAAAACTgCATGCCAgCcTCCACTCCTTGG-AATAATTAAATGACATGACGTGCCTGAgg
||||||||||||*|||| |||||||| | ||||||||||||||||||||||||*||||
AAGTATCAATCAAAACTACATGCCAACGTCCACTCCTTGGAAATAATTAAATGACATGACGTGCCTGATT
|||||||||||| |||| |||||||| | ||||||||||||||||||||||||||| |||| |||||||
AAGTATCAATCAgAACTgCATGCCAgCcTCCACTCCTTGGAAATAATTAAATGACgT-ACtTGCCTGATT
||||||||||||*||||*| |||||||||| |||||||||||||||||||||| *||||| | | |||||
AAGTATCAATCAgAACTgCgTGCCAgCcTCCACTCCTTGGAAATAATTAAATGAagTGACGTaCtTGATT


         OTF-1              GATA
TTTTtttttttctTccTGCACTGcgATTTGCATCaGCTGAAGGAATTTcTCTTtggTCCTGAgGCt -919
||||    *   |  *||||*| |||||||| |||||||||||| |||| |||*|||*|| -1170
TTTTCAGCTGG-TGATGCACTGTAATTTGCATCTGCTGAAGGAATTTATCTTAAGTCCTGAAGCCCAGCCA
|||||| || | ||| ||||||||||| |||||*||||||||| |||*||
TTTTCAGTCGGGTaAaGCACCGTgATTTGCATCTGCTGAAGGcAcTATCTTAAGTCtTGAgGCg -1328
|||||||**||*|*|*|||||* ||||||||||||||||||| ||        | |      *
TTTTCAGtcGGg-aAaGCACCcaTgATTTGCATCTGCTGAAGGAATTctaaTcAttaatatcttga -1337


E-box                                                        MEF-2
CTTGAGACAACTGAGGTGATTTTTCTGCTCTGCTTTTGCTCATGCGGATGGTGCGTTATTGTTAAACACA   Human


      GGAgcAAgTGCcTCATTCTGtAgCCTACTC
      ***   ** ***  ********  * *******
AAAGTGGACTAATTGCTTCATTCTGCAACCTACTCCGTGAAGAAAGCTGCTCTTCTTTGTGAAGAGAATA
```

Figure 4. Nucleotide sequence alignment of SERCA2 gene 5′-regulatory regions. The identity in nucleotide sequence of 1.58 kb of SERCA2 regulatory sequences among human, rabbit, rat and mouse species is indicated by a *vertical line* (|). An asterisk (*) indicates similarity only between two sequences. The consensus DNA sequences for various regulatory elements are shown in gray areas, and ERSE *is boxed*. The 5′-non-translated sequence of the first exon is in bold letters. MacVector 6.5.3, Blast NCBI, and Genomatix MatInspector Professional 5.1 were used to align sequences and to identify putative DNA binding motifs.

```
                                                   -975                       SRE/CArG
TGTTCATGTTTTGTTCATGAATTCCATGCAATTTCCCATCCCCTTGTTAAGTAATGTAGCTTCTTTATAT   Human
                 EcoRI                              ||| || |||||||||
                                        -1004     ctccgTGTgGCcTCTTTATAT    Rat
                                                  |||*||*||||||||||
                                        -1015 TGTgGCcTCTTTATAT             Mouse
```

```
SRE/CArG  -944                              -905    E-box
TGGCAAAATTCCCTTTATCTTGCTGTGACCTGCGCTTTGTCCTCCCGAGCAGAGCAAATCATCTGTGGTT
|||||||||||| |*|||                            || |**||*|||||||
TGGCAAAATTaCgTTcca -966                       CAcAaCATaTGTGGTT
||||||||||*|*|| **                            || |* ||*|||||||
TGGCAAAATTaCCTTgcat -981                      CAgATgATCTGTGGTT
```

```
        -875
TAAGAGCAGCTTTGGATTCAAGTCCCCTTTTCTCCTGTCGAGGGAAGTGAGTCTATGAAATGGCCTTCAT   Human
|||||  || |||||***  *** * ********** * * ********
TAAGAatAGaTTTGGATTgAAGgCtCCTTTTCTCCcaTtGgGGGAAGTGAaag -869
|||||**||*|||||
TAAGAatAGaTTTGG   -919
```

```
CTGAAAGCCACAGCGAAGCACCTCCTAGCCCAAGTCTAGCTGCTGTGTGGCAGCTCCAGCGGCGTGAACT
```

```
              GATA/Nkx2.5                   MEF-2            G+A
GTGACTGCCCTGCAGACACCTATCAAGCGCTGCGTCAGCTATTAATAATAAAATCAACTCTTCTCCCTCC
```

```
AP-2             -661
CCCCCGCGAGGGGGGTTCCCTCGTCAGGGCCCAGAACCCGCTGGGGAAGAATCGGGGCTGGCGTGCGAAG
                 ||  |||  |||| |||||||||| |||||||  |  ||||||||  || |  |
           -706  CCctGTCgGGGCaCAGAACCCGCaGGGGAAGgA--AGGGCTGGtGTttG--G
                 |**|||*||||*||||||||||*||||||*| *|||||||*||**| |
           -728  tCctGTCgGGGCaCAGAACCCGCaGGGGAAGgA--AGGGCTGGtGTttG--G
```

```
        AP-2                                E-box
GAGCTGGCGGCAGGGGGTGTAGGATGCGGTGTTCCCGAGGCGACAGATGAAGGATTTGGGTTGTGTGGGA
*  |||  ||||  ||||||| |||||||||||||||||||||||| | ||| || |||||||||
GgGCTttCGGCtGGGGGTGTgGGATGCGGTGTTCCCGAGGCGACAGATGAgcGcTTTtGGcTGTGTGGGA
**|||**||||*||||||||*|||||||||||||||||||||||||**|*|||*|*|||||||||
agGCTttCGGCtGGGGGTGTgGGATGCGGTGTTCCCGAGGCGACAGATGAgcGcTTTtGGcTGTGTGGGA
```

```
        M-CAT                                    SRE/CArG
AGTGAACTGCGGAATTCCTCCCCTTGGTTTCTGAGGGGGGCTCTGAAGGAGCCAGATTAGGATGCAGAGC
|| |||||||||||||||||||||||| |||||||||||||||||| | ||||||||||||||||
AGgGAACTGCGGAATTCCTCCCCTTGGTtgCTGAGGGGGGCTCTGAAGGAG--AcATTAGGATGCAGAGC
||*||||||||||||||||||||||||*|||||||||||||||||| |*|||||||||||||||
AGgGAACTGCGGAATTCCTCCCCTTGGTtgCTGAGGGGGGCTCTGAAGGAG--AcATTAGGATGCAGAGC
         EcoRI
```

```
        RXR/TRE-1                                 -410
GCAGCCCGGGCGACCGAGGGCGAGGAGGCGAGCCAAGGACATCAGCCCGAGGGCGCCTCGAGACGCCCCG
| ||| || |  || ||||||  |||||| ||||||||||||| ||| *|**| ********
aCgGCtCGcaCtgCCcAGGGCGcGGAGGcaAGCCAAGGACAcCAGtCCctG -456
*|*||*||**|**|*|*|||||*||||||*|||||||||||||*|||* |**| ********
ACgGCtCGcaCtgCCcAGGGCGcGGAGGcaAGCCAAGGACAcCAGtgCGAGcGCGCCTCG -469
```

Figure 4. Continued

```
CGTGGACCGCGCTCCCAGCTCCTCGGCCTCGCCTTCCAACCATCCGCCCACCGGCCCCAGAGCAGCGTGC
                                                                           Human
CCACTGTGAGCGCCCCACCCTGCGTCTGCAGGTGGGTGGGTCAGAGAACCGCAGGCACAGAAGAGGGTAC
                                                                    Kpn1
                  -236                        TRE-3          Sp1 I
         cccggggCCgCaGCCAGCatCGCGcggGgcGCGCGCGCGG-CTCGATCCGGGTTCCTgGGGGCGGtGC   Rabbit
         SmaI  ** * ******    |||| **|  *||||||||| |||||||||||||||| |||||||| ||
CCAGCTTCCCCTCCGCCAGCCCCGCGACCGCGGCGCGCGCGGCCTCGATCCGGGTTCCTAGGGGCGGCGC   Human
                        |||| * |  ||||||||||||||||||||| || |||||||||
            -237    tgCGCGcgCaCacCGCGCGCGGCCTCGATCCGGGTTaCTgGGGGCGGCGC   Rat
                    **||| | * ||*||||||||||||| ||||||||*|*||||||||| ||||
            -236    CgCGCacagGCGcCGCGCGCGGCCTCGATCCGGGTTCCTgGGGGgcGCGC   Mouse

   G+A   Sp1 II                                    G+A        G+A
GCGGGAGGGGGCGGGGCCTGCGCGGCgGCGTGG-CGCgAG-CGCGC-GGA-GGAGGGcGCCGGGgGGAGGG
||||||||*|||||||||||||||||*||||||||| |||*** ||||| *|* ||||||||||||||||||
GCGGGAGGGGGCGGGGCCTGCGCGGCAGCGTGGGCGCCAGGCGCGGGA-GGAGGGAGCCGGGAGGAGGG
|| ||||||| |||||||||||||| ||||*||||||||* |||||||| |||||| ||||||||||
GCGGGAGGCGGCGGGGCCTGC-CGGCAGCGTGGGCGCgcaGCGCGCGcGcgGGAGGGcGCCGGG-GGAGGG
|| ||||||| |||||||||||| |||* |||||||||* |||||||*|***||||||||| ||||||||||
GCGGGAGGaGGCGGGGCCTGC-tGGCg-GCGTGGGCGCgtGCGCGCGcGcggGGAGGGcGCCGG-AGGAGGG

                                            ERSE
GGCGGGGCCGCGCCGCCCGCGCCGCGCTGGGCGCTCTCGGCCAATGAGCGGCGTCCACATGCCGCGGCaG
|||||||||||||||||||||||||||||*|||||||||||||||||||||||||||||| |||||||| |
GGCGGGGCCGCGCCGCCCGCGCCGCGCTGGGCGCTCTCGGCCAATGAGCGGCGTCCACATGCCGCGGCGG
|||||||||||||||||||||||||||||||||||| |||||||||||||||||||||||||
GGCGGGGCCGCGCCGCCCGCGCCGCGCTGGGCtCTCTCGGCCAATGAGCGGCGTCCACATGCCGCGGCGG
|||||||||||||||||||||||||||||*||||||||||||||||||||||||||||| |||||| ||||
GGCGGGGCCGCGCCGCCCGCGCCGCGCTGGGCtCTCTCGGCCAATGAGCGGCGTCCACATGCCC--GCGG
Sp1 III      Sp1 IV                    CAAT-box      E-box/USF

      G+A            TATA-box/A+T-rich      +1
CGGCCGAgAGGGGAGGCAGCGGCCGATAAAT-CTATTAGAGCAGCCGCCGCGGAGCCGTCCCCGACGCCAC
|||||| |||||||||||||||*|||||||| |||||||||||||*|||||||||||||||||||||||
CGGCGAAAGGGGAGGCAGCGGCCGATAAATGCTATTAGAGCAGCCGCCGCGGAGCCGTCCCCGACGCCAC
|||||| ||||||||||||||||||| ||||||||||||||||*|||||||||||||||||||||||||
CGGCCGAgAGGGGAGGCAGCGGCgGATAAATGCTATTAGAGCAGCCtCCGCGGAGCCGTCCCCGACGCCAC
|||||||*|||||||||||||||||* ||||||||||||||||*|||||||||||||||||||||||
CGGCCGAgAGGGGAGGCAGCGGCgGATAAATGCTATTAGAGCAGCCtCCGCGGAGCCGTCCCCGACGCCAC
```

Figure 4. *Continued*

families of repeated sequences (L2, Alu, CAAAA, MER, MIR, LIMB, etc.) are located upstream from position −1.7 kb interspersed in a continuous manner for more than 40 kb. The third important observation is that the rabbit 5′-flanking sequence only shares homology with the mouse, rat and human sequences in the first and third regions, but there is no homology between positions −250 and −1170 bp of the rabbit sequence [6]. Therefore, one could speculate that the rabbit SERCA2 regulatory region could be modulated in different manner.

Functional studies of SERCA2-promoter-luciferase constructs

In order to analyze DNA regions which regulate the transcriptional activity of the human SERCA2 gene in cardiac myocytes, constructs containing −2529, −1741,

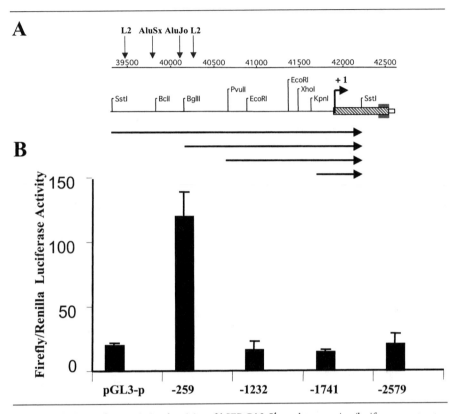

Figure 5. Design and transcriptional activity of hSERCA2 5'-regulatory region/luciferase constructs. **Panel A.** Restriction mapping of the 5'-regulatory region of the human SERCA2 gene is indicated. Deletion constructs containing −259, −1232, −1741 and −2579 are indicated with arrows. The transcription initiation site is indicated with (+1). The positions of the repeat sequences L2 and Alu are shown with arrows on top of the bar indicating the nucleotide position in the genomic clone RPC 13-305I20. **Panel B.** Neonatal rat cardiac myocytes were transfected with SERCA2/Luc constructs using Lipofectamine as described under Methods. The transcriptional activity of the hSERCA2/Luciferase constructs is shown as the normalized ratio of Firefly/Renilla luciferase activities (mean+/−S.D.). The pGL3-promoter plasmid was used to compare relative transcriptional strength.

−1232, −259 bp of 5'-flanking region were transiently transfected into neonatal rat cardiomyocytes (Figure 5A). The shortest construct containing the proximal conserved promoter region showed the maximal activity, 3- to 5-fold higher than constructs containing at least −1.2 kb of regulatory region (Figure 5B). These results indicate that the proximal regulatory region is necessary and sufficient for cardiac muscle specific expression. It is also apparent that the region located between −225 and −1232 bp contains regulatory elements that modulate the expression of the gene in negative fashion such as GATA, SRE and M-CAT. There was no significant difference in transcriptional activity among constructs containing -1.2, -1.7, and -2.5 kb of 5′-flanking sequence.

DISCUSSION

SERCA2a and SERCA2b mRNAs are produced by alternative splicing

Alternative mRNA splicing is an essential process that regulates developmental stage and/or tissue specific gene expression. This process can generate two or more mRNAs from a single pre-mRNA. Alternative splicing patterns can be classified as retained intron, selecting internal donor or acceptor sites, mutually exclusive exon, and cassette exon. For instance, the SERCA1 gene by a mechanism of mutually exclusive exon splicing produces two transcripts that encode two developmentally regulated isoforms expressed in fast-twitch skeletal muscle, the SERCA1a (adult isoform) and SERCA1b (neonatal isoform) (1,2). In contrast, the SERCA2 gene by a splicing mechanism of internal intron donor site selection produces the SERCA2a and SERCA2b isoforms (4). Therefore, if exon 20 is not spliced at the internal GT intron donor site, the mRNA produced is for the ubiquitous SERCA2b isoform. Although the mechanism involved for tissue specific splicing of SERCA2 pre-mRNA is not fully understood, it is interesting to note that the 3′ acceptor sites located in the 3′-region of intron 20 have consensus sequences for known intronic splicing suppressors (ISS) 5′-ACCUUGA-3′, 5′-UUCUCU-3′ and 5′-UUCCUU-3′ (Figure 3B) (13). The same reversed 5′-AGUUCCA-3′ element is also present in the alternatively spliced exon 9 of the F1 ATP synthase gamma subunit gene, and it has been shown to be essential for muscle specific exon exclusion *in vivo* (13). The 5′-region of SERCA2 exon 21 has a purine-rich sequence that matches exactly with the consensus sequence for an exonic splicing enhancer (ESE) element (5′-AAUGAAA-3′) recently described for the F1 ATP synthase gamma subunit gene (14). This putative ESE is located in the 5′ region of exon 21 downstream from the putative ISS sequences located in the boundary of intron 20 with exon 21 (Figure 3B), and may play a key role for splice site selection in alternative splicing to produce SERCA2a mRNA. Therefore, it could be speculated that the putative ESE present in exon 21 binds trans-acting regulatory factors present in cardiac and slow-twitch skeletal muscle, thus, overcoming the influence of the suppressor elements present in intron 20 and favoring splicing that allows inclusion of exon 21 in the SERCA2a mRNA transcript. Regarding the identity of the trans-acting factors involved in muscle specific splicing it has been reported that the polypyrimidine tract-binding protein (PTB) is able to bind to ISS sequences similar to those present in the 3′ flanking junction region of intron 20 of the hSERCA2 gene (Figure 3B) (15). Thus, it is possible that PTB functions as part of a constitutive exon selection mechanism. However, it does not seems to be the regulatory factor determining factor for muscle specific alternative splicing, because its ubiquitous expression (15). To date, the role of other splicing factors (such as hnRNP H) that are expressed in muscle tissue has to be examined for the SERCA2 splicing and experimental work is necessary to identify the proteins that bind these sequences.

Sequence and functional analysis of the proximal SERCA2 promoter

Functional studies have shown that the proximal promoter region of the SERCA2 gene is sufficient to regulate the expression of the SERCA2 gene during myogenic differentiation of the mouse skeletal cell lines C_2C_{12} and Sol8 (6,16). This region also confers high transcriptional activity in cardiomyocytes (10). Although, the proximal promoter region is necessary and sufficient for muscle specific expression, other distal sequences contained within 1.5 kb of regulatory region are probably important for regulated expression of the gene during cardiac hypertrophy. Among the DNA cis-elements present in the distal promoter region are potential binding sites for: GATA-4, -5, -6, Nkx-2.5/Csx, octamer factor-1 (OTF-1), upstream stimulatory factor (USF), myogenic enhancer factor-2 (MEF-2), serum response factor (SRF), PPAR/RXR, AP-2, and thyroid hormone receptors, as well as E-box and M-CAT sequences. In Sol8 cells, an E-box/A+T-rich element located in the distal 5'-regulatory region of the rabbit SERCA2 gene has been suggested to contribute to the muscle specific expression of this gene (17). Therefore, it appears that the entire functional 5'-regulatory region of the SERCA2 gene is most likely confined within the 1.5 kb upstream from the transcription initiation site. The functional analysis presented in this study is in agreement with previous reports and suggest that regulatory elements necessary for SERCA2 expression in cardiac muscle are located within 1.2 kb of 5'-flanking region.

Thyroid hormone and stress agents modulate SERCA2 transcription

The SERCA2 gene expression is up regulated by thyroid hormones (7,10–12,18). Three TREs have been described in the rat SERCA2 gene. TRE-1 is located upstream from the proximal promoter in second conserved region of homology (−481 to −456 bp), TRE-2 is located in the region that does not share high homology (−310 to −287 bp) whereas TRE-3 is located within the proximal 225 bp of promoter sequence (−219 to −194 bp) (Figure 4) (11–12). TRE-1 and TRE-3 are also present in the mouse, rabbit and human genes (8–10). TRE-1 is a direct repeat of two half sites separated by four nucleotides that can be contacted preferably by the monomeric form of TR-alpha1, homodimers of TR-beta or by heterodimers TR-alpha/RXR. In addition, retinoic acid can also stimulate the SERCA2 gene expression by a mechanism that do not involve the complete TRE-1 but only the 5'-half site. In contrast, TRE-2 and TRE-3 are inverted palindromes of two half sites separated by 4 or 6 nucleotides which can bind homodimers of TR-alpha1 or TR-beta (10–12). Further, it has been shown for rat and rabbit SERCA2 promoter/reporter fusion gene constructs containing the proximal 500 bp of regulatory region that can be trans-activated by TR isoforms alpha-1 and beta-1 (10–12). Using the rat heart-derived cell line H9c2 it has been demonstrated that the transcription factor MEF2a increases the transcription of the rat SERCA2 gene induced by the TR-alpha1 and TR-beta1 (12). Recently, it was reported that TR-alpha1, TR-alpha2 and TR-beta1 follow different changes in the pattern of expression in physiological vs. pathological cardiac hypertrophy (19). The three TR subtypes are down regulated in pressure overload animal models and in cultured cardiomyocytes treated with phenylephrine (19). In contrast, TR-beta1 was up regulated in cardiomyocytes in culture treated with triiodothyronine or in exercise induced cardiac hypertrophy (19). These findings explain, at least in part, why a decreased SERCA2 expression is observed in certain cardiac hypertrophy models, in spite of normal circulating levels of thyroid hormones.

SERCA2 expression can be induced by endoplasmic reticulum (ER) stress agents such as intracellular Ca^{2+} depletion or by agents that affect glycosylation of proteins like tunicamycin, dithiothreitol, or L-azetidine-2-carboxylic acid (20–22). A recent study has shown that the proximal SERCA2 promoter region contains a functional consensus endoplasmic reticulum stress responsive elements (ERSE) that is active in response to Ca^{2+} depletion (22). The ERSE present in the SERCA2 promoter (CCAATN9CCACA) could bind NF-Y/CBF, YY-1, and ERSF (Figure 4). The same study demonstrated that ATF6 transactivates the expression of the rat SERCA2 gene, and it has been proposed that ATF6 could interact with NF-Y and also make contact with the 5'-CCACA-3' sequence of the ERSE, although this sequence differs from the consensus sequence 5'-CCACG-3'. The 5'-CCACA-3' sequence is part of the proximal E-box/USF element and may play an important role in the basal and regulated expression of this gene. It is interesting to speculate that ATF6 may not bind directly to that sequence but rather interact with another factor(s) that actually binds to the E-box/USF sequence (5'-CACATG-3') that is part of the ERSE. Finally, it is not known if the ERSE present in the SERCA2 gene responds to other stress agents in addition to calcium depletion, including increasing or decreasing transcription of the gene by glucose deprivation increasing or decreasing the transcription of the gene.

SERCA2 expression is down regulated in cardiac hypertrophy and failure

Many research groups have documented that in animal models of cardiac hypertrophy and patients with heart failure the mRNA expression of SERCA2 is decreased (18,23,24). Recently, it has been demonstrated that the decreased SERCA2 mRNA levels arise from a reduced gene transcription (25–27). The Sp1-factor mRNA levels as well as the Sp1-factor binding activity has been shown increased in pressure overloaded (PO) hearts (28,29). Sp1 has been reported to be necessary for induction of the skeletal alpha-actin in pressure overload cardiac hypertrophy (28). Recently, it was reported that two proximal Sp1 binding sites within the SERCA2 promoter (Sp1 I and Sp1 III) are responsible for the Sp1 mediated transcriptional inhibition observed in pressure overload cardiac hypertrophy (Figure 4) (29). Recent evidence also suggests that activation of the p38-MAPK pathway may participate in the down regulation of SERCA2 gene transcription in response to a hypertrophic growth of the heart (30). It can, therefore, be suggested that a decreased SERCA2 expression leads to a dysregulation of cardiac myoplasmic free $[Ca^{2+}]$, and ultimately to activation of NF-AT pathway of cardiac hypertrophy. NF-

AT3 when dephosphorylated is able to interact with GATA-4 binding to its consensus sequence thereby affecting the transcriptional activity of target genes. Thus, there is a possibility that GATA binding sites in the SERCA2 promoter are involved in down-regulating SERCA2 expression during cardiac hypertrophy.

It has been reported that in doxorubicin (DXR) induced cardiomyopathy SR Ca^{2+} transport is decreased, as well as the SERCA2 mRNA levels and gene transcriptional activity (31,32). DXR induced cardiomyopathy can be prevented by a specific inhibitor of p44/42 MAPK. ANF, beta-myosin heavy chain, Egr-1, and TAFII250 expression were increased by DXR treatment (31,32). Egr-1 is a nuclear phosphoprotein with three zinc fingers that bind to the GC-rich element (CGC CCCCGC) and can modulate transcription through repressive and activating domains that involves also competition with Sp1 (31). A G+C-rich sequence is present in the Egr-1 gene and the proximal promoter of the SERCA2 genes (Figure 4). Transfection assays located the DXR responsive element within the proximal SERCA2 promoter region, and over-expression of Egr-1 decreased the transcriptional activity of the SERCA2 gene (31). These findings suggested that reactive oxygen species mediate their transcriptional effect on the SERCA2 gene *via* p44/42 MAPK and Egr-1. To date, other transcriptional mechanisms influencing the SERCA2 gene in pathologic conditions are incompletely understood.

ACKNOWLEDGMENTS

This work was supported by grants from the Dirección General del Personal Académico, UNAM and from CONACyT, México.

REFERENCES

1. Brandl CJ, deLeon S, Martin DR, MacLennan DH. 1987. Adult forms of the Ca2+ATPase of sarcoplasmic reticulum. Expression in developing skeletal muscle. J Biol Chem 262:3768–3774.
2. Korczak B, Zarain-Herzberg A, Brandl CJ, Ingles CJ, Green NM, MacLennan DH. 1988. Structure of the rabbit fast-twitch skeletal muscle Ca2+-ATPase gene. J Biol Chem 263:4813–4819.
3. MacLennan DH, Brandl CJ, Korczak B, Green NM. 1985. Amino-acid sequence of a $Ca^{2+} + Mg^{2+}$-dependent ATPase from rabbit muscle sarcoplasmic reticulum, deduced from its complementary DNA sequence. Nature 316:696–700.
4. Lytton J, Zarain-Herzberg A, Periasamy M, MacLennan DH. 1989. Molecular cloning of the mammalian smooth muscle sarco(endo)plasmic reticulum Ca^{2+}-ATPase. J Biol Chem 264:7059–7065.
5. Kovacs T, Felfoldi F, Papp B, Paszty K, Bredoux R, Enyedi A, Enouf J. 2001. All three splice variants of the human sarco/endoplasmic reticulum Ca^{2+}-ATPase 3 gene are translated to proteins: a study of their co-expression in platelets and lymphoid cells. Biochem J 358:559–568.
6. Zarain-Herzberg A, MacLennan DH, Periasamy M. 1990. Characterization of rabbit cardiac sarco(endo)plasmic reticulum Ca^{2+}-ATPase gene. J Biol Chem 265:4670–4677.
7. Rohrer DK, Hartong R, Dillmann WH. 1991. Influence of thyroid hormone and retinoic acid on slow sarcoplasmic reticulum Ca^{2+}-ATPase and myosin heavy chain alpha gene expression in cardiac myocytes: Delineation of cis-active DNA elements that confer responsiveness to thyroid hormone but not to retinoic acid. J Biol Chem 266:8638–8646.
8. Wankerl M, Boheler KR, Fiszman MY, Schwartz K. 1996. Molecular cloning of the human cardiac sarco(endo)plasmic reticulum Ca^{2+}-ATPase (SERCA2) gene promoter. J Mol Cell Cardiol 28: 2139–2150.
9. Ver Heyen M, Reed TD, Blough RI, Baker DL, Zilberman A, Loukianov E, Van Baelen K, Raeymaekers L, Periasamy M, Wuytack F. 2000. Structure and organization of the mouse Atp2a2 gene encoding the sarco(endo)plasmic reticulum Ca2+-ATPase 2 (SERCA2) isoforms. Mamm Genome 11:159–163.

10. Zarain-Herzberg A, Marques J, Sukovich D, Periasamy M. 1994. Thyroid hormone receptor modulates the expression of the rabbit cardiac sarco (endo) plasmic reticulum Ca^{2+}-ATPase gene. J Biol Chem 269:1460–1467.

11. Hartong R, Wang N, Kurokawa R, Lazar MA, Glass CK, Apriletti JW, Dillmann WH. 1994. Delineation of three different thyroid hormone-response elements in promoter of rat sarcoplasmic reticulum Ca^{2+}-ATPase gene. Demonstration that retinoid X receptor binds 5' to thyroid hormone receptor in response element 1. J Biol Chem 269:13021–13029.

12. Moriscot AS, Sayen MR, Hartong R, Wu P, Dillmann WH. 1997. Transcription of the rat sarcoplasmic reticulum Ca^{2+}-adenosine triphosphatase gene is increased by 3,5,3'-triiodothyronine receptor isoform-specific interactions with the myocyte-specific enhancer factor-2a. Endocrinology 138: 26–32.

13. Hayakawa M, Sakashita E, Ueno E, Tominaga S, Hamamoto T, Kagawa Y, Endo H. 2002. Muscle-specific exonic splicing silencer for exon exclusion in human ATP synthase gamma-subunit pre-mRNA. J Biol Chem 277:6974–6984.

14. Ichida M, Hakamata Y, Hayakawa M, Ueno E, Ikeda U, Shimada K, Hamamoto T, Kagawa Y, Endo H. 2000. Differential regulation of exonic regulatory elements for muscle-specific alternative splicing during myogenesis and cardiogenesis. J Biol Chem 275:15992–16001.

15. Carstens RP, Wagner EJ, Garcia-Blanco MA. 2000. An intronic splicing silencer causes skipping of the IIIb exon of fibroblast growth factor receptor 2 through involvement of polypyrimidine tract binding protein. Mol Cell Biol 19:7388–7400.

16. Baker DL, Dave V, Reed T, Periasamy M. 1996. Multiple Sp1 binding sites in the cardiac-slow twitch muscle sarcoplasmic reticulum Ca2+-ATPase gene promoter are required for expression in Sol8 muscle cells. J Biol Chem 271:5921–5928.

17. Baker DL, Dave V, Reed T, Misra S, Periasamy M. 1998. A novel E box/AT-rich element is required for muscle-specific expression of the sarcoplasmic reticulum Ca^{2+}-ATPase (SERCA2) gene. Nucleic Acids Res 26:1092–1098.

18. Nagai R, Zarain-Herzberg A, Brandl CJ, Fujii J, Tada M, MacLennan DH, Alpert NR, Periasamy M. 1989. Regulation of myocardial Ca^{2+}-ATPase and phospholamban mRNA expression in response to pressure overload and thyroid hormone. Proc Natl Acad Sci USA 86:2966–2970.

19. Kinugawa K, Yonekura K, Ribeiro RC, Eto Y, Aoyagi T, Baxter JD, Camacho SA, Bristow MR, Long CS, Simpson PC. 2001. Regulation of thyroid hormone receptor isoforms in physiological and pathological cardiac hypertrophy. Circ Res 89:591–598.

20. Caspersen C, Pedersen PS, Treiman M. 2000. The sarco/endoplasmic reticulum calcium-ATPase 2b is an endoplasmic reticulum stress-inducible protein. J Biol Chem 275:22363–22372.

21. Wu KD, Bungard D, Lytton J. 2001. Regulation of SERCA Ca2+ pump expression by cytoplasmic Ca2+ in vascular smooth muscle cells. Am J Physiol Cell Physiol 280:C843–C851.

22. Thuerauf DJ, Hoover H, Meller J, Hernandez J, Su L, Andrews C, Dillmann WH, McDonough PM, Glembotski CC. 2001. Sarco/endoplasmic reticulum calcium ATPase-2 (SERCA2) expression is regulated by ATF6 during the endoplasmic reticulum stress response: Intracellular signaling of calcium stress in a cardiac myocyte model system. J Biol Chem 276:48309–48317.

23. Lehnart SE, Schillinger W, Pieske B, Prestle J, Just H, Hasenfuss G. 1998. Sarcoplasmic reticulum proteins in heart failure. Ann NY Acad Sci 853:220–230.

24. Qi M, Shannon TR, Euler DE, Bers DM, Samarel AM. 1997. Down regulation of the sarcoplasmic reticulum Ca^{2+}-ATPase during progression of left ventricular hypertrophy. Am J Physiol 41: H2416–H2424.

25. Ribadeau Dumas A, Wisnewsky C, Boheler KR, Ter Keurs H, Fiszman MY, Schwartz K. 1997. The sarco(endo)plasmic reticulum Ca2+-ATPase gene is regulated at the transcriptional level during compensated left ventricular hypertrophy in the rat. C R Acad Sci III 320:963–969.

26. Takizawa T, Arai M, Yoguchi A, Tomaru K, Kurabayashi M, Nagai R. 1999. Transcription of the SERCA2 gene is decreased in pressure-overloaded hearts: A study using in vivo direct gene transfer into living myocardium. J Mol Cell Cardiol 12:2167–2174.

27. Aoyagi T, Yonekura K, Eto Y, Matsumoto A, Yokoyama I, Sugiura S, Momomura S, Hirata Y, Baker DL, Periasamy M. 1999. The sarcoplasmic reticulum Ca^{2+}-ATPase (SERCA2) gene promoter activity is decreased in response to severe left ventricular pressure-overload hypertrophy in rat hearts. J Mol Cell Cardiol 4:919–926.

28. Sack MN, Disch DL, Rockman HA, Kelly DP. 1997. A role for Sp and nuclear receptor transcription factors in a cardiac hypertrophic growth program. Proc Natl Acad Sci USA 94:6438–6443.

29. Takizawa T, Arai M, Tomaru K, Baker DL, Periasamy M, Kurabayashi M. 2001. Transcription factor

Sp1 is critical for the transcriptional activity of sarcoplasmic reticulum Ca^{2+}-ATPase (SERCA2) gene in pressure-overloaded heart: A study using in vivo direct gene transfer into living myocardium. Circulation 104:II-137.

30. Andrews C, Ho PD, Dillmann WH, Glembotski CC, McDonough PM. 2001. Activation of the MKK6-p38-MAPK pathway in cardiac myocytes prolongs the decay phase of the contractile calcium transient, downregulates SERCA2 expression, and activates NF-AT-dependent gene expression in contraction-dependent manner. Circulation 104:II-136.

31. Arai M, Yoguchi A, Takizawa T, Yokoyama T, Kanda T, Kurabayashi M, Nagai R. 2000. Mechanism of doxorubicin-induced inhibition of sarcoplasmic reticulum Ca(2+)-ATPase gene transcription. Circ Res 86:8–14.

32. Saadane N, Alpert L, Chalifour LE. 1999. TAFII250, Egr-1, and D-type cyclin expression in mice and neonatal rat cardiomyocytes treated with doxorubicin. Am J Physiol 276:H803–H814.

Index